Practical Haematology

Sir John V. Dacie MD (Lond) FRCPath FRS
Emeritus Professor of Haematology, University of London,
Royal Postgraduate Medical School, London

S. M. Lewis BSc MD (Cape Town) DCP (Lond) FRCPath
Emeritus Reader in Haematology, University of London, Senior Research Fellow, Royal
Postgraduate Medical School and Consultant Haematologist,
Hammersmith Hospital, London

SEVENTH EDITION

CHURCHILL LIVINGSTONE
EDINBURGH LONDON MELBOURNE AND NEW YORK 1991

CHURCHILL LIVINGSTONE
Medical Division of Longman Group UK Limited

Distributed in the United States of America by Churchill
Livingstone Inc., 1560 Broadway, New York, N.Y. 10036, and
by associated companies, branches and representatives
throughout the world.

First Edition 1950
Second Edition 1956
    Italian Edition 1957
Third Edition 1963
    Spanish Edition 1963
Fourth Edition 1968
    Spanish Edition 1970
    Italian Edition 1972
Fifth Edition 1975
    Japanese Edition 1980
Sixth Edition 1984
    Italian Edition 1986
    Spanish Edition 1987
Seventh Edition 1991

ISBN 0-443-03952-6

British Library Cataloguing in Publication Data
Dacie, Sir, John V. (John Vivian) 1912-
    Practical haematology. -7th ed.
    1. Man. Blood. Diagnosis. Laboratory techniques
    I. Title II. Lewis, S. M. (Shirley Mitchell)
    616.15075

Library of Congress Cataloging in Publication Data
Dacie, John V. (John Vivian), Sir.
    Practical haematology/Sir John V. Dacie. S.M. Lewis.—7th ed.
        p.   cm.
    Includes bibliographical references.
    Includes index
    ISBN 0-443-03952-6
    1. Blood--Examination. 2. Hematology—Technique.
I. Lewis, S. M. (Shirley Mitchell) II. Title.
    [DNLM: 1. Blood.   2. Diagnosis, Laboratory.
3. Hematologic Diseases—diagnosis. QY 400 D118p]
RB45.D24   1990
616.07'561—dc20
DNLM/DLC
for Library of Congress   90–1980
                                            CIP

Produced by Longman Singapore Publishers Pte Ltd
Printed in Singapore

Practical Haematology

Preface

With each edition, *Practical Haematology* has expanded progressively in size, reflecting the major developments which have occurred, year by year, since 1950, in the laboratory aspects of haematology. In the six years which have elapsed since the 6th edition there have been significant changes in diagnostic procedures and profound changes in laboratory organization, especially with the advent of automated instruments of increasing sophistication. It is, however, appreciated that there are many laboratories with limited resources which still depend mainly on simple technology. Taking this into account, we have included, for instance, a description of the use of haemocytometer counting chambers as well as that of automated blood cell counting systems. Where appropriate, simple screening tests have been described alongside more complex quantitative assays.

In referring to special reagents, test kits and apparatus we have indicated the manufacturers (generally in the UK) from which our supplies have been obtained. However, in many cases equivalent material can be obtained from other sources.

The previous edition has been closely scrutinized; obsolete techniques have been omitted but the amount of important material added has meant that the size of the book has had to be further increased. We have, however, retained our original aim. In addition to serving as a practical bench manual, each test that is described is accompanied by an explanation of the principle involved, its reliability and clinical significance, causes of error in the test and in its interpretation and the advantages (and limitations) of the method or methods which we have chosen to describe. Special attention has been paid to standardization, quality control and other aspects of quality assurance. In essence, the book is dedicated to good laboratory practice.

We are indebted to our collaborators. They comprise five contributors to the 6th edition (M. Brozovic, D. Catovsky, E.E. Lloyd, A. Waters and J.M. White) and six new contributors (D.W. Dawson, E.H. Jones, L. Luzzatto, I. Mackie, G.W. Marsh, M. Worwood), all of whom have given valued help in the chapters which deal with aspects of practical haematology in which they have special knowledge and experience. It is sad to report the death of Dr George Marsh shortly after he had completed a draft of Chapter 15.

We are also indebted to other colleagues who have given us advice on various sections of the text, and we have also obtained valuable guidance from individual members of the expert panels of the International Committee for Standardization in Haematology, in addition to referring extensively to the recommendations which have been published by that Committee. The photomicrographs of blood films new to this edition have been taken for us with great skill by Mr W. F. Hinks. Finally, we should like to thank Mrs Pramila Marwaha for secretarial assistance, and the Publishers for doing their best to expedite the appearance of this new edition.

John Dacie
Mitchell Lewis

Contributors

Milica Brozovic MD FRCPath
Consultant Haematologist, Central Middlesex
Hospital, London

Daniel Catovsky DSc (Med) FRCP FRCPath
Professor of Haematology, Royal Marsden Hospital,
London

D. W. Dawson MB FRCP(Ed) FRCPath
Consultant Pathologist, North Manchester General
Hospital, Manchester

A. V. Hoffbrand MA DM FRCP FRCPath DSc
Professor of Haematology, Royal Free School of
Medicine and Honorary Consultant Haematologist,
Royal Free Hospital, London

E. H. Jones BSc PhD
Lecturer at the Institute of Cancer Research,
London

E. E. Lloyd FIMLS
Principal Medical Laboratory Scientific Officer,
Haematology/Blood Transfusion, Department of
Haematology, Royal Postgraduate Medical School,
Hammersmith Hospital, London

L. Luzzato MD FRCP FRCPath
Professor of Haematology, Royal Postgraduate
Medical School, Hammersmith Hospital, London

Ian J. Mackie BSc FIMLS
Lecturer in Haematology, University College and
Middlesex School of Medicine, The School of
Pathology, Middlesex Hospital, London

G. W. Marsh MD (deceased)
Former Consultant Haematologist, The North
Middlesex Hospital, London

A. H. Waters PhD FRCPath FRCP
Professor of Haematology, University of London,
St Bartholomew's Hospital, London

J. M. White MD(Sheffield) MRCPath
Formerly Director of Pathology, Corniche
Hospital, Abu Dhabi

M. Worwood PhD FRCPath
Reader in Haematology, University of Wales
College of Medicine and Honorary Principal
Scientific Officer, South Glamorgan Health
Authority

Contents

Units of measurement

In keeping with recommendations of the World Health Organization, the International Committee for Standardization in Haematology and other international authorities we have used the Système International (SI) for expressing quantities and units (p. 541). In this system the basic unit of volume is the litre; and in keeping with the recommended convention haemoglobin is expressed in g/l.

1. Collection and handling of blood

Venous blood is preferred for most haematological examinations. Peripheral samples can be almost as satisfactory for some purposes if a free flow of blood is obtained (see p. 6), but this procedure should be avoided, if possible, in any patient considered to carry a risk of transmissible disease.

VENOUS BLOOD

This is best withdrawn from an antecubital vein by means of a dry glass syringe. If available, a disposable plastic syringe should be used. The needles should not be too fine or too long; those of 19 or 20 SWG★ are suitable, and short needles with shafts about 15 mm long are particularly valuable for use in children. The skin should be cleaned with 70% alcohol (e.g. isopropanol) and allowed to dry before being punctured.

When a series of samples is required or when the blood sampling is to be followed by a transfusion, it is convenient to collect the blood by means of a butterfly needle connected to a length of plastic tubing attached to the patient's arm by adhesive tape. If a large volume of blood is required, and a large syringe is not available, a needle of larger bore, e.g. 16 SWG★, provided with a short length of plastic tubing should be used; with this equipment 100 ml of blood or more can be easily withdrawn.

Except in the case of very young children it should be possible with practice to obtain venous blood even from patients with difficult veins. Suc-cessful venepuncture may be facilitated by keeping the subject's arm warm, applying to the upper arm a sphygmomanometer cuff kept at approximately diastolic pressure and smacking the skin over the site of the vein. In obese patients it may be easier to use a vein on the dorsum of the hand, after warming it by immersion in warm water. When the hand is dried and the fist clenched, veins suitable for puncture will usually become apparent. If the veins are very small, a 23 SWG★ needle should be used and this should enable at least 2 ml of blood to be obtained satisfactorily. Vein punctures in the dorsum of the hand tend to bleed more readily than at other sites. The arm should be elevated after withdrawal of the needle and pressure should be applied for several minutes before an adhesive dressing is placed over the puncture site.

If possible, congestion should be completely avoided so as to prevent haemoconcentration. In practice, it is usually necessary to use a tourniquet. This should be loosened once the needle has been inserted into the vein. The piston of the syringe should be withdrawn slowly and no attempt made to withdraw blood faster than the vein is filling. After detaching the needle, the blood should be delivered carefully from the syringe into a container, and if it is desired to prevent coagulation it should be

---

★The nearest equivalent American gauges and diameters are as follows: 16 SWG = 14 (1.625 mm); 19 SWG = 18 (1.016 mm); 20 SWG = 19 (0.914 mm); 23 SWG = 22 (0.610 mm).

promptly and thoroughly but gently mixed with anticoagulant.

Ideally, blood films should be made immediately the blood has been withdrawn. For this it is convenient to deliver a small drop of blood directly on to a glass slide. In practice, blood samples are often collected by the clinical staff and sent to the laboratory after a variable delay. Films should be made in the laboratory from such blood as soon as is practicable. After carefully and thoroughly mixing it, a glass capillary can be used to sample the blood and to deliver a drop of the right size on to a slide so that films can be made.

The differences between films made of fresh blood (no anticoagulant) and anticoagulated blood are dealt with on p. 4. It is convenient to use as containers for blood samples disposable glass or plastic flat-bottomed tubes fitted with caps; except for coagulation studies, the choice between glass and plastic is a matter of availability or personal preference. Because of the possibility of infection of personnel when blood has leaked from the container or when removing the cap causes an aerosol discharge of the contents, it is essential to use containers designed to minimize these risks. Design requirements for this and other specifications have been described in a number of national and international standards, e.g. those of the British Standards Institution (BS 4851), the International Organization for Standardization (ISO 4822) and the European Committee for Clinical Laboratory Standards.[4]

The most common disposable containers available from commercial sources contain dipotassium or tripotassium or disodium EDTA as anticoagulant and are marked at the 2.5 or 5 ml level to indicate the correct amount of blood to be added (see p. 3). Containers are also available containing trisodium citrate, heparin or acid citrate dextrose.

Haemolysis can be avoided or minimized by using clean apparatus, withdrawing the blood slowly, not using too fine a needle, delivering the blood gently into the receiver and avoiding frothing during the withdrawal of the blood and subsequent mixing with the anticoagulant.

Evacuated containers have been designed to be used in conjunction with a double-ended needle for collecting blood without the need for a syringe. The vacuum should ensure that the container will fill to the prescribed volume when the needle is inserted and the seal is broken. The containers are invariably made of glass as they must maintain their vacuum during storage before use, and they have an expiry date. Design requirements have been specified by the European Committee for Clinical Laboratory Standards[4] and by the US National Committee for Clinical Laboratory Standards.[11] With a special adaptor it is possible to fill several tubes in succession from one venepuncture.

SERUM

Blood collected in order to obtain serum should be delivered into sterile tubes or screw-capped bottles and allowed to clot undisturbed for 1–2 h at 37°C. When the blood has firmly clotted and the clot has started to retract, the sample may be left in a refrigerator overnight at 4°C, so that clot retraction may become complete under conditions unfavourable for the growth of bacteria. If the clot fails to retract, it may be gently detached from the wall of the container by means of a platinum wire or sealed Pasteur pipette. If it is roughly treated, lysis is certain to follow. However, exactly how serum should be obtained depends also on what it is required for. For instance, if complement is to be estimated, the serum should be separated and then frozen at −20°C or below with the minimum of delay.

When serum is required urgently or when both serum and cells are required, as in the investigation of certain types of haemolytic anaemia, the sample can be defibrinated. This can be simply performed by placing the blood in a receiver such as a conical flask containing a central glass rod on to which small pieces of glass capillary have been fused (Fig. 1.1). The blood is whisked around the central rod by moderately rapid rotation of the flask. Coagulation is usually complete within 5 min, most of the fibrin collecting upon the central rod. When fibrin formation seems complete, the defibrinated blood may be centrifuged and serum obtained quickly and in relatively large volumes. Blood defibrinated in this way should not undergo any visible degree of lysis. The morphology of the red cells and the leucocytes is well preserved.

If cold agglutinins are to be titrated, the blood must be kept at 37°C until the serum has separated, and if cold agglutinins are known to be present in

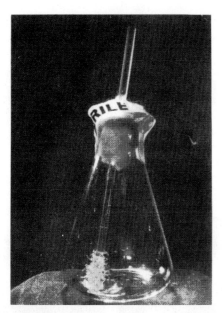

Fig. 1.1 Flask for defibrinating 10–50 ml of blood. The glass rod has had some small pieces of drawn-out glass capillary fused to its lower end.

high concentration it is best to bring the patient to the laboratory and to collect blood into a previously warmed syringe and then to deliver the blood into containers which have been kept warm at 37°C. When filled the containers should be promptly replaced in the 37°C water-bath. In this way it is possible to obtain serum free from haemolysis even when cold antibodies are present capable of causing agglutination at temperatures as high as 30°C. A practical way of warming the syringe is to place it in its container for 10 min in an oven at approximately 50°C or for 30 min or so in a 37°C incubator. When the clot has retracted in the sample and clear serum has been expressed, the serum is removed by a Pasteur pipette and transferred to a tube which has been warmed by being allowed to stand in a water-bath. It is then rapidly centrifuged so as to rid it of any suspended red cells.

BIOHAZARDOUS SPECIMENS

See p. 24.

ANTICOAGULANTS

For various purposes a number of different anticoagulants are available.

Ethylenediamine tetra-acetic acid (EDTA)

The sodium and potassium salts of EDTA are powerful anticoagulants and they are especially suitable for routine haematological work. EDTA acts by its chelating effect on the calcium molecules in blood. To achieve this requires a concentration of 1.2 mg of the anhydrous salt per ml of blood (c 4 μmol). The anticoagulant of choice is the dipotassium salt at a concentration of 1.50 ± 0.25 mg/ml of blood. At this concentration the tripotassium salt produces some shrinkage of red cells which results in a 2–3% decrease in PCV.[14]

Excess of EDTA, irrespective of which of its salts, affects both red cells and leucocytes, causing shrinkage and degenerative changes. EDTA in excess of 2 mg/ml of blood may result in a significant decrease in packed cell volume (PCV) and increase in mean cell haemoglobin concentration (MCHC).[8,12] The platelets are also affected; excess of EDTA causes them to swell and then disintegrate, causing an artificially high platelet count as the fragments are large enough to be counted as normal platelets. Care must therefore be taken to ensure that the correct amount of blood is added, and that by repeated inversions of the container the anticoagulant is thoroughly mixed in the blood added to it. The dipotassium salt is very soluble (1650 g/l) and is to be preferred on this account to the disodium salt which is considerably less soluble (108 g/l).[7] Rapid solution of the EDTA can be ensured by coating the container with a thin film of the salt.

The dilithium salt of EDTA is equally effective as an anticoagulant,[13] and its use has the advantage that the same sample of blood can be used for chemical investigation. However, it is less soluble than the dipotassium salt (160 g/l).

EDTA is not suitable for use in the investigation of coagulation problems and should not be used in the estimation of prothrombin time.

Trisodium citrate

100–120 mmol/l trisodium citrate (32 g/l $Na_3C_6H_5O_7.2H_2O$) is the anticoagulant of choice in coagulation studies. Nine volumes of blood are added to 1 volume of the sodium citrate solution and immediately well mixed with it. Sodium citrate is also the anticoagulant most widely used in the estimation of the sedimentation rate (ESR); for this 4 volumes of venous blood are diluted with 1 volume of the sodium citrate solution.

Heparin

This may be used at a concentration of 10–20 iu per ml of blood. Heparin is an effective anticoagulant and does not alter the size of the red cells; it is a good dry anticoagulant when it is important to reduce to a minimum the chance of lysis occurring after blood has been withdrawn. However, heparinized blood should not be used for making blood films as it gives a faint blue colouration to the background when the films are stained by Romanowsky dyes. This is especially marked in the presence of abnormal proteins. Heparin is the best anticoagulant to use for osmotic fragility tests; otherwise it is inferior to EDTA for general use and should not be used for leucocyte counts as it tends to cause the leucocytes to clump.

EFFECTS OF ANTICOAGULANTS ON BLOOD-CELL MORPHOLOGY

If blood is allowed to stand in the laboratory before films are made, degenerative changes occur. The changes are not solely due to the presence of an anticoagulant for they also occur in defibrinated blood.

Irrespective of anticoagulant, films made from blood which has been standing for not more than 1 h at room temperature (18–25°C) are not easily distinguished from films made immediately after collection of the blood. By 3 h changes may be discernible and by 12–18 h these become striking. Some but not all neutrophils are affected; their nuclei may stain more homogeneously than in fresh blood, the nuclear lobes may become separated and the cytoplasmic margin may appear ragged or less well defined; small vacuoles appear in the cytoplasm (Fig. 1.2). Some or many of the large mononuclears develop marked changes; small vacuoles appear in the cytoplasm and the nucleus undergoes irregular lobulation which may almost amount to disintegration (Fig. 1.3). Some of the lymphocytes, too, undergo a similar type of change: a few vacuoles may be seen in the cytoplasm and

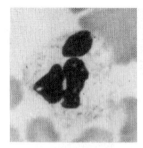
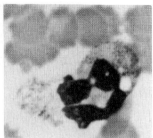

Fig. 1.2 Effect of storage on leucocyte morphology. Photomicrographs of polymorphonuclear neutrophils in a film made from EDTA-blood after 18 h at 20°C.

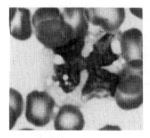
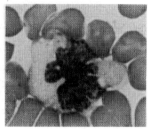

Fig. 1.3 Effect of storage on leucocyte morphology. Photomicrographs of monocytes in a film made from EDTA-blood after 18 h at 20°C.

the nucleus may undergo major budding so as to give rise to nuclei with two or three lobes (Fig. 1.4). Other lymphocyte nuclei may stain more homogeneously than usual.

The red cells (of normal blood at least) are little affected by standing for up to 6 h at room temperature (18–25°C). Longer periods lead to progressive crenation and sphering (Figs. 1.5 and 8.50).

The cells in defibrinated blood undergo degenerative changes at about the same rate as those in EDTA blood, but with an excess of EDTA (p. 3)

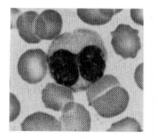
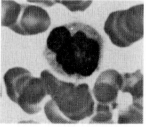

Fig. 1.4 Effect of storage on leucocyte morphology. Photomicrographs of lymphocytes in a film made from EDTA-blood after 18 h at 20°C.

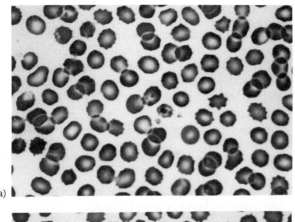

(a)

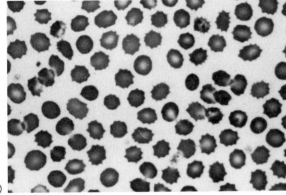

(b)

Fig. 1.5 Effect of storage on red cell morphology.
Photomicrographs of red cells in films made from blood after storage at 20°C in different concentrations of dipotassium EDTA. (a) 24 h at 1.3 mg/ml; (b) 12 h at 3.5 mg/ml.

a marked degree of crenation occurs within a few hours.

All the above changes are retarded but not abolished in blood kept at 4°C. Their occurrence underlines the importance of making films as soon as possible after withdrawal. But delay of up to 1–3 h or so is certainly permissible.

The practice of making films of blood before it is added to the anticoagulant is to be commended, especially when screening for lead toxicity, as the granules of punctate basophilia may stain less obviously in anticoagulated blood. In fresh blood films, however, the platelets usually clump and it is less easy to estimate the platelet count from inspection of the films. Such films are nevertheless of particular value in investigating patients suspected of suffering from purpura, as in certain rare conditions, the absence of platelet clumping is a useful pointer to the diagnosis (see p. 112).

MODE OF ACTION OF ANTICOAGULANTS

EDTA and sodium citrate remove calcium which is essential for coagulation. Calcium is either precipitated as insoluble oxalate (crystals of which may be seen in oxalated blood) or bound in a non-ionized form. Heparin works in a different way; it neutralizes thrombin by inhibiting the interaction of several clotting factors in the presence of a plasma co-factor, antithrombin III. Sodium citrate or heparin can be used to render blood incoagulable before transfusion. For better long-term preservation of red cells for certain tests and for transfusion purposes citrate is used in combination with dextrose in the form of acid-citrate-dextrose (ACD), citrate-phosphate-dextrose (CPD) or Alsever's solution (see p. 535).

EFFECTS OF STORAGE OF BLOOD BEFORE QUANTITATIVE ESTIMATIONS ARE PERFORMED

Regardless of the anticoagulant, certain changes take place when blood is allowed to stand in vitro at room temperature (18–25°C), although they are less marked in blood in ACD, CPD or Alsever's solution than in EDTA blood. The red cells start to swell, with the result that the MCV increases, osmotic fragility and prothrombin time slowly increase and the sedimentation rate decreases; the leucocyte and platelet counts gradually fall.[2] There is no significant change in MCV if the blood is kept overnight at 4°C.[2,9] Other changes, too, take place more slowly at this temperature, so that for many purposes blood may safely be allowed to stand overnight in the refrigerator if precautions against freezing are taken. Nevertheless, it is best to count leucocytes and especially platelets within 2 h. Reticulocyte counts decrease only slightly when the blood is kept in either EDTA or ACD anticoagulant for 24–48 h at 4°C or at 20°C. Nucleated red cells disappear from the blood specimen within 1–2 days at these temperatures.[1] The advisability of making films as soon as possible has already been stressed.

Haemoglobin remains unchanged for days, provided that the blood does not become infected, shown by turbidity or discolouration of the specimen.

The importance of effectively mixing blood after collection, particularly if it has been stored and is cold and viscid, cannot be over-emphasized. If cold, the blood should first be allowed to warm up to room temperature, then mixed, preferably by rotation, for at least 2 min. The difficulty of mixing stored blood adequately is a strong point in favour of performing blood counts without delay.

'CAPILLARY' (PERIPHERAL) BLOOD

Capillary blood is liable to give erroneous results, and should be used only when it is not possible to obtain venous blood. Furthermore, there is greater likelihood of contamination and risk of transmission of disease than with venesection. The blood can be obtained from an ear-lobe or finger of an adult or from the heel of an infant. A free flow of blood is essential, and only the very gentlest squeezing is permissible; ideally, large drops of blood should exude slowly but spontaneously. If it is necessary to squeeze firmly in order to obtain blood, the results are unreliable. If the poor flow is due to the part being cold and cyanosed, too high figures for red cell count, Hb content and leucocyte count are usually obtained.

The discrepancies between peripheral and venous samples are more marked if the ear-lobe rather than the finger is chosen as the site for puncture.[3,10] However, if the ear is rubbed well (with a piece of lint or cotton wool) until it is pink and warm, a good spontaneous flow of blood can be obtained from most patients if sterile lancets are used as prickers. Under these circumstances the figures for red cell count, Hb content and leucocyte count approximate closely to those of venous blood.

Ear-lobe puncture is carried out as follows. Rub the ear with lint until warm. Then prick it to a depth of 2–3 mm with a sterile lancet into the ear-lobe by a single stabbing action. Wipe away the first few drops and collect the sample when the blood is flowing spontaneously, usually in about 30 s. A separate lancet must be used for each patient.

When a finger is used this should be the distal digit of the 3rd or 4th finger on its palmer surface, about 3–5 mm lateral from the nail bed, or on its dorsal surface proximal to the nail bed.

Heel blood

Satisfactory samples can be obtained in infants by a deep puncture using a steel lancet, but only if the heel is really warm—it may be necessary to bathe it in hot water. Appropriate sites are the lateral or medial parts of the plantar surface of the heel. The central plantar area and the posterior curvature should not be punctured in small infants to avoid the risk of injury to the underlying tarsal bones.

COLLECTION OF CAPILLARY BLOOD FOR QUANTITATIVE STUDIES

The usual procedure is to use a micropipette to draw up the correct amount of blood (usually 20 µl). An alternative method is to use disposable capillary tubes cut to size so as to contain the exact volume of blood when completely filled. The capillary tube is filled by capillarity and then dropped into a tube containing the appropriate amount of diluent solution. A potential disadvantage is the presence of contaminating blood on the outside of the capillary where it has been in contact with the source. Such blood is difficult to wipe off without causing the loss of a portion of the blood contained within the capillary. In another system (Unopette) the calibrated capillary, which is to be completely filled with blood, is attached by a special holder directly to a reservoir containing the pre-measured volume of diluent*.[5]

As an alternative method the capillary can be connected to a rubber teat and its contents can then be discharged into the diluent by squeezing the teat**. These methods are particularly suitable for use by the bedside or in the 'field', as less technical skill is required to draw up the correct amount of blood than in the micropipette method.

DIFFERENCES BETWEEN 'CAPILLARY' AND VENOUS BLOOD

It is probable that the PCV, red-cell count and Hb content of venous blood and capillary blood are not quite the same, even if the latter is freely flowing.

*Becton Dickinson Ltd.
**e.g. Drummond Microcaps or 'Volupettes', Scientific Supplies Co. Ltd.

It is likely that freely flowing blood obtained by skin puncture is more nearly arteriolar in composition than is capillary blood. Indeed, the PCV, red cell count and Hb content of true capillary blood are significantly less than those of venous blood.[6] This results in the venous PCV being significantly greater than the 'whole body' PCV, a difference which is of significance in the calculation of total blood volume from an estimation of plasma or red cell volume (see p. 365).

The platelet count appears to be higher in venous than in capillary blood—this may be due to adhesion of platelets to the site of the skin puncture. Leucocyte counts are probably identical, but only if the peripheral blood is freely flowing—if the ear is cold, the capillary count may be much higher than the venous count.[10] Neutrophils especially tend to accumulate in the ear-lobe if the blood is not free-flowing.

REFERENCES

[1] BAER, D. M. and KRAUSE, R. B. (1968). Spurious laboratory values resulting from simulated mailing conditions. *American Journal of Clinical Pathology*, **50**, 111.

[2] BRITTIN, G. M., BRECHER, G., JOHNSON, C. A. and ELASHOFF, R. M. (1969). Stability of blood in commonly used anticoagulants. *American Journal of Clinical Pathology*, **52**, 690.

[3] BRÜCKMANN, G. (1942). Blood from the ear lobe: preliminary report. *Journal of Laboratory and Clinical Medicine*, **27**, 487.

[4] European Committee for Clinical Laboratory Standards (1984). *Standard for Specimen Collection Part 1: Blood Containers*. ECCLS Document Vol 1, No. 1, 1–6. Beuth Verlag, Berlin.

[5] FREUNDLICH, M. H. and GERARDE, H. W. (1963). A new, automatic, disposable system for blood counts and hemoglobin, *Blood*, **21**, 648.

[6] GIBSON, J. G. 2nd, SELIGMAN, A. M., PEACOCK, W. C., AUB, J. C., FINE, J. and EVANS, R. D. (1964). The distribution of red cells and plasma in large and minute vessels of the normal dog, determined by radioactive isotopes of iron and iodine. *Journal of Clinical Investigation*, **25**, **848**.

[7] HADLEY, G. G. and WEISS, S. P. (1955). Further notes on use of salts of ethylenediamine tetraacetic acid (EDTA) as anticoagulants. *American Journal of Clinical Pathology*, **25**, 1090.

[8] LAMPASSO, J. A. (1965). Error in hematocrit value produced by excessive ethylenediaminetetraacetate. *American Journal of Clinical Pathology*, **44**, 109.

[9] LAWRENCE, A. C. K., BEVINGTON, J. M. and YOUNG, M. (1975). Storage of blood and the mean corpuscular volume. *Journal of Clinical Pathology*, **28**, 345.

[10] LUCEY, H. C. (1950). Fortuitous factors affecting the leucocyte count in blood from the ear. *Journal of Clinical Pathology*, **3**, 146.

[11] National Committee for Clinical Laboratory Standards (1976). *Standard for Evacuated Tubes for Blood Specimen Collection*, 2nd edn. NCCLS, Villanova, Pa.

[12] PENNOCK, C. A. and JONES, K. W. (1966). Effect of ethylene-diamine-tetraacetic acid (dipotassium salt) and heparin on the estimation of packed cell volume. *Journal of Clinical Pathology*, **19**, 196.

[13] SACKER, L. S., SAUNDERS, K. E., PAGE, B. and GOODFELLOW, M. (1959). Dilithium sequestrene as an anticoagulant. *Journal of Clinical Pathology*, **12**, 254.

[14] VAN ASSENDELFT, O. W. and PARVIN, R. M. (1988). Specimen collection, handling and storage. In *Quality Assurance in Haematology*. Eds. S. M. Lewis and R. L. Verwilghen, p. 5. Baillière Tindall, London.

2. Reference ranges and normal values

A number of factors affect haematological values in apparent health. These include:

1. The sex, age, occupation, body build, ethnic background and environment, especially altitude.
2. The physiological conditions under which the specimens are obtained, including the subject's diet, his posture when the sample was taken, whether ambulant or confined to bed.
3. The technique and timing of specimen collection, transport and storage.
4. Variation in the analytical methods used.

Furthermore, it is difficult to be certain in any survey of a population for the purposes of obtaining data from which normal ranges may be constructed that the 'normal' subjects are completely healthy and do not have mild chronic infections, parasitic infestations or nutritional deficiencies.

The borderline between health and ill-health is indefinite; so it is with haematological values, for the normal and abnormal undoubtedly overlap. For instance, a value well within the recognized normal range may be definitely pathological in a particular subject, e.g. a total leucocyte count of $10.0 \times 10^9/l$ is abnormal for a man whose count usually ranges between 4.0 and $6.0 \times 10^9/l$. For these reasons the concept of 'normal values' and 'normal ranges' is being replaced by 'reference values' and 'reference limits' in which the variables are defined when establishing the values for the reference population in a particular test.[25] The ultimate goal is to have a data bank of reference values which take account of the physiological variables mentioned above, so that an individual's result can be expressed and interpreted relative to a comparable normal. Such data are at present available for only a limited number of haematological tests, mainly for red cell indices.[29]

REFERENCE RANGES

A reference range for a population can be established from measurements on a relatively small number of subjects (see below) if they are assumed to be representative of the population as a whole.[19,25,49] The conditions for obtaining samples from the individuals must be standardized and data should be analysed separately for different variables such as individuals in bed or ambulant, smokers or non-smokers. The samples should be collected at about the same time of day, preferably in the morning before breakfast; the last meal should have been eaten not later than 9 p.m. on the previous evening and at that time alcohol should have been restricted to one bottle of beer or an equivalent amount of other alcoholic drink.[26]

STATISTICAL PROCEDURE[27]

A reasonably reliable estimate can be obtained with 40 values although a larger number, 120 or more, is preferable.[40] It is usually assumed that the data will fit a specified type of pattern, either symmetric (Gaussian) or asymmetric with a skewed distribution (non-Gaussian) (p. 543). If the data (x_1, x_2 etc.) fit a Gaussian distribution the arithmetic mean ($\bar{x}$) and SD may be calculated as described on p. 543.

Alternatively, a frequency histogram is plotted (Fig. 2.1). Taking the modal value (see p. 543) and the calculated SD as reference points, a Gaussian curve is superimposed. From this curve practical reference limits can be determined even if the original histogram included outlying results from some subjects not belonging to the normal population. Limits representing the 95% range (reference interval) are calculated from arithmetic mean ±2 SD (or more accurately ±1.96 SD). When there is

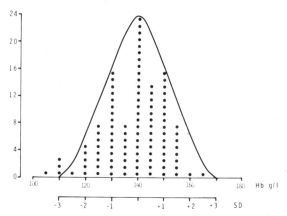

Fig. 2.1 Example of establishing a reference range. Data of haemoglobin measurements in a population, with Gaussian curve superimposed.

a log normal (skew) distribution of measurements, the range to − 2SD may extend below zero (Fig. 2.2). To avoid this anomaly the data should be converted to their logarithms by means of log-tables or a calculator with the appropriate facility. The mean and SD are calculated in the usual way (p. 543); the figures are then converted to their

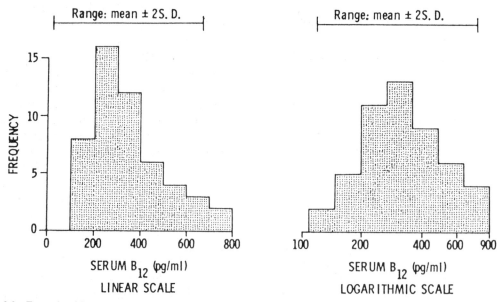

Fig. 2.2 Example of log normal distribution. Data of vitamin B_{12} measurements in a population. Left: arithmetic scale; Right: geometric scale. Arithmetic mean 343 pg/ml and SD 161 pg/ml; 2 SD range would thus be 21–665 pg/ml. When the data are converted to their logarithms as described on p. 543, the geometric mean is 308 pg/ml, and a 2 SD range is 121–783 pg/ml. Reproduced with permission from J. M. England (1975) *Medical Research: A Statistical and Epidemiological Approach*, p. 20, Churchill Livingstone, Edinburgh.

antilogs in order to express the data in the original scale.

The data given in Table 2.1 provide a rough guide to so-called normal values which are applicable to most healthy individuals. The data have been derived from various sources, including observations from the authors' own laboratory and personal communications. The range of ± 2 SD from the mean indicates the limits which should cover 95% of normal subjects; 99% of normal subjects will be included in a range of ± 3 SD.

A 'normal range' has been given without SD, when the distribution of the data is too skew to provide a Gaussian curve or when the data are too scanty for analysis.

PHYSIOLOGICAL VARIATION

PHYSIOLOGICAL VARIATION IN Hb CONTENT, PCV AND RED CELL COUNTS

It is well known that there is considerable variation in the red cell count and Hb content at different periods of life. At birth the Hb is higher than at any period subsequently (Table 2.1). The red cell count is high immediately after birth[5,12,32] and values for Hb greater than 200 g/l, red cell count higher than $6.0 \times 10^{12}/l$ and PCV of 0.65 are encountered frequently when the cord is tied late after delivery. Probably it is the cessation of pulsation of the umbilical artery in the cord as well as the uterine contractions which result in the blood contained in the placenta re-entering the infant's circulation. After the immediate post-natal period the Hb falls fairly steeply to a minimum of about 100 g/l at about the 3rd month.[5,12,32] The red cell count and PCV also fall, though less steeply and the cells become hypochromic with the development of 'physiological' iron-deficiency anaemia.

In the neonate the mean MCHC is 300 g/l with a SD of 27 g/l; it does not alter significantly during the first 3 yr but the SD diminishes. The mean MCV is 120 fl in the neonate, 100 at 2 months, 95 at 3 months and within the adult range by 3 yr.

The Hb content and red cell count normally rise gradually to almost adult levels by the time of puberty; thereafter the levels in women tend to be significantly lower than those of men.[22,29] Factors influencing the difference between men and women include a hormonal influence on haemopoiesis and menstrual blood loss; the extent to which the latter is a significant factor is not clear, as a loss of up to 100 ml of blood with each period does not appear to cause a fall in Hb although it results in lower levels of serum iron.[11,21] Moreover, arrest of menstruation by oral contraceptives causes an increase in serum iron without affecting the haemoglobin level.[6]

In normal pregnancy there is an increase in erythropoietic activity. However, at the same time an increase in plasma volume occurs and this results in a fall in Hb and red cell count.[8,30] The level returns to normal about a week after delivery. Serum ferritin falls in early pregnancy and usually remains low throughout pregnancy even when supplementary iron is given.[23]

In old age the Hb is reported to fall; in one study this was found to be, in men, to a mean level of 134 g/l at 65, 129 g/l at 75 and 122 g/l at over the age of 85.[44] Lesser differences have been recorded by others.[22,29] By contrast, in older women the level tends to rise, so that a sex difference of 20 g/l in younger age groups is reduced to 10 g/l or less in old age.[11,37] There is a concomitant increase in serum iron although serum ferritin levels remain higher in men than in women.[33] The MCHC remains remarkably constant at all ages, in both men and women.

In addition to the permanent effects of age and sex, there seem to be transient fluctuations, the significance of which is often difficult to assess. Muscular activity, if at all strenuous, unquestionably raises the red cell count and Hb, presumably largely due to the re-entry into the circulation of cells previously sequestered in shut-down capillaries and to an extent to reduction in plasma volume; increases in red cells amounting to 0.5 ×

Table 2.1   Haematological values for normal individuals expressed as mean + 2 SD (95% range)

Red cell count
Men	$5.5 \pm 1.0 \times 10^{12}/l$
Women	$4.8 \pm 1.0 \times 10^{12}/l$
Infants (full-term cord blood)	$6.0 \pm 1.0 \times 10^{12}/l$
Children, 3 months	$4.0 \pm 0.8 \times 10^{12}/l$
Children, 1 yr	$4.4 \pm 0.8 \times 10^{12}/l$
Children, 3–6 yr	$4.8 \pm 0.7 \times 10^{12}/l$
Children, 10–12 yr	$4.7 \pm 0.7 \times 10^{12}/l$

Haemoglobin
Men	155 ± 25 g/l*
Women	140 ± 25 g/l
Infants (full-term cord blood)	165 ± 30 g/l
Children, 3 months	115 ± 20 g/l
Children, 1 yr	120 ± 15 g/l
Children, 3–6 yr	130 ± 10 g/l
Children, 10–12 yr	130 ± 15 g/l

Packed cell volume (PCV; haematocrit value)
Men	0.47 ± 0.07 (l/l)
Women	0.42 ± 0.05 (l/l)
Infants (full-term, cord blood)	0.54 ± 0.10 (l/l)
Children, 3 months	0.38 ± 0.06 (l/l)
Children, 3–6 yr	0.04 ± 0.04 (l/l)
Children, 10–12 yr	0.41 ± 0.04 (l/l)

Mean cell volume (MCV)
Adults	86 ± 10 fl
Infants (full-term, neonates)	120 fl (mean)
Children, 3 months	95 fl (mean)
Children, 1 yr	78 ± 8 fl
Children, 3–6 yr	84 ± 8 fl
Children, 10–12 yr	84 ± 7 fl

Mean cell haemoglobin (MCH)
Adults	29.5 ± 2.5 pg
Children, 3 months	29 ± 5 pg
Children, 1 yr	27 ± 4 pg
Children, 3–6 yr	27 ± 3 pg
Children, 10–12 yr	27 ± 3 pg

Mean cell haemoglobin concentration (MCHC)
Adults and children	325 ± 25 g/l
Infants (full-term, neonates)	300 ± 27 g/l

Red cell diameter (mean values)
Adults (dry films)	6.7–7.7 μm

Red cell density

1092–1100 g/l

Reticulocyte count
Adults and children	0.5–2.5% (c 50–100 $\times 10^9/l$)
Infants (full-term, cord blood)	2–6% (mean 150 $\times 10^9/l$)

Blood volume
Red cell volume, men	30 ± 5 ml/kg
women	25 ± 5 ml/kg
Plasma volume	45 ± 5 ml/kg
Total blood volume	70 ± 10 ml/kg

Red cell life-span

120 ± 30 days

Leucocyte count
Men	$7.5 \pm 3.5 \times 10^9/l$
Infants (full-term, 1st day)	$18 \pm 8 \times 10^9/l$
Infants, 1yr	$12 \pm 6 \times 10^9/l$
Children, 4–7 yr	$10 \pm 5 \times 10^9/l$
Children, 8–12 yr	$9 \pm 4.5 \times 10^9/l$

Table 2.1 (*Continued*)

Differential leucocyte count	
Adults:	
Neutrophils	$2.0–7.5 \times 10^9/l(40–75\%)$
Lymphocytes	$1.5–4.0 \times 10^9/l(20–45\%)$
Monocytes	$0.2–0.8 \times 10^9/l(2–10\%)$
Eosinophils	$0.04–0.4 \times 10^9/l(1–6\%)$
Basophils	$0.02–0.1 \times 10^9/l(1\%)$
Infants (1st day):	
Neutrophils	$5.0–13.0 \times 10^9/l$
Lymphocytes	$3.5–8.5 \times 10^9/l$
Monocytes	$0.5–1.5 \times 10^9/l$
Eosinophils	$0.1–2.5 \times 10^9/l$
Basophils	$0.02–0.1 \times 10^9/l$
Infants (3 days):	
Neutrophils	$1.5–7.0 \times 10^9/l$
Lymphocytes	$2.0–5.0 \times 10^9/l$
Monocytes	$0.3–1.1 \times 10^9/l$
Eosinophils	$0.2–2.0 \times 10^9/l$
Basophils	$0.02–0.1 \times 10^9/l$
Children (6 yr):	
Neutrophils	$2.0–6.0 \times 10^9/l$
Lymphocytes	$5.5–8.5 \times 10^9/l$
Monocytes	$0.7–1.5 \times 10^9/l$
Eosinophils	$0.3–0.8 \times 10^9/l$
Basophils	$0.02–0.1 \times 10^9/l$
Platelet count	$150–400 \times 10^9/l$
Bleeding time (Ivy's method)	2–7 min
(Template method)	2.5–9.5 min
Prothrombin time	11–16 s
Partial thromboplastin time (PTTK)	30–40 s
Prothrombin-consumption index	0–10%
Plasma fibrinogen	1.5–4.0 g/l
Fibrinogen titre	⩾128
Plasminogen	80–120 u/dl
Euglobulin lysis time	90–240 min
Antithrombin III	75–125 u/dl
β-thromboglobulin	<50 ng/ml
Platelet factor 4	<10 ng/ml
Protein C	70–140%
Protein S	70–140%
Heparin co-factor II	55–145%

Osmotic fragility (at 20°C and pH 7.4)

NaCl(g/l)	Before incubation % lysis	After incubation for 24 h at 37°C % lysis
2.0	100	95–100
3.0	97–100	85–100
3.5	90–99	75–100
4.0	50–95	65–100
4.5	5–45	55–95
5.0	0–6	40–85
5.5	0	15–70
6.0	0	0–40
6.5	0	0–10
7.0	0	0–5
7.5	0	0
8.0	0	0
8.5	0	0

Median corpuscular fragility (MCF) (g/l NaCl)

4.0–4.45	4.65–5.9

Table 2.1 *(Continued)*

Autohaemolysis (37°C)	
48 h, without added glucose	0.2–4.0%
48 h, with added glucose	0–0.5%
Cold-agglutinin titre (4°C)	<64
Serum iron	13–32 µmol/l
	(0.7–1.8 mg/l)
Total iron-binding capacity	45–70 µmol/l
	(2.5–4.0 mg/l)
Transferrin	2.0–3.0 g/l
Ferritin	
Adults	15–300 µg/l
Children	15–140 µg/l
Serum vitamin B_{12} (as cyanocobalamin)	160–760 ng/l
Serum folate	3–20 µg/l
Red cell folate	160–640 µg/l
Plasma haemoglobin	10–40 mg/l
Serum haptoglobin (Hb-binding)	0.3–2.0 g/l
Sedimentation rate (Westergren, 1h at 20 ± 3°C)	
(upper limits)	
Men 17–50 yr	10 mm
>50 yr	12–14 mm
Women 17–50 yr	12 mm
Women >50 yr	19–20 mm
Plasma viscosity	
(25°C)	1.50–1.72 mPa/s
(37°C)	1.16–1.33 mPa/s
Heterophile (anti-sheep red cell) agglutinin titre	<80
After absorption with guinea-pig kidney	<10

*Throughout the book Hb is expressed in g/l, i.e. g/dl × 10.

10^{12}/l and in Hb to 15 g/l may be observed. Posture, too, appears to cause transient alterations in the plasma volume, and thus in Hb and PCV. There is a small but significant increase as the posture changes from lying to sitting especially in women[17] and, conversely, change from walking about to lying down results in a 5–10% fall in the Hb and PCV. This occurs within 20 min, after which time, the PCV is stabilized at the lower level.[14,34] Consistently similar findings have also been reported by Eisenberg in a study of 25 subjects.[13] He also showed that the position of the arm during venous sampling affected the magnitude of the increase in PCV; it was 2–4% lower when the arm was held at the atrial level instead of being dependent.

It is not clear whether emotion or light exercise raises the red cell count or Hb significantly above the base line observed with the subject at rest; the effects may be small enough to be submerged in the technical errors of estimation.[45] Athletes tend to have slightly lower Hb levels than non-athletes, with significantly higher total red cell volume which is partly obscured by a concomitant increase in plasma volume.[4] Diurnal variation is usually slight[15] but fluctuations as much as 15% have been reported;[46] in most cases the Hb was highest in the morning and lowest in the evening, the mean difference being about 8%.

It has been suggested that seasonal variations also occur, but the evidence for this is conflicting.[39,42] There may be an ethnic difference in red cell indices; lower levels of Hb and MCV have been reported in Africans and West Indians living in Britain, not related to nutritional status.[20]

The effect of altitude is to raise the Hb and increase the number of circulating red cells; the magnitude of the polycythaemia depends on the degree of anoxaemia.[24] At an altitude of 2 km (c 6500 ft) the Hb is c 10 g/l higher than at sea level; at 3 km (c 10 000 ft) it is c 20 g/l higher. Corresponding increases occur at intermediate altitudes. These increases appear to be due both to increased erythropoiesis as a result of the anoxic stimulus and to the decrease in plasma volume which occurs at high altitudes.[31,38] Smokers have slightly higher Hb values and PCV.[28,48] This is probably in consequence of the accumulation of carboxyhaemoglobin in the blood. After a single cigarette the carboxyhaemoglobin level increases by about 1%,[41] and in heavy smokers the carboxyhaemoglobin may constitute c 4–5% of the total haemoglobin.[18] There may be polycythaemia.[43]

PHYSIOLOGICAL VARIATIONS IN THE TOTAL LEUCOCYTE COUNT[22,45]

The effect of age is indicated in Table 2.1; at birth the neutrophil polymorphonuclears predominate, reaching a peak of c 13.0 × 10^9/l at 12 h and then falling to a mean of c 4.0 × 10^9/l over the next 2–3 days, at which level the count remains steady. The lymphocytes fall during the first 3 days of life to a low level of c 2.0–2.5 × 10^9/l and then rise up to the 10th day;[51] after this time they are the predominant cell (up to about 60%) until the 5th–7th yr when they give way to the neutrophils. There are slight sex differences; the total leucocyte count and the neutrophil count may be slightly higher in women than men.[16] After the menopause the counts fall in women so that they tend to become lower than in men of similar age.[10,11,16]

People differ considerably in their leucocyte counts. Some tend to maintain a relatively constant level over long periods of time;[3] others have counts which may vary by as much as 100% at different times. In some subjects there appears to be a rhythm, occurring in cycles of 14–23 days, and in women this may be related to some extent to the menstrual cycle.[36] Some forms of oral contraception have been reported to raise the leucocyte count.[16] There is also diurnal variation which differs on an hour-to-hour basis as well as from day to day;[45] it affects the total leucocyte count as well as all the individual cell types. The minimum count is found in the morning with the subject at rest; the maximum in the afternoon. Random activity may raise the count slightly; strenuous exercise causes rises of up to 30 × 10^9/l, chiefly due, it is thought, to liberation into the blood stream of neutrophils formerly sequestered in shut-down capillaries and in the spleen. Large number of lymphocytes also enter the blood stream during strenuous exercise.

Adrenaline injection causes an increase in the leucocyte count; here, too, increases in the numbers of all major types of leucocytes (and platelets) occur.[7] The rise has been thought to be a reflection of the extent of the reservoir of mature blood cells present not only in the bone marrow and spleen but also in other tissues and organs of the body. Emotion may possibly cause an increase in the leucocyte count in a similar way. The effect of ingestion of food is uncertain. Cigarette smoking causes a significant increase in the leucocyte count.[9,22,48] A moderate leucocytosis of up to 15 × 10^9/l is common during pregnancy, with the peak about 8 weeks before parturition. The count returns to normal levels a week or so after delivery.[10] The rise in leucocytes is due to neutrophilia.

Diurnal variation of the eosinophil count is especially marked.[45] The height of the count is controlled at least in part by the adrenal cortex, increased adrenocortical activity leading to a fall in the number of circulating eosinophils; diurnal fluctuations parallel diurnal glucocorticoid fluctuation.

The environment may influence the leucocyte count. Thus in tropical Africa there is a tendency for a reversal of the neutrophil:lymphocyte ratio, with the low total leucocyte counts.[50] This may be partly due to endemic parasitic and protozoal disease; however, genetics are also likely to play a part as significantly lower leucocyte counts, especially neutrophils, have been observed in Africans living in Britain.[2] In some tropical areas reactive eosinophilia or monocytosis is sufficiently common to be regarded as a reference value for that population.

PHYSIOLOGICAL VARIATION IN THE PLATELET COUNT

There may be a sex difference; thus, in women the count has been reported to be about 20% higher than in men.[47] A fall in the platelet count may occur in women at about the time of menstruation and there is some evidence of a cycle with a 21–35 day rhythm.[35] There is no evidence that oral contraceptives affect the platelet count. There is a variation during the course of a day as well as from day to day.[45] Within the wide normal range there are no significant ethnic differences but in healthy West Indians and Africans platelet counts may on average be 10–20% lower than those in Europeans living in the same environment.[1] There are no obvious age differences; at birth and in the first few weeks of infancy, however, the platelet count tends to be at the lower level of the adult normal range, rising to adult values at about 6 months.

Refinement of present-day blood-counting systems has produced remarkably increased precision, so that even small differences in successive measurements may be significant. It is thus most important to establish and understand the limits of physiological variation etc. for the various tests. With this proviso, present-day blood count data can now provide sensitive indications of minor abnormalities which may be important in clinical interpretation and health screening.

REFERENCES

[1] BAIN, B. J. and SEED, M. (1986). Platelet count and platelet size in healthy Africans and West Indians. *Clinical and Laboratory Haematology,* **8,** 43.

[2] BAIN, B. J., SEED, M. and GODSLAND, I. (1984). Normal values for peripheral blood white cell counts in women of four different ethnic origins. *Journal of Clinical Pathology,* **37,** 188.

[3] BOOTH, K. and HANCOCK, R. E. T. (1961). A study of the total and differential leucocyte counts and haemoglobin levels in a group of normal adults over a period of two years. *British Journal of Haematology,* **7,** 9.

[4] BROTHERHOOD, J., BROZOVIC, B. and PUGH, L. G. C. (1975). Haematological status of middle and long distance runners. *Clinical Science and Molecular medicine,* **48,** 139.

[5] BURMAN, D. (1972). Haemoglobin levels in normal infants aged 3 to 24 months and the effect of iron. *Archives of Diseases in Childhood,* **47,** 261.

[6] BURTON, J. L. (1967). Effect of oral contraceptives on haemoglobin, packed cell volume, serum-iron and total iron-binding capacity in healthy women. *Lancet,* **i,** 978.

[7] CHATTERJEA, J. B., DAMESHEK, W. and STEFANINI, M. (1953). The adrenalin (epinephrin) test as applied to hematologic disorders. *Blood,* **8,** 211.

[8] CHESLEY, L. C. (1972). Plasma and red cell volumes during pregnancy. *American Journal of Obstetrics and Gynecology.* **112,** 440.

[9] CORRE, F., LELLOUCH, J. and SCHWARTZ, D. (1971). Smoking and leucocyte counts; results of an epidemiological survey. *Lancet,* **ii,** 632.

[10] CRUICKSHANK, J. M. (1970). The effects of parity on the leucocyte count in pregnant and non-pregnant women. *British Journal of Haematology,* **18,** 531.

[11] CRUICKSHANK, J. M. and ALEXANDER, M. K. (1970). The effect of age, parity, haemoglobin level and oral contraceptive preparations on the normal leucocyte count. *British Journal of Haematology,* **18,** 541.

[12] DEMARSH, Q. B., ALT, H. L., WINDLE, W. F. and HILLIS, D. S. (1941). The effect of depriving the infant of its placental blood. *Journal of American Medical Association,* **116,** 2568.

[13] EISENBERG, S. (1963). The effect of posture and position of the venous sampling site on the hematocrit and serum protein concentration. *Journal of Laboratory and Clinical Medicine,* **51,** 755.

[14] EKELUND, L. G., EKLUND, B. and KAIJSER, L. (1971). Time course for the change in hemoglobin concentration with change in posture. *Acta Medica Scandinavica,* **190,** 335.

[15] ELWOOD, P. C. (1962). Diurnal haemoglobin variation in normal male subjects. *Clinical Science,* **23,** 379.

[16] ENGLAND, J. M. and BAIN, B. J. (1976). Total and differential leucocyte count. *British Journal of Haematology,* **33,** 1.

[17] FELDING, P., TRYDING, N., HYLTOFT PETERSEN, P. and HORDER, M. (1980). Effects of posture on concentration of blood constituents in healthy adults: practical application of blood specimen collection procedures recommended by the Scandinavian Committee on Reference Values. *Scandinavian Journal of Clinical and Laboratory Investigation,* **40,** 615.

[18] GALEA, G. and DAVIDSON, R. J. L. (1985). Haematological and haemorheological changes associated with cigarette smoking. *Journal of Clinical Pathology,* **38,** 978.

[19] GARBY, L. (1970). The normal haemoglobin level (Annotation). *British Journal of Haematology,* **19,** 429.

[20] GODSLAND, I. F., SEED, M., SIMPSON, R., BROOM, G., WYNN, V. (1983). Comparison of haematological indices between women of four ethnic groups and the effect of oral contraceptives. *Journal of Clinical Pathology,* **36,** 184.

[21] HALLBERG, L., HOGDAHL, A. M., NILSSON, L. and RYBO, G. (1966). Menstrual blood loss and iron deficiency. *Acta Medica Scandinavica,* **180,** 639.

[22] HELMAN, N. and RUBENSTEIN, L. S. (1975). The effects of age, sex and smoking on erythrocytes and leukocytes. *American Journal of Clinical Pathology,* **63,** 35.

[23] HOWELLS, M. R., JONES, S. E., NAPIER, J. A. F., SAUNDERS, K. and CAVILL, I. (1986). Erythropoiesis in pregnancy. *British Journal of Haematology,* **64,** 595.

[24] HURTADO, A., MERINO, C. and DELGADO, E. (1945). Influence of anoxemia on the hemopoietic activity. *Archives of Internal Medicine,* **75,** 284.

[25] International Committee for Standardization in Haematology (1981). The theory of reference values. *Clinical and Laboratory Haematology,* **3,** 369.

[26] International Committee for Standardization in Haematology (1982). Standardization of blood specimen collection procedures for reference values. *Clinical and Laboratory Haematology,* **4,** 83.

[27] International Federation of Clinical Chemistry. (1984). The theory of reference values. Part 5. Statistical treatment of collected reference values. Determination of reference limits. *Clinica Chimica Acta,* **137,** 97F.

[28] ISAGER, H. and HAGERUP, L. (1971). Relationship between cigarette smoking and high packed cell volume and haemoglobin levels. *Scandinavian Journal of Haematology,* **8,** 241.

[29] KELLY, A. and MUNAN, L. (1977). Haematologic profile of natural populations: red cell parameters. *British Journal of Haematology,* **35,** 153.

[30] LARGE, R. D. and DYNESIUS, R. (1973). Blood volume changes during normal pregnancy. *Clinics in Haematology,* **2,** 433.

[31] LEVIN, N. W., METZ, J., HART, D., van HEERDEN, D. R., BOARDMAN, R. G. and FARBER, S. A. (1960). The blood volume of healthy adult males resident in Johannesburg (altitude 5740 feet). *South African Journal of Medical Sciences*, **28**, 132.

[32] MATOTH, Y., ZAIZON, R. and VARSANO, I. (1971). Post-natal changes in some red cell parameters. *Acta Paediatrica Scandinavica*, **60**, 317.

[33] MATTILA, K. S., KUUSELA, V., PELLINIEMI, T. T., RAJAMAKI, A., KAIHOLA, H. L. and JUVA, K. (1986). Haematological laboratory findings in the elderly; influence of age and sex. *Scandinavian Journal of Clinical and Laboratory Investigation*, **46**, 411.

[34] MOLLISON, P. L. (1983). *Blood Transfusion in Clinical Medicine*, 7th edn., p. 77. Blackwell Scientific Publications, Oxford.

[35] MORLEY, A. (1969). A platelet cycle in normal individuals. *Australasian Annals of Medicine*, **18**, 127.

[36] MORLEY, A. (1973). Correspondence. *Blood*, **41**, 329.

[37] MYERS, A. M., SAUNDERS, C. R. G. and CHALMERS, D. G. (1968). The haemoglobin level of fit elderly people. *Lancet*, **ii**, 261.

[38] MYHRE, L. D., DILL, D. B., HALL, F. G. and BROWN, D. K. (1970). Blood volume changes during three-week residence at high altitude. *Clinical Chemistry*, **16**, 7.

[39] NATVIG, H., BJERKEDAL, T. and JONASSEN, O. (1963). Studies on hemoglobin values in Norway. III. Seasonal variations. *Acta Medica Scandinavica*, **174**, 351.

[40] REED, A. H., HENRY, R. J. and MASON, W. B. (1971). Influence of statistical method used on the resulting estimate of normal range. *Clinical Chemistry*, **17**, 275.

[41] RUSSEL, M. A. H., WILSON, C., COLE, P. V., IDLE, M. and FEYERABEND, C. (1973). Comparison of increases in carboxyhaemoglobin after smoking 'extramild' and 'non mild' cigarettes. *Lancet*, **ii**, 687.

[42] SAUNDERS, C. (1965). Some erythrocyte parameters on a cross section of U. K. A. E. A. employees. *Laboratory Practice*, **14**, 1390.

[43] SMITH, J. R. and LANDOW, S. A. (1978). Smoker's polycythemia. *New England Journal of Medicine*, **298**, 6.

[44] SMITH, J. S. and WHITELAW, D. M. (1971). Hemoglobin values in aged men. *Canadian Medical Association Journal*, **105**, 816.

[45] STATLAND, B. E., WINKEL, P., HARRIS, S. C., BURDSALL, M. J. and SAUNDERS, A. M. (1978). Evaluation of biologic sources of variation of leukocyte counts and other hematologic quantities using very precise automated analyzers. *American Journal of Clinical Pathology*, **69**, 48.

[46] STENGLE, J. M. and SCHADE, A. L. (1957). Diurnal-nocturnal variations of certain blood constituents in normal human subjects: plasma iron, siderophilin, bilirubin, copper, total serum protein and albumin, haemoglobin and haematocrit. *British Journal of Haematology*, **3**, 117.

[47] STEVENS, R. F. and ALEXANDER, M. K. (1977). A sex difference in the platelet count. *British Journal of Haematology*, **37**, 295.

[48] TIBBLIN, E., BENGTSSON, C., HALLBERG, L. and LENNARTSSON, J. (1979). Haemoglobin concentration and peripheral blood cell counts in women. The population study of women in Goteborg, 1968–1969. *Scandinavian Journal of Haematology*, **22**, 5.

[49] VITERI, F. E., DE TUNA, V. and GUZMAN, M. A. (1972). Normal haematological values in the Central American population. *British Journal of Haematology*, **23**, 189.

[50] WOODLIFF, H. J., KATAAHA, P. K., TIBALEKA, A. K. and NZARO, E. (1972). Total leucocyte count in Africans. *Lancet*, **ii**, 875.

[51] XANTHOU, M. (1970). Leucocyte blood picture in healthy full-term and premature babies during neonatal period. *Archives of Disease in Childhood*, **45**, 242.

3. Laboratory organization

The essential function of the haematology laboratory is to provide information which will help in diagnosis and clinical management of patients. The tests which are used should be selected on the basis of their relevance and their reliability, taking into account the technical skill which they demand and the cost of labour and materials which are necessary for their performance. To achieve an efficient and effective service good management is essential. The requirements for this include:

1. Adequate records of test results and workload
2. Quality assurance
3. Optimal use of resources
4. Careful selection of equipment to be purchased
5. Inspection and maintenance of equipment
6. Provision of congenial working conditions and protection of laboratory staff against health risks and hazard when handling specimens and using equipment.

The reliability of laboratory tests also depends on the way in which the blood is collected (see Chapter 1) as well as correct labelling, proficient delivery to the laboratory and correct storage of specimens before the tests are performed.

DOCUMENTATION OF LABORATORY DATA

It is essential that adequate records are kept. The processing, storage and retrieval of data can be facilitated, especially in large laboratories, by a computer (see below). Alternatively, by using a filing card on which the results of tests are recorded serially it is possible to see at a glance whether there has been any change in a patient's blood values (Fig. 3.1). The trend of a blood count is even better appreciated when the figures are plotted as a time-related graph, and this is of special value in assessing the effects of therapy on the blood picture (Fig. 3.2). An arithmetical scale should be used for haemoglobin, reticulocytes and red cell counts, while leucocyte and platelet counts are best recorded on a logarithmic scale. On the horizontal scale of the chart illustrated in Figure 3.2 each small square represents 1 day, and there are prominent vertical lines every 7 days.

USE OF COMPUTERS

Two systems are available: on-line and off-line. In the on-line system the results of laboratory tests are entered into the computer store as they become available and reports are printed out automatically; they are updated continuously and cumulative reports can be produced, together with the results

19

USE OF HAEMATOLOGICAL TECHNIQUES IN CLINICAL WORK

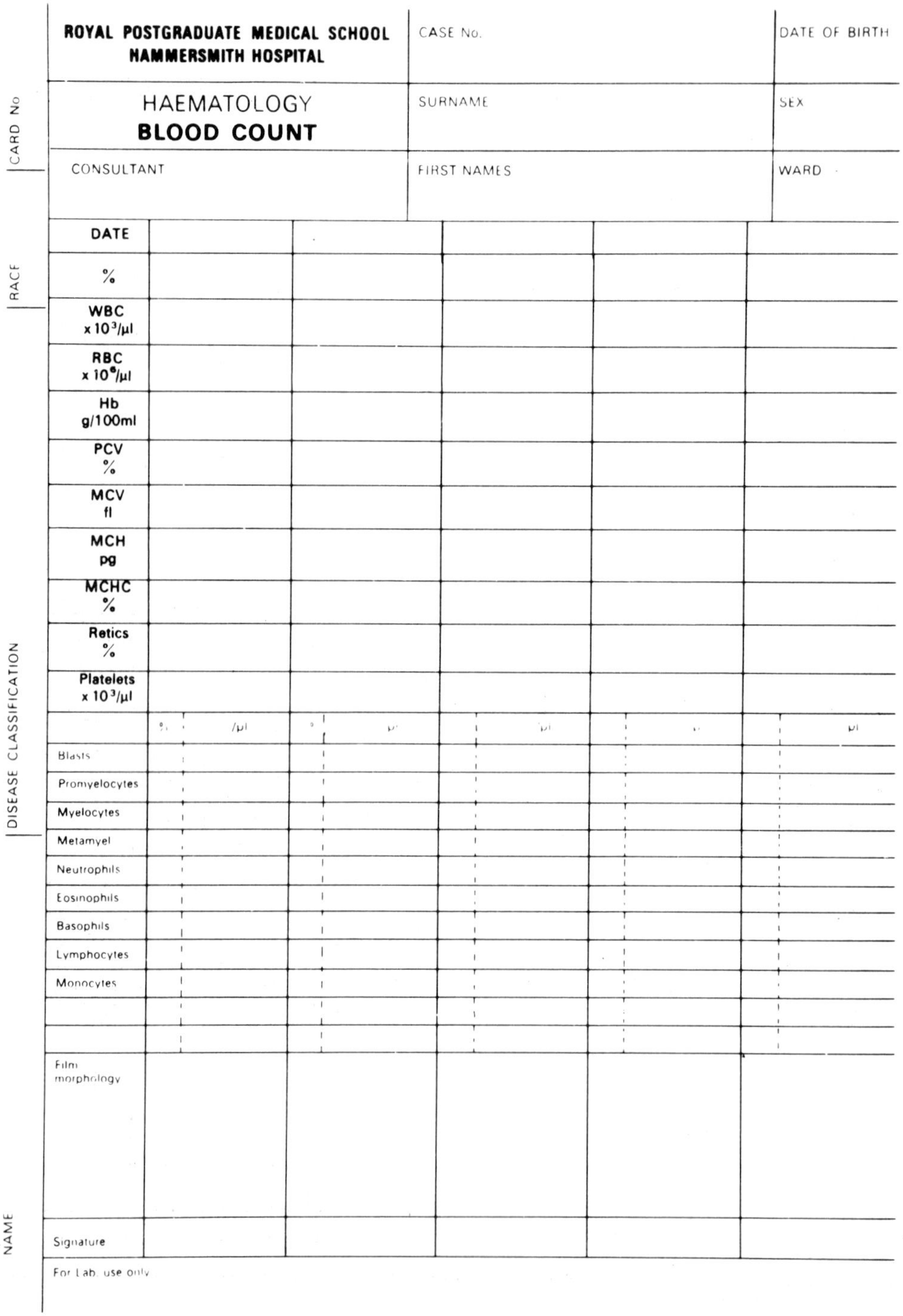

ROYAL POSTGRADUATE MEDICAL SCHOOL **HAMMERSMITH HOSPITAL**	CASE No.	DATE OF BIRTH
HAEMATOLOGY **BLOOD COUNT**	SURNAME	SEX
CONSULTANT	FIRST NAMES	WARD

CARD No — RACE — DISEASE CLASSIFICATION — NAME

DATE					
%					
WBC $\times 10^3/\mu l$					
RBC $\times 10^6/\mu l$					
Hb g/100ml					
PCV %					
MCV fl					
MCH pg					
MCHC %					
Retics %					
Platelets $\times 10^3/\mu l$					
	% /µl	% µl	% µl	% µl	% µl
Blasts					
Promyelocytes					
Myelocytes					
Metamyel					
Neutrophils					
Eosinophils					
Basophils					
Lymphocytes					
Monocytes					
Film morphology					
Signature					

For Lab. use only

Fig. 3.1 Example of blood-count record card. As used at Royal Postgraduate Medical School before introduction of a computer method for data presentation.

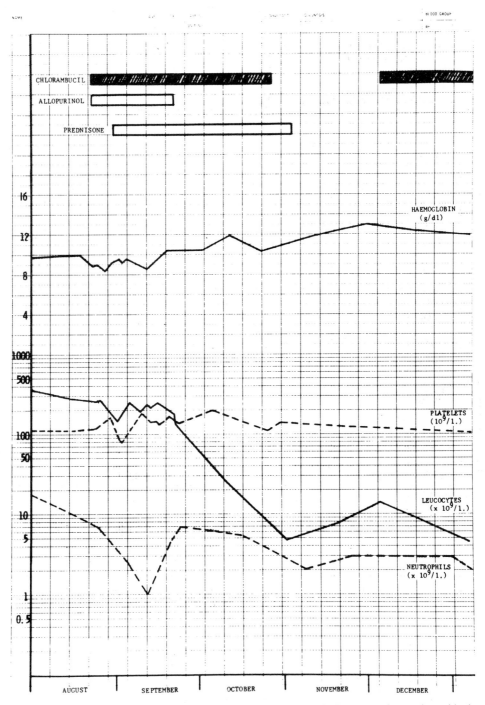

Fig. 3.2 Haematology chart for recording blood-count data as a time-related graph. The course in a patient with chronic lymphocytic leukaemia is illustrated.

of all other tests performed on the same patient. Reports can be displayed on a video-display unit (VDU) or typed by teletype printer in the laboratory or in wards or other sites away from the laboratory.

As a rule processing of blood counts is practical only by an on-line system capable of handling the high volume of work which this entails.

By interphasing the computer with the cell counter, results can be entered automatically into the computer store for processing. This also provides a powerful tool for continuous quality control by testing the constancy of the mean results of red cell indices (see p. 34).

When only off-line facilities are available, the data are processed at intervals throughout the day, depending on the availability of the computer, which will, as a rule, be shared by other users.

The scope of a computer's performance depends, essentially, on the time it takes to respond to an enquiry or instruction and its storage capacity. The time taken to answer an enquiry or to allow the next entry to be handled is a crucial factor in the acceptability of a system. A consistent delay of more than 2–3 s may become intolerable in a busy laboratory. For a laboratory with a workload of up to 1000 tests a day, a core store of at least 16 K (K = 1024 locations) is necessary. A complete system to include all tests in a busy laboratory might require a capacity of 56–120 K. Even so, in most cases, only 2–3 months of cumulative reports can be stored for ready access.

In recent years various programs have been developed for clinical laboratories. Their uses and limitations in haematological work have been described in a number of reviews.[1,3,4] In blood transfusion departments they are useful for recording information on blood groups of patients and donors, and on the use of blood and blood products both for the patients' records and for blood bank stock control.[5,8,13]

Bar coding on the labels attached to specimen containers allows the specimens to be identified by an analyser equipped with a bar-code recorder and for their identity to be included automatically in the reports of the test results.

Computers also have a useful role in laboratory management for monitoring expenditures and calculating the cost of different tests,[2] and for maintaining workload records (see below).

WORKLOAD RECORDS

Effective management requires the controlled use of the laboratory. An important aspect of this control is to relate each test to its cost, taking account of the cost of reagents, disposable materials, capital cost and maintenance of equipment, use of computer facilities as well as the time taken to perform the test and the level of technical skill required. No method for cost analysis is applicable to all laboratories, but a number of systems have been proposed which provide useful guidelines.[2,6,12]

MAINTENANCE OF EQUIPMENT

All equipment in the laboratory should be inspected at regular intervals and specific maintenance procedures carried out as indicated in Table 3.1. Full service is usually undertaken by the manufacturer; other procedures will normally be within the competence of the laboratory staff.

INSTRUMENT EVALUATIONS

Before selecting an instrument in preference to others which are available it is necessary to assess the claims for each by their manufacturers and to decide which is most likely to serve the needs of a particular laboratory. Protocols suitable for evaluating blood cell counters and other haematology analysers have been published by the International Committee for Standardization in Haematology.[10,11] The following are included in an evaluation:

1. Verification of instrument requirements for space, and services.
2. Extent of technical training required to operate the instrument.
3. Clarity and usefulness of instruction manual.
4. Assessment of safety (mechanical, electrical, microbiological and chemical).
5. Determination of
   (a) linearity;
   (b) precision;
   (c) carry over;
   (d) accuracy by comparison with measurement by definitive or reference methods;

Table 3.1 Scheme for inspection and maintenance of equipment

Type of apparatus	Type of maintenance	Frequency
Pipettes	Calibrate	When first used
	Check tip	Each time used
Autodiluters/pipettes	Check calibration	Weekly
Photometers and	Check calibration	Daily before use
spectrophotometers	Prepare calibration graph	6-monthly
	Stability	6-monthly
	Full service	*
Cell counter	Clean with bleach**	Weekly or more frequently
	Rinse glassware	Weekly
	Grease seals	Monthly
	Check calibration	Daily or when control is unsatisfactory
	Full Service	*
Centrifuge	Clean and disinfect	Weekly or more frequently
	Check speed	6-monthly
	Check times and locks	6-monthly
	Full service	*
pH meter	Two-point calibration	Daily
	Full service	*
Temperature-controlled instruments (water-baths, incubators, centrifuges, refrigerators)	Record upper and lower temperature extremes	Daily
Microscope	Keep free of dust	Daily
	Clean lenses	Daily
	Full service	*
Safety cabinet	Air flow	Weekly
	Full service	*

*According to manufacturer's recommendations
**e.g. Sodium hypochlorite solution with 5% available chlorine.

(e) comparability with an established method used in the laboratory;

(f) sensitivity (i.e. determination of the smallest change in analyte* concentration which gives a measured result);

(g) specificity (i.e. extent of errors caused by interfering substances).

6. Throughput time and number of specimens that can be processed within a normal working day.
7. Cost per test.
8. Reliability of the instrument when in routine use and adequacy of service and maintenance provided.
9. Staff acceptability, impact on laboratory organization and level of technical expertise required to operate the instrument.

*i.e. the substance which is being measured.

As a rule this type of evaluation is carried out by a reference laboratory on behalf of a national consumer organization or Government Health Agency.

After an instrument has been purchased and installed it is necessary for the individual user to ensure that the specific instrument is satisfactory. This requires a less extensive check of performance with regard to precision, linearity, carry over and comparability.

Precision

Carry out appropriate measurements 10–20 times consecutively on three or more specimens, selected in the pathological range so as to include a low, a high and normal concentrate of the analyte or analytes. Calculate standard deviation (SD) and coefficient of variation (CV) as derived on p. 543.

Linearity

This demonstrates the effects of dilution.

Prepare a specimen with a high concentration of the analyte to be tested, e.g. packed cells for haemoglobin and red cell count, buffy layer for leucocytes and platelets. As accurately as possible make a series of dilutions in plasma so as to obtain ten samples with evenly spaced concentration levels between 10% and 100%. Measure each sample and calculate the means. Plot results on arithmetic graph paper. All points should fall on a straight line which should pass through the zero of the horizontal and vertical axes. Inspection of the graph will show whether there is linearity throughout the range or whether it is limited to part of the range. Linearity can also be assessed by calculating the expected value for measurements from its dilution. The actual results should lie within the limits of CV obtained from the analysis of precision (see above). The red cell indices MCV, MCH and MCHC should not be affected by dilution of the specimen and a horizontal line (zero slope) should be obtained for these.

Carry over

This indicates the extent to which a measurement of an analyte in a specimen is likely to be affected by the preceding specimen.

Measure a specimen with a high concentration in triplicate, immediately followed by a specimen with a low concentration of the analyte.

$$\text{Carry over (\%)} = \frac{l_1 - l_3}{h_3 - l_3} \times 100,$$

where l_1 and l_3 are the results of the first and third measurements of the samples with a low concentration and h_3 is the third measurement of the sample with a high concentration.

Comparability

This tests whether the new instrument (or method) gives results which agree satisfactorily with those obtained with an established procedure, e.g. that in routine use in the laboratory. At least 100 specimens should be measured alternatively or in batches by the two procedures. Whilst the specimens should in general be unselected it may be necessary to augment them with specimens which will provide information on the extreme limits of the pathological range and on the effects of interfering substances (e.g. in hyperbilirubinaemia, lipaemia, paraproteinaemia).

Results can be analysed by two procedures:

1. If the result obtained by the instrument under test is p and by the established method is q, determine p − q, and then plot the data on arithmetic graph paper, with q on the horizontal axis and p − q on the vertical axis. If the methods are comparable the points will lie close to the horizontal axis.

2. Analyse the data statistically by paired t-test (p. 543) to determine whether differences between the measurements are significant.

LABORATORY SAFETY

Two aspects need to be considered:

1. Handling of biohazardous specimens
2. Exposure to reagents which are toxic or potentially carcinogenic

Handling of biohazardous specimens[7,9]

All material of human origin should be regarded as capable of transmitting infections, and must be handled carefully to avoid contamination. Mouth pipetting is forbidden and no eating, drinking or smoking should be permitted in the laboratory working area. In addition, specimens of blood, bone marrow and other materials from patients suffering from hepatitis or AIDS as well as blood found to contain hepatitis B antigens or antibodies or HIV antibody are biohazardous. Other high risk specimens include those from patients who have previously received multiple transfusions of untested blood or blood products and drug addicts. When blood is collected from such patients, special precautions must be taken to avoid contamination, e.g. by wearing plastic or rubber gloves, promptly disposing of syringe, needle, dressing etc., and by decontaminating any spillage which may occur.

When handling the specimens:

1. Use a separate room if possible or at least a dedicated part of the laboratory and carry out all manual procedures in a microbiological safety cabinet.
2. Wherever possible use disposable plastic containers instead of glassware. Do not use broken or chipped glassware and take great care not to prick yourself with sharp-pointed instruments such as scissors or needles.
3. Wear close-fitting plastic or rubber gloves, wear glasses or goggles and a disposable plastic apron over the normal laboratory protective clothing.
4. Keep the bench area clear of all equipment other than that required for the immediate procedure.
5. Centrifuge specimens only in sealed centrifuge buckets to minimize droplets or aerosol spray.
6. Immediately after completion of the work disinfect the working area with freshly prepared 1% sodium hypochlorite (e.g. Chloras, Domestos); soak pipettes in 2.5% solution for 30 min or longer, and for blood spillage use a 10% solution.★
7. After using automated blood cell counters or other automated equipment, disinfect them by flushing several times with 10% sodium hypochlorite solution or with glutaraldehyde, freshly diluted to 2% in 3 g/l sodium bicarbonate, followed by thorough rinsing in water. Only glutaraldehyde should be used in instruments with a metal surface as hypochlorite causes corrosio...
8. Place all material for disposal in ... bags for transport without spillage t... autoclave.
9. In case of accidental skin puncture wash th... affected part gently in running tap water without scrubbing.

Reagents

A number of reagents used in haematological tests contain chemicals which are extremely toxic (e.g. potassium cyanide) or potentially carcinogenic (e.g. benzidine). However, in the amounts required in test reagents the risk from these substances is negligible when used with reasonable care under normal working conditions. The reagents should be prepared from the hazardous substances only by experienced workers; the following precautions should be observed:

1. Store the chemical in a secure place with restricted access.
2. Weigh the desired amount of chemical in a fume cupboard with a minimum inward air velocity of 0.8 m/s at the opening.
3. Wear plastic or rubber gloves and protective clothing.

Radiation hazard

Radiation protection when using radionuclides is described in Chapter 21.

★Commercial products usually contain 10% (10^4 ppm) available chlorine.

REFERENCES

[1] ARDERN, J. C., HEROD. E., HYDE, K., URMSTON, A., MacIVER, J. E. (1982). Microcomputer data handling for the Phoenix system. *Clinical and Laboratory Haematology*, **4**, 299.

[2] BROUGHTON, P. M. G. and WOODFORD, F. P. (1983). Benefits of costing in the clinical laboratory. *Journal of Clinical Pathology*, **36**, 1028.

[3] BULL, B. S. and KORPMAN, R. A. (1986). Computer systems: design and management. In *Automation and Quality Assurance in Haematology*. Eds. R. M. Rowan and J. M. England, p. 178. Blackwell Scientific Publications, Oxford.

[4] CLARKE, A. A., COLEMAN, S. J., PRALL, A. and WOOTTON, I. D. P. (1980). Data processing in pathology laboratories: the extension of the Phoenix system into haematology. *Clinical and Laboratory Haematology*, **2**, 63.

[5] CLARK, I. R., PAREKH, J., PETERS, M., FREW, I. and IBBOTSON, R. N. (1984). Hospital blood bank laboratory data processing system. *Journal of Clinical Pathlogy*, **37**, 1157.

[6] College of American Pathologists (1977). *Laboratory Workload Recording Method*, 4th edn. CAP, Skokie, I11.

[7] Department of Health and Social Security (1978). *Code of Practice for the Prevention of Infection in Clinical Laboratories and Post-mortem Room*. HMSO, London.

[8] GUNSON, H. H. (1986). Blood transfusion automation and data processing. In *Automation and Quality Assurance in Haematology*. Eds. R. M. Rowan and J. M. England, p. 251. Blackwell Scientific Publications, Oxford.

[9] Health Services Advisory Committee (1985). *Safety in Health Service Laboratories: Hepatitis B*. HMSO, London.

[10] International Committee for Standardization in Haematology (1978). Protocol for type testing equipment and apparatus used for haematological analysis. *Journal of Clinical Pathology*, **31**, 275.

ial Committee for Standardization in
ology (1983). Protocol for evaluation of automated
cell counters. *Clinical and Laboratory Haematology*,
59.

ENNER, D. W. (1982). The workload recording method: a
management tool for the clinical laboratory. *Human*

Pathology, **13**, 393.

[13] REICH, L. M., MITCHELL, M. J. B., JAMBOIS, W. H.,
HOFFER, J. L., REPS, D. N. and MAYER, K. (1983). A
computer system designed for a hospital transfusion service.
Transfusion, **23**, 316.

4. Quality assurance

Quality assurance in the haematology laboratory is intended to ensure the reliability of the laboratory tests. In this context, account must also be taken of proficiency in collection, labelling, delivery and storage of specimens before the tests are performed, and efficiency of recording and reporting of results.

A quality assurance programme has two separate aspects, namely, internal quality control and external quality assessment. Internal quality control is based on monitoring various aspects of the haematology test procedures that are performed in the laboratory. It includes measurements on specially prepared materials, and repeated measurements on routine specimens, as well as statistical analysis, day by day, of data obtained from the tests which have been routinely carried out. Internal quality control is intended to ensure that there is continual evaluation of the reliability of the work of the laboratory and control is exercised over the release of test results. External quality assessment is the objective evaluation by an outside agency of performance by a number of laboratories on material which is supplied specially for the purpose; this is usually organized on a national or regional basis. Analysis of performance is retrospective.

The objective of a quality assurance programme is to achieve precision and accuracy. Accuracy refers to the closeness of the estimated value to that considered to be true. Precision refers to the reproducibility of a result, accurate or inaccurate. Inaccuracy and/or imprecision occurs as a result of improper standards or reagents, incorrect instrument calibration, or poor technique, e.g. consistently faulty dilution or the use of a method that gives a reaction that is incomplete or not specific for the test. Precision can be controlled by replicate tests, check tests on previously measured specimens and statistical evaluation of results. Accuracy can, as a rule, be checked only by the use of reference materials which have been assayed by independent methods of known precision. In general, reference materials are either assayed samples that can be measured alongside each batch of routine specimens without being identifiable during the test or standard preparations handled in a special way. It is important to distinguish between reference standards that are used for instrument calibration and fresh or preserved blood used for quality control. In some cases the same material may serve both functions, but it is important that their different purposes are appreciated.

REFERENCE PREPARATIONS: HAEMOGLOBIN AND BLOOD CELLS

Haemoglobin

The availability of an international reference preparation[8] has contributed to improved accuracy of Hb measurement. In several countries working standards are prepared which conform to the international reference preparation and the appropriate national authority certifies that this is so.

For quality assurance, blood of attested Hb content is valuable. Because such blood can be kept only for a short time, it cannot be used as an alternative to a haemiglobincyanide (HiCN) standard. Both whole blood and lysates are of use, as differences in results obtained with these preparations help to distinguish errors due to incorrect dilution from those due to inadequate mixing or failure of a reagent to bring about complete lysis. Whole-blood reference samples should be introduced into a batch of blood samples and all the samples assayed together.

Red cells

Reference preparations for the red cell count are essential for the calibration of electronic particle counters, especially automated systems which can be adjusted arbitrarily. This means that to obtain a true result the machine has to be calibrated using a reference preparation with assigned values of known accuracy (p. 43).

Natural blood, collected into EDTA, is of no value as a reference preparation because of its short life in the laboratory. Blood will, however, keep for a few weeks at 4°C if acid citrate dextrose (ACD) or citrate phosphate dextrose (CPD) has been added to it. Even so, the MCV slowly increases and some of the red cells are slowly lost, with the result that the blood cannot be regarded as a reference material, although it can be used as a control to check the precision and reliable functioning of a cell counting system over relatively short periods of time.[13]

Attempts have been made to provide suitably sized particles in stable suspension as substitutes for normal blood cells. These include spherical latex particles and glutaraldehyde-fixed red cells.[14] The cells can be permanently stabilized by fixation,

especially in glutaraldehyde solution. The glutaraldehyde causes the red cells to shrink in size immediately and the shrinking process continues for 3–4 days. Thereafter, the cells remain constant in size and shape, and the results of cell counts and the cell size distribution remain the same for months or even years. Unfortunately, there are, nevertheless, disadvantages in using these cells as a cell reference preparation: in most counting systems, natural (fresh) red blood cells become spherical when diluted, whereas the fixed red cells remain biconcave discs; they are too inflexible and have different flow properties so that they cannot be used to calibrate an instrument for subsequent measurement of natural blood.[16,18] Latex spheres are now available in a series of defined sizes between 2 and 12 µm in diameter, and some of these preparations may prove suitable for use as primary reference materials for sizing red cells provided that a reliable 'shape factor' can be established.[14]

Platelets

Glutaraldehyde or formaldehyde

Fixed platelets provide a useful reference preparation for platelet counting, as they retain their natural shape when diluted. It is, however, important to ensure that the method does not result in aggregation and irreversible clumping of the platelets.

Leucocytes

Three types of material are suitable as reference materials for leucocyte counts:

1. Leucocytes concentrated from human blood and fixed in the following solution:[19]
   Glacial acetic acid 42 mg
   Sodium sulphate 7 g
   Sodium chloride 7 g
   Water to 1 litre.
2. Glutaraldehyde-fixed turkey or chicken erythrocytes resuspended in leucocyte-free mammalian whole blood.[13]

3. Latex particles 5–6 μm in diameter.[14]

Leucocytes undergo changes when a fresh blood sample is diluted for measurement in an automated counting system. These size changes are not paralleled in the reference materials. They are thus unsuitable as standards for leucocyte sizing and for differential counts based on the identification of cells by difference in size.

Other analytes

These will be referred to in the sections where the tests are described. International preparations are, as a rule, biological material, available from the World Health Organization, with assigned values of activity. They include preparations for erythropoietin, blood group sera, thromboplastins and several other coagulation factors.[22] These preparations are not freely available for routine use but are intended to act as standards for assigning values to commercial (or laboratory produced) 'secondary standards' or calibrators.

In some countries national standards are available, while in Europe the Bureau of Reference (BCR)* of the EEC is establishing a number of reference materials.

QUALITY CONTROL MATERIAL FOR BLOOD COUNTS

The best material for internal quality control procedures for haemoglobin, red cell and leucocyte counts is human, horse or donkey blood collected into ACD or CPD (see p. 535) and passed through a blood-infusion set to remove any clots. For different aspects of the blood count preserved blood, stabilized red cells or a lysate are used. One unit of blood (500 ml) will be sufficient to provide about 75 ml of lysate or 200 ml of resuspended stabilized cells. For platelets a special collection procedure is required.

When human blood is used, it should, if possible, first be checked to ensure that it is hepatitis-B antigen and AIDS-antibody negative. If this information is not available it should be handled in the same way as a patient's sample (see p. 24).

PREPARATION OF PRESERVED BLOOD[21]

Collect a unit of blood into a blood transfusion donor bag containing ACD or CPD. Run the blood through a transfusion-giving set into a sterile 2 1 round-bottomed flask. The contents of the flask must be mixed continuously** throughout the subsequent steps and every effort must be made to minimize bacterial contamination by careful technique.

Adjust the red cell count and leucocyte count as required:

1. To increase the red cell count, let the cells settle over exit vents of the pack and then run them into the flask with a minimum of plasma.

2. To lower the red cell count, add compatible plasma or a solution containing 1.5 volumes of ACD and 10 volumes of 9 g/l NaCl.

3. To raise the leucocyte count, add fixed avian cells (p. 30).

4. To lower the leucocyte count, pass blood through a leucocyte filter.† Add 10^6 units of benzyl penicillin and 1 g of streptomycin per 500 ml total volume. With continuous mixing** dispense into sterile containers and cap tightly. Store at 4°C. Assign values for Hb, red cell and leucocyte counts and PCV by 10 replicate measurements using the system on which the material will be used. The CV should not exceed 2%. Check dispensing by repeated counts on five randomly selected tubes. Before analysis, mix a sample on a roller mixer or continuously by hand for 5 min before opening. Unopened vials of human blood should keep in good condition for about 3 weeks at 4°C, horse blood for up to 3 months.[13]

---

*Bureau Communautaire de Référence, Rue de la Loi 200, B-1049 Brussels, Belgium.
** A mixing unit which is particularly suitable is available.[4,20]
† e.g. Sepacel R-500 (Ashahi Medical Co., Tokyo).

PREPARATION OF LYSATE

Collect blood as described above into a blood transfusion donor bag. Centrifuge at c 2000 g for 20 min and remove the plasma aseptically. Add an equal volume of 9 g/l NaCl (saline), mix well, transfer to a sterile centrifuge bottle and re-centrifuge; discard the supernatant and the buffy coat. Repeat the saline wash three times to ensure complete removal of the plasma, leucocytes and platelets. Add to the washed cells half their volume of carbon tetrachloride, cap and then shake vigorously on a mechanical shaker or vibrator for 1 h. Then keep overnight at 4°C to allow the lipid/cell debris to form a semi-solid interface between the carbon tetrachloride and lysate. On the following day, centrifuge at c 2500 g for 20 min, remove the upper lysate layers and pool them in a clean bottle.

Using gentle water-pump suction, filter the lysate through Whatman No. 1 filter paper in a Büchner funnel. Repeat filtration using Whatman No. 42 filter paper, changing the paper whenever the filtration slows down. It is important not to overload the funnel with lysate. To each 70 ml of lysate add 30 ml of glycerol. Mix well; if it is necessary to lower the Hb concentration, add 30% glycerol in saline. To each 500 ml of glycerol-lysate add 10^6 units of benzyl penicillin and 1 g of streptomycin. Mix well and dispense aseptically into sterile containers* and cap tightly.

Assign a value for Hb concentration by the spectrophotometric method (p. 38); carry out 10 replicate tests, taking samples at random from several tubes of the batch. The CV should be less than 2%. Stored at 4°C, the product should maintain its assigned value for several months.

PREPARATION OF STABILIZED ERYTHROCYTES[21]

Sterility must be maintained throughout the procedure. Centrifuge blood at c 2000 g for 20 min and remove the plasma aseptically. Add an equal volume of 0.15 mol/l phosphate buffer, pH 7.4 (p. 538); mix and transfer to a sterile centrifuge bottle; re-centrifuge and discard the supernatant and buffy coat. Repeat the wash and centrifugation twice. To the washed cells, add 10 times their volume of glutaraldehyde fixative (0.25% in 0.15 mol/l phos-

phate buffer, pH 7.4). Leave overnight at 4°C. On the next day shake vigorously to ensure complete resuspension. Mix on a mechanical mixer for 1 h. To check that fixation has been complete centrifuge 2–3 ml of the suspension, discard the supernatant and add water to the deposit. If lysis occurs, the stock glutaraldehyde requires replacement.

When fixation is complete (i.e. after 18 h exposure), centrifuge the suspension at c 2000 g for 10 min and discard the supernatant. Add an equal volume of water to the fixed cell deposit, resuspend and mix by stirring and shaking; re-centrifuge at c 2000 g for 10 min and discard the supernatant; repeat twice. Resuspend the fixed cells in an appropriate volume of aqueous glycine (125 g/l) and mix well by vigorous shaking; place on a mechanical shaker for 24 h to break up microclumps. The addition of a few 8 mm diameter glass beads helps in this process. Add 10^6 units of benzyl penicillin and 1 g of streptomycin for every 500 ml of suspension. Mix well for at least 20 min and then, with continuous mixing in a mixing unit (p. 29) or constant mixing by hand, dispense into sterile containers with two or three 3 mm glass beads. Cap tightly and seal with plastic tape.**

Establish the cell count by 10 replicate measurements by visual counting or electronic cell counting (p. 42). Fixed cells should only be used in fully automated systems after manual pre-dilution. Check dispensing by repeated counts on five randomly selected tubes. The CV should be less than 3%. For use, resuspend by vigorous shaking by hand or on a vortex mixer for 1 min and then mix on a rotary mixer for at least 10 min before opening the tube. The cells in unopened vials should be stable for several years.

PREPARATION OF 'PSEUDO-LEUCOCYTES'[21]

Stabilized chicken and turkey red cells are suitable for use as 'pseudo-leucocytes' in preserved blood: 25 ml of blood collected into ACD (p. 535) are sufficient. The procedure for preparation is the

---

*γ-irradiated containers are available from most laboratory suppliers. Autoclaving and dry heat sterilization distorts some containers and caps, subsequently causing leakage when filled.
**e.g. Viskrings (Viscose Development Co. Ltd., Croydon, Surrey, UK).

same as for stabilized human red cells (p. 30). Before use, resuspend by vigorous shaking by hand followed by mechanical mixing until no clumps remain at the base of the container. Transfer the required volume of suspension to a sample of human preserved blood or lysate (p. 29), mix well and dispense as already described. Although a 'pseudo-leucocyte' cell concentrate (c 2.5×10^{12}/l) is unsuitable for direct use in fully automated systems, no problems occur when it is diluted in preserved blood, or added to a lysate for the simultaneous control of leucocyte count and Hb or after it has been prediluted manually in 9 g/l NaCl. Establish the cell count by five replicate measurements on two vials from the batch by visual counting (p. 55) or by an electronic cell counter (p. 54). Check the dispensing by repeated counts on 5–10 randomly selected tubes. The CV should be less than 5%.

PREPARATION OF PLATELET CONTROL

Reagents

Alsever's solution. p. 535.

EDTA: 100 g/l in Alsever's solution. This reagent can be kept at 4°C for 6 months.

Diluent: Isoton II (Coulter).

Fixative: 2 ml of 40% formaldehyde in 100 ml of Alsever's solution.

Platelet-rich plasma: Collect one or more units of blood into plastic bags containing ACD or CPD anticoagulant (see p. 00). Centrifuge the bags at 200 g for 10 min; transfer the supernatant plasma containing platelets from each into a transfer pack or another plastic bag. When reconstituted (see below), one unit of normal blood should provide 500 ml of platelet suspension containing c 70–80 $\times 10^9$ platelets per 1 or 250 ml containing c 150 $\times 10^9$ platelets per l.

Method

Add one unit of platelet-containing plasma to each of a series of 150 ml glass bottles containing 1 ml of EDTA solution. Leave at 37°C in a water bath for 1 h to allow the platelets to disaggregate.

Check the disaggregation by passing a small sample from each bottle through a blood counting system set for platelet counts and with a facility for analysing size distribution curves, or by visual inspection of a diluted sample in a haemocytometer chamber. If aggregation is still present leave in the water bath for another 1 h.

Dispense 200 ml of fixative into each of a series of plastic bottles, and into each add the platelet-containing plasma from one glass bottle. Leave at room temperature for about 48 h.

Centrifuge the plastic bottles at c 50 g for 10 min at room temperature.

Distribute the platelet-rich supernatants from each plastic bottle equally into two sterile 500 ml glass bottles. Fill the bottles with Alsever's buffer.

Centrifuge the bottles three times at c 750 g for 30 min at room temperature, resuspending the platelets in Alsever's buffer. After the third wash, remove the buffer and resuspend the platelets in 10 ml of fresh buffer. Mix well.

Transfer the contents of the two bottles into a single glass container or mixing flask (p. 29) and add 500 ml or 250 ml (see above) of Isoton or similar diluent. Add antibiotics (see p. 29). Carefully mix and dispense into sterile containers. Cap and seal with plastic tape (see p. 30).

The preparations will last in a satisfactory condition for at least a year if stored at 4°C.

Assign values by 10 replicate measurements on two samples from the batch by visual counting (p. 55) or by electronic counter (p. 57). To check dispensing, repeated counts should be done on five randomly selected samples. The CV should be less than 3%.

QUALITY CONTROL FOR BLOOD COUNT ANALYSERS

The method described below provides a suitable preparation for control of total red cell, leucocyte and platelet counting by electronic counts, as well as haemoglobin. It should be stable for c 3 weeks if kept at 4°C.

Method

Collect a unit of human blood into CPD anticoagulant (p. 535). Carry out the subsequent procedure no later than one day after collection.

Filter the blood through a blood transfusion recipient set into a 500 ml glass bottle.

Add 1 ml of 40% formaldehyde. Mix well by inverting and then leave on a roller mixer for 1 h.

Leave at 4°C for 7 days, mixing by inverting a few times each day. At the end of this period of storage mix well on a roller mixer for 20 min and then with constant mixing by hand dispense in 2 ml volumes into sterile containers.

Cap tightly and seal with plastic tape. Store at 4°C. Before use mix the vials on a roller mixer for 10–20 min at room temperature. Establish the count for each parameter by 10 replicate measurements on each instrument for which it is intended as a control.

Standard deviation of control specimens

If a value is assigned to a specimen a number of times, the dispersion of results around the mean will indicate the error of reproducibility. This can be expressed as the standard deviation (SD). Subsequently, 95% of results on the same specimen should be within ±2 SD and 99.7% within ±3 SD. Thus, by chance alone 1 in 20 of the measurements might be expected to fall outside ±2 SD but only 1 in 333 outside ±3 SD. If the measurements are more widely dispersed this indicates an error in the test.

To determine the SD, 10–20 identical tests are carried out on samples of the specimen. The standard deviation is then calculated as shown on p. 543.

Calculating the coefficient of variation (CV) provides an alternative way of expressing the dispersion of results. The advantage of the CV is that it relates the SD to the level of the measurements. It is calculated as shown on p. 543.

Control Chart[5,7]

Charts have been used in the laboratory, especially for clinical chemistry, for many years.[12] Samples of the control specimen are included with every batch of patients' specimens and the results checked on a control chart. To check precision it is not necessary to know the exact value of the control specimen. If, however, its value has been determined reliably by a reference method, the same material can also be

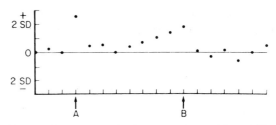

Fig. 4.1 Control chart. At time A a value outside +2 SD occurred as a result of pipetting error. At time B several values had occurred consecutively on one side of the mean, due to deterioration of a reagent. When this was remedied the test was satisfactory.

used to check accuracy or to calibrate an instrument. If possible, controls with high, low and normal values should be used. It is advisable to use at least one control sample per batch even if the batch is very small. As the controls are intended to simulate random sampling, they must be treated exactly like the patients' specimens. The results obtained with the control samples can be plotted on a chart as described below.

The mean value and SD of the control specimen should be first calculated. Using arithmetical graph paper a horizontal line is drawn to represent the mean (as a base) and on an appropriate scale of quantity and unit, lines representing +2 SD and −2 SD are drawn above and below the mean (Fig. 4.1). The results of successive control sample measurements are plotted. The following indicate a fault in technique or in the instrument used:

- Two or more results on or outside the +2 SD and −2 SD limits.
- Consecutive values rising.
- Consecutive values falling.
- Consecutive values on one side of the mean (Fig. 4.1).

CUMULATIVE SUM METHOD [(cusum) 1,7,17]

The CUSUM is the running total of the difference between each measurement and the established mean of the control tests. Taking the plus and minus signs into account it provides another way to display the data obtained in the precision test. It can indicate more sensitively than a control chart a faulty technique or instrument, and it is especially useful for detecting a change in performance due to drift, a consistent error in one direction (bias) or a slight progressive drift away from the original mean.

As a rule, when results fall outside 2 SD of the mean the test is considered to be unreliable. However, the size of change that the test is designed to detect (i.e. sensitivity of analysis) can be varied for the individual test, taking account of the clinical significance of changes in result.

Graphical presentation of CUSUM

Establish the mean value and SD of the control specimen as for the control chart (p. 32). Subtract this mean value from each subsequent observed value for the control specimen and plot the difference on arithmetical graph paper (Fig. 4.2).

Random changes tend to cancel each other out, so that, if the observed values are close to the established mean value, with only random differences, some of the differences will be positive and some negative: the CUSUM will then oscillate around zero, and the charted data will form an approximately horizontal line. Consistent differences in values will result in all the values being either above or below the zero line, or in a change in the slope of the plotted line; the differences become significant if they reach 2 SD of the mean. The scale used for plotting the results should be such that each unit on the horizontal axis (e.g. 1 day) corresponds in scale to 2 SD on the vertical axis.

Numerical analysis of CUSUM[7]

Method

1. Establish mean and SD of the control preparation; decide on the minimum significant change which should be detected, usually 2 SD.

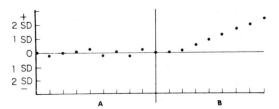

Fig. 4.2 CUSUM chart. A illustrates a satisfactory performance; B indicates a small consistent error.

2. Calculate the following values for the control:
   Upper reference value (URV) = m + 1 SD*
   Lower reference value (LRV) = m − 1 SD*
   Where m = mean
   Decision interval (DI) = 2.6 SD*

3. Analyse a sample of the control after every 10–20 patient samples. Start with the CUSUM as zero, and begin to record results only if the measured value of the control falls outside URV or LRV. If so, record the difference between the result (x) and the appropriate reference value (i.e. x − URV or LRV − x) for a positive score.

4. With each subsequent test add the difference between the result and the same reference value to the previous CUSUM score (observing the sign) to give the new CUSUM.

If the CUSUM changes direction but its value does not exceed the opposite reference value, stop recording it. Restart the calculation only if the value again falls outside one of the reference values.

If on the other hand the CUSUM changes sign and this causes the result to lie outside the opposite reference value, there has been an abrupt calibration shift or a sporadic 'blunder'. A repeat test on further samples of the control specimen may help to elucidate the cause.

If the CUSUM exceeds the decision interval (i.e. 2.6 SD), a significant change in accuracy has probably occurred. Check and correct calibration and then start a new CUSUM as described above.

DUPLICATE TESTS ON PATIENTS' SPECIMENS

This provides another way of checking the precision of routine work.[3] Test ten consecutive specimens in duplicate. Calculate the differences between the pairs of results and derive the SD (p. 543). In all instances the duplicate tests should not differ from each other by more than 2 SD. This method is not sensitive to gradual drift nor will it detect incorrect calibration.

Check tests are similar to duplicate tests but specimens are used that have been measured originally in an earlier batch. The two tests should agree with each other within 2 SD. This procedure

---

*or higher value if this is too narrow in practice.

will detect any deterioration of apparatus and re-agents which may have developed between tests, if it is certain that the earlier specimen has not altered.

USE OF NORMAL HAEMATOLOGICAL DATA FOR QUALITY CONTROL

In healthy individuals, the blood count data remain virtually constant day by day, subject only to the physiological changes already discussed (p. 11). It is possible to use observations on healthy individuals for quality control in routine laboratory work by analysing the results of blood counts from 5–10 healthy subjects at intervals and calculating means and SD for MCV, MCH and MCHC (p. 51). On each occasion the mean should not vary by more than 2 SD and the SDs themselves should remain constant. Significant difference in mean indicates a constant error, e.g. incorrect calibration; random errors will result in an increase in SD although the mean may be unaffected.

USE OF PATIENT DATA FOR QUALITY CONTROL

In medium to large hospitals with a large number (i.e. several hundred) of patients investigated each day, there should be no significant day-to-day variability in the means of their red cell indices obtained by an automated blood counter provided that the population of patients remains stable and that samples from a particular clinical source are not processed all in the same set thus disproportionately influencing the mean. Assuming that the sample population is stable, any significant change in the means of the red cell indices will indicate a change in instrument calibration or a drift due to a fault in its function.

To start this programme it is first necessary to assay samples from at least 500 patients in an automated blood counter and to establish the means of MCV, MCH and MCHC. Then, using an algorithm proposed by Bull,[10] and a computer, it is possible to analyse the result on successive batches of 20 specimens. By plotting these results ($\overline{X}_B$) on a graph any drift from the three indices can be readily recognized and used to identify instrument faults[2] (Fig. 4.3).

The algorithm is now incorporated in some automated blood counters. This method appears to be as accurate and as precise as the use of preserved blood controls.[11] It is particularly useful in validating successive batches of calibrators.

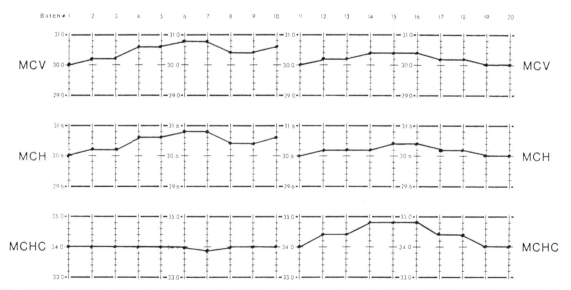

Fig. 4.3 Example of quality control based on patients' data: synchronous changes in MCV and MCH caused by partial blockage of aperture (Batches 1–10) and synchronous changes in MCV, MCH and MCHC caused by bubbles (Batches 11–20). The plots are mean results in batches of 20 tests.
Reproduced with permission from Bull, B. S. and Korpman, R. A. (1982). Interlaboratory quality control using patients' data. *Methods in Hematology*, **4**, 121.

EXTERNAL QUALITY ASSESSMENT[6,9,15,21]

External Quality Assessment (EQA) is an important supplement to the internal control system used by an individual laboratory. Even when all possible precautions are taken to achieve accuracy and precision in the laboratory, errors arise which are only detectable by objective external assessment. The principle is that the same material is sent from a national or regional centre to a large number of laboratories. All the laboratories send results back to the centre where they are analysed and the median or mean and SD are calculated. An individual laboratory can then compare its performance in the survey with that of other laboratories and with its own previous performance. A 'deviation index' can be calculated, i.e. the difference between the individual laboratory's result and the mean (calculated from the results of all laboratories) related to the SD.

Deviation Index

$$= \frac{\text{Actual results} - \text{weighted mean or median for test}\star}{\text{Weighted SD}\star}$$

A deviation index (score) of less than 0.5 denotes excellent performance; a score between 0.5 and 1.0 is satisfactory and a score between 1.0 and 2.0 is still acceptable. A score above 2.0 indicates that there is a defect requiring attention.

In addition to providing guidance on the laboratory's general level of performance, a major purpose of EQA is to achieve harmonization or concordance between laboratories. Specimens used for surveys must remain stable during transit. In general material used for internal quality control (p. 29) is suitable for EQA surveys. However, some blood cell counters handle preserved blood differently from routine specimens and even if correctly calibrated different types of counters may differ in their responses to EQA samples; it may thus be necessary to analyse results separately for different groups of instruments. When there are unexplained differences in counts on EQA samples with different instruments in a laboratory, counts should be made on fresh EDTA blood samples with the different instruments in order to check their comparative performance.

ROUTINE QUALITY ASSURANCE PROGRAMME: A SUMMARY

The procedures which should be included in a comprehensive programme will vary with the tests undertaken, the instruments used (especially if these include a fully-automatic counting system), the size of the laboratory and the numbers of specimens handled, the computer facilities available and the amount of time which can be devoted to the programme. Some at least of the following must be carried out:

Calibration of instruments (at intervals; some daily, others weekly): by means of reference preparations and standards; e.g. HiCN reference preparations, preserved blood (in ACD), stabilized blood-cell standards, calibrators with certified values.

Tests on control specimens (daily): control sample with each batch of specimens; control chart; CUSUM; duplicate measurements on patients' specimens (5 or more).

Statistical analysis of patient data (daily): mean of MCV, MCH, MCHC.

Interlaboratory (EQA) surveys (at intervals; usually monthly or 3-monthly).

Correlation assessment (at all times): by means of cumulative report forms (see p. 19); blood film appearances and numerical data; clinical state.

★ Weighted results are obtained by recalculation of the mean after excluding results outside ± 3 SD. When distribution is non-Gaussian, the median should be used rather than the mean and the results weighted by excluding those outside 25th–75th percentiles.

REFERENCES

[1] BISSELL, A. F. (1982). Statistical foreword. *Methods in Hematology*, **4**, 1.

[2] BULL, B. S. and KORPMAN, R. A. (1982). Interlaboratory quality control using patients' data. *Methods in Hematology*, **4**, 121.

[3] CARSTAIRS, K. C., PETERS, E. and KUZIN, E. J. (1977). Development and description of the 'random duplicates' method of quality control for a hematology laboratory. *American Journal of Clinical Pathology*, **67**, 379.

[4] CHAPPELL, D. A., and WARD, P. G. (1978). Safe and sterile mixer for biological fluids. *Laboratory Equipment Digest*, **16**, 75.

[5] ENGLAND, J. M. (1984). Internal quality control and calibration. In *Automation and Quality Assurance in Haematology*. Eds. J. M. England and R. M. Rowan, p. 8–17. Blackwell Scientific Publications, Oxford.

[6] European Committee for Clinical Laboratory Standards (1986). *Standard for Quality Assurance, Part 5: External Quality Assessment in Haematology*. ECCLS Document, Volume 3, No. 1 Beuth Verlag, Berlin.

[7] European Committee for Clinical Laboratory Standards (1987). *Standard for Quality Assurance, Part 4: Internal Quality Control in Haematology*. ECCLS Document. Vol. 4, No. 2. Beuth Verlag, Berlin.

[8] International Committee for Standardization in Haematology (1978). Recommendations for reference methods of haemoglobinometry in human blood (ICSH Standard EP 6/2: 1977) and specifications for international haemiglobincyanide reference preparation (ICSH Standard EP 6/3: 1977). *Journal of Clinical Pathology*, **31**, 139.

[9] KOEPKE, J. A. (1986). In *Automation and Quality Assurance in Haematology*. Eds. J. M. England and R. M. Rowan, p. 62–83. Blackwell Scientific Publications, Oxford.

[10] KORPMAN, R. A. and BULL, B. S. (1976). The implementation of a robust estimator of the mean for quality control on a programmable calculator or a laboratory computer. *American Journal of Clinical Pathology*, **65**, 252.

[11] LEVY, W. C., BULL, B. S. and KOEPKE, J. A. (1986). The incorporation of red blood cell index mean data into quality control programs. *American Journal of Clinical Pathology*, **86**, 193.

[12] LEVY, S. and JENNINGS, E. R. (1950). The use of control charts in the clinical laboratory. *American Journal of Clinical Pathology*, **20**, 1059.

[13] LEWIS, S. M. (1975). Standards and reference preparations. In *Quality Control in Haematology*. Eds. S. M. Lewis and J. F. Coster, p. 79. Academic Press, London.

[14] LEWIS, S. M. (1981). The philosophy of value assignment. In *Advances in Hematological Methods: The Blood Count*. Eds. O. W. van Assendelft and J. M. England, p. 231. CRC Press, Florida.

[15] LEWIS, S. M. (1986). External quality assessment in Europe. In *Automation and Quality Assurance in Haematology*, Eds. J. M. England and R. M. Rowan, p. 18. Blackwell Scientific Publications, Oxford.

[16] RICHARDSON JONES, A. (1982). Counting and sizing of blood cells using aperture-impedance systems. In *Advances in Hematological Methods: The Blood Count*. Eds. O. W. van Assendelft and J. M. England, p. 50. CRC Press, Boca Raton.

[17] RICKETTS, C. (1982). Intralaboratory quality control using control samples. *Methods in Hematology*, **4**, 151.

[18] THOM, R. (1972). Hemocytometry: method and results by improved electronic blood-cell sizing. In *Modern Concepts in Hematology*. Eds. G. Izak and S. M. Lewis, p. 91. Academic Press, New York.

[19] TORLONTANO, G. and TATA, A. (1972). Stable standard suspension of white blood cells suitable for calibration and control of electronic counters. In *Modern Concepts in Hematology*. Eds. G. Izak and S. M. Lewis, p. 230. Academic Press, New York.

[20] WARD, P. G. CHAPPELL, D. A. FOX, J. G. C. and ALLEN B. V. (1975). Mixing and bottling unit for preparing biological fluids used in quality control. *Laboratory Practice*, **24**, 577.

[21] WARD, P. G., WARDLE, J. and LEWIS, S. M. (1982). Standardization for routine blood counting—the role of interlaboratory trials. *Methods in Hematology*, **4**, 102.

[22] World Health Organization (1984). *Biological substances: International Standards Reference Preparations and Reference Reagents*. WHO, Geneva.

5. Basic haematological techniques

ESTIMATION OF HAEMOGLOBIN

The Hb content of a solution may be estimated by several methods: by measurement of its colour, by its power of combining with oxygen or carbon monoxide and by its iron content. The clinical methods to be described are all colour or light-intensity matching techniques, which measure at the same time with different degrees of efficiency any proportion of inert pigments, i.e. methaemoglobin (Hi) or sulphaemoglobin (SHb), that may be present. The oxygen-combining capacity of blood is 1.34 ml O_2 per g Hb. Ideally, as a functional estimation of Hb, measurement of oxygen capacity should be carried out, but this is hardly practicable in clinical work. It gives results at least 2% lower than the other methods because a small proportion of inert pigment is probably always present. The iron content of Hb can be estimated accurately,[86] but again the method is impracticable for routine purposes. Estimations based on iron content are generally taken as authentic, but iron bound to inactive pigment is included. Iron content is converted into Hb content by assuming the following relationship: 0.347 g iron = 100 g Hb.[34]

MEASUREMENT OF HAEMOGLOBIN USING A PHOTOELECTRIC COLORIMETER

In the following section three procedures will be described and their merits and disadvantages discussed:

1. The cyanmethaemoglobin (haemiglobincyanide (HiCN) method.
2. The oxyhaemoglobin (HbO_2) method.
3. The alkaline-haematin method.

There is little to choose in accuracy between the methods, although the alkaline-haematin procedure is probably less accurate than the others. A major advantage of the HiCN method is the availability of a stable and reliable reference preparation. Sahli's

37

acid-haematin method is less accurate than any of the methods mentioned above as the colour which develops is unstable and begins to fade almost immediately after it reaches its peak.

Collection of blood samples for determination of haemoglobin

Venous blood or free-flowing capillary blood added to any solid anticoagulant can be used. The concentration of anticoagulant is not critical. Measurements can be carried out on blood that has been stored at 4°C for several days, provided it has not become obviously infected; but the blood must be allowed to warm up to room temperature and be well mixed before it is sampled.

HAEMIGLOBINCYANIDE (CYANMETHAEMOGLOBIN) METHOD

The basis of the method is dilution of blood in a solution containing potassium cyanide and potassium ferricyanide.[16] Hb, Hi and HbCO (but not SHb) are converted to HiCN. The absorbence of the solution is then measured in a photoelectric colorimeter at a wavelength of 540 nm or with a yellow-green filter (e.g. Ilford 625).

Diluent

This is based on Drabkin's cyanide-ferricyanide solution.[16] The original Drabkin reagent had a pH of 8.6. The following modified solution, which has a pH of 9.6, is less likely to cause turbidity from precipitation of plasma proteins; it consists of potassium ferricyanide 200 mg, potassium cyanide 50 mg, water to 1 litre.

The above solution reacts relatively slowly, and the diluted blood must stand for at least 15 min to ensure complete conversion of Hb. The following further modification, as recommended by the International Committee for Standardization in Haematology,[34] results in a shorter conversion time (3–5 min), although it has the disadvantage that the presence of a detergent causes some degree of frothing:

  Potassium ferricyanide 200 mg
  Potassium cyanide 50 mg
  Potassium dihydrogen phosphate 140 mg

Non-ionic detergent 1 ml
Water to 1 litre.

The pH should be 7.0–7.4. Suitable non-ionic detergents include Nonidet P40 (Sigma), Nonic 218 (Pennsalt Chemicals), Quolac Nic 218 (Unibasic) and Triton X-100 (Rohm and Haas).

The diluent should be clear and pale yellow in colour. When measured against water as blank in a photoelectric colorimeter at a wavelength of 540 nm, absorbence must be zero. If stored at room temperature in a brown borosilicate glass bottle, the solution keeps for several months. It must not be allowed to freeze, as this can result in its decomposition.[87] The reagent must be discarded if it becomes turbid, or if the pH is found to be outside the 7.0–7.4 range or if it has an absorbence other than zero at 540 nm against a water blank.

Haemiglobincyanide (HiCN) reference preparation

With the advent of HiCN as a stable solution other standards have become outmoded. The International Committee for Standardization in Haematology has defined specifications on the basis of a molecular weight of 64 458 and a millimolar coefficient extinction of 44.0.*[34] These specifications have been widely adopted; in Britain they have been incorporated into a British Standard (BS 3985: 1966) for a HiCN solution for photometric haemoglobinometry, and a WHO International Standard has been established.

Solutions of HiCN are stable for at least several years. Reference solutions that conform to the international specifications are available commercially. They contain 550–850 mg Hb per litre and the exact concentration is indicated on the label. The solution is dispensed in 10 ml sealed ampoules, and, to ensure that contamination is avoided, any unused solution should be discarded at the end of the day on which the ampoule is opened. In use, the reference solution is regarded as a dilution of whole blood, and the original Hb concentration that it represents is obtained by multiplying the figure stated on the label by the dilution to be applied to the blood sample. Thus, if the standard solution contains 600 mg Hb per litre, it will have the same

---

* i.e. the absorbence of a solution containing 4×55.8 mg of Hb iron per litre at 540 nm.

optical density as that of a blood sample containing 120 g Hb per litre diluted 1 in 200, or as one containing 150 g Hb per litre diluted 1 in 250.*

The HiCN reference preparation is intended primarily for direct comparison with blood which is also converted to HiCN. It can also be used for the standardization of a whole-blood standard in the HbO_2 method and for the calibration of Gibson and Harrison's standard used in the alkaline-haematin method (see p. 40).

Method

Add 20 µl of blood to 4 ml of diluent. Stopper the tube containing the solution and invert it several times. After being allowed to stand at room temperature for a sufficient period of time to ensure the completion of the reaction (3–5 min, see above), the solution of HiCN is ready to be compared with the standard and a reagent blank in a spectrophotometer at 540 nm or in a photoelectric colorimeter with a suitable filter.** Open an ampoule of HiCN standard (brought to room temperature if previously stored in a refrigerator) and measure the absorbence of the solution in the same spectrophotometer or photoelectric colorimeter against the blank. The standard should be discarded at the end of the day and during the day must be kept in the dark. The absorbence of the test sample must be measured within 6 h of its being diluted.

Calculation

$$\text{Hb g/l} = \frac{^\dagger A^{540} \text{ of test sample}}{A^{540} \text{ of standard}} \times \text{conc. of standard}$$
$$\times \frac{\text{dilution factor (e.g. 201).}}{1000}$$

---

*Within the SI system many measurements are now expressed in terms of substance concentration, using the mole as unit. For clinical purposes, there are practical advantages in continuing to express Hb in mass concentration, i.e. as g/1; if substance concentration is used, the monomer should be the elementary entity used in calculation.[85]
**e.g. Ilford 625, Wratten 74 or Chance 0 Gr 1.
†i.e. absorbence; formerly called optical density. In some instruments, measurements are read as percentage transmittance.

Preparation of standard curve and standard table

When many blood samples are to be tested it is convenient to read the results from a standard curve or table relating absorbence readings to Hb concentration in g/1 for the individual instrument. These can be prepared as follows.

Open an ampoule of HiCN reference solution (brought to room temperature) and measure in the same photometer as is to be used for the subsequent haemoglobinometry the absorbence or transmittance of the solution against a blank of cyanide-ferricyanide reagent. Make readings with the same standard solution diluted with the reagent 1 in 2, 1 in 3, 1 in 4, etc. Translate the Hb value of the solutions into terms of g/1, as described above. If the readings record absorbence, plot them on linear graph paper using arithmetical scales, with absorbence as ordinates (vertical scale). If the readings are in percentage transmittance, use semilogarithmic paper with the transmittance recorded on the vertical (log) scale. As Lambert-Beer's law is valid for HiCN, the points should fit a straight line that passes through the origin. This provides a check that the calibration of the photometer is linear (assuming that the standard has been correctly diluted). From the standard curve it is possible to construct a table of readings and corresponding Hb values. The table may be more convenient than the graph when large numbers of measurements are made. Prepare a calibration curve whenever a new photometer is put into use.

It is important that the performance of the instrument should not vary and that its calibration remains constant in relation to Hb measurements. To ensure this, the reference preparations should be measured at frequent intervals, preferably with each batch of blood samples.

The main advantages of the HiCN method for Hb determination are that it allows direct comparison with the HiCN standard and that the readings need not be made immediately after dilution; it also has the advantage that all forms of Hb, except SHb, are readily converted to HiCN. The use of KCN in the preparation of Drabkin's solution is a potential hazard but the diluent itself, containing only 50 mg of KCN per litre, is relatively innocuous; 600–1000 ml would have to be swallowed to produce serious effects. As already referred to, a possible disadvantage is that the diluted blood has to stand for a period of time to ensure complete conversion of the Hb. Also, the rate of conversion of blood containing COHb is markedly slowed. This difficulty can be overcome by prolonging the reaction time to 30 min.[78]

Abnormal plasma proteins or a high leucocyte count may result in turbidity when the blood is diluted in the cyanide-ferricyanide reagent. The turbidity can be avoided by centrifuging the diluted sample or by increasing the concentration of potassium dihydrogen phosphate to 33 mmol/l (4.0 g/l).[50]

OXYHAEMOGLOBIN METHOD

This is the simplest and quickest method for general use with a photoelectric colorimeter. Its advantages is that it is not possible to prepare a stable HbO_2 standard. The reliability of the method is not affected by a moderate rise in plasma bilirubin but it is not satisfactory in the presence of HbCO, Hi or SHb.

Method

Wash 20 µl of blood into 4 ml of 0.4 ml/l ammonia (sp gr 0.88) contained in a tube provided with a tightly fitting stopper. Mix by inverting the tube several times. The solution of HbO_2 is then ready for matching in the colorimeter at 540 nm or with a yellow-green filter (e.g. Ilford 625). If the absorbence of the Hb solution exceeds 0.7, dilute the blood further with an equal volume of water.

Standard

At a dilution of 1 in 200, blood containing 146 g Hb/l, placed in a 1 cm cell, gives an extinction coefficient of 0.475, using a yellow-green filter (Ilford 625, Wratten 74 or Chance 0 Gr 1) or at 540 nm. A neutral grey filter of 0.475 density (Ilford or Chance) can, therefore, be used as a 146 g/l standard.

Colorimeters and light filters unfortunately differ sufficiently one from the other to make it essential to check the chosen standard at frequent intervals against a HiCN reference preparation in the colorimeter in which it is going to be used. It is probably preferable to use a new fresh whole-blood sample each day as a secondary standard after measuring its Hb content by the HiCN method. Preserved blood (p. 29) or lysate (p. 30) can be used instead.

As originally used, a disadvantage of the HbO_2 method was the tendency for the solution of HbO_2 to fade.[68] This has been found to be due to the high dilution of the solution and the unnecessary high pH, resulting from the use of 1 g/l sodium carbonate solution or relatively strong ammonia solution as diluent. However, using 0.4 ml/l ammonia, the solution appears to be stable for a day or more at room temperature.

ALKALINE-HAEMATIN METHOD

The alkaline-haematin method is a useful ancillary method under special circumstances as it gives a true estimate of total Hb even if HbCO, Hi or SHb is present. A true solution is obtained and plasma proteins and lipids have little effect on the development of colour, although they cause turbidity unless the blood and alkali are quickly and thoroughly mixed.

A disadvantage of the method is that certain forms of Hb are resistant to alkali denaturation, in particular Hb F and Hb Bart's (see p. 240), but this can be overcome by heating the solution in a boiling water-bath for 4 min. In normal circumstances the method is more cumbersome and less accurate than the HiCN or HbO_2 methods, and is thus unsuitable for use as a routine method.

Two methods will be described:

1. The standard method[12] using Gibson and Harrison's standard.[23]
2. The acid-alkali method.

Standard method

Add 50 µl of blood to 4.95 ml of 0.1 mol/l NaOH and heat in a boiling water-bath for exactly 4 min. Cool the sample rapidly in cold water and when cool match against the standard in a photoelectric colorimeter at 540 nm or using a yellow-green filter (e.g. Ilford 625).

Standard

This is a mixture of chromium potassium sulphate, cobaltous sulphate and potassium dichromate in aqueous solution. The solution is equal in colour to a 1 in 100 dilution of blood containing 160 g Hb per litre.

It is essential to heat the standard along with the test sample. Only after heating, which alters the ionization of the salts it contains, does the ability of the standard to absorb green light approximate closely to that of alkaline haematin. A fresh sample of standard should be heated on each occasion and then discarded.

Acid-alkali method

A disadvantage of the alkaline-haematin method, as previously described, is that the solution of Hb in alkali has to be heated to ensure complete denaturation. This procedure can be omitted if the blood is collected first into acid and, after standing for 20–30 min, sufficient alkali is added to neutralize the acid and convert the acid haematin into alkaline haematin.

Wash 50 µl of blood into 4.0 ml of 0.1 mol/1 HC1 and mix immediately. After the tube has stood for 20–30 min, add 0.95 ml of 1 mol/1 NaOH and invert the tube several times. After a further 2 min, measure the test sample in a photoelectric colorimeter at 540 nm or with a yellow-green filter (e.g. Ilford 625) employing as a standard heated Gibson and Harrison's standard (see above) or a grey filter or solution[73] previously calibrated against blood of known Hb content treated by acid and then alkali as described above.

OTHER METHODS OF HAEMOGLOBINOMETRY

Direct-reading haemoglobinometers

These instruments have a built-in filter and a scale calibrated for direct reading of haemoglobin in g/dl or g/l. They are generally based on the oxyhaemoglobin method but a number of instruments are now available which are standardized for the cyanmethaemoglobin method, with a light-emitting diode of appropriate wavelength.* The calibration of this type of instrument should be checked regularly to ensure maintenance of accuracy and precision, using HiCN reference solutions or a secondary standard of preserved blood (p. 29) or lysate (p. 30).

Spectrophotometry

The Hb content of blood can be determined accurately by spectrophotometry. The blood is diluted suitably (1 to 200 or 1 to 250) with cyanideferricyanide reagent (see p. 38) and the absorbence is measured at 540 nm. The Hb content is calculated as follows:

Concentration (g/l)

$$= \frac{A^{540}\text{HiCN} \times 64\,500 \times \text{dilution factor}}{44.0 \times d \times 1000},$$

where A^{540}HiCN = absorbence of the solution at 540 nm, 64 500 = molecular weight of Hb (derived from 64 458), dilution = 201 when 20 µl of blood are diluted in 4 ml of reagent, 44.0 = millimolar extinction coefficient, d = layer thickness in cm, and 1000 = conversion factor for mg to g.

The spectrophotometric method gives a direct measurement of the Hb content of the diluted blood. Calibration of the spectrophotometer should be checked from time to time by verifying that it gives an accurate value for the HiCN standard. Slight deviations from the expected A^{540}HiCN value for the standard may be used to correct the results of test samples for a bias in measurement.[34]

THE TOTAL RED CELL COUNT

The ease, speed and precision with which a red cell count can be obtained by electronic cell counters have increased enormously their diagnostic value. Some instruments are limited to particle counting; others have inter-related systems by means of which the size of cells can be measured, so as to provide values for PCV and MCV; Hb as well, can be

---

*e.g. HemoCue (HemoCue AB, Helsingborg)

determined on the same samples, thus also providing values for MCH and MCHC.

Visual counting is, however, still a necessary procedure in laboratories which do not possess electronic counters and, also, in many laboratories for platelet counts and leucocyte counts.

COUNTING RED CELLS WITH ELECTRONIC COUNTERS

In recent years many different electronic counters have become available. In general they are based on one of the following principles.

Aperture impedance method

This method, first described by Coulter in 1956,[13] depends on the fact that blood is a poor conductor of electricity, whereas certain diluents are good conductors. This difference forms the basis of the Coulter Counter System and is also used in the Sysmex(Toa) counters and in several other counters that have been marketed in recent years.

For a cell count, blood is highly diluted in a buffered electrolyte solution. An external vacuum initiates movement of a mercury siphon which causes a measured volume of the sample to flow through an aperture tube of specific dimensions,

e.g. 100 µm in diameter and 70 µm in length. By means of a constant source of electricity a direct current is maintained between an electrode in the sample beaker and one inside the aperture tube. As a blood cell is carried through the orifice of the aperture tube, it displaces some of the conductive fluid and increases the electrical resistance. This produces a corresponding change in potential between the electrodes, which lasts as long as the cell passes through the aperture tube, and assumes the shape of a pulse. The amplitude of the pulse is proportional to cell volume. The pulses are displayed on an oscilloscope screen, the volume of the cells being indicated by the height of the pulses. The pulses are led to a threshold circuit provided with an amplitude discriminator for selecting the minimal pulse height that will be counted (Fig. 5.1). The process by which the size of the pulses is used to obtain MCV is described on p. 51.

Light scattering

A diluted red cell suspension flows through a chamber so that the cells pass a focused light source in single file; the beam of light is scattered by the cells and converted by a detector into pulses with magnitude proportional to the size of the cells. The

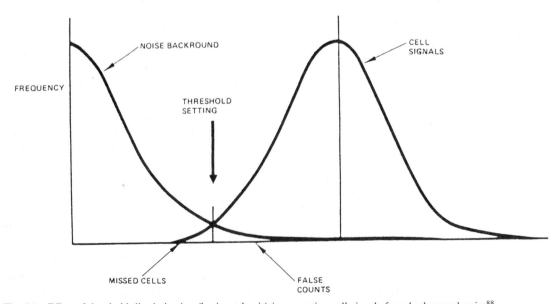

Fig. 5.1 Effect of threshold discrimination (horizontal axis) in separating cell signals from background noise[88].

pulses pass to an electronic system where they accumulate and are counted. Non-coherent tungsten light has been used (e.g. in the Technicon H6000) but newer instruments such as the Technicon H1 and Ortho ELT systems employ a high intensity coherent laser beam which has the advantage of greater depth of focus and less diffusion of the light.

In choosing an instrument for a particular laboratory, account has to be taken of the daily workload, the rate at which specimens are received by the laboratory, and whether the laboratory is concerned primarily with health care screening or with providing a diagnostic service. For a small laboratory all its needs may be satisfied by a simple single-channel cell counting instrument which requires manual dilution of each sample, together with a haemoglobinometer. On the other hand, for large laboratories dealing with 300 or more blood samples daily, automated instruments designed specifically for a routine screening procedure, including platelet counting and differential leucocyte counts, are more suitable (see p. 58).

Detailed discussions of the physical and other aspects of electronic cell counting are beyond the scope of this book; they can be found in a number of other publications.[58,76] Nor will the actual use of the various instruments be described here, as detailed instructions for assembly and operation are supplied by the manufacturers. A number of reports on the evaluation of various instruments have been published in journals and other reports are available in the UK from the NHS Procurement Directorate of the Department of Health.

RELIABILITY OF ELECTRONIC COUNTERS

Electronic blood-cell counters vary considerably in ease of maintenance both from the mechanical and electronic standpoints. Because large numbers of cells can be enumerated, replicate counts correspond closely, and the CV should only be a fraction of that of counts done visually on 500–1000 cells. Electronic counters thus have a very great potential advantage over visual methods of counting blood cells. Not only can many thousands of cells be counted, but the actual time of counting (10–100 s according to the type of machine, is also far less

than that necessary for even a perfunctory visual count. However, the recorded count on the same sample may vary from instrument to instrument and even with different models of the same instrument.[45,80] This is likely to be due to incorrect setting of the threshold discrimination, variation in counting volume or flow rate, or the use of orifice tubes of different dimensions. Other factors include coincidence counts for which adequate correction may not be made, dead-time of the electrical circuit, air bubbles being counted as cells, recirculation of cells around the orifice of the aperture tube, and adhesion of cells to the surface of the container in which the blood is diluted.

It may not be possible to recognize the existence of erroneous results when measurements are carried out on a single machine, as the error may be constant in the particular instrument. The only adequate method of checking is to use a reference preparation to calibrate the instrument (p. 28) and, at frequent intervals, quality assurance procedures to check on precision and accuracy (see p. 35). Auto-agglutinated blood, due to the presence of high-thermal-amplitude cold agglutinins may give erroneously low counts. However, the discrepancy should be obvious when the red cell count is compared with PCV and Hb content. There will be a spuriously high MCV and the cause of the error will be identified when a blood film is examined.

Discrimination threshold

In order to separate background noise from pulses generated by cells and, conversely, not to exclude any signals due to cells, it is necessary to set the threshold of the counter by adjusting the aperture current and pulse amplification (see below). Many modern counters are precalibrated by the manufacturer, especially systems integrating cell counting and sizing.

Calibration

A simple method is to dilute a fresh blood sample (for red cell or leucocyte counting as appropriate) and to carry out successive counts on the suspension whilst the lower threshold control is moved incrementally from its maximum to minimum position.

At the maximum setting the count should be zero or close to zero, and the counts will rise as the amplitude is reduced. The counts at each setting are plotted on arithmetic graph paper (Fig. 5.2). The correct threshold setting is at the far left of the horizontal part of the graph before the line begins to slope. It is important to check that the setting selected for normal red cells is also valid for microcytic cells.

The threshold can be defined more precisely for any individual sample by means of a pulse height analyser linked to the counting system. The lower threshold is correctly set if beyond this point there are less than 0.5% of the counts at the peak (mode) of the pulse size distribution curve (Fig. 5.1).

Coincidence counts

Errors of coincidence can be detected by carrying out a series of measurements of various dilutions of the specimen, plotting the data on graph paper and then extrapolating the graph to the base line for the true value.[71]

Sheath flow

In some systems the diluted blood is injected into a sheath of fluid as it flows into the sensing zone. This induces the cells to pass through the centre of the sensing zone in single file, and free of distortion. This process is also referred to as hydrodynamic focusing. Another device is a 'sweep flow'; this is a directed stream of diluent that sweeps cells and debris away from the aperture, thus preventing cells from being recounted and debris from being counted as cells.

Diluent

The composition of the diluent is critical. For counters based on the impedance method pH, temperature and rate of ionization have to be standardized and remain constant, for changes influence the electrical field and may lead to artefactual alterations in the size, shape and stability of the blood cells in the diluent. Using the diluent prescribed by the manufacturer is especially important for cell sizing measurements.[81] For aperture imped-

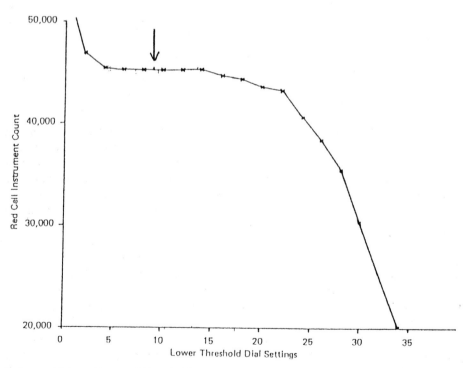

Fig. 5.2 Method to establish working conditions of cell counters. The correct setting of the threshold (at arrow) is intended to exclude noise pulses without loss of the signal pulses produced by the blood cells.

ance counters, a modified Eagle's solution, under the trade name Isoton, was originally recommended by Coulter Electronics. This contained azide, which is a potentially explosive substance.

Modifications of that reagent (Isoton II and III) are recommended by Coulter Electronics for use in different models of the Coulter systems; similarly, other instrument manufacturers recommend diluents in accordance with their own specifications. Adherence to a standard diluent is less important for red cell counting in simple single channel counters, provided that the solution has a pH of 7.0–7.5 and osmolarity 340 ± 10 mmol. [39]

Physiological saline (9 g/1 NaC1), or phosphate buffered saline (Appendix, p. 538), which have the advantages of simplicity and ready availability, can be used as a red cell diluent, provided that the counts are performed immediately after dilution in order to avoid errors due to sphering. Another reason for counting immediately after dilution is to avoid loss of counts due to settling of the red cells.

The solution used for dilution must, as far as possible, be particle-free. Commercial solutions of saline (for intravenous use) are generally suitable; with other solutions it may be necessary to remove dust particles by filtration through a 0.22 or 0.45 μm micropore filter. The diluent should give a background count of less than 50 particles in the measured volume. For instruments in which several measurements are carried out consecutively on a single blood sample, the diluent includes a reagent to lyse the red cells (for the leucocyte count) and to convert Hb to HiCN. Apart from the reagents specified by the manufacturers, a diluent containing potassium cyanide and potassium ferricyanide together with ethylhexadecyldimethyl ammonium bromide can be used.[2,64]

COUNTING RED CELLS BY VISUAL MEANS

Make a 1:200 dilution of blood in formal-citrate solution. This is most conveniently done by washing 20 μl of blood taken into a micropipette into 4 ml of diluting fluid contained in a glass or plastic 75 × 12 mm tube. After sealing the tube with a tightly fitting rubber or plastic bung, mix the diluted blood in a mechanical mixer or by hand for at least 2 min by tilting the tube through an angle

of about 120° combined with rotation, thus allowing the air bubble to mix the suspension.

Fill a clean dry counting chamber, with its cover-glass already in position, without delay. This is simply accomplished with the aid of a Pasteur pipette or a length of stout capillary glass tubing which has been allowed to take up the suspension by capillarity. Care should be taken that the counting chamber is filled in one action and that no fluid flows into the surrounding moat. Leave the chamber undisturbed on a bench for at least 2 min for the cells to settle, but not much longer, for drying at the edges of the preparation initiates currents which cause movement of the cells after they have settled. The bench must be free of vibrations and the chamber not exposed to draughts or to direct sunlight or other sources of heat. It is important that the cover-glass should be of a special thick glass and perfectly flat, so that when laid on the counting chamber, diffraction rings are seen. The cover-glass should be of such a size that when placed correctly on the counting chamber the central ruled areas lie in the centre of the rectangle to be filled with the cell suspension. The preparation must be discarded and the filling procedure repeated using another clean dry chamber if any of the following filling defects occur:

1. Overflow into moat.
2. Chamber area incompletely filled.
3. Air bubbles anywhere in chamber area.
4. Any debris in chamber area.

The type of counting chamber used and the arrangement of the rulings are matters of personal preference and availability. The Neubauer and improved Neubauer chambers have been the commonest types in general use. The visibility of the rulings is as important as the accuracy of calibration.

Count the cells using a 4 mm dry objective and × 6 or × 10 eyepieces. It is important to count as many cells as possible, for the accuracy of the count is increased thereby (see below); 500 cells should be considered the absolute minimum. With a Neubauer chamber (Figs. 5.3 and 5.4), count the cells in 4 or 8 horizontal rectangles of 1 mm × 0.05 mm (80 or 160 small squares) or in 5 or 10 groups of 16 small squares, including the cells which touch the bottom and left-hand margins of the small squares.

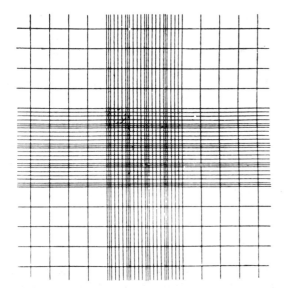

Fig. 5.3 Neubauer counting chamber. The total ruled area is 1 mm × 3 mm; the central ruled area is 1 mm × 1 mm. In the central area 16 groups of 16 small squares are separated by triple rulings.

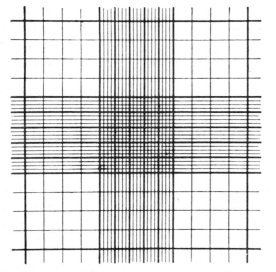

Fig. 5.4 Improved Neubauer counting chamber. The central area consists of 25 groups of 16 small squares separated by closely ruled triple lines (which appear as thick black lines in the photograph).

Calculation

Red cell count (per 1)

$$= \frac{\text{No. of cells counted}}{\text{Volume counted (\mu l)}} \times \text{dilution} \times 10^6.$$

Thus, when the cells in 80 small squares of an improved Neubauer chamber are counted (total volume = 0.02 μl) and the blood is diluted 1:200, the red cell count will be:

$$\frac{N}{0.02} \times 200 \text{ per } \mu l \text{ or } \frac{N}{0.02} \times 200 \times 10^6 \text{ per l.}$$

Red cell diluting fluid

A solution of 10 ml of 40% formalin, made up to 1 litre with 32 g/l trisodium citrate is recommended. The solution is simple to prepare; it keeps well and does not need to be sterilized. The red cells maintain their normal disc-like form and are not agglutinated. The cells are well preserved and counts may be performed several hours after the blood has been diluted.

Occasionally, when the patient's blood is auto-agglutinated, as in some cases of auto-immune haemolytic anaemia, it is advantageous to use as a diluting fluid 32 g/l trisodium citrate solution without the addition of formalin. Auto-agglutination may disperse and enable a count to be carried out in the absence of formalin which appears to prevent, (?) by its fixing action, the clumps of agglutinated cells from breaking up.

Range of red cell counts in health
(see p. 12)

ERRORS OF VISUAL RED CELL COUNTING

The errors associated with the count are of two main kinds: those due to inaccurate apparatus, indifferent technique or unrepresentative nature of the blood counted ('technical' errors) and that due to the distribution of the suspension of red cells in the counting chamber—the 'inherent' or 'field' error. The former errors can be minimized by careful technique, the latter error can be diminished by counting a large number of cells.

Technical errors

These include bad sampling of the blood due to an inadequate flow from a skin puncture; the prolonged use of a tourniquet; insufficient mixing of venous blood which has sedimented after collection; inaccurate pipetting and the use of badly calibrated pipettes or counting chambers; inadequate mixing of the red cell suspension; faulty filling of the counting chamber, and careless counting of cells within the chamber.

It is essential that the accuracy of the apparatus be known so that, if necessary, appropriate correction factors can be applied. The British Standard for Haemocytometer and Particle Counting Chambers (BS 748: 1982) specified a tolerance of dimensions which provides reasonable accuracy. But even so, the chance summation of all the tolerances for different parts of the apparatus in a single counting chamber would result in an error as large as $\pm$ 7%. The exact chamber depth depends also on the cover-glass, which should be free from bowing and sufficiently thick so as not to bend when pressed on the chamber. It must be free from scratches, and even the smallest particle of dust may cause unevenness in its lie on the chamber.

Bulb diluting pipettes are not recommended; they are difficult to calibrate and easily broken. The volumes of blood used are unnecessarily small and the pipettes are difficult to label and handle. In particular, filling the counting chamber so that the exact amount of fluid is delivered from the pipette is an art difficult to master. 20 μl pipettes are relatively inexpensive and easy to calibrate. By the use of 4 ml of diluting fluid in a glass or plastic tube provided with a tightly fitting rubber or plastic bung, a suspension easy to label and handle is obtained, and with a little practice a perfect filling of the counting chamber can regularly be accomplished with the aid of a fine Pasteur pipette or stout glass capillary.

The accuracy of 20 μl pipettes may be checked, after careful cleaning, by filling them to the mark with clean mercury, expelling the mercury and weighing it.[67] 20 μl of mercury weigh 272 mg; 50 μl weigh 680 mg. It is convenient to draw up the mercury to the mark in the pipette by attaching to the pipette a small length of pressure tubing, one end of which has been closed. The measured column of mercury is then expelled on to a previously weighed watch-glass and weighed in a balance sensitive to a difference of 1 mg.

Automatic diluter units are useful. These consist of a dual metering system which enables a volume of diluent and the appropriate volume of blood to be dispensed consecutively into a tube. A variety of automatic diluting systems are now available which have good accuracy and precision. Hand-held semi-automatic microsamplers with a detachable tip (e.g. Eppendorf, Oxford, Labora) are designed to operate as 'to deliver' pipettes.

Pipetting errors apply to all tests which involve dilution of the blood sample and they also occur with autodiluters which are liable to error with viscid fluids and when the delivery volume of the unit is not correctly adjusted. The inherent error, discussed below, is unique to counting.

Inherent error

The distribution of cells in a counting chamber is of an irregular (random) pattern even in a perfectly mixed sample. However, the pattern of distribution conforms to a definite type. Theoretical considerations indicate that variation between the numbers of red cells which settle in areas similar in size should conform to a Poisson distribution (see p. 543) and that the deviation of the distribution of the number of cells in areas of equal size should be given by $\sqrt{\lambda}$ where λ is the total number of cells in each area. However, the movement of the cells in the chamber during the filling process causes them to collide and this influences their distribution which thus differs from the theoretical expectation of the variance.[49] This is given instead by $\sigma = 0.92 \sqrt{\lambda}$. This means that if a counting chamber is filled with a red cell suspension so that the number of cells in an area (say 80 small squares) is 100, σ would be 9.2. Then, if it were possible to count the number of cells in each of 100 similar areas, in 95 areas the number of cells encountered would range between 82 and 118, i.e. 100 $\pm$ 2 σ; in the remaining five areas the counts would be outside this range.

Clearly, this random distribution has a very important bearing on the accuracy of visual blood counts, for no amount of mixing will minimize the inherent variation in numbers between area and area.

The ratio σ/λ is the variation of the *distribution* of cells and this calculated as a percentage gives a convenient way of expressing the inherent error of blood counts.

Table 5.1 Error of the visual red-cell count

No. of small squares counted	No. of cells counted (λ)	$(0.92 \times \sqrt{\lambda})$	Range (95%) $\lambda \pm 2\sigma$	Calculated red cell count ($\times 10^{12}/1$)	Count variation %
80	560	22	516–604	5.16–6.04	3.9
160	1120	31	1058–1182	5.29–5.91	2.8
320	2240	44	2152–2328	5.38–5.82	2.0
640	4480	62	4356–4604	5.44–5.75	1.4

Shows how the inherent error of red-cell counting may be reduced by counting large numbers of red cells.

By contrast to σ, standard deviation (SD) and coefficient of variation (CV) are measures of variance between each result (see p. 543). The inherent error can be reduced only by counting more cells in a preparation. The calculations set out in Table 5.1 demonstrate that, in theory, the count varies in proportion to the square root of the number of cells counted, i.e. if four times the number of cells are counted, the variation is halved. For example, if the imaginary (ideal) figures given in Table 5.1 are studied, it will be seen that 19 out of 20 counts based on the number of cells in 80 small squares will lie within the wide range of 5.16 to $6.04 \times 10^{12}1$. If the cells in 320 small squares are counted, the range will be considerably narrower— 5.38 to $5.82 \times 10^{12}/l$. Causes of error of red cell counts include personal bias from fore-knowledge of what the result should be, selection of counting areas and uneven distribution of cells within the counting chamber due to the momentum given to the cells as the chamber is filled.[61]

The method of making serial counts and taking the mean has been widely (perhaps unconsciously) used as a means of reducing the error of the red cell count. If a sufficient number of counts are done, the truth is likely to reveal itself; and there is also a chance that errors in technique will cancel each other out.

Clearly, the errors of blood counting by visual means are very considerable. That due to the random distribution of the cells in the counting chamber can be reduced by counting the cells in a larger area, as already mentioned (see Table 5.1), but in ordinary laboratory practice there is rarely time to count carefully the cells in more than 160 small squares—about 1000 cells in a normal count. The practice of making counts in duplicate is a good one, but does not necessarily increase accuracy: it is always possible that the second count will be further from the truth than the first, due to the random distribution of cells. It is better to repeat a count using a second chamber and pipette than to count double the number of cells in a single filling of the counting chamber.

DETERMINATION OF PACKED CELL VOLUME (PCV OR HAEMATOCRIT VALUE)

Haematocrit (literally 'blood separation') tubes are in daily use in many haematological laboratories where automated blood-count systems are not available, as the measurement of the PCV can be used as a simple screening test for anaemia. In addition, in conjunction with accurate estimations of Hb and red cell count, knowledge of the PCV enables the calculation of 'absolute' values (see p. 51). Furthermore, it can be used as a reference method for calibrating automated blood count systems.[36] The two methods of direct measurement of PCV that are in current use are :

1. A macro-method using Wintrobe tubes.
2. A micro-method using capillary tubes.

MACRO-METHOD (WINTROBE'S METHOD)

Wintrobe tubes, 2.5–3 mm in general diameter and about 110 mm in length, calibrated at 1 mm intervals to 100 mm, are employed. They hold about 1 ml of blood.

Method

Collect venous blood with minimal stasis and render it incoagulable by EDTA at a concentration of c 1.5 mg/ml or by heparin at a concentration of 15–20 iu/ml. Dipotassium EDTA is to be preferred to the tripotassium salt as the latter produces some shrinkage of red cells which results in a 2–3% decrease in PCV.

Mix the blood carefully by repeated inversion and fill the haematocrit tube at once to the 100 mm mark by means of a glass capillary pipette. Centrifuge the tube at 2000–2300 g for 30 min.*

The height of the column of red cells is taken as the PCV (the volume occupied by the red cells expressed as a fraction of the total volume of the blood). Above the red cells and not included in the figure for the PCV will be seen a greyish-red layer of leucocytes and above this, just below the plasma, a thin creamy layer of platelets. These comprise the 'buffy coat'.

Range for packed cell volume in health
(see p. 52)

Accuracy of macro-method

This is a potentially accurate method with reproducibility c 1%. However, a number of technical factors can lead to significant inaccuracies. These include:

1. Specimen handling.
2. The tubes.
3. Centrifugation and trapped plasma.

Specimen handling. Apart from inaccuracies due to delay in setting up the tests, failure to mix the samples of blood adequately or incomplete filling or faulty reading, EDTA anticoagulant in excess of 1.5 mg/ml of blood may lead to cell

---

*i.e. at a speed of 3000 rpm in a centrifuge of 22.5 cm radius or at a speed of 3800 rpm in a centrifuge of 15 cm radius (see p. 541).

shrinkage. The degree of oxygenation of the blood also affects the result, as the PCV of venous blood is c 2% higher than that of fully aerated blood (which has lost CO_2 and taken up O_2). Storage of blood leads to changes in PCV. Although these changes take place relatively slowly and can be delayed by keeping the blood at 4° C, the measurement of PCV should be carried out with as little delay as possible, and preferably not longer than 6 h after collecting the blood.

Tubes. Variation in bore is the main cause of error. In tubes which conform to the British Standard for Apparatus for Measurement of Packed Red Cell Volume (BS 4316: 1968) the bore is 2.55 mm and it does not vary by more than ± 2% of the mean throughout.

Centrifugation. The aim is to achieve complete packing of the red cells. In addition to the centrifugal force applied, the speed of packing depends upon the density and the size of the cells, the viscosity of the suspending fluid and the relative densities of cells and fluid.

Centrifugation for 30 min at c 2000 g (within the capacity of most laboratory centrifuges) is sufficient to pack the red cells of an anaemic patient to a constant volume. With PCVs of about the normal range (0.36–0.54), an additional 30 min centrifuging will reduce the apparent red cell volume by c 1%, whilst in polycythaemia, with a PCV exceeding 0.55, the further packing resulting from the prolonged centrifugation may amount to as much as 3% (e.g. a reduction in PCV from 0.60 to 0.58). The reason for these discrepancies is that the effective mean radius of the centrifuge (the distance from the spindle of the centrifuge to the mid-point of the packed cell mass) is greater with a low PCV than with a normal PCV. With an abnormally high PCV the effective mean radius of the centrifuge is less than with blood of a normal PCV. As the centrifugal force applied to the contents of the tube is a function of the speed of rotation and the effective radius of the centrifuge, the effective centrifugal force is greater with a low PCV than with a high PCV.

Under the usual conditions of the test procedure, trapped plasma may account for about 2.5–3% of the apparent red cell column in normal blood and even more in certain abnormal conditions, notably polycythaemia, iron deficiency, thalassaemia, spherocytosis and sickle-cell disease. While this is not a serious problem in routine clinical practice, it must be taken into account when a high degree of accuracy is required, for example, when estimating blood volume or for calibrating automated blood counters. It is possible to correct for trapped plasma using radioactive human serum albumin as an indicator of the amount that has been trapped.[36]

MICRO-METHOD

The use of capillary tubes of much smaller diameter and capacity than Wintrobe tubes is very convenient as a routine procedure in clinical work. The centrifuge used with capillary tubes provides a centrifugal force of c 12 000 g and 3–5 min centrifugation results in a constant PCV. When the PCV is greater than 0.5, it may be necessary to centrifuge for a further 5 min. When packing is as complete as possible the column of cells will appear translucent. The amount of trapped plasma is less than with the Wintrobe method. Garby and Vuille reported a mean of 1.3% (range 1.1–1.5%).[22] Pearson and Guthrie reported a slightly higher amount with normal blood (mean 1.53%, SD 0.166)[54] and other authors have reported values of 2–3%.[20] Plasma trapping is increased in macrocytic anaemias,[20] spherocytosis, thalassaemia, hypochromic anaemias and sickle-cell anaemia;[54] it may be as high as 20% in sickle-cell anaemia if all the cells are sickled.[20]

Method

Capillary tubes 75 mm in length and having an internal diameter of about 1 mm are required. They can be obtained plain or coated inside with 2 iu of heparin. The latter type are suitable for the direct collection of capillary blood. Plain tubes are used for anticoagulated venous blood.

Allow the blood to enter the tube by capillarity, leaving at least 15 mm unfilled. Then seal the tube by a plastic seal, e.g. Cristaseal (Hawksley, Lancing, Sussex) or by heating the dry end of the tube rapidly in a fine flame, e.g. the pilot light of a Bunsen burner, combined with rotation. After centrifugation for 5 min, measure the PCV using a reading device.

Accuracy of micro-method

The inaccuracies due to specimen handling described for the macro-method apply equally to this method. Variation of the bore of the tubes may, too, cause serious errors if they are not manufactured within the narrow limits of precision that conform to defined standards, e.g. British Standard for apparatus for Measurement of Packed Red Cell Volume (BS 4316: 1968).

Other errors unique to the micro-method are due to difficulty in heat-sealing the lower end of the tube so as to obtain a flat base and difficulties in reading. To avoid errors in reading with the special reading device, a magnifying glass should be used. Alternatively, the ratio of red cell column to whole column (i.e. red cells plus plasma) can be calculated from measurements obtained by placing the tube against arithmetic graph paper or against a ruler. In routine practice it is not customary to correct for trapped plasma. But when accuracy is of especial importance, e.g. when the PCV is required for calculating blood volume or for calibrating an automated counter, the amount of trapped plasma should be determined using radioactive human serum albumin as an indicator[54] or the observed PCV should be reduced by a 2% correction factor when the PCV is less than 0.5. When it is more than 0.5, centrifugation should be continued for a further 5 min and 3% should be deducted from the observed reading.[35]

MEASUREMENT OF PACKED CELL VOLUME FROM MEAN CELL VOLUME AND RED CELL COUNT

With some electronic counters PCV can be derived indirectly from the red cell count and MCV. The PCV obtained by this method is frequently 1.5–3% lower than the micro-haematocrit value. This is because errors due to trapped plasma and inadequate oxygenation are eliminated. On the other hand, the accuracy of derived PCV measurements may be influenced by the shape of the red cells in the diluting medium and their orientation in the sensing zone, by other blood constituents and by the calibration settings of the instrument as described on p. 43. Applying a calibration correction to the instrument settings in order to achieve comparability with PCV by centrifugation does not take into account the extent to which plasma trapping varies in different blood specimens.

MEASUREMENT AND CALCULATION OF SIZE OF RED CELLS

ABSOLUTE VALUES

The mean cell volume (MCV), mean cell Hb (MCH) and mean cell Hb concentration (MCHC) have been referred to as 'absolute' values. These values, calculated from the results of the red cell count, Hb concentration and PCV have been widely used in the classification of anaemia.

With fully automated counting systems absolute values are measured simultaneously with the red cell count. MCV is calculated either from the mean height or a selected span of the pulses generated during the red cell count or from the sum of the pulse heights divided by the number of pulses which are generated during the count. Hb is measured as HiCN in a standard procedure; PCV is deduced from the red cell count and MCV; MCH is deduced from the Hb and red cell count; whilst MCHC is calculated from the measured Hb and the deduced PCV. The relationship of pulse height to cell volume is obtained automatically by comparison of the pulse derived from blood cells to voltages which are generated by calibration material. The accuracy of using this procedure is limited by differences in the shapes adopted by fresh blood cells and calibrator (e.g. stabilized blood or latex spheres) as they pass the sensing zone of the counter. Thus, a correction factor is required for comparing the preparations; this 'shape factor' is about 1.2 for fixed biconcave cells and 1.5 for fixed spheres.[20]

Red cell flexibility is also an important determinant of pulse sizes; thus when red cells are relatively inflexible, because of a membrane defect, this will result in greater differences in the measurement of MCV and MCHC between manual and automated methods than with normal red cells.[20] The recorded MCV is also affected by any delay in carrying out the test and the tonicity of the diluent.

MCV and PCV are also affected by alteration in plasma osmolarity as a result of hyperglycaemia and ketosis in diabetes,[21,32] cold agglutinins[66] and warm auto-antibodies.[82]

Calculation of mean cell volume (MCV)

If the PCV and the number of red cells per litre (or μl) are known, the MCV can be calculated:

e.g. if the PCV is 0.45, 1 litre of blood contains 0.45 l of red cells. Therefore, if there are 5×10^{12} red cells per litre, they occupy a volume of 0.45 l.

$$\text{Therefore, volume of 1 cell} = \frac{0.45}{5 \times 10^{12}}$$

$$= 90 \text{ fl.}$$

In practice, the PCV (0.45) is divided by the red cell count in millions per μl (5.0) and multiplied by 1000. The answer is expressed in femtolitres (fl).

Calculation of mean cell haemoglobin (MCH)

This can be calculated if the Hb and red cell count are known:

e.g. if there are 150 g of Hb per litre of blood, and if there are 5×10^{12} red cells per litre, the mean cell Hb is

$$\frac{150}{5 \times 10^{12}} = \frac{3}{10^{11}} \text{ g} = 30 \text{ picograms (pg)}.$$

Calculation of mean cell haemoglobin concentration (MCHC)

This can be calculated if the Hb per litre of blood and PCV are known:

e.g. if there are 150 g per litre of blood, of PCV 0.45, the MCHC is

$$150 \div 0.45 = 333 \text{ g/l.}$$

RANGE OF 'ABSOLUTE' VALUES

The range of normal 'absolute' values varies slightly depending on whether they are based on automated measurements (and the type of counter used) or on the PCV as determined by centrifuging blood at approximately 1500 *g* or at 2000–2300 *g* for 30 min, or by the micro-method at a much higher *g,* or whether the PCV has been 'corrected' for trapped plasma. In practice, the differences are small and without clinical significance except in iron-deficiency anaemia and thalassaemia and in polycythaemia[26] in which the PCV is significantly lower by some automated counters than by micro-haematocrit. This results in an automated MCHC which is less abnormally low than is the MCH. The normal range given below is based on micro-haematocrit data *not corrected for trapped plasma.* Measurements by electronic counters should be within this range but may differ slightly, depending on the calibration of the individual counter. Their SD should be smaller.

Normal adults (mean ± 2 SD)

Mean cell volume (MCV) = 86 ± 10 fl.
Mean cell haemoglobin (MCH) = 29.5 ± 2.5 pg.
Mean cell haemoglobin concentration (MCHC) = 325 ± 25 g/l.

In disease

1. In macrocytic anaemias:
    MCV increased up to about 150 fl (rarely higher).
    MCH increased up to about 50 pg (rarely higher).
    MCHC normal or diminished.
2. In microcytic hypochromic anaemias:
    MCV diminished to 50 fl (rarely lower).
    MCH diminished to 15 pg (rarely lower).
    MCHC diminished to 220 g/l (rarely lower).

ACCURACY OF THE CALCULATION OF 'ABSOLUTE' VALUES

A danger attached to the calculation of 'absolute' values from visual blood count measurements is that the observer may delude himself into a false sense of their accuracy, particularly when the results are expressed to one place of decimals, as has sometimes unjustifiably been done.

Until the advent of electronic cell counters the only measurement which could be relied upon was the MCHC calculated from the relatively accurate Hb and PCV measurements. MCVs and MCHs based on visual red cell counts were relatively inaccurate and of less clinical value.

Electronic cell counters can give highly repro-ducible values for MCV and MCH, but their accuracy is limited by variable shape factors and red cell flexibility as described above (p. 50) as well as by differences in values assigned to the materials used to calibrate them. Nonetheless, they are reliable aids to recognizing minor degrees of macrocytosis or to diagnosing iron deficiency at an early stage.[15,43,75]

Accurate measurement of MCV and MCH may help to discriminate between iron deficiency and β-thalassaemia trait, and a number of formulae using these measurements have been elaborated. Two simple ones are

$$\text{MCV (fl)} \div \text{red cell count } (\times 10^{12}/\text{l})$$

and

$$\text{MCV}^2 \text{ (fl)} \times \text{MCH (pg).}$$

These formulae discriminate between the two con-ditions better than does measuring MCH or MCHC alone.[11] The following more complicated formula also seems to be useful:

$$\text{MCV (fl)} - \text{RBC } (\times 10^{12}/\text{l}) - (0.5 \times \text{Hb (g/l)} - k,$$

where k is a constant factor, dependent on the instrument calibration: a negative result points to β-thalassaemia.[19] An analogous calculation has been shown to be useful in detecting β-thalassaemia trait.[28] Another useful measurement is the red cell distribution width (RDW) (p. 54). A low MCV with a normal RDW suggests β-thalassaemia trait; a low MCV with an increased RDW indicates iron deficiency.[6,41]

RED CELL SIZE DISTRIBUTION

RED CELL DIAMETERS

Normally, even in health, a population of red cells can be seen to vary appreciably in size, and it was largely owing to the work of Price-Jones[55] that this normal variation was measured and recorded. He showed that if the diameters of a large number of red cells were measured and the cells grouped together in classes according to their diameters, the frequency-distribution curve of diameters was of the 'normal' type. Price-Jones applied statistical methods to his data and calculated limits of normal variation; and he also showed that characteristic deviations from normal were encountered in various types of anaemia. This work excited great interest and at one time the drawing of a Price-Jones curve was considered to be an almost essential step in the investigation of any obscure case of anaemia—although the labour expended contributed nothing to the understanding of the case and merely placed on paper what was to be seen by inspection of a stained film!

The measurement of red cell diameters in dried films is a highly artificial method; not only do cells shrink on drying, but their diameters also vary appreciably artefactually in different parts of a dried film. An area of film where the cells are neither distorted nor shrunken has therefore to be found before measurements can be made. Moreover, in anaemias such as severe pernicious anaemia it is extremely difficult, if not impossible, to measure accurately the diameters of the poikilocytes likely to be present. There is little doubt but that the laborious Price-Jones method of measuring the diameter of individual red cells in dried films is less accurate than was at one time supposed. The method is now obsolete.

Measurement of red cell diameter with an eye-piece micrometer

The method has the advantages of directness and simplicity and can be quickly applied to stained blood films.

The scale of the eye-piece micrometer has to be calibrated in relation to the objective, eye-piece and tube-length employed, before it can be used. This is best done using a slide on which a scale, usually 1 mm in 0.01 mm (10 µm) intervals, has been engraved. Alternatively, the calibrations on a counting chamber can be utilized (the side of the smallest square is 0.05 mm in length).

It is convenient to have a conversion scale kept near the microscope, e.g. using a 2 mm objective and × 6 eye-pieces: 5.0 divisions = 6.6 µm, 5.5 divisions = 7.2 µm, 6.0 divisions = 7.9 µm, 6.5 divisions = 8.5 µm, etc.

The diameters of red cells can be measured to about 0.5 µm without difficulty with the aid of the eye-piece micrometer. The method is useful, although minor degrees of deviation from the normal will not be detected. Nevertheless, in practice, it is possible by measuring a few representative cells to confirm or refute a visual impression of abnormality. This does not mean that the observer should search for the largest or smallest cells to measure, for a few as large as 9 µm or as small as 6 µm may be seen in dried films of normal blood. It is much more significant to find an unusually high proportion of cells of 8.5 µm than a few outside these limits.

Range of red cell diameters in health (MCD)

Price Jones dry films[55], 6.7–7.7 µm (mean 7.2 µm).

Houchin, Munn and Parnell[33], cells in rouleaux 8.1–8.7 µm (mean 8.4 µm.

Westerman, Pierce and Jensen,[83] cells in rouleaux 8.3–9.1 µm (mean 8.7 µm); isolated cells 8.6 µm (mean).

Normal range for red cell surface area

Houchin, Munn and Parnell,[33] 128–144 µm^2 (mean 134 µm^2).

Westerman, Pierce and Jensen,[83] 132–160 µm^2 (mean 145 µm^2).

RED CELL VOLUMES

As the MCV is only a measure of the mean red cell volume, its measurement may miss a small but possible significant degree of microcytosis or macrocytosis and the presence of anisocytosis. It is now possible to obtain volume distribution curves using automated counters. Curves obtained in this way are more sensitive than are the conventional red cell indices for studying, for example, the early response to therapy in iron deficiency and megaloblastic anaemias, identifying multiple deficiency states or a dimorphic red cell population and discounting the confusing presence of (normal) transfused cells in the blood of a patient whose own cells are abnormal. The patterns of curves which occur in various conditions and their interpretation are illustrated in monographs by Rowan[58] and Bessman.[5]

RED CELL DISTRIBUTION WIDTH (RDW)

This is a sensitive measurement of red cell aniso-cytosis, with potential value for discriminating between different causes of anaemia (see p. 52). It is expressed either as the SD (fl) or CV (%) of the MCV after excluding the tail of the size distribution curve. In the Coulter counter it is reported as CV, with a normal range of 11.5–14.5%; in the Sysmex (Toa) counter as SD with a normal range of 30–50 fl. Unfortunately, in addition to confusion because of the different methods used to express RDW, insufficient account has been taken of artefactual changes in red cell size measurements, including the effect of anticoagulant, specimen storage, diluent and instrument errors; as a result widely different normal values have been reported for RDW, the CV ranging between 7.4 and 13.4%.[5,6,57,58] Nonetheless, measurement of RDW is useful in distinguishing between iron deficiency (high RDW) and thalassaemia (normal RDW) provided that the method is standardized and each laboratory establishes its own normal reference range.

LEUCOCYTE COUNTS

TOTAL COUNTS BY ELECTRONIC METHODS

To get rid of the red cells before the leucocytes are counted, a lytic agent is required which destroys the red cells without affecting the ability of the leucocytes to be counted and reduces red cell stroma to a residue which causes no detectable response on the counting system. The manufacturers of counters recommend their own specified reagents; their use is essential when the leucocyte count is combined with an automated differential count (see p. 69). For a total leucocyte count on a simple single-channel counter, the following fluid appears to be satisfactory:

Cetavlon 20g
10% formaldehyde (in 9 g/l NaCl (saline) 2 ml
Glacial acetic acid 16 ml
Sodium citrate 14 g
NaCl 6 g
Water to 1 litre.

Dilute 20 μl of blood in 10 ml of saline, and add 2 drops of the above solution. Lysis is instanta-neous. The count is stable for at least 40 min and the background count is low.

Saponin has also been used as a lytic agent but it does not cause complete lysis of the red cells, the leucocytes swell and the background count is relatively high. With Zaponin (Coulter), Zapoglobin (Coulter), Lyse S (Coulter), Stromatolyser (Toa) and similar commercial products, the cytoplasm shrinks down to the nucleus. Thus, when calibrating the counter the same lytic agent and diluent should be used subsequently for routine counts. The principle of calibration is similar to that for red cells (p. 43). Threshold selection and avoiding coincidence are easier than with red cells.

It is important to know the counter's upper limit of reliability; with high counts (e.g. above 40 $\times 10^9$/l) the sample may need to be diluted further. Difficulties occur with nucleated red cells which are included with the leucocytes, and errors may occasionally be produced by platelet clumps and fibrin strands, present probably as a result of faulty specimen collection.[29] Erroneously high counts have been reported in cryoglobulin-aemia.[27]

TOTAL COUNTS BY VISUAL METHOD

Make a 1 in 20 dilution of blood by adding 20 μl of blood to 0.38 ml of diluting fluid in a 75 × 10 mm glass or plastic tube. Bulb pipettes are not recommended (see p. 47). After tightly corking the tube, mix the suspension by rotating in a cell-suspension mixer for at least 1 min. Fill the Neubauer counting chamber by means of a Pasteur pipette or stout glass capillary, as for red cell counts (p. 45).

The red cells are lysed by the diluting fluid (see below, but the leucocytes remain intact, their nuclei staining deep violet-black. View the preparation using a 4 mm objective and × 6 eyepieces or a 16 mm objective and ×6 or × 10 eyepieces. Count at least 100 cells in as many 1 mm^2 areas (0.1 μl in volume) as may be necessary— the ruled area in an improved Neubauer chamber consists of 9 of these areas.

Calculation

$$\text{Count (/l)} = \frac{\text{No. of cells counted}}{\text{volume counted (μl)}} \times \text{dilution} \times 10^6.$$

Thus, if N cells are counted in 0.1 μl, then the leucocyte count per litre

$$= N \times 10 \times \text{(dilution)} \times 10^6$$

$$= N \times 200 \times 10^6/l$$

$$(= N \times 200 \text{ per μl}).$$

Diluting fluid

2% (20 ml/l) acetic acid coloured pale violet with gentian violet.

Range of the total leucocyte count in health
(see p. 12)

Error of the total leucocyte count

The factors causing errors in counting leucocytes by the visual method are the same as in counting red cells. As many leucocytes as possible should be counted; 100 cells is a reasonable and practical figure for visual counts. The inherent distribution error (σ) of a 100-cell count is approximately $\sqrt{100}$ = 10, and the count variation is thus 10% (see p. 48); 95% of counts of mean value 100 would thus lie within the range of 100 ± 2σ = 80–120. Translated into actual results, this means that 95% of observed counts on a blood of true value 5.0×10^9 cells per litre would lie within the range 4.0–6.0.

Fortunately, error in the leucocyte count is not nearly as important as error in red cell counts; even an error as high as 20% does not matter much—the difference between 5.0 and 6.0×10^9 cells per litre is of little practical significance. The error can be reduced by counting more cells, and with high counts this can be accomplished without the expenditure of much extra time. If 400 cells are counted, the error is reduced to 5%.

Other potential causes of error include mistaking dirt or clumped red cell debris for leucocytes and the clumping of leucocytes. The latter—usually several leucocytes stuck to debris—seems to occur particularly in heparinized blood, especially when the concentration of hepatin exceeds 25 iu per ml of blood. The clumps are most frequently seen in blood which has been allowed to stand for several hours before undertaking the count.

PLATELET COUNTS

The platelet count is an important component of the blood count. Electronic counting systems have greatly improved counting precision but visual methods are still used extensively. A visual direct method is described which is suitable for moderately low normal to high counts. A method is also described using plasma, which is valuable when the count is low.

VISUAL METHOD FOR WHOLE BLOOD[8,47]

The diluent consists of 1% aqueous ammonium oxalate in which the red cells are lysed. There is a possibility that red cell debris may be mistaken for platelets but with some experience this should not cause any difficulties. The method is recommended in preference to that using formal-citrate as diluent, which leaves the red cells intact and is more likely to give incorrect results, when the platelet count is low.

Reagent

10 g/l ammonium oxalate. Not more than 500 ml should be made at a time, using scrupulously clean glassware and fresh glass-distilled or de-ionized water. The solution should be filtered through a micropore filter (0.22 μm) and kept at 4°C. For use, a small part of the stock is refiltered and dispensed in 1.9 ml volumes in 75 × 12 mm tubes.

Method

Collect blood into a dry plastic syringe using a short needle of 19 or 20 SWG. It is essential that the puncture is a clean one and that the blood flows into the syringe with the minimum of suction. Detach the needle from the syringe and deliver the requisite amount of blood without frothing into a vessel containing EDTA. Mix gently and without delay. If the collection of blood has been satisfactory, the dilution of the blood may be postponed for 3–4 h.

It is convenient to make a 1 in 20 dilution of the blood in the diluent by adding 0.1 ml of blood to 1.9 ml of the diluent. Mix the suspension on a mechanical mixer for 10–15 min.

Fill a Neubauer counting chamber with the suspension, using a stout glass capillary or Pasteur pipette. Place the counting chamber in a moist Petri dish and leave untouched for at least 20 min to give time for the platelets to settle.

Examine the preparation with the 4 mm objective and × 6 or × 10 eyepieces. The platelets appear under ordinary illumination as small (but not minute) highly refractile particles, if viewed with the condenser racked down; they are usually well separated and clumps are rare if the blood sample has been skilfully collected. They are more easily seen with the phase-contrast microscope. A special thin-bottomed (1 mm) counting chamber is best for optimal phase-contrast effect.

The number of platelets in one or more areas of 1 mm^2 should be counted. The total number of platelets counted should always exceed 200.

Calculation

$$\text{Count (/l)} = \frac{\text{No. of cells counted}}{\text{Volume counted (μl)}} \times \text{dilution} \times 10^6.$$

Thus if N be the number of platelets counted in an area of 1 mm^2 (0.1 μl in volume), the number of platelets per litre of blood

$$= \text{N} \times 10 \times 20 \text{ (dilution)} \times 10^6$$

$$= \text{N} \times 200 \times 10^6/\text{l}$$

$$(= \text{N} \times 200 \text{ per μl}).$$

MODIFIED METHOD USING PLASMA IN PLACE OF WHOLE BLOOD

This method is basically the same as that described in the preceding paragraphs. However, instead of diluting whole blood, plasma is used; this enables low platelet counts (even as low as 10×10^9/l) to be carried out reliably. The EDTA blood is allowed to stand at room temperature (18–25°C) until a few mm of plasma are visible. Make a 1 in 10 dilution of the plasma by adding 0.1 ml of plasma to 0.9 ml of diluting fluid. Mix for 1 min, and then fill the counting chamber and let the preparation stand in a damp chamber for 20 min or even longer for all the platelets to settle before counting.

Calculation

$$\text{Count (/l)} = \frac{\text{No. of cells counted}}{\text{Volume counted (μl)}} \times \text{dilution} \times (1 - \text{PCV}) \times 10^6.$$

Thus, if N be the number of platelets counted in an area of 1 mm^2 (0.1 μl in volume), the number of platelets per litre of blood

$$= \text{N} \times 10 \times 10 \text{ (dilution)} \times (1 - \text{PCV}) \times 10^6/\text{l}$$

$$= \text{N} \times 100 \times (1 - \text{PCV}) \times 10^6/\text{l}$$

$$(= \text{N} \times 100 \times (1 - \text{PCV}) \text{ per μl}).$$

The result is adjusted by multiplying by (1 − PCV) to allow for the fact that the count is carried out on plasma, not on whole blood.

PLATELET COUNTS ON PERIPHERAL BLOOD

Platelet counts can be carried out on finger or ear-prick blood but the results are less satisfactory than those carried out on venous blood. Peripheral-blood counts are significantly lower than venous and less constant[9] and a variable number of platelets are probably lost at the site of the skin puncture.

PLATELET COUNTS BY ELECTRONIC METHODS

Electronic instruments with appropriate threshold calibration can be used for counting platelets. Their reliability may be affected by errors connected with the instrument and its calibration and the tendency of platelets to aggregate, and by the presence in the diluent of particles which may be little smaller than platelets, and by overlap in size between large platelets and small red cells. Reference materials are now available to ensure correct instrument calibration (p. 28). Identification of platelets in whole blood requires a degree of resolution which is only available in the modern counters which have been developed in recent years.[56] These use a narrow aperture and require some form of hydro-dynamic focusing or sweep-flow (see p. 44). Platelet counting by simple aperture-impedance instruments requires the separation of red cells from the platelet-containing plasma. A method which has been used extensively is based on the gravitational sedimentation of blood.[10] This method is liable to error due to variation in the level of the supernatant plasma at which the sample is removed.[46] The differential centrifugation method described below overcomes this source of error, and is recommended.

DIFFERENTIAL CENTRIFUGATION METHOD[14]

Diluting fluid

Pour 60 ml of 32.8% sodium metrizoate solution, sp gr 1.200 (± 0.001) into a clean dry 150 ml glass bottle. Add 60 ml of Isoton II (Coulter Electronics) and mix well for 10 min on a roller mixer. Filter through a 0.22 micropore filter. Store at 4° C in the dark.

Method

Pour 10 ml of the fluid into a plastic 25 ml container. Add 0.1 ml of a well-mixed sample of EDTA blood, using a clean dry pipette. Mix the blood with the fluid by rolling the tube in the palms of the hands for 30 s. Then centrifuge for 3 min at 2000 *g*. Remove approximately 8 ml of the red-cell-free supernatant into a clean plastic container. Re-mix for 30 s before removing 0.2 ml and diluting in 10 ml of Isoton II for electronic counting. By this procedure the original whole blood sample has been diluted 1:5151.

If a larger volume of blood is available, platelet-containing plasma can be obtained by sedimentation alone. Layer *c* 1 ml of EDTA blood on top of 1 ml of the separating fluid in a plastic tube of 8 mm internal diameter and leave to stand vertically on the bench. Sufficient plasma will usually be available within 10–15 min.

A sedimentation method that is suitable for use with small volumes of blood is described below.

SEDIMENTATION METHOD

Prepare sedimentation tubes from small bore plastic (polyvinyl chloride, PVC) tubing, internal diameter 2 mm, as follows: seal the tubing every 8 cm (by means of a blood-bank tubing sealer) and then cut through at the seals and midway between them in order to form segments 4 cm in length, sealed at one end.* Dip the open end of a tube into a container of EDTA blood, and then gently squeeze the tube so that *c* 0.1 ml of the blood is sucked into the tube to a level above the open end. Then wipe the open end clean and place the tube with the sealed end up in a rack at an angle of 45°. Allow the sedimentation to proceed for sufficient time to provide an adequate amount of plasma. This usually takes 10–50 min. Then cut the tube through with scissors at or above the junction of red cells and plasma, and invert the upper part so that any residual red cells will sediment rapidly through the plasma. Take a volume of the plasma layer into a capillary pipette and deliver into an appropriate

---

* or available from Coulter Electronics Ltd.

volume of diluent for subsequent platelet counting. Correct the result of the count for PCV as described on p. 56.

Normal range of platelet count

In health there are approximately $150-400 \times 10^9$ platelets per litre of blood. Some studies have reported an upper limit of $500 \times 10^9/l$.[1,25] The counts in individual subjects have been reported as being relatively constant,[8,65] although there is some evidence of a diurnal variation. There may also be a sex difference (see p. 15); in women there is cycling with a slightly lower count at about the time of menstruation.[52]

The use of EDTA as anticoagulant has removed the one former major difficulty in platelet counting—namely, clumping of the platelets. In some cases, however, a concentration of 1.5 mg/ml fails to prevent this. It should, nevertheless, not be used at a concentration greater than c 2 mg/ml, for the platelets then tend to swell and disrupt, producing an erroneously high count. Accuracy in visual counting can be achieved only by the most careful regard to detail, particularly with respect to the cleanliness of the preparation, and by experience, which alone can help in deciding what is and what is not a platelet. As already mentioned, the use of phase-contrast microscopy helps considerably in recognizing and counting platelets.

With the visual method the coefficient of variation (CV) is 8–10%. By electronic counting better reproducibility is obtained and a CV of 3–4% is possible. With fully-automated counters the inter-laboratory CV is c 6%, partly caused by inter-instrument variability.

MEASUREMENT OF PLATELET VOLUME

Some automated systems measure platelet volume distribution. Normally platelet volume is distributed in a log-normal way.[53] In EDTA blood the mean platelet volume (MPV) is c 8–9.5 fl,[59] median volume being slightly less. Several studies have illustrated the potential value of these measurements.[5,7,59] Thus, platelet volume appears to be positively correlated with platelet aggregation and other tests of function.[42] On the other hand, volume and count are normally inversely correlated. This is generally, however, not true of platelet disorders: thus, it may be possible to distinguish between various causes of thrombocytopenia on the basis of inappropriately high or low MPV for the level of platelet count. It should be noted, however, that platelet volume is seriously affected by the method of collection, type of anticoagulant used and the time that has elapsed between collection and counting.[25,48,72,74]

In EDTA blood the MPV increases during the first 2 hours and is then stable for about 8 hours. An anticoagulant comprising EDTA dissolved in ACD is said to delay platelet size changes for several hours.[72]

The importance of a standardized procedure and a correctly calibrated instrument cannot be over-emphasized.

AUTOMATED HAEMATOLOGY

The introduction of a comprehensive automated system usually means that the laboratory has to be re-organized to ensure efficient and effective use of the expensive equipment. In selecting a system, it is important to assess how it will fulfil the requirements of the laboratory. Account must be taken of the rate at which the equipment can operate. At present between 50 and 120 specimens can be handled per hour by different instruments: clearly, therefore, the slower machines would be inadequate for a laboratory with a daily workload of 500 specimens or more. The cost of reagents and other materials must be ascertained, as reagents supplied specifically for the instrument are often more expensive, and are required in larger amounts, than those used in manual techniques. Their bulk, too, may create a storage problem. The availability of services (water, compressed air, drainage) has to be considered; also whether a controlled environment is required, and the effect of the instrument on the environment in terms of vibration, noise and heat production. Also to be considered are the training required and the extent to which this is provided by the manufacturer, and the maintenance and repair service provided by the manufacturer or agent.

Guidelines have been published to help the choice of an instrument suitable for the needs of an individual laboratory and also to assess its performance, as compared with the claims of the manufacturer, when it has been installed and is being used in routine practice.[37,63]

Results of blood counts by automated systems may include histograms of the size distribution of each type of blood cell. Their interpretation requires skill and experience; they provide a new dimension in haematological diagnosis which complements microscopic morphology. A number of papers and some recent reviews illustrate the patterns in health and in various abnormal conditions.[5,58]

Examples of reports obtained with different systems are illustrated in Figs. 5.5–5.7.

CALIBRATION OF AUTOMATED BLOOD CELL COUNTERS

The preserved blood and other stable control preparations described in Chapter 4 can also be used to calibrate automated blood cell counters. However, these preparations may respond in an automated counter differently to fresh blood; it is thus necessary first to assign comparable blood count values to these preparations by the following indirect procedure.[18,38]

1. Collect a 5 ml blood sample in EDTA from each of 3 normal subjects with MCHC 32–34 g/dl and MCV 80–95 fl.

2. Keep at room temperature (c 20°C) and test within 4 h. Immediately before testing mix each of the samples well by gently inverting the container 20 times.

3. Carry out the blood count measurements as follows:

> Hb by haemiglobincyanide method (p. 38); calculate mean of 2 measurements.
> PCV by microhaematocrit method (p. 50); calculate mean of 4 tubes.

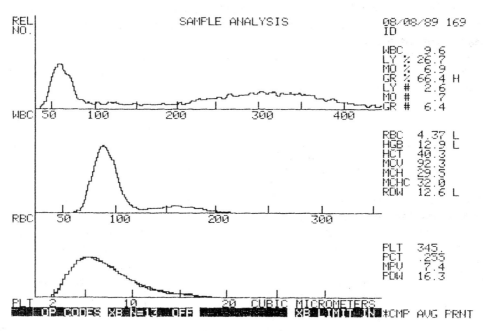

Fig. 5.5 Blood count report from Coulter S plus IV counter.

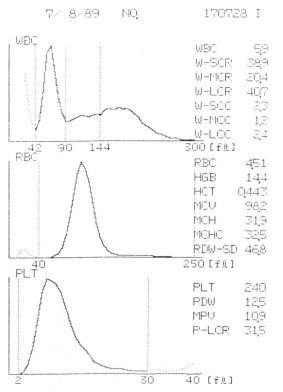

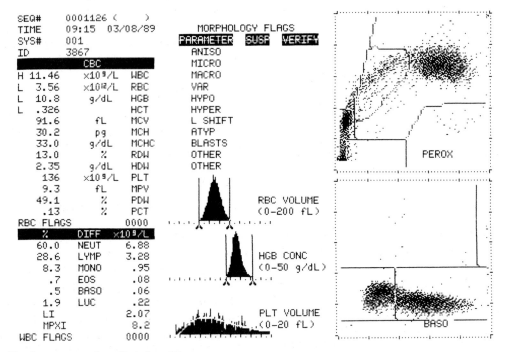

7/ 8/89	NO.	170728 I

WBC

WBC	59
W-SCR	389
W-MCR	204
W-LCR	407
W-SCC	23
W-MCC	12
W-LCC	24

42 90 144   300 [fL]

RBC

RBC	451
HGB	144
HCT	0.443
MCV	98.2
MCH	31.9
MCHC	325
RDW-SD	46.8

40   250 [fL]

PLT

PLT	240
PDW	12.5
MPV	10.9
P-LCR	31.5

2   30   40 [fL]

Fig. 5.6 Blood count report from Sysmex E 5000 counter.

RBC by a single-channel aperture-impedance counter (p. 42); calculate mean of 2 dilutions, each counted twice

MCV, MCH and MCHC by calculation

WBC by a single-channel aperture impedance counter (p. 54); mean of 2 dilutions, each counted twice

Platelet count as described on p. 55; mean of 2 dilutions.

4. Measure the fresh blood samples and the preserved material (calibrator) on the automated blood cell counter (A). Obtain the mean of two measurements for each blood count component. From the ratios of fresh blood to calibrator assign corrected values to the calibrator by the following calculation:

Corrected calibrator value =

$$A_C \times \sqrt[3]{\frac{D_{F1}}{A_{F1}} \times \frac{D_{F2}}{A_{F2}} \times \frac{D_{F3}}{A_{F3}}},$$

where A_C = measurement of calibrator by automated counter

A_F = measurement of the fresh bloods (1, 2 and 3) by automated counter

D_F = direct measurements of the fresh bloods (1, 2 and 3).

SEQ#	0001126 (	)
TIME	09:15 03/08/89
SYS#	001
ID	3867

	CBC	
H 11.46	×10⁹/L	WBC
L 3.56	×10¹²/L	RBC
L 10.8	g/dL	HGB
L .326		HCT
91.6	fL	MCV
30.2	pg	MCH
33.0	g/dL	MCHC
13.0	%	RDW
2.35	g/dL	HDW
136	×10⁹/L	PLT
9.3	fL	MPV
49.1	%	PDW
.13	%	PCT
RBC FLAGS		0000

%	DIFF	×10⁹/L
60.0	NEUT	6.88
28.6	LYMP	3.28
8.3	MONO	.95
.7	EOS	.08
.5	BASO	.06
1.9	LUC	.22
	LI	2.07
	MPXI	8.2
WBC FLAGS		0000

MORPHOLOGY FLAGS

PARAMETER	SUSP	VERIFY
ANISO		
MICRO		
MACRO		
VAR		
HYPO		
HYPER		
L SHIFT		
ATYP		
BLASTS		
OTHER		
OTHER		

PEROX

RBC VOLUME (0-200 fL)

HGB CONC (0-50 g/dL)

PLT VOLUME (0-20 fL)

BASO

Fig. 5.7 Blood count report from Technicon HI counter.

Considerable care is required to ensure that the initial measurements on the fresh blood are as accurate as possible. Dilutions should be made with individually calibrated pipettes and grade A volumetric flasks. The cell counter should be calibrated as described on p. 42, with a signal to noise ratio of greater than 100:1, and the count corrected for coincidence. Details of procedures to be used are described by the International Committee for Standardization in Haematology.[38]

THE RETICULOCYTE COUNT

Reticulocytes are juvenile red cells; they contain remnants of the ribosomes and the ribonucleic acid which were present in larger amounts in the cytoplasm of the nucleated precursors from which they were derived. Ribosomes have the property of reacting with certain basic dyes such as azure B, brilliant cresyl blue or New methylene blue to form a blue precipitate of granules or filaments. This reaction takes place only in vitally-stained unfixed preparations. The most immature reticulocytes are those with the largest amount of precipitable material; in the least immature only a few dots or short strands are seen. Stages of maturation can be identified by their morphological features.[24]

If a blood film is allowed to dry and is afterwards fixed with methanol, reticulocytes appear as red cells staining diffusely basophilic if the film is stained with basophilic dyes. Complete loss of basophilic material probably occurs as a rule in the blood stream and, particularly, in the spleen[4] after the cells have left the bone marrow.[62] The ripening process is thought to take 2–3 days, of which about 24 h are spent in the circulation.

The number of reticulocytes in the peripheral blood is a fairly accurate reflection of erythropoietic activity, assuming that the reticulocytes are released normally from the bone marrow, and that they remain in circulation for the normal period of time. These assumptions are not always valid as an increased erythropoietic stimulus leads to premature release into the circulation. The maturation time of these so-called 'stress' or stimulated reticulocytes may be as long as 3 days. In such cases, it is possible to deduce the reticulocyte maturation time and calculate a 'corrected' reticulocyte count by using plasma-iron turnover data.[30,31] Nevertheless, adequate information is usually obtained from a simple reticulocyte count recorded as a percentage of the red cells or preferably, if the red cell count is known, expressed as absolute numbers.

A TECHNIQUE FOR THE RETICULOCYTE COUNT

Better and more reliable results are obtained with New methylene blue in the author's experience than with brillant cresyl blue. New methylene blue stains the reticulo-filamentous material in reticulocytes more deeply and more uniformly than does brilliant cresyl blue, which varies from sample to sample in its staining ability. Purified azure B is a satisfactory substitute for New methylene blue; it has the advantage that the dye does not precipitate[51] and it is available in pure form.[84] It is used in the same concentration and the staining procedure is the same as with New methyene blue.

Staining solution

Dissolve 1.0 g of New methylene blue (CI 52030)* or azure B thiocyanate (p. 79) in 100 ml of iso-osmotic phosphate buffer pH 7.4 (p. 538).

Method

Deliver 2 or 3 drops of the dye solution into a 75 × 10 mm glass or plastic tube by means of a Pasteur pipette. Add 2–4 volumes of the patient's EDTA blood to the dye solution and mix. Keep the mixture at 37°C for 15–20 min. Resuspend the red cells by gentle mixing and make films on glass slides in the usual way. When dry, examine the films without fixing or counterstaining.

---

*New methylene blue is chemically different from methylene blue which is a poor reticulocyte stain.

The exact volume of blood to be added to the dye solution for optimal staining depends upon the red cell count. A larger proportion of anaemic blood, and a smaller proportion of polycythaemic blood, should be added than of normal blood. In a successful preparation the reticulo-filamentous material should be stained deep blue and the non-reticulated cells stained diffusely shades of pale greenish blue.

Films should not be counterstained. The reticulo-filamentous material is not better defined after counterstaining and precipitated stain overlying cells may cause confusion. Moreover, Heinz bodies will not be visible in fixed and counterstained preparations. If the stained preparation is examined under phase contrast, both the mature red cells and reticulocytes are well defined. By this technique late reticulocytes characterized by the presence of remnants of filaments or threads are readily distinguished from cells containing inclusion bodies. Satisfactory counts may be made on blood that has been allowed to stand (unstained) for as long as 24 h, although the count will tend to fall slightly after 6–8 hours.f

Counting reticulocytes

An area of film should be chosen for the count where the cells are undistorted and where the staining is good. A common fault is to make the film too thin; however, the cells should not overlap. To count the cells, use the 2 mm oil-immersion objective and if possible eyepieces provided with an adjustable diaphragm. If eyepieces with an adjustable diaphragm are not available, a paper or cardboard diaphragm, in the centre of which has been cut a small square with sides about 4 mm in length, can be inserted into an eyepiece and used as a less convenient substitute.

The counting procedure should be appropriate to the number of reticulocytes present. Very large numbers of cells have to be surveyed if a reasonably accurate count is to be obtained when only small numbers of reticulocytes are present.[62] When the count is less than 10% a convenient method is to survey successive fields until at least 100 reticulocytes have been counted and to count the total cells in at least ten fields in order to determine the average number of cells per field.

Calculation

Number of reticulocytes in n fields = x
Average number of cells per field = y
Total number of cells in n fields = n × y

$$\text{Reticulocyte percentage} = \frac{x}{n \times y} \times 100\%$$

Absolute reticulocyte count = % × RBC ($\times 10^{12}$/l).

It is essential that the reticulocyte preparation be well spread to ensure an even distribution of cells in successive fields.

When the reticulocyte count exceeds 10% only a relatively small number of cells will have to be surveyed to obtain a standard error of 10%.*

An alternative method is based on the principle of 'balanced sampling', using a Miller ocular.** This is an eyepiece giving a square field, in the corner of which is a second ruled square, one-ninth the area of the total square. Reticulocytes are counted in the large square and the total number of cells in the small square. The number of fields which should be surveyed to obtain a desired degree of accuracy depends on the proportion of reticulocytes (Table 5.2).

Table 5.2   Accuracy of reticulocyte counts with Miller ocular

| Reticulocytes | | Standard error (σ) | | |
%	Proportion (p)	2%	5%	10%
1	.01	27500	4400	1100
2	.02	13600	2180	550
5	.05	5280	845	210
10	.10	2500	400	100
25	.25	835	135	35

Columns 3–5 indicate the total number of red cells to be counted **in the small squares** so as to give the required standard error at different reticulocyte levels. It is derived from $\sigma = \sqrt{\dfrac{p(1-p)}{\lambda}}$, where

$p = \dfrac{\text{number of reticulocytes in n large squares}}{\text{number of red cells in n small squares} \times f}$

f = ratio of large to small squares (i.e. 9), and
λ = approximate total number of cells in n large squares

It is essential that the reticulocyte preparation be well spread and well stained. Other important factors which affect the accuracy of the count are the visual acuity and patience of the observer and

---

* Standard error $(\sigma) = \sqrt{\dfrac{p(1-p),}{\lambda}}$ where p is the proportion of reticulocytes and λ is the total number of cells surveyed.
** e.g. Graticules Ltd, Morley Road, Tonbridge, Kent.

the quality and resolving power of the microscope. The most accurate counts are carried out by a conscientious observer who has no knowledge of the supposed reticulocyte level, thus eliminating the effect of conscious or unconscious bias.

The decision as to what is and what is not a reticulocyte may be difficult, as the most mature reticulocytes contain only a few dots or threads of reticulo-filamentous material. Fortunately, in well-stained preparations, viewed under the light micro-. scope, the Pappenheimer (iron-containing) type of granular material—usually present as a single small dot, less commonly as multiple dots—stains a darker shade of blue than does the reticulo-filamentous material of the reticulocyte. As described above, phase contrast will help to distinguish them. If there is any doubt, Pappenheimer's bodies can be identified by overstaining the film for iron by Perls's reaction (see p. 116).

HbH undergoes denaturation in the presence of brilliant cresyl blue or New methylene blue, resulting in round inclusion bodies which stain greenish-blue (Fig. 9.6, p. 120). These can be clearly differentiated from reticulo-filamentous material (Fig. 5.8).

Heinz bodies are also stained by New methylene blue, but they stain a lighter shade of blue than the reticulo-filamentous material of reticulocytes (Figs. 9.4 and 9.5, p 119).

Reticulocytes can be counted by fluorescent microscopy.[40,77] Add 1 volume of acridine orange solution (50 mg/100 ml of 9 g/1 NaCl) to 1 volume of blood. Mix gently for 2 min; make films on glass slides, dry rapidly and examine in a fluorescent microscope.

RNA gives an orange-red fluorescence whilst nuclear material (DNA) fluoresces yellow. However, the method is not suitable for routine use for reticulocyte counting. Although the amount of fluorescence is proportional to the amount of RNA, the brightness and colour of the fluorescence fluctuates and the preparation quickly fades when

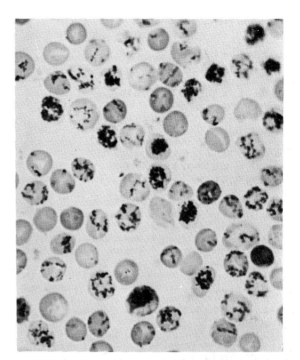

Fig. 5.8 Photomicrographs of reticulocytes in haemolytic anaemia. Stained supravitally by New methylene blue. See also Fig. 9.7, p. 120.

exposed to light; also, it requires a special fluorescent microscope.

Fluorescent staining combined with flow cytometry has been developed as a method for automated reticulocyte counting.[60,69,79] This has the potential advantage that a large number of cells are counted, giving much better statistical reliability, especially with low reticulocyte counts, and the possibility of identifying minor changes in erythropoiesis in a patient on treatment.[70]

Range of reticulocyte count in health

Adults and children 0.5–2.5%.
Infants (full term, cord blood) 2–6%.

In absolute numbers the normal reticulocyte count in health is about 50–100 × 10^9/1.

REFERENCES

[1] BAIN, B. J. (1985). Platelet count and platelet size in males and females. *Scandinavian Journal of Haematology*, **35,** 77.
[2] BALLARD, B. C. D. (1972). Lysing agent for the Coulter S. *Journal of Clinical Pathology*, **25,** 460.
[3] BAYNES, R. D., FLAX, H., BOTHWELL, T. H., BEZWODA, W.

R., ATKINSON, P. and MENDELOW, B. (1986). Red blood cells distribution width in the anemia secondary to tuberculosis. *American Journal of Clinical Pathology*, **85,** 226.
[4] BERENDES, M. (1973). The proportion of reticulocytes in the

erythrocytes of the spleen as compared with those of circulating blood, with special reference to hemolytic states. *Blood*, **14**, 558.

[5] BESSMAN, J. D. (1986). *Automated Blood Counts and Differentials: A Practical Guide.* John Hopkins University Press, Baltimore.

[6] BESSMAN, J. D., GILMER, P. R. and GARDNER, F. H. (1983). Improved classification of anemias by MCV and RDW. *American Journal of Clinical Pathology*, **80**, 322.

[7] BESSMAN, J. D., WILLIAMS, L. J. and GILMER, P. R. (1982). Platelet size in health and hematologic disease. *American Journal of Clinical Pathology*, **78**, 150.

[8] BRECHER, G. and CRONKITE, E. P. (1950). Morphology and enumeration of human blood platelets. *Journal of Applied Physiology*, **3**, 365.

[9] BRECHER, G., SCHNEIDERMAN, M. and CRONKITE, E. P. (1953). The reproducibility and constancy of the platelet count. *American Journal of Clinical Pathology*, **23**, 15.

[10] BULL, B. S., SCHNEIDERMAN, M. and BRECHER, G. (1965). Platelet counts with the Coulter counter. *American Journal of Clinical Pathology*, **44**, 678.

[11] CHALEVELAKIS, G., TSIROYANNIS, K., HATZIIOANNOU, J. and ARAPAKIS, G. (1984). Screening for thalassaemia and/or iron deficiency: evaluation of some discrimination functions. *Scandinavian Journal of Clinical and Laboratory Investigation*, **44**, 1.

[12] CLEGG, J. W. and KING, E. J. (1942). Estimation of haemoglobin by the alkaline haematin method. *British Medical Journal*, **ii**, 329.

[13] COULTER, W. H. (1956). High speed automatic blood cell counter and cell size analyser. *Proceedings of National Electronics Conference*, **12**, 1034.

[14] COUSINS, S. and LEWIS, S. M. (1982). A rapid and accurate differential centrifugation method for platelet counts. *Journal of Clinical Pathology*, **35**, 114.

[15] DAVIDSON, R. J. L. and HAMILTON, P. J. (1978). High mean red cell volume: its incidence and significance in routine haematology. *Journal of Clinical Pathology*, **31**, 493.

[16] DRABKIN, D. L. and AUSTIN, J. H. (1932). Spectrophotometric studies: spectrometric constants for common haemoglobin derivatives in human, dog and rabbit blood. *Journal of Biological Chemistry*, **98**, 719.

[17] ELLIOT, W. G. and WOOD, J. A. (1969). A concentrated stromalytic solution for electronic leukocyte counts. *American Journal of Clinical Pathology*, **51**, 298.

[18] ENGLAND, J. M., CHETTY, M. C., GARVEY, B. et al (1982). Value assignment to quality control materials. In *Advances in Hematological Methods: The Blood Count.* Eds. O. W. van Assendelft and J. M. England, p. 239. CRC Press, Boca Raton, Florida.

[19] ENGLAND, J. M. and FRASER, P. M. (1973). Differentiation of iron deficiency from thalassaemia trait. *Lancet*, **i**, 1514.

[20] ENGLAND, J. M., WALFORD, D. M. and WATERS, D. A. W. (1972). Reassessment of the reliability of the haematocrit. *British Journal of Haematology*, **23**, 247.

[21] EVAN-WONG, L. and DAVIDSON, R. J. (1983). Raised Coulter mean corpuscular volume in diabetic ketoacidosis, and its underlying association with marked plasma hyperosmolarity. *Journal of Clinical Pathology*, **36**, 334.

[22] GARBY, L. and VUILLE, J. C. (1961). The amount of trapped plasma in a high speed micro-capillary haematocrit centrifuge. *Scandinavian Journal of Clinical and Laboratory Investigation*, **13**, 642.

[23] GIBSON, Q. H. and HARRISON, D. C. (1945). An artificial standard for use in the estimation of haemoglobin. *Biochemical Journal*, **39**, 490.

[24] GILMER, P. R. and KOEPKE, J. A. (1976). The reticulocyte: an approach to definition. *American Journal of Clinical Pathology*, **66**, 262.

[25] GRAHAM, S. S., TRAUB, B. and MINK, I. B. (1987). Automated platelet-sizing parameters in a normal population. *American Journal of Clinical Pathology*, **87**, 365.

[26] GUTHRIE, D. L. and PEARSON, T. C. (1982). PCV measurement in the management of polycythaemia patients. *Clinical and Laboratory Haematology*, **4**, 257.

[27] HAENEY, M. R. (1976). Erroneous values for the total white cell count and ESR in patients with cryoglobulinaemia. *Journal of Clinical Pathology*, **29**, 894.

[28] HEGDE, U. M., WHITE, J. M., HART G. H. and MARSH, G. W. (1977). Diagnosis of β-thalassaemia trait from Coulter Counter's indices. *Journal of Clinical Pathology*, **30**, 884.

[29] HENDERSON, S. J. and WOOD, J. K. (1986). Factors producing error in the total leucocyte count as measured on the Coulter Counter S Plus IVD. *Clinical and Laboratory Haematology*, 1986, **8**, 341.

[30] HILLMAN, R. S, (1969). Characteristics of marrow production and reticulocyte maturation in normal man in response to anemia. *Journal of Clinical Investigation*, **48**, 443.

[31] HILLMAN, R. S. and FINCH, C. A. (1969). The misused reticulocyte. *British Journal of Haematology*, **17**, 313.

[32] HOLT, J. T., DEWANDLER, M. J. and ARVAN, D. A. (1982). Spurious elevation of the electronically determined mean corpuscular volume and hematocrit caused by hyperglycemia. *American Journal of Clinical Pathology*, **77**, 561.

[33] HOUCHIN, D. N., MUNN, J. I. and PARNELL, B. L. (1958). A method for the measurement of red cell dimensions and calculation of mean corpuscular volume and surface area. *Blood*, **13**, 1185.

[34] International Committee for Standardization in Haematology (1978). Recommendations for reference method for haemoglobinometry in human blood and specifications for international haemiglobincyanide reference preparation. *Journal of Clinical Pathology*, **31**, 139.

[35] International Committee for Standardization in Haematology (1980). Recommended methods for measurement of red-cell and plasma volume. *Journal of Nuclear Medicine*, **21**, 793.

[36] International Committee for Standardization in Haematology (1980). Recommendations for reference method for determination by centrifugation of packed cell volume of blood. *Journal of Clinical Pathology*, **33**, 1.

[37] International Committee for Standardization in Haematology (1983). Protocol for evaluation of automated blood cell counters. *Clinical and Laboratory Haematology*, **6**, 69.

[38] International Committee for Standardization in Haematology; Expert Panel on Cytometry (1988). The assignment of values to fresh blood used for calibrating automated blood cell counters. *Clinical and Laboratory Haematology*, **10**, 203.

[39] International Committee for Standardization in Haematology (1990). Selected methods for red cell and white cell enumeration by semi-automated single channel instruments. In preparation.

[40] JAHANMEHR, S. A. H., HYDE, K., GEARY, C. G., CINKOTAI, K. I. and MacIVER, J. E. (1987). Simple technique for fluorescence staining of blood cells with acridine orange. *Journal of Clinical Pathology*, **40**, 926.

[41] JOHNSON, C. S., TEGOS, C. and BEUTLER, E. (1983). Thalassemia minor: routine erythrocyte measurements and differential from iron deficiency. *American Journal of Clinical Pathology*, **80**, 31.

[42] KARPATKIN, S. (1978). Heterogeneity of human platelets. VI. Correlation of platelet function with platelet volume, *Blood*, **51**, 307.

[43] KLEE, G. G., FAIRBANKS, V. F., PIERRE, R. V. and O'SULLIVAN, M. B. (1976). Routine erythrocyte measurement in diagnosis of iron-deficiency anemia and thalassemia minor. *American Journal of Pathology*, **66**, 870.

[44] LEWIS, S. M. (1972). Cell counting—enumeration of blood cells and bacteria. In *Biomedical Technology in Hospital Diagnosis*. Eds. A. T. Elder and D. W. Neill, p. 211. Pergamon Press, Oxford.

[45] LEWIS, S. M. (1986). External Quality Assessment in Europe: In *Automation and Quality Assurance in Haematology*. Eds. R. M. Rowan and J. M. England, p. 118. Blackwell Scientific Publications, Oxford.

[46] LEWIS, S. M., SKELLY, J. V. and COUSINS, S. (1981). Automated platelet counting—a re-evaluation of the sedimentation method. *Clinical and Laboratory Haematology*, **3**, 215.

[47] LEWIS, S. M., WARDLE, J., COUSINS, S. and SKELLY, J. V. (1979). Platelet counting—development of a reference method and a reference preparation. *Clinical and Laboratory Haematology*, **1**, 227.

[48] LIPPI, U., SCHINELLA, M., MODENA, N. and NICOLI M. (1987). Unpredictable effects of K_3 EDTA on mean platelet volume. *American Journal of Clinical Pathology*, **87**, 391.

[49] MAGATH, T. B., BERKSON, J. and HURN, M. (1936). The error of determination of the erythrocyte count. *American Journal of Clinical Pathology*, **6**, 568.

[50] MATSUBARA, T., OKUZONO, H. and SENBA, U. (1979). Modification of Van Kampen-Zijlstra's reagent for the hemiglobincyanide method. *Clinica Chimica Acta*, **93**, 163.

[51] MARSHALL, P. N., BENTLEY, S. A. and LEWIS, S. M. (1976). Purified azure B as a reticulocyte stain. *Journal of Clinical Pathology*, **29**, 1060.

[52] MORLEY, A. (1969). A platelet cycle in normal individuals. *Australasian Annals of Medicine*, **18**, 127.

[53] PAULUS, J. M. (1975). Platelet size in man. *Blood*, **46**, 321.

[54] PEARSON, T. C. and GUTHRIE, D. L. (1982). Trapped plasma in microhematocrit. *American Journal of Clinical Pathology*, **78**, 770.

[55] PRICE-JONES, C. (1933). *Red Blood Cell Diameters*. Oxford University Press, London.

[56] RICHARDSON JONES, A. (1982). Counting and sizing of blood cells using aperture-impedance systems. In *Advances in Hematological Methods: The Blood Count*. Eds. O. W. van Assendelft and J. M. England, p. 49. CRC Press, Boca Raton, Florida.

[57] ROBERTS, G. T. and EL BADAWI, S. B. (1985). Red blood cell distribution width index in some hematologic diseases. *American Journal of Clinical Pathology*, **83**, 222.

[58] ROWAN, R. M. (1983). Blood cell volume analysis—a new screening technology for the haematologist. Albert Clark, London.

[59] ROWAN, R. M. and FRASER, C. (1982). Platelet size distribution analysis. In *Advances in Hematological Methods: The Blood Count*. Eds. O. W. van Assendelft and J. M. England, p. 125. CRC Press, Boca Raton, Florida.

[60] SAGE, B. H., O'CONNELL, J. P. and MERCOLINO, T. J. (1983). A rapid, vital staining procedure for flow cytometric analysis of human reticulocytes. *Cytometry*, **4**, 222.

[61] SANDERS, C. and SKERRY, D. W. (1961). The distribution of blood cells on haemocytometer counting chambers with special reference to the amended British Standards Specification 748 (1958). *Journal of Clinical Pathology*, **48**, 298.

[62] SEIP, M, (1953). Reticulocyte studies: the liberation of red blood corpuscles from the bone marrow into the peripheral blood and the production of erythrocytes elucidated by reticulocyte investigations. *Acta Medica Scandinavica*, Suppl. 282.

[63] SHINTON, N. K., ENGLAND, J. M. E. and KENNEDY, D. A. (1982). Guidelines for the evaluation of instruments used in haematological laboratories. *Journal of Clinical Pathology*, **35**, 1095.

[64] SKINNIDER, L. F. and MUSGLOW, E. (1972). A stromatolysing and cyanide reagent for use with the Coulter Counter Model S. *American Journal of Clinical Pathology*, **57**, 537.

[65] SLOAN, A. W. (1951). The normal platelet count in man. *Journal of Clinical Pathology*, **4**, 37.

[66] SOLANKI, D. L. and BLACKBURN, B. C. (1985). Spurious red blood cell parameters due to serum cold agglutinins: observations on Ortho ELT-8 cell counter. *American Journal of Clinical Pathology*, **83**, 218.

[67] STEVENSON, C. F. SMETTERS, G. W. and COOPER, J. A. D. (1951). A gravimetric method for the calibration of hemoglobin micropipets. *American Journal of Clinical Pathology*, **21**, 489.

[68] SUNDERMAN, F. W., MacFATE, R. P., MacFADZEAN, D., STEVENSON, G. F. and COPELAND, B. E. (1953). Symposium on clinical hemoglobinometry. *American Journal of Clinical Pathology*, **23**, 519.

[69] TANKE, H. J. ROTHBARTH, P. H., VOSSEN, J. M. J. J., KOPER, G. J. M. and PLOEM, J. S. (1983). Flow cytometry of reticulocytes applied to clinical hematology. *Blood*, **61**, 1091.

[70] TANKE, H. J., VAN VIANEN, P. H., EMILIANI, F. M. F., NEUTEBOOM, I., deVOGEL, N. and TATES, A. D. (1986). Changes in erythropoiesis due to radiation or chemotherapy as studied by flow cytometric determination of peripheral blood reticulocytes. *Histochemistry*, **84**, 544.

[71] THOM, R. (1981). Calibration in haematology: In *New Approaches to Laboratory Medicine*. Ed. S. B. Rosalki. Ernst Giebeler, Darmstadt.

[72] THOMPSON, C. B., DIAZ, D. D., QUINN, P. G., LAPINS, M., KURTZ, S. R. and VALERI, C. R. (1983). The role of anticoagulation in the measurement of platelet volumes. *American Journal of Clinical Pathology*, **80**, 327.

[73] THOMPSON, L. C. (1946). An inorganic grey solution. *Transactions of the Faraday Society*, **42**, 663.

[74] THREATTE, G. A., ADRABOS, C., EBBE, S. and BRECHER, G. (1984). Mean platelet volume: the need for a reference method. *American Journal of Clinical Pathology*, **81**, 769.

[75] UNGER, K. W. and JOHNSON, D. (1974). Red blood cell mean corpuscular volume: a potential indicator of alcohol usage in a working population. *American Journal of Medical Sciences*, **267**, 281.

[76] VAN ASSENDELFT, O. W. and ENGLAND, J. M. (eds.) (1981). *Advances in Hematological Methods: The Blood Count*. CRC Press, Boca Raton, Florida.

[77] VANDER, J. B., HARRIS, C. A. and ELLIS, S. R. (1963). Reticulocyte counts by means of fluorescence miscroscopy. *Journal of Laboratory and Clinical Medicine*, **62**, 132.

[78] Van Kampen, E. J. and Zijlstra, W. G. (1983). Spectrophotometry of hemoglobin and hemoglobin derivatives. *Advances in Clinical Chemistry*, **23,** 199.

[79] Vaughan, W. P., Hall, J., Johnson, K., Dougherty, C. and Pebbles, D. (1985). Simultaneous reticulocyte and platelet counting on a clinical flow cytometer. *American Journal of Hematology*, **18,** 385.

[80] Ward, P. G., Wardle, J. and Lewis, S. M. (1982). Standardization for routine blood count—the role of interlaboratory trials. *Methods in Hematology*, **4,** 102.

[81] Wardle, J., Ward, P. G. and Lewis, S. M. (1985). Response of various blood counting systems to CPD-AI preserved whole blood. *Clinical and Laboratory Haematology*, **7,** 245.

[82] Weiss, G. B. and Bessman, J. D. (1984). Spurious automated red cell values in warm autoimmune hemolytic anemia. *American Journal of Hematology*, **17,** 433.

[83] Westerman, M. P., Pierce, L. E. and Jensen, W. N. (1961). A direct method for the quantitative measurement of red cell dimensions. *Journal of Laboratory and Clinical Medicine*, **57,** 819.

[84] Wittekind, D. and Schulte, E. (1987). Standardized Azure B as a reticulocyte stain. *Clinical and Laboratory Haematology*, **9,** 395.

[85] World Health Organization (1977). The SI for the health professions, WHO, Geneva.

[86] Zijlstra, W. G. and van Kampen, E. J. (1960). Standardization of hemoglobinometry. I. The extinction coefficient of hemiglobincyanide at $\lambda = 540$ mμ: ε^{540}HiCN. *Clinica Chimica Acta*, **91,** 339.

[87] Zweens, J., Frankena, H. and Zijlstra, W. G. (1979). Decomposition on freezing of reagents used in the ICSH recommended method for the determination of total haemoglobin in blood; its nature, cause and prevention. *Clinica Chimica Acta*, **91,** 339.

[88] Groner, W. and Epstein, E. (1982). Counting and sizing of blood cells using light scattering. *Advances in Haematological Methods: The Blood Count*. Eds O.W. van Assendelft and J. M. England, p. 77. CRC Press, Boca Raton, Florida.

6. Differential leucocyte count

Differential leucocyte counts are usually performed on blood films which are prepared on slides by the spread or 'wedge' technique. Unfortunately, even in well-spread films the distribution of the various cell types is not totally random (see below). To overcome this, a spin preparation method has been proposed by means of which the cells are evenly distributed on the slide as a monolayer.[14,24] The disadvantage of this procedure in a busy laboratory is the longer time required for preparing the slides; also, it requires special equipment.

For a reliable differential leucocyte count on films spread on slides the film must not be too thin and the tail of the film should be smooth. To achieve this the film should be made with a rapid movement using a smooth glass spreader (see p. 75). This should result in a film in which there is some overlap of the red cells, diminishing to separation near the tail, and in which the leucocytes in the body of the film are not too badly shrunken. If the film is made too thinly, or if a rough-edged spreader is used, many of the leucocytes, perhaps even 50% of them, accumulate at the edges and in the tail (Fig. 6.1). Moreover, a gross qualitative irregularity in distribution is the rule: polymorphonuclear neutrophils and monocytes predominate at the margins and the tail, and lymphocytes in the middle of the film (Fig. 6.2). This separation probably depends upon differences in stickiness, size and specific gravity among the different classes of cells.

Various systems of performing the differential count have been advocated. The problem is to overcome the differences in distribution of the various classes of cells, which are probably always present to a small extent even in well made films. No system of counting will compensate for the gross irregularities in distribution in a badly made film. It is a waste of time to attempt a differential count on such a film and, if this is attempted, futile to count only the cells in the centre of the film, where lymphocytes probably predominate, and to neglect altogether the tail, where most of the neutrophils lie. If the film had been well made, and many leucocytes are present in the body of the film

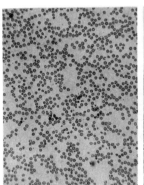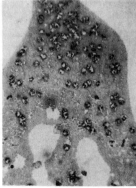

Fig. 6.1 Centre (left) and tail (right) of a badly made blood film. The centre of the film is almost devoid of leucocytes; in the tail neutrophils, particularly, are present in large numbers. × 100.

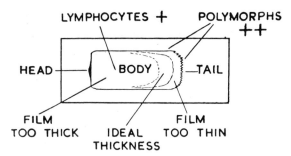

Fig. 6.2 Schematic drawing of a blood film made on a slide. The film has been spread from left to right. An indication is given of the way the leucocytes are distributed (see text).

and there is no great accumulation at the tail, the following technique of counting is recommended.

VISUAL COUNTING

Count the cells using a 4 mm dry or 3.7 mm oil-immersion lens, in a strip running the whole length of the film. Avoid the lateral edges of the film. Inspect the film from the head to the tail, and if less than 100 cells are encountered in a single narrow strip, examine one or more additional strips until at least 100 cells have been counted. Each longitudinal strip represents the blood drawn out from a small part of the original drop of blood when it has spread out between the slide and spreader (Fig. 6.3). If all the cells are counted in such a strip, the differential totals will approximate closely to the true differential count. This technique is liable to error if cells in the thick part of the film cannot be identified; also it does not allow for any excess of

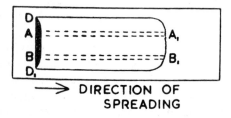

Fig. 6.3 Schematic drawing illustrating the longitudinal method of performing differential leucocyte counts. The original drop of blood spreads out between spreader and slide (D–D_1). The film is made in such a way that representative strips of films, such as A–A_1 and B–B_1 are formed from blood originally at A and B, respectively. In order to perform an accurate differential count, all the leucocytes in one or more strips, such as A–A_1 and B–B_1, should be inspected and classified.

neutrophils and monocytes at the edges of the film, but this preponderance is slight in a well made film and in practice makes little difference to the result.

The above technique is easy to carry out; with high counts ($10-30 \times 10^9$ cells per litre) a short, 2–3 cm, film is desirable. In patients with very high counts (as in leukaemia) the method has to be abandoned and the cells should be counted in any well spread area where the cell types are easy to identify. Other systems of counting, such as the 'battlement' count,[19] seem to be more elaborate and have no advantage.

Most workers find it possible to remember accurately the differential counts of small groups of 20 to 25 cells, writing the results on paper when each small group has been surveyed. However, a multiple manual register is a help in recording the results of a count. With some sophisticated electronic registers, the differential count is entered directly into a computerized data processor alongside the results of the automated blood count.

The observed differential count depends not only on artefactual differences in distribution due to the process of spreading, but also on 'random' distribution; together they are by far the most important cause of unreliable differential counts.[10] Distribution of the counts of a major cell population is Gaussian; that of a minor population is a Poisson distribution (see p. 543). In practical terms the random distribution means that, if a total of 100 cells are counted, with a true neutrophil proportion of 50%, the range (± 2 SD) within which 95% of the counts will fall, is of the order of $\pm 14\%$, i.e. 36–64% neutrophils.

A 200-cell count can provide a more accurate estimate; in the above example, the ± 2 SD range will be about 40–60%. In a 500-cell count the range would be reduced to 44–56% neutrophils. In the case of a minor population, if the true count is 3% in a 100-cell differential count, in 95 out of 100 counts, the count would range between 0% and 6%, whilst a true count of 10% is likely to be counted as anything between 5% and 15%. Even 500-cell counts are little better for accurate counting of cells present in low percentages, but if abnormal cells are present in small numbers they are more likely to be detected when 200–500 cell counts are performed than with a 100-cell count.[26] In practice a 200-cell count is recommended as a routine procedure.

Reporting the differential leucocyte count

The differential count, expressed as the percentage of each type of cell, should be related to the total leucocyte count and the results reported in absolute numbers ($\times 10^9$/l). Nucleated red cells are not included; these are recorded as numbers per 100 leucocytes. Myelocytes and metamyelocytes, if present, are included separately from neutrophils. Band (stab) cells are generally counted as neutrophils but it may be useful to record them separately. They normally constitute less than 6% of the neutrophils; an increase may point to an inflammatory process even in the absence of an absolute leucocytosis.[21]

AUTOMATED DIFFERENTIAL LEUCOCYTE COUNTING

Automated systems for differential leucocyte counting have had a major influence on the organization of laboratories where they are in use. Whether they are able to replace manual counts entirely, or should be used only for screening those which are expected to be normal, is a matter of debate. A 'flagging' system to identify abnormal specimens which require a visual count is essential.

Three methods have been developed:
cell size analysis,
flow cytochemistry and
high resolution pattern recognition.

Cell size analysis[4,16,29]

Based on early observation by England and collegues[11,13] on size differences of lymphoid and myeloid cells in saponin-based lysing reagents, equipment for limited differential leucocyte counting in aperture-impedance systems has been developed (e.g. Coulter S Plus IV; Toa (Sysmex) E5000). The leucocytes can be classified into three main groups on the basis of their size after suitable dilution (see p. 000).

Small cells, 30–60 fl, correspond to lymphocytes; medium sized cells, up to 150 fl, represent the monocytes, eosinophils and basophils and reactive lymphocytes; and cells larger than 150 fl the neutrophils, myelocytes and metamyelocytes; unusually large lymphocytes will also be counted in the largest category. Instruments differ in the way in which the size discriminators are set and the data of size distribution are processed; consequently, eosinophils and basophils are included amongst the largest cells by Coulter S Plus IV, and as intermediate-sized cells by Sysmex E5000.

In general, however, the results with the two instruments are consistent,[25] and the instrument results correlate well with manual counts for granulocytes and normal lymphocytes. The instruments are, however, unreliable when atypical lymphoid cells are present, as in lymphoproliferative conditions and in infants and neonates.[2,8,28] Monocyte counts are poorly correlated. Thus, this method of automatic counting cannot replace manual counting with respect to accuracy; the method is, however, a very rapid one, with good reproducibility.

More advanced versions of these instruments are now available which give a more accurate classification of the different cells.

In the Coulter VCS, cell size analysis by aperture impedance is supplemented by light scatter and high frequency conductivity to provide clear discrimination between lymphocytes, monocytes, neutrophils, eosinophils and basophils. In the Sysmex NE8000, radiofrequency is used to obtain information on nuclear size and density which, together with cell sizing, enables the different cells to be identified.

Continuous flow cytochemistry

The prototype machine was the Technicon Hemalog D;[20] this was followed by the H6000,[27,32] and more recently by the H1. In this process the blood streams into one channel where the alkaline peroxidase reaction (4-chloro-1-naphthol with hydrogen peroxide as substrate at a high pH) takes place and into a second channel in which heparin-containing granules of basophils are stained with alcian blue. Stained cells are classified as small or large. From the permutations of size, whether stained or unstained and, if stained, the intensity of staining reaction, the cells are differentiated into neutrophils, eosinophils, basophils, lymphocytes, monocytes and 'large unstained cells'. The last group includes blast cells and atypical mononuclears; these are also specifically flagged to indicate that a film should be examined. The major advantage of the system is that 10 000 cells are counted in 1 min, thus providing high precision and a rapid result. There is a small number of discrepancies when comparison is made with classification based on traditional morphology.[6,15,18] A comparison with counts by aperture-impedance has shown only small overlaps between the different classes of cells, but the Technicon system is more sensitive in detecting blast cells in acute leukaemia[17] and in discriminating between several different types of cells that are included together as mononuclears in the Coulter S Plus IV.[7]

Pattern recognition

This is an adaptation of traditional differential leucocyte counting and, although it uses sophisticated computer technology for the pattern recognition, its basis is classification of cells by their morphological features in Romanowsky-stained films. These are scanned under a microscope by a high resolution photosensor which generates electronic signals corresponding to various features of the cells (e.g. size, shape, periphery, texture, granularity, nuclear-cytoplasmic ratio) and compares them with patterns of cells in the computer's memory. Thus, the reliability of the instrument in identifying cells will depend on how and to what extent it has been instructed; moreover, it is dependent on the staining of the test slides being similar to that of the original training set.

Although a number of systems have been developed, few of these are now available commercially (e.g. Leitz Hematrak; Microx Omron Analyser, Hitachi 8200). The main limitations have been the extent to which they are dependent on an operator's supervision when a count is being carried out and the speed of performance which in the different systems is rather slow, a 500-cell count taking from 2 to 6 min.

EOSINOPHIL COUNTS BY A COUNTING-CHAMBER METHOD

Although total eosinophil counts can be roughly calculated from the total and differential leucocyte counts, the staining properties of eosinophils make it possible to count them directly and more accurately in a counting chamber.

The principles underlying the counting-chamber or 'wet' eosinophil count were reviewed by Spiers.[33] Ideally, the diluent should stain the eosinophil granules brightly and distinctly and at the same time lyse the red cells and all other types of leucocytes.

Diluting fluids for eosinophil counts

The acetone group of diluents, introduced by Dunger,[9] contain:

1. An acid dye, such as eosin or phloxine.
2. Water to lyse the red cells and rupture the leucocyte membranes (the eosinophils seem more resistant than other leucocytes in this respect).
3. Acetone to inhibit the lytic action of water on the leucocytes according to the proportion used—about 5–10% seems to be the most useful concentration.

In later modifications of Dunger's diluent small amounts of a detergent[9] or alkali[33] were added to accelerate the staining of the eosinophil granules.

Method

Add 20 µl of EDTA blood to 0.38 ml of diluting fluid to give a 1 in 20 dilution. Mix the suspension for not longer than 30 s, and then fill the counting chamber using a stout glass capillary or Pasteur pipette. The eosinophils may be counted as soon as they have settled or the count may be postponed for up to 30 min or so if the counting chamber is placed in a moist chamber (a Petri dish with cover containing a pledget of damp cotton wool).

Counting chamber

A chamber with the Fuchs-Rosenthal ruling is suitable. The ruled area in a Fuchs-Rosenthal chamber is a 4 mm square (Fig. 6.4) and the chamber is 0.2 mm in depth (area 16 mm^2 and volume 3.2 μl)*. With counts at the upper limit of the normal range (see below) the whole ruled area should be surveyed and the total number of eosinophils recorded. With lower counts several fillings of the counting chamber should be surveyed. It is convenient to use a 16 mm objective and × 10 eyepieces. In a good clean preparation the eosinophils should be easily identified; their granules stain deep red and the cells containing them should be intact.

As in ordinary leucocyte counts the accuracy of the count is largely determined by the number of cells counted. In a serious investigation 100 cells should be looked upon as the minimum, the counting chamber being filled several times, if necessary. The CV due to the random distribution of the cells is c 10% in a 100-cell count.

Calculation

$$\text{Count (/l)} = \frac{\text{No of cells counted}}{\text{Volume counted (μl)}}$$
$$\times \text{ dilution } \times 10^6.$$

Thus, if N eosinophils are counted in 3.2 μl, then the total eosinophil count per litre

$$= \frac{N \times 20 \text{ (dilution)}}{3.2} \times 10^6$$

$$= N \times 6.25 \times 10^6/l$$

$$(= N \times 6.25 \text{ per μl}).$$

*A modified version is also available in which the ruled area is a 3 mm square, total area 9 mm^2.

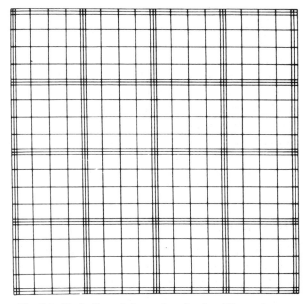

Fig. 6.4 Fuchs-Rosenthal counting chamber. The total ruled area is 4 mm × 4 mm, divided into 16 large squares, 1 mm × 1 mm, each containing 16 small squares.

Diluting fluid

Aqueous eosin (200 g/l) 10 ml
Acetone 10 ml
Water 80 ml.

The fluid will keep for 2–3 weeks at 4°C. It must be filtered before use.

Eosinophils slowly disintegrate in the diluting fluid and the count should not be delayed for more than 30 min. It is probably best to fill the counting chamber as soon as the blood is diluted and to avoid prolonged mixing, for in this way, clumping of eosinophils may be prevented.[3]

Range of eosinophil count in health
40–440 × 10^6/l[23,30]

There is normally considerable diurnal variation in the eosinophil count and differences amounting to as much as 100% have been recorded. The lowest counts are found in the morning (10 a.m. to noon) and the highest at night (midnight to 4 a.m.).[5,30,34] Muehrcke et al.[23] found that the counts of 42 healthy but fasting young males conformed to a log-normal distribution.

BASOPHIL COUNTS BY A COUNTING-CHAMBER METHOD

Alcian blue stains basophil granules specifically and at a low pH the contrast between the stained basophils and other (unstained) leucocytes is excellent.[12]

Diluting fluid

Solution A. EDTA 1 g/l in 9 g/l NaCl.
Solution B. Cetyl pyridinium chloride monohydrate
0.76 g
Lanthanum chloride $6H_2O$ 7g
NaCl 9g Tween 20 2.1 ml
Alcian blue 8 GX (CI 74240) 1.43 g
Water to 1 litre.
Solution C. HCl 1 mol/l.

Method[12]

Dilute 0.1 ml of EDTA blood with 0.4 ml of Solution A. Add 0.45 ml of Solution B; mix gently for 1 min. Add 0.05 ml of Solution C; mix gently for a few seconds and then fill a Fuchs-Rosenthal counting chamber, using a stout glass capillary or Pasteur pipette.

Leave for 5–10 min in a moist chamber (a Petri dish with cover containing a pledget of damp cotton wool). Count the stained cells in the whole ruled area.

Calculation

$$\text{Count (/l)} = \frac{\text{No of cells counted}}{\text{Volume counted (µl)}} \times \text{dilution} \times 10^6.$$

Thus, if N cells are counted in the entire chamber, (i.e. 3.2 µl),

$$\text{count/l} = \frac{N \times 10}{3.2} \times 10^6$$

$$= N \times 3.13 \times 10^6/l$$

$$(= N \times 3.13 \text{ per µl}).$$

Range of basophils in health 20–50 $\times 10^6/l$[31]

Gilbert and Ornstein[12] reported a 95% distribution in normal subjects of 10–80 $\times 10^6/l$. There are no age or sex differences although serial counts have shown lower levels during ovulation.[22]

REFERENCES

[1] BAIN, B. J. (1986). An assessment of the three population differential count on the Coulter Model S Plus IV. *Clinical and Laboratory Haematology*, **8**, 347.

[2] BAIN, B., DEAN A. and BROOM, G. (1984). The estimation of the lymphocyte percentage by the Coulter Counter Model S Plus III. *Clinical and Laboratory Haematology*, **6**, 273.

[3] BERGSTRAND, C. G., HELLSTRÖM, B. and JOHNSSON, B (1950). Remarks on the technique of eosinophil counting. *Scandinavian Journal of Clinical and Laboratory Investigation*, **2**, 341.

[4] BESSMAN, J. D. (1986). *Automated blood counts and differentials: a practical guide.* Johns Hopkins University Press, Baltimore.

[5] BEST W. R. and SAMSTER M (1951). Variation and error in eosinophil counts of blood and bone marrow. *Blood*, **6**, 61.

[6] CAIRNS, J. W., HEALY, M. J. R., STAFFORD, D. M., VITEK, P. and WATERS, D. A. W. (1977). Evaluation of the Hemalog D differential leucocyte counter. *Journal of Clinical Pathology*, **30**, 997.

[7] CLARK, P. T., HENTHORN, J. S. and ENGLAND, J. M. (1985). Differential white cell counting on the Coulter Counter Model S Plus IV (Three population) and the Technicon H6000: A comparison by simple and multiple regression. *Clinical and Laboratory Haematology*, **7**, 335.

[8] COX, C. J., HABERMANN, T. M., PAYNE B. A., KLEE, G. G. and PIERRE R. V. (1985). Evaluation of the Coulter Counter Model S Plus IV. *American Journal of Clinical Pathology*, **84**, 297.

[9] DUNGER, R. (1910). Eine einfache Methode der Zählung der eosinophilen Leukozyten und der praktische Wert dieser Untersuchung. *Münchener medizinische Wochenschrift*, **57**, 1942.

[10] ENGLAND, J. M. (1979). Prospect for automated differential leucocyte counting in the routine laboratory. *Clinical and Laboratory Haematology*, **1**, 263.

[11] ENGLAND, J. M., DOWN, M. C., BASHFORD, C. C. and SABRY-GRANT, R. (1976). Differential leukocyte-counts on Coulter Counter Model S. *Lancet*, **i**, 1134.

[12] GILBERT, H. S. and ORNSTEIN, L. (1975). Basophil counting with a new staining method using Alcian blue. *Blood*, **46**, 279.

[13] HUGHES JONES, N. C., ENGLAND, J. M., NORLEY, I. and YOUNG, J. M. S. (1974) Differential leucocyte counts by volume distribution analysis. *British Journal of Haematology*, **28**, 148.

[14] INGRAM, M. and MINTER, F. M. (1969). Semiautomatic preparation of coverglass blood smears using a centrifugal device. *American Journal of Clinical Pathology*, **51**, 214.

[15] KOEPKE, J. A. (1978), *Differential leukocyte counting: CAP Conference Aspen, 1977*. College of American Pathologists, Skokie, Illinois.

[16] KOEPKE, J. A., ROSS, D. and BULL, B. S. (1984) (Eds.). The white blood cell differential. *Blood Cells*, **11** (1 and 2), 1–339.

[17] LAI, A. P., MARTIN, P. J., RICHARDS, J. D. M., GOLDSTONE, A. M. and CAWLEY, J. C. (1986). Automated leucocyte differential counts in acute leukaemia: A comparison of the Hemalog D, H6000 and Coulter S-Plus IV. *Clinical and Laboratory Haematology*, **8**, 33.

[18] LEWIS, S. M. (1981). Automated differential leukocyte counting: present status and future trends. *Blut*, **43**, 1.

[19] MACGREGOR, R. G., SCOTT RICHARDS, W. and LOH, G. L. (1940). The differential leucocyte count. *Journal of Pathology and Bacteriology*, **51**, 337.

[20] MANSBERG, H. P., SAUNDERS, A. M. and GRONER, W. (1974). The Hemalog D white cell differential system. *Journal of Histochemistry and Cytochemistry*, **22**, 711.

[21] MATHY, K. A. and KOEPKE, J. A. (1974). The clinical usefulness of segmented vs. stab neutrophil criteria for differential leucocyte counts. *American Journal of Clinical Pathology*, **61**, 947.

[22] METTLER, L. and SHIRWANI, D. (1974). Direct basophil count for timing ovulation. *Fertility and Sterility*, **25**, 718.

[23] MUEHRCKE, R. C., ECKERT, E. L. and KARK, R. M. (1952). A statistical study of absolute eosinophil cell counts in healthy young adults using logarithmic analysis. *Journal of Laboratory and Clinical Medicine*, **40**, 161.

[24] NOURBAKHSH, M., ALWOOD, J. G., RACCIO, J. and SELIGSON, D. (1978). An evaluation of blood smears made by a new method using a spinner and diluted blood. *American Journal of Clinical Pathology*, **70**, 885.

[25] PIERRE, R. V., PAYNE, A., LEE, W. K., HYMA, B. A., MELCHERT, L. M. and SCHEIDT, R. M. (1987). Comparison of four leukocyte differential methods with the National Committee for Clinical Laboratory Standards (NCCLS) Reference Method. *American Journal of Clinical Pathology*, **87**, 201.

[26] ROCK, W. A., MIALE, J. B. and JOHNSON, W. D. (1984). Detection of abnormal cells in white cell differentials: comparison of the HEMATRAK automated system with manual methods. *American Journal of Clinical Pathology*, **81**, 233.

[27] ROSS, D. W. and BARDWELL, A. (1980). Automated cytochemistry and the white cell differential in leukaemia. *Blood Cells*, **6**, 455.

[28] ROSS, D. W., WATSON, J. S., DAVIS, P. H. and TRACY, S. L. (1985). Evaluation of the Coulter three-part differential screen. *American Journal of Clinical Pathology*, **84**, 481.

[29] ROWAN, R. M. (1983). *Blood cell volume analysis. A new screening technology for the haematologist*. Albert Clark, London.

[30] RUD, F. (1947). The eosinophil count in health and mental disease. *Acta Psychiatrica et Neurologica (København)*, Suppl., **40**.

[31] SHELLEY, W. B. and PARNES, H. M. (1965). The absolute basophil count. Technique and significance. *Journal of American Medical Association*, **192**, 368.

[32] SIMSON, E. (1984). *Hematology beyond the microscope*. Technicon Instruments Corp., Tarrytown, N. Y.

[33] SPIERS, R. S. (1952). The principles of eosinphil diluents. *Blood*, **7**, 550.

[34] UHRBRAND, H. (1958). The number of circulating eosinophils: normal figures and spontaneous variations. *Acta Medica Scandinavica*, **160**, 99.

7. Preparation and staining methods for blood and bone-marrow films

PREPARATION OF BLOOD FILMS ON SLIDES

Blood films can be made on glass slides or cover-glasses. The latter have the single possible advantage of a more even distribution of the leucocytes, but in every other respect slides are to be preferred. Unlike cover-glasses, slides are not easily broken; they are simple to label and when large numbers of films are to be dealt with, slides will be found much easier to handle.

Good films may be made in the following manner, using clean slides (p. 540) wiped free from dust immediately before use.

Place a small drop of blood in the centre line of a slide about 1 or 2 cm from one end. Then, without delay, place a glass slide with a smooth edge, which is trimmed to a width of *c* 2 cm, at an angle of 45° to the slide and move it back to make contact with the drop. The drop should spread out quickly along the line of contact of the spreader with slide. The moment this occurs, spread the film by a rapid, smooth, forward movement of the spreader.

The drop should be such a size that the film is 3 or 4 cm in length (Fig. 7.1). The ideal thickness is such that there is some overlap of red cells throughout much of the film's length, but separation and lack of distortion towards the tail of the film (see p. 67). The leucocytes should be easily recognizable throughout the length of the film, although possibly with some difficulty in the thicker part at the head of the film. (The preparation of films of aspirated bone marrow is described on p. 160.)

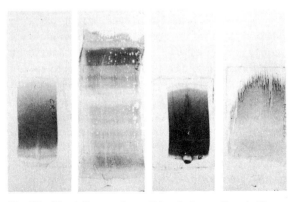

Fig. 7.1 Blood films made on slides. Left: a well-made film. Left centre: a film which is too long, too wide, grossly irregular in thickness and which has been made on a greasy slide. Right centre: a film which is too thick. Right: a film which has been spread with an irregularly-edged spreader and which shows long tails (see also Fig. 6.1). (Slightly reduced).

75

Spin method

This is an automated method by which 1 or 2 drops of blood, placed in the centre of a glass slide are briefly spun at high speed in a special centrifuge (e.g. Hemaspinner;* Cytospin**); the blood spreads on the slide in a monolayer. By this method leucocytes and platelets are distributed uniformly and free of distortion.[24,33] The red cells show a tendency to become distorted, but this can be overcome by diluting 2 volumes of blood with 1 volume of 9 g/1 NaCl immediately prior to putting the blood on the slide.[24]

Labelling blood films

A recommended method is to write the name of the patient and the date or a reference number in pencil (graphite) on the film itself. It will not be removed by staining. A paper label should be affixed to the slide later. In some computerized laboratories bar-coded specimen identification labels are used.

Bone-marrow films

The method for preparation of films from aspirated bone marrow is described on p. 160. They should be made without delay. Some films should be fixed in the appropriate fixatives for special staining (Chapters 9 and 10): others should be fixed and stained with a Romanowsky stain as described below.

STAINING BLOOD AND BONE-MARROW FILMS

Romanowsky stains are universally employed for staining blood films as a routine, and very satisfactory results may be obtained. As far as possible films should be stained as soon as they have dried in the air; they certainly should not be left unfixed for more than a few hours. If the films are left unfixed for a day or more, it will be found that the background of dried plasma stains a pale blue which is impossible to remove without spoiling the staining of the blood cells. Sometimes staining has to be postponed for up to several days, as when films are sent to the laboratory by post. It is advisable to fix such films before despatch if possible; even so, the results are likely to be less satisfactory than with freshly made films.

The remarkable property of the Romanowsky dyes of making subtle distinctions in shades of staining, and of staining granules differentially, depends on two components, namely, azure B (trimethylthionin) and eosin Y (tetrabromo-fluorescein).[20,34] The main cause of capricious staining is the presence of other dyes such as azure A, azure C, methyl violet etc. Some commercial stains contain as many as 10 different dyes identifiable by chromatography, and a variable amount of each in different batches of the same stain.[21] The stains also contain a variable amount of metal salts which influences staining characteristics.[21] Some commercial preparations of eosin Y are also impure,[22,29] but this has a less critical effect on their staining properties.[35] Other factors which affect the results are the staining time, dye concentration, ratio of azure B to eosin Y and the pH of the staining solution.

The original Romanowsky combination was polychrome methylene blue and eosin. Several of the stains now used routinely which are based on azure B also include methylene blue, but the need for this is debatable. Its presence in the stain is thought by some to enhance the staining of nucleoli and polychromatic red cells; in its absence normal neutrophil granules tend to stain heavily and may resemble 'toxic granules' in conventionally stained films.[19]

As indicated above, variation in staining is likely to be due to contaminants in the commercial dyes, and a simple combination of pure azure B and

---

* Beckman Instruments
** Shandon Southern Products Ltd.

eosin Y is preferable to the more complex stains.[34,36] Amongst the Romanowsky stains now in use, Jenner's is the simplest and Giemsa's the most complex. Leishman's stain, which occupies an intermediate position, is still widely used in the routine staining of blood films, although the results are inferior to those obtained by the combined Jenner-Giemsa method. Wright's stain, which is widely used in North America, gives results which are similar to those obtained with Leishman's stain.

A pH to the alkaline side of neutrality accentuates the azure component at the expense of the eosin and vice versa. A pH of 6.8 is usually recommended for general use, but to some extent this depends on personal preference. (When looking for malaria parasites a pH of 7.2 is recommended in order to see Schüffner's dots.) To achieve a uniform pH, 50 ml of 66 mmol/l Sörensen's phosphate buffer (p. 79) may be added to each 1 litre of the water used in diluting the stains and washing the films.

The mechanism by which certain components of a cell's structure stain with particular dyes and other components fail to do so, although staining with other dyes, depends on complex differences in binding of the dyes to chemical structures and interactions between the dye molecules. Azure B in dimer form is bound to anionic molecules, e.g. phosphate groups of DNA, and eosin Y is bound as a monomer to cationic sites on proteins.

As soon as the dyes are bound, either electron interaction occurs with dye–dye aggregation[34] or the eosin Y molecule is intercalated between the azure B molecules and the complex is held together by charge effect.[23] Thus, the acidic groupings of the nucleic acids and proteins of the cell nuclei and primitive cytoplasm determine their uptake of the basic dye azure B, and, conversely, the presence of basic groupings on the Hb molecule results in its affinity for acidic dyes and its staining by eosin. The granules in the cytoplasm of neutrophil leucocytes are weakly stained by the azure complexes. Eosinophilic granules contain a spermine derivative with an alkaline grouping which stains strongly with the acidic component of the dye, whereas basophilic granules contain heparin which has an affinity for the basic component of the dye.

STAINING METHODS

May-Grünwald-Giemsa's stain

Dry the films in the air, then fix by immersing in a jar of methanol for 10–20 min. For bone marrow films leave for 20–25 min in the methanol. Transfer to a staining jar containing May-Grünwald's stain freshly diluted with an equal volume of buffered water. After the films have been allowed to stain for c 15 min, transfer them without washing to a jar containing Giemsa's stain freshly diluted with 9 volumes of buffered water. After staining for 10–15 min, transfer the slides to a jar containing buffered water, rapidly wash in three or four changes of water and finally allow to stand undisturbed in water for a short time (usually 2–5 min) for differentiation to take place. This may be controlled by inspection of the wet slide under the low power of the microscope; with experience the naked-eye colour of the film is often a good guide. The slides should be transferred from one staining solution to the other without being allowed to dry. As the intensity of the staining is affected by any variation in the thickness of a film, it is not easy to obtain uniform staining throughout a film's length.

When differentiation is complete, stand the slides upright to dry. When thoroughly dry, cover the films by a rectangular No. 1 cover-glass, using for this purpose a mountant, which is miscible with xylol.* For a temporary mount, cedar-wood oil may be used.

The cover-glass should be sufficiently large to overlie the whole film, including both the edges and the tail. If a neutral mounting medium is used the staining should be preserved for at least 5–10 yr if kept in the dark. Although it is probable that stained films keep best unmounted, there are objections to this course: it is almost impossible to keep the slides free from dust and from being scratched, and in the absence of a cover-glass the observer is tempted to examine the film solely with the oil-immersion objective, a practice which is to be deprecated.

As an alternative to a neutral mountant and cover-glass, the slide may be covered with a layer of polystyrene or acrylic resin in solvent.** This has

---

*e.g. Gurr DPX Mountant (B D H)
**Acrylek (Fisons Ltd); Trycolac (Aerosol Marketing & Chemical Co. Ltd.)

the advantage of speedy application and rapid drying. However, the resin tends to gather dust and finger-marks which are less easily removed than from glass.

The May-Grünwald-Giemsa staining method described above is designed for staining a number of films at the same time. Single slides may be stained by flooding the slide with a combined fixative and staining solution (e.g. Leishman's stain).

A relatively prolonged fixation, at least 10 min, is required for good staining; particularly is this so in staining films of bone marrow. It is important to ensure that the methanol used as fixative is completely water-free. As little as 4% water may affect the appearance of the films and a higher water content causes gross changes (Figs. 7.2, 7.3).

The diluted stains usually retain their staining powers sufficiently well for several batches of slides

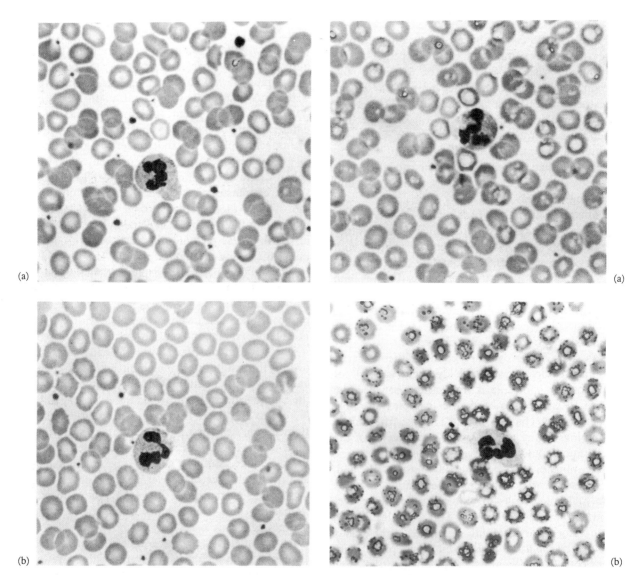

(a)

(b)

(a)

(b)

Fig. 7.2 Blood film appearances following methanol fixation. Photomicrographs of Romanowsky-stained blood films which have been fixed in methanol containing (a) 1% water and (b) 3% water. The red cells and leucocytes are well fixed.

Fig. 7.3 Blood film appearances following methanol fixation. Photomicrographs of Romanowsky-stained blood films which have been fixed in methanol containing (a) 4% water and (b) 10% water. In (a) the red cells are poorly fixed; in (b) they are very badly fixed.

to be stained in them. They must be made up freshly each day, and it is probably best to stain the day's films all at the same time, or if this is not possible in consecutive batches. There is no need to filter the stains before use unless a deposit is present.

Jenner-Giemsa's stain

Jenner's stain may be substituted for May-Grünwald's stain in the above described technique. The results are little less satisfactory. The stain is used with 4 volumes of buffered water and the films, after being fixed in methanol, are immersed in it for approximately 4 min before being transferred to the Giemsa's stain. They should be allowed to stain in the latter solution for 7–10 min. Differentiation is carried out as described above.

Leishman's stain

Dry the film in the air and flood the slide with the stain. After 2 min add double the volume of water and stain the film for 5–7 min. Then wash it in a stream of buffered water until it has acquired a pinkish tinge (up to 2 min). After the back of the slide has been wiped clean, set it upright to dry.

Preparation of solutions of Romanowsky dyes

May-Grünwald's stain. Weigh out 0.3 g of the powdered dye and transfer to a conical flask of 200–250 ml capacity. Add 100 ml of methanol and warm the mixture to 50°C. Allow the flask to cool to c 20°C and shake several times during the day. After standing for 24 h, filter the solution. It is then ready for use, no ripening being required.

Jenner's stain. Prepare a 5 g/l solution in methanol in exactly the same way as descibed above for May-Grünwald's stain.

Giemsa's stain. Weigh 1 g of the powdered dye and transfer to a conical flask of 200–250 ml capacity. Add 100 ml of methanol and warm the mixture to 50°C; keep at this temperature for 15 min with occasional shaking, then filter the solution. It is then ready for use, but will improve on standing.

Buffered water. Make up 50 ml of 66 mmol/l Sörensen's phosphate buffer to 1 litre with water (see p. 539). An alternative buffer may be prepared from buffer tablets which are available commercially. Solutions of the required pH are obtained by dissolving the tablets in water.

Automatic staining machines are available which enable large batches of slides to be handled. As a rule, staining is of a uniform high standard, but, to achieve this, reliable stains are required and the cycle time has to be carefully controlled.

It is especially important to have consistent staining with automated differential leucocyte counters that are based on pattern recognition. These are programmed to identify cells stained by the specified method, but other stains, e.g. May-Grünwald-Giemsa can be used provided that the staining process is appropriately adapted.[26]

STANDARDIZED ROMANOWSKY STAIN

The following stain is based on the use of pure dyes, and is a slightly modified version of the method published by the International Committee for Standardization in Haematology (ICSH) as a tentative standard.[15] It has the advantage of being standardized; it thus ensures consistent results from batch to batch.

Reagents

Stock solution. Dissolve 750 mg of pure azure B, tetrafluoroborate or thiocynate, (CI 52010) in 75 ml of dimethylsulphoxide (DMSO) at c 37°C. Dissolve 100 mg of eosin Y acid (CI 45380) in 25 ml of DMSO at c 37°C. When both dyes are completely dissolved, add the eosin Y solution to the azure B solution and stir well. This stock solution should remain stable for several months if kept at room temperature in the dark. DMSO will crystallize below 18°C. If necessary, allow it to redissolve before use.

Fixative. Mix 1 volume of stock solution with 15 volumes of methanol.

Staining solution. Immediately before use dilute 1 volume of the stock solution with 15 volumes of HEPES buffer, pH 6.5–6.6 (p. 538). This solution is stable for about 8 h.[4]

Method

Fix films for 3 min in fixative. Leave the slides in the diluted stain for 10 min. Rinse in phosphate buffer solution pH 5.8 (p. 538) for 1 min. Then rinse with water, air dry and mount. For bone marrow films, fix for 5 min and leave the slides in the stain for 15–20 min.

The staining solution should be renewed at intervals when several batches of films are being stained in succession. Loss of staining power is usually due to precipitation of the eosin Y and this will result in the nuclei staining blue instead of purple.

RAPID STAINING METHOD

Field's method[11,12,13] was introduced to provide a quick method for staining thick films for malaria parasites (see below). With some modifications it can be used fairly satisfactorily for the rapid staining of thin films.

Stains

Stain A (polychromed methylene blue).

Methylene blue 1.3 g
Disodium hydrogen phosphate
   (Na_2HPO_4. $12H_2O$) 12.6 g
Potassium dihydrogen phosphate (KH_2PO_4)
   6.25 g
Water 500 ml.

Dissolve the methylene blue and the disodium hydrogen phosphate in 50 ml of water. Then boil the solution in a water-bath almost to dryness in order to 'polychrome' the dye. Add the potassium dihydrogen phosphate and 500 ml of freshly boiled water. After stirring to dissolve the stain, set aside the solution for 24 h before filtering. Filter again before use. The pH is 6.6–6.8.

Azure B may be added to the methylene blue in the proportion of 0.5 g of azure B to 0.8 g of methylene blue. In this case the dyes can be dissolved directly in the phosphate buffer solution.

Stain B (eosin).

Eosin 1.3 g
Disodium hydrogen phosphate
   (Na_2HPO_4. $12H_2O$) 12.6 g

Potassium dihydrogen phosphate (KH_2PO_4)
   6.25 g
Water 500 ml.

Dissolve the phosphates in warm freshly boiled water, and then add the dye. Filter the solution after standing for 24 h.

Method of staining

Fix the film for 10–15 seconds in methanol. Pour off the methanol and drop on the slide 12 drops of diluted Stain B (1 volume of stain to 4 volumes of water). Immediately, add 12 drops of Stain A. Agitate the slide to mix the stains. After 1 min rinse the slide in water, then differentiate the film for 5 s in phosphate buffer at pH 6.6, wash the slide in water and then place it on end to drain and dry. Two-stage stains of this type are also available commercially (e.g. Diff-Quick, Harleco).

Standardized stain

The standardized stain (p. 79) can also be used for rapid staining of individual slides.
   Fixative (p. 79).
   Staining solution. Immediately before use dilute 1 volume of stock stain (p. 79) with 25 volumes of HEPES buffer pH 6.5 (p. 538).

Method

Cover the slide with fixative solution. Decant after 3 min. Without rinsing, cover the slide with staining solution for 3–6 min. Rinse in water, air dry and mount.

MAKING AND STAINING THICK BLOOD FILMS

Thick blood films are widely used in the diagnosis of malaria. A relatively large volume of blood may be scrutinized in a short time and parasites seen even if present in very small numbers. Methods of staining have been reviewed by Field and Sandosham.[13] Field's method of staining[11,12] is quick and usually satisfactory, but the method is not practical for staining large numbers of films; for this purpose the Giemsa method is more suitable. Both methods will be described.

Making thick films

Make a thick film by placing a small drop of blood in the centre of a slide and spread it out with a corner of another slide to cover an area about four times its original area. The correct thickness for a satisfactory film will have been achieved if, with the slide placed on a piece of newspaper, small print is just visible.

Allow the film to dry thoroughly for at least 30 min at 37°C before attempting to stain it. Alternatively, leave the slide on the top of a microscope lamp, where the temperature is 50°–60°C, for *c* 7 min. Absolutely fresh films, although apparently dry, often wash off in the stain.

Field's method[11,12,13]

The preparation of the stains is described on p. 80. Dip the slide with the dried but otherwise unfixed film on it into Stain A for 1–2 s. Rinse it in buffered water (pH 6.8–7.0) until the stain ceases to flow from the film (5–10 s). Dip into Stain B for 1 s and then rinse rapidly in buffered water for 10 s. Shake off excess water and leave the slide upright to dry. Do not blot.

Giemsa's stain

Dry the films thoroughly as above, immerse the slides for 20–30 min in a staining jar containing Giemsa's stain freshly diluted with 15–20 volumes of buffered water. Gently wash the films with buffered water. Stand the slides upright to dry. Do not blot.

Sometimes the films are ov stain or spoilt by the envelope being visible. These defects either by soaking the stained and few minutes in 9 g/l NaCl or by in the first instance in Giemsa's ...uch has been diluted in buffered 9 g/l NaCl, pH 6.8, instead of water.[31]

Relative value of thick and thin films in the diagnosis of malaria

Thick films are extremely useful when parasites are scanty, but the identification of the parasites is less easy than in thin films. Mixed infections may be missed and there may be doubt as to the identification of any particular object. However, an experienced observer should be able to find and recognize with certainty parasites in badly stained thick films, whilst in a well stained film parasites should be easily recognized even by beginners. Five min spent in examining a thick film is equivalent to about 1 h spent in traversing a thin film. Rapid screening can also be carried out by fluorescent microscopy at low magnification, as malaria parasites fluoresce intensely with acridine orange.[17,32]

Study of thin films enables an exact diagnosis as to the species to be made. Seldom, if ever, should there be any doubt as to whether or not an object is a malarial parasite if the film has been well stained.

Thick films, if well stained, are also useful when there is severe leucopenia. It is possible to perform differential counts (or at least to estimate the proportion of polymorphonuclear to mononuclear cells) much more rapidly and more accurately than in thin films made from the same blood.

EXAMINATION OF BLOOD CELLS IN PLASMA

The examination of a drop of blood sealed between a slide and cover-glass is sometimes of considerable value.

The preparation may be examined in several ways; by ordinary illumination, by dark-ground or by Nomarski (interference) illumination. Chemically clean slides and cover-glasses (p. 540) must be used and the blood allowed to spread out thinly between them. If the glass surfaces are free from dust, the blood will spread out spontaneously, and pressure, which is undesirable, should not be necessary. The edges of the preparation may be sealed with a melted mixture of equal parts of petroleum jelly and paraffin wax.

cells

Rouleaux formation is usually seen in varying degrees in 'wet' preparations of whole blood and has to be distinguished from auto-agglutination.

Rouleaux formation versus auto-agglutination

The distinction between rouleaux formation and auto-agglutination is sometimes a matter of considerable difficulty, particularly when, as not infrequently happens, rouleaux formation is superimposed on agglutination. The rouleaux, too, may be notably irregular in haemolytic anaemias characterized by spherocytosis, while the clumping due to massive rouleaux formation of normal type may closely simulate true agglutination.

'Pseudo-agglutination' due to massive rouleaux formation may be distinguished from true agglutination in two ways:

1. By noting that the red cells, although forming parts of larger clumps, are mostly arranged side by side as in typical rouleaux.
2. By adding 3–4 volumes of 9 g/l NaCl to the preparation. Pseudo-agglutination due to massive rouleaux formation should either disperse completely or transform itself into typical rouleaux. The addition of saline to blood which has undergone true agglutination may cause the agglutination to break up somewhat, but a major degree of it is likely to persist and typical rouleaux will not be seen.

Anisocytosis and poikilocytosis can be recognized in 'wet' preparations of blood, but the tendency to crenation and the formation of rouleaux tend to make observations on shape changes rather difficult. Such changes can best be studied in a wet preparation after fixation. For this freshly collected heparinized or EDTA blood is diluted in 10 volumes of iso-osmotic phosphate buffer, pH 7.4 (see p. 538) and immediately fixed with an equal volume of 0.3% glutaraldehyde in iso-osmotic phosphate buffer, pH 7.4. After standing for 5 min one drop of this suspension is added to 4 drops of glycerol and 1–2 drops are placed on a glass slide which is then sealed.[37]

The sickling of red cells in 'wet' preparations of blood is described on p. 234.

Parasites

Wet preparations of blood are suitable for the detection of microfilariae and the spirochaetes of relapsing fever. The presence of small numbers of the latter is revealed by occasional slight agitation of groups of red cells.

Leucocytes

The motility of leucocytes can be readily studied in heparinised blood if the microscope stage can be warmed to c 37°C. Usually only the granulocytes show significant progressive movements.

Leucocytes can also be examined under dark-ground illumination or phase-contrast microscopy, either unstained or after supravital staining with neutral red or Janus green dyes, or with fluorescent dyes such as acridine orange or auramine.

It seems doubtful whether supravital staining or the use of the phase-contrast, interference or fluorescent microscope helps in the day-to-day problems of diagnostic haematology, and no attempt will be made to describe the appearances of cells viewed by these methods. Excellent photographs of cells viewed with the phase-contrast microscope were given by Bessis.[2] Cell shape and surface structures are particularly well demonstrated by means of Nomarski interference microscopy.[2,3] Kosenow[18] and Jackson[16] illustrated the appearances of leucocytes which had taken up fluorescent dyes.

SEPARATION AND CONCENTRATION OF BLOOD CELLS

A number of methods are available for the concentration of leucocytes or abnormal cells when they are present in only small numbers in the peripheral blood. Concentrates are most simply prepared from the buffy coat of centrifuged blood.

Making a buffy-coat preparation

Defibrinate venous blood in a flask and then centrifuge a sample for 15 min in a Wintrobe haematocrit tube at 3000 rpm (1500 *g*). Remove the supernatant serum carefully with a fine pipette, and with the same pipette deposit the platelet and underlying leucocyte layers on to one or two slides. Emulsify the buffy coat in a drop of the patient's serum and then spread the films. Allow them to dry in the air and then fix and stain in the usual way.

When leucocytes are scanty or if many slides are to be made, it is worth while centrifuging the blood twice; first, *c* 5 ml are centrifuged and a haematocrit tube is then filled from the upper cell layers of this sample.

As an alternative to centrifugation, the blood may be allowed to sediment, with the help of sedimentation-enhancing agents such as fibrinogen, dextran, gum acacia, Ficoll (Pharmacia) or methyl cellulose.[5,8] Bøyum's reagent[6,7] (methylcellulose and sodium metrizoate) is particularly suitable for obtaining leucocyte preparations with minimal red cell contamination. Sodium metrizoate can also be used to obtain platelet preparations (p. 57).

Most methods of separation affect to some extent subsequent staining properties, chemical reactions and the viability of the separated cells.

The buffy coat

It is well known that atypical or primitive blood cells circulate in small numbers in the peripheral blood in health. Thus, atypical mononuclear cells, metamyelocytes and megakaryocytes may be found. Even promyelocytes, blasts and nucleated red cells may occasionally be seen, but only in very small numbers. Efrati and Rozenszajn[9] described a method for the quantitative assessment of the numbers of atypical cells in normal blood and gave figures for the incidence of megakaryocyte fragments (e.g. mean 21.8 per 1 ml of blood) and of atypical mononuclears and metamyelocytes and myelocytes. In cord blood the incidence of all types of primitive cells is considerably greater.[10]

In disease, leaving the leukaemias and allied disorders out of consideration, abnormal cells may be seen in buffy-coat preparations in much larger numbers than in films of whole blood. For instance,

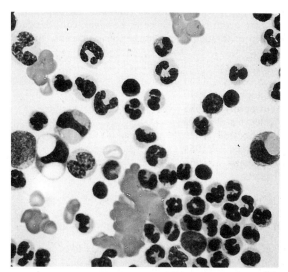

Fig. 7.4   Film of buffy coat. Erythrophagocytosis in autoimmune haemolytic anaemia.

megakaryocytes and immature cells of the granulocyte series are found in relatively large numbers in disseminated carcinoma.[28] Megaloblasts so found may help in the diagnosis of a megaloblastic anaemia. Erythrophagocytosis may be conspicuous in cases of anto-immune haemolytic anaemia (Fig. 7.4), and in systemic lupus erythematosus a few LE cells may be found—this is, however, not the best way to demonstrate LE cells.

It is rash to attempt an accurate differential count on buffy-coat concentrates as the different leucocytes tend to sediment under the influence of gravity at different rates and form layer upon layer. However, in leucopenia there is a fairly satisfactory correlation between the buffy-coat differential count and the standard method.[27]

SEPARATION OF SPECIFIC CELL POPULATIONS

Differences in density of cells can be used to separate individual cell types, using gradient solutions of selected specific gravity.[1,7,8] These include an erythrocyte-aggregating polysaccharide (Ficoll, Pharmacia), polyvinyl pyrrolidone (PVP)-coated silica gel (Percoll, Pharmacia), and sodium metrizoate (e.g. Isopaque, Nycomed). Mixtures of Ficoll with sodium metrizoate (Lymphoprep, Nycomed), sodium metrizoate with methyl cellulose and aqueous buffered solutions of sodium metrizoate (e.g. Nycodenz, Nycomed) will provide media of selected densities. In this way it is possible to separate cell populations with reasonable purity. The median values for the main haemopoietic cells are given below. There is, however, considerable overlap in the density ranges between adjacent types of cells.[7,8,25]

Erythrocytes	1100
Eosinophils	1090
Neutrophils	1085
Myelocytes	1075
Lymphocytes	1070
Monocytes	1064
Myeloblasts	1062
Platelets	1035

Isolation of tumour cells from blood

The methods used for demonstrating tumour cells in circulating blood involve elimination of the red cells and differential sedimentation or filtration of the leucocytes. Fleming and Stewart[14] assessed several methods critically and concluded that differential separation was to be preferred for routine use. They recommended a slight modification of the silicone flotation method of Seal.[30] Positive identifications are seldom made except in advanced cancer when the diagnosis is usually only too obvious.

REFERENCES

[1] ALI, F. M. K. (1986). *Separation of Human Blood and Bone Marrow Cells.* John Wright, Bristol.

[2] BESSIS, M. (1973). *Living Blood Cells and their Ultrastructure.* Springer-Verlag, Berlin.

[3] BESSIS, M. and THIÉRY, J. P. (1957). Les cellules du sang vues au microscope à interférences (Système Nomarski). *Revue d'Hématologie,* **12,** 518.

[4] BINS, M., HUIGES, W. and HALIE, M. R. (1985). Stability of azure B-eosin Y staining solutions. *British Journal of Haematology,* **59,** 73.

[5] BLOEMENDAL, H. (Ed.) (1977). *Cell Separation Methods.* Elsevier-North Holland, Amsterdam.

[6] BØYUM, A. (1964). Separation of white blood cells. *Nature* (London), **204,** 793.

[7] BØYUM, A. (1984). Separation of lymphocytes, granulocytes and monocytes from human blood using iodinated density gradient media. *Methods in Enzymology,* **108,** 88.

[8] CUTTS, J. H. (1970). *Cell separation: Methods in Hematology.* Academic Press, New York.

[9] EFRATI, P. and ROZENSZAJN, L. (1960). The morphology of buffy coat in normal human adults. *Blood,* **16,** 1012.

[10] EFRATI, P., ROZENSZAJN, L. and SHAPIRA, E. (1961). The morphology of buffy coat from cord blood of normal human newborns. *Blood,* **17,** 497.

[11] FIELD, J. W. (1940–41). The morphology of malarial parasites in thick blood films. Part IV. The identification of species and phase. *Transactions of the Royal Society of Tropical Medicine and Hygiene,* **34,** 405.

[12] FIELD, J. W. (1941–42). Further notes on a method of staining malarial parasites in thick films. *Transactions of the Royal Society of Tropical Medicine and Hygiene,* **35,** 35.

[13] FIELD, J. W. and SANDOSHAM, A. A. (1964). The Romanowsky stains—aqueous or methanolic? *Transactions of the Royal Society of Tropical Medicine and Hygiene,* **58,** 164.

[14] FLEMING, J. A. and STEWART, J. W. (1967). A critical and comparative study of methods of isolating tumour cells from the blood. *Journal of Clinical Pathology,* **20,** 145.

[15] International Committee for Standardization in Haematology (1984). ICSH reference method for staining of blood and bone marrow films by azure B and eosin Y (Romanowsky stain). *British Journal of Haematology,* **57,** 707.

[16] JACKSON, J. F. (1961). Supravital blood studies, using acridine orange fluorescence. *Blood,* **17,** 643.

[17] JAHANMEHR, S. A. H., HYDE. K., GEARY, C. G., CINKOTAL, K. I. and MACIVER, J. E. (1987). Simple technique for fluorescence staining of blood cells with acridine orange. *Journal of Clinical Pathology,* **40,** 926.

[18] KOSENOW, K. (1956). Lebende Blutzellen im Fluoreszenz und Phasenkontrastmikroscop. *Bibliotheca Haematologica (Basel),* Fasc 4.

[19] MARSHALL, P. N. (1977). Methylene blue-azure B-eosin as a substitute for May-Grünwald-Giemsa and Jenner-Giemsa stains. *Microscopica Acta,* **79,** 153.

[20] MARSHALL, P. N. (1978). Romanowsky-type stains in haematology. *Histochemical Journal,* **10,** 1.

[21] MARSHALL, P. N., BENTLEY, S. A. and LEWIS, S. M. (1975). An evaluation of some commercial Romanowsky stains. *Journal of Clinical Pathology,* **28,** 680.

[22] MARSHALL, P. N. BENTLEY, S. A. and LEWIS, S. M. (1975). A procedure for assaying commercial samples of eosin. *Stain Technology,* **50,** 107.

[23] MARSHALL, P. N. and GALBRAITH, W. (1984). On the nature of the purple coloration of leucocyte nuclei stained with Azure B-Eosin Y. *Histochemical Journal,* **16,** 793.

[24] NOURBAKHSH, M., ATWOOD, J. G., RACCIO, J. and SELIGSON, D. (1978). An evaluation of blood smears made by a new method using a spinner and diluted blood. *American Journal of Clinical Pathology,* **70,** 885.

[25] OLOFSSON, T., GÄRTNER, I. and OLSSON, I. (1980). Separation of human bone marrow cells in density gradients of polyvinyl pyrrolidone coated silica gel (Percoll). *Scandinavian Journal of Haematology,* **24,** 254.

[26] PENTILLA, I. M., MAHLAMÄKI, E., MONONEN, I. and KÄRKKÄINEN, P. (1985). Adaptation of the May-Grünwald-Giemsa staining method for automated differential counting of blood leucocytes by a Hematrak analyser. *Scandinavian Journal of Haematology,* **34,** 274.

[27] PFLIEGER, H., GAUS, W. and DIETRICH, M. (1979). Differential blood counts from cell concentrates. A comparison with routine differential blood counts. *Acta Haematologica,* **61,** 150.

[28] ROMSDAHL, M. M., McGREW, E. A., McGRATH, R. G. and VALAITIS, J. (1964). Hematopoietic nucleated cells in the peripheral venous blood of patients with carcinoma. *Cancer* (Philadelphia), **17,** 1400.

[29] SCHENK, E. A., CHURUKIAN, C., WILLIS, C. and STOTZ, E. (1983). Staining problems with eosin Y: a note from the Biological Stain Commission. *Stain Technology,* **58,** 377.

[30] SEAL, S. H. (1959). Silicone flotation: a simple quantitative method for the isolation of free-floating cancer cells from the blood. *Cancer* (Philadelphia), **12,** 590.

[31] SHUTE, P. and MARYON, M. (1960). *Laboratory Technique for the Study of Malaria*, p. 9. Churchill, London.

[32] SODEMAN, T. M. (1970). The use of fluorochromes for the detection of malaria parasites. *American Journal of Tropical Medicine*, **19,** 40.

[33] WENK, R. E. (1976). Comparison of five methods for preparing blood smears. *American Journal of Medical Technology*, **42,** 71.

[34] WITTEKIND, D., (1979). On the nature of Romanowsky dyes and the Romanowsky Giemsa effect. *Clinical and Laboratory Haematology*, **1,** 247.

[35] WITTEKIND, D. (1985). Standardization of dyes and stains for automatic cell pattern recognition. *Analytic and Quantitative Cytology*, **7,** 6.

[36] WITTEKIND, D. H., KRETSCHMER, V. and SOHMER, I. (1982). Azure B-eosin Y stain as the standard Romanowsky-Giemsa stain. *British Journal of Haematology*, **51,** 391.

[37] ZIPURSKY, A., BROWN, E., PALKO, J. and BROWN, E. J. (1983). The erythrocyte differential count in newborn infants. *American Journal of Pediatric Hematology and Oncology*, **5,** 45.

8. Blood-cell morphology in health and disease

Examination of a fixed and stained blood film is an essential part of a haematological investigation, and it cannot be emphasized too strongly that for the most to be made out of the examination the films must be well spread, well stained and examined systematically. Details of the recommended technique of examination are given below. It is clearly impossible to include in a book of this size and scope a comprehensive atlas of blood-cell morphology. However, the most important red cell abnormalities, as seen in fixed and stained films, are described and illustrated in black and white, and some notes on their significance and importance in diagnosis are added. Leucocyte and platelet abnormalities are described more briefly. Only a few illustration of leucocytes are included, as many photomicrographs, especially in colour, would be essential to illustrate adequately the morphological features of even a selection of the abnormalities met with in disorders which affect the leucocytes. These are better dealt with in a specialized atlas.

Unless otherwise stated the photomicrographs have been enlarged to $c \times 700$ to illustrate red cells and when appropriate to $c \times 1200$ to show fine detail.

TECHNIQUE OF EXAMINATION OF BLOOD FILMS

The point has already been made that blood films must be well spread, well fixed and well stained and examined systematically. It is useless to place a drop of immersion oil anywhere on the film and then to examine it straightaway using the high-power 2 mm objective.

First, the film should be covered with a cover-glass using a neutral medium as mountant. Next, it should be inspected under a low magnification (with a 16 mm objective) in order to get an idea of the quality of the preparation and of the number, distribution and staining of the leucocytes, and to find an area where the red cells are evenly distributed and are not distorted.

Having selected a suitable area, a 4 mm objective or 3.5 mm oil-immersion objective should then be used. A much better appreciation of variation in red cell size, shape and staining can be obtained with these objectives than with the 2 mm oil-immersion lens. The latter in combination with $\times 6$ eyepieces should be reserved for the final examination of unusual cells and for looking at fine details such as cytoplasmic granules, punctate basophilia, etc.

As the diagnosis of the type of anaemia or abnormality present usually depends upon a comprehension of the whole picture which the film presents, the red cells, leucocytes and platelets should all be systematically examined.

RED CELL MORPHOLOGY

In *health*, the red blood cells vary relatively little in size and shape (Fig. 8.1). In well spread dried films the great majority of cells have round smooth contours and have diameters within the comparatively narrow range (mean $\pm$ 2SD) of 6.0 to 8.5 μm. They stain quite deeply with the eosin component of Romanowsky dyes, particularly at the periphery of the cell in consequence of the cell's normal biconcavity. A small but variable proportion of cells in well made films (usually less than 10%) are definitely oval rather than round and a very small percentage may be contracted and have an irregular contour or appear to be cells which have lost part of their substance as the result of fragmentation. There may be a very occasional pyknocyte or schistocyte (see p. 95 and p. 98). According to Marsh the percentage of 'pyknocytes' and schistocytes in normal blood does not exceed 0.1% and the proportion is usually considerably less than this;[12] in normal full-term infants the proportion is higher, 0.3–1.9%,[12] and in premature infants still higher, up to 5.6%.[12]

Normal and pathological red cells are subject to considerable distortion in the spreading of a film and, as already referred to, it is imperative to scan films carefully to find an area where the red cells are least distorted before attempting to examine the cells in detail. Such an area can usually be found towards the tail of the film, although not actually at the tail. Rouleaux often form rapidly in blood after withdrawal from the body and may be conspicuous even in films made at a patient's bedside. They are particularly noticeable in the thicker parts of a film, which have dried more slowly. Ideally, red cells should be examined in an area in which little or no rouleaux have formed, but the film in the chosen area must not be so thin as to cause red cell distortion. The very different appearances of different areas of the same blood film are illustrated in Figs. 8.2–8.4. The area illustrated in Fig. 8.2. could clearly be the best for looking at red cells critically.

The advantages and disadvantages of examining red cells suspended in plasma have been referred to briefly in Chapter 7 (p. 81). By this means red cells can be seen in the absence of artefacts produced by drying, and abnormalities in size and shape can be better and more reliably appreciated than in films of blood dried on slides. However, the ease and rapidity with which dried films can be made, and their permanence, confer to the conventional dried-film technique an overwhelming advantage in routine studies.

In *disease*, abnormality in the red cell picture stems from four main causes:

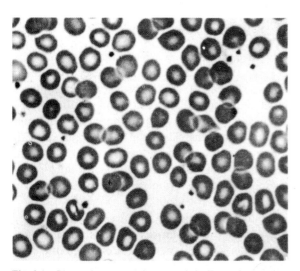

Fig. 8.1 Photomicrograph of a blood film. Film of a healthy adult.

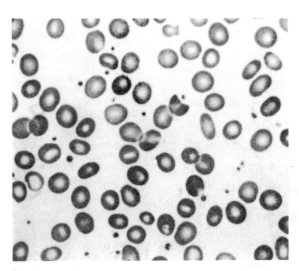

Fig. 8.2 Photomicrograph of a blood film. Ideal thickness for examination.

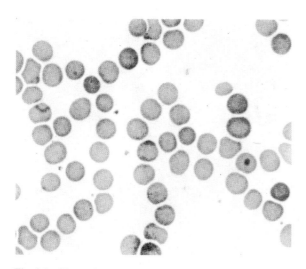

Fig. 8.3 Photomicrograph of a blood film. Film too thin. From same slide as Fig. 8.2.

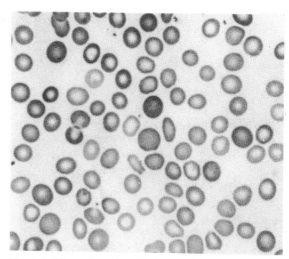

Fig. 8.5 Photomicrograph of a blood film. Shows a moderate degree of anisocytosis and anisochromasia.

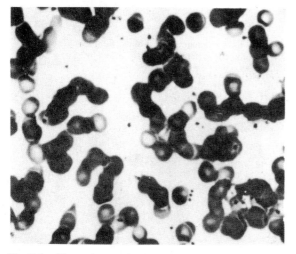

Fig. 8.4 Photomicrograph of a blood film. Film too thick. From same slide as Fig. 8.2.

1. Abnormal erythropoieses which may be effective or ineffective.
2. Inadequate haemoglobin formation.
3. Damage to, or changes affecting, the red cells after leaving the bone marrow.
4. Attempts by the bone marrow to compensate for anaemia by increased erythropoiesis.

These processes result, respectively, in the following abnormalities of the red cells:

1. Increased variation in size and shape (*anisocytosis* and *poikilocytosis*).
2. Reduced or unequal haemoglobin content (*hypochromasia* or *anisochromasia*).
3. *Spherocytosis*, irregular contraction or fragmentation *(schistocytosis)*.
4. Signs of immaturity (*polychromasia, punctate basophilia* and *erythroblastaemia*).

INCREASED VARIATION IN SIZE AND SHAPE

Anisocytosis (*ἄνισός*, unequal) **and poikilocytosis** (*πόικιλός*, varied)

These are non-specific features of almost any blood disorder. The terms imply more variation in size than is normally present (Fig. 8.5). Anisocytosis may be due to the presence of cells larger than normal (*macrocytosis*) or cells smaller than normal (*microcytosis*); frequently both macrocytes and microcytes are present together (Fig. 8.6).

Macrocytes

Classically found in megaloblastic anaemias (Fig. 8.7), but they are also present in aplastic anaemia (and other dyserythropoietic anaemias). In one rare form of congenital dyserythropoietic anaemia (Type III), some of the macrocytes may be exceptionally large (Fig. 8.8). Another cause of macrocytosis is chronic liver disease. In this condition the

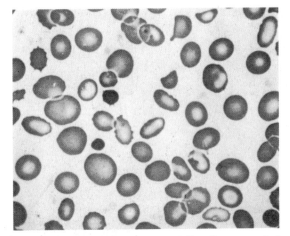

Fig. 8.6 Photomicrograph of a blood film. Shows a marked degree of anisocytosis caused by the presence of both microcytes and macrocytes.

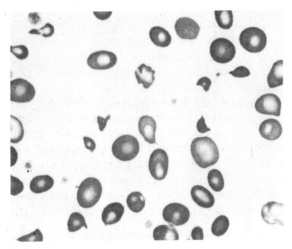

Fig. 8.7 Photomicrograph of a blood film. Shows macrocytes, poikilocytes and cell fragments (schistocytes), and extreme anisocytosis.

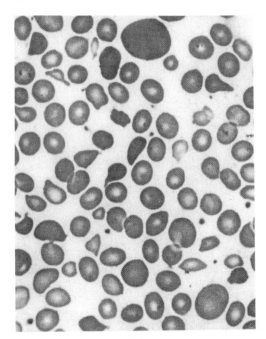

Fig. 8.8 Photomicrograph of a blood film. Congenital dyserythropoietic anaemia Type III. Shows unusually large macrocytes.

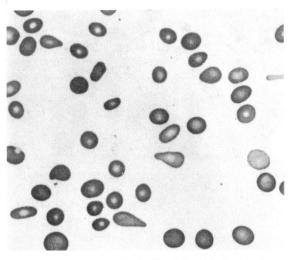

Fig. 8.9 Photomicrograph of a blood film. Myelosclerosis. Shows poikilocytosis and moderate anisocytosis.

red cells tend to be fairly uniform in size and shape. Macrocytosis also occurs whenever there is increased erythropoiesis, because of the presence of reticulocytes. These are identified by their staining slightly basophilically in routinely stained films, giving rise to polychromasia (p. 105) and their presence can be easily confirmed by special stains (e.g. New methylene blue).

Microcytes

Result from fragmentation of normally sized red cells (normocytes) or macrocytes, as occurs with many types of abnormal erythropoiesis, e.g. megaloblastic anaemia (Fig. 8.7). Microcytes are formed as such, or result from fragmentation, in iron-deficiency anaemia (Fig. 8.14) and thalassaemia (Fig. 8.17). In haemolytic anaemias, microcytes result from the process of spherocytosis or from fragmentation (Figs. 8.19–8.32).

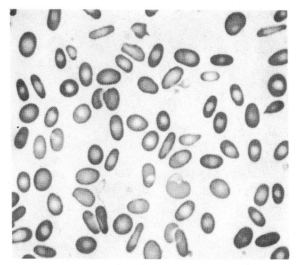

Fig. 8.10 Photomicrograph of a blood film. Myelosclerosis. Almost all the cells are elliptical or oval. (cf. Fig. 8.11).

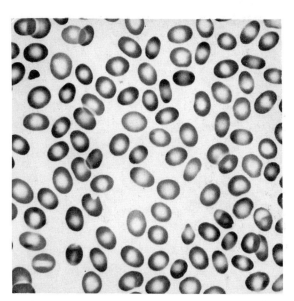

Fig. 8.12 Photomicrograph of a blood film. Hereditary ovalocytosis. The majority of the cells are oval; a few are moderately elliptic.

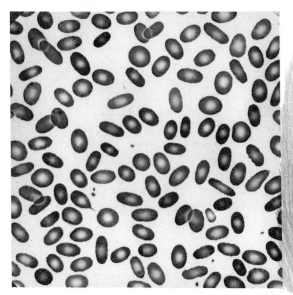

Fig. 8.11 Photomicrograph of a blood film. Hereditary elliptocytosis. Almost all the cells are elliptical.

Poikilocytes

Produced in many types of abnormal erythropoiesis, e.g. megaloblastic anaemia, iron-deficiency anaemia, thalassaemia, myelosclerosis; they also result from damage to circulating red cells, as in microangiopathic haemolytic anaemia. Poikilocytosis (and anisocytosis) are illustrated in Figs. 8.7, 8.9, 8.17 and 8.28–8.31.

Elliptocytosis

In disease many more oval or elliptical red cells may be found than in health. Elliptical or oval cells are thus frequent in megaloblastic anaemias and in hypochromic anaemias (Fig. 8.14); they may, too, be conspicuous in myelosclerosis (Fig. 8.10). The highest percentages are found in hereditary elliptocytosis (Fig. 8.11) and hereditary ovalocytosis (Fig. 8.12), in which 90% or more of the adult red cells may be markedly elliptical or oval, and in the South-East Asia variant of hereditary ovalocytosis (SEAHO) (Fig. 8.13). Remarkably, the reticulocytes in the above conditions are round in contour; that is to say, the cell assumes an abnormal shape only in the late stages of maturation.

INADEQUATE HAEMOGLOBIN FORMATION

Hypochromasia (υπόρ, under)

Present when red cells stain unusually palely. (In doubtful cases it is wise to compare the staining of the suspect film with that of a normal film stained at the same time.) There are two possible causes: a lowered haemoglobin concentration and abnormal

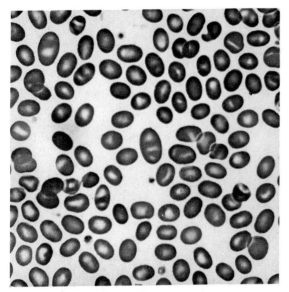

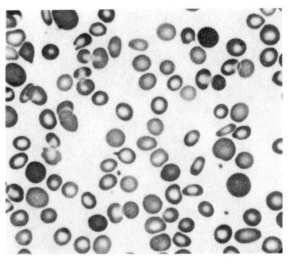

Fig. 8.15 Photomicrograph of a blood film. Iron-deficiency anaemia. Shows anisochromasia following treatment with iron. A macrocytic and orthochromic population contrasts with a microcytic and hypochromic one (dimorphic picture).

Fig. 8.13 Photomicrograph of a blood film. South-East Asian hereditary ovalocytosis. Some cells show a duplicated central pallor.

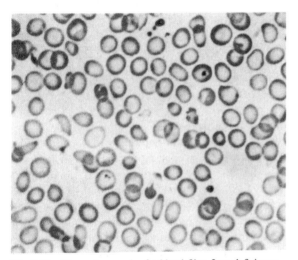

Fig. 8.14 Photomicrograph of a blood film. Iron-deficiency anaemia. Shows a marked degree of hypochromasia, microcytosis and anisocytosis, and a few poikilocytes and cell fragments.

thinness of the red cells. A lowered haemoglobin concentration results from impaired haemoglobin synthesis. This may stem from failure of haem synthesis—iron deficiency is a very common cause (Fig. 8.14), sideroblastic anaemia a rare cause—or failure of globin synthesis as in the thalassaemias (Fig. 8.17). Haemoglobin synthesis may also be

interfered with by infections. It cannot be too strongly stressed that a hypochromic blood picture does not necessarily mean iron deficiency, although this is the most common cause. In iron deficiency the red cells are characteristically hypochromic and microcytic, but the extent of these abnormalities depends on the severity; hypochromasia may be overlooked if the Hb exceeds 100 g/l. In homozygous β-thalassaemia, the abnormalities are greater than in iron deficiency at the same level of Hb (cf. Figs. 8.14 and 8.17), but it may not be possible to distinguish heterozygous β-thalassaemia from iron deficiency by the blood film (cf. Figs. 8.14 and 8.16).

Anisochromasia

Some but not all of the red cells stain palely. It can be seen in several circumstances; in a patient with an iron-deficiency anaemia responding to iron therapy (Fig. 8.15), after the transfusion of normal blood to a patient with a hypochromic anaemia, and in sideroblastic anaemia (Fig. 8.18). Such blood pictures have been referred to as 'dimorphic'.

Hyperchromasia (υπέρ, over)

Unusually deep staining of the red cells may be seen in macrocytosis when the red cell thickness is

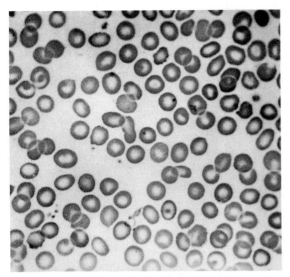

Fig. 8.16 Photomicrograph of a blood film. β-thalassaemia trait.

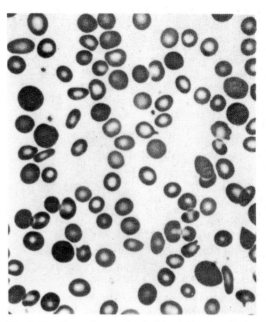

Fig. 8.18 Photomicrograph of a blood film. Acquired sideroblastic anaemia. Shows marked anisocytosis and anisochromasia (cf. Fig. 8.15).

DAMAGE TO RED CELLS AFTER FORMATION

Spherocytosis (σφαιρα, a sphere)

Spherocytes are cells which are more spheroidal (i.e. less disc-like) than normal red cells. Their diameter is less and their thickness greater than normal. Only in extreme instances are they almost spherical in shape. Spherocytes may result from genetic defects of the red cell membrane as in hereditary spherocytosis (Figs. 8.19 and 8.20), from the interaction between immunoglobulin- or complement-coated red cells and phagocytic cells, as in ABO haemolytic disease of the newborn (Fig. 8.21) and auto-immune haemolytic anaemia (Figs. 8.22 and 8.23) and from the action of bacterial toxins, e.g. *Cl. welchi* lecithinase (Fig. 8.24).

Spherocytes typically appear perfectly round in contour in stained films; they have to be carefully distinguished from 'spherical forms' or 'crenated spheres' (Fig. 8.52), the end-result of crenation or acanthocytosis (see p. 102). 'Spherical forms' can develop as artefacts especially in blood which has been allowed to stand before films are spread. In

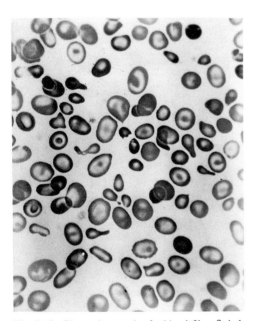

Fig. 8.17 Photomicrograph of a blood film. β-thalassaemia major. Shows hypochromasia, anisochromasia and anisocytosis, and numerous poikilocytes and cells fragments.

increased and the haemoglobin concentration normal, as in neonatal blood and megaloblastic anaemias, and in spherocytosis in which the red-cell thickness is greater than normal and the MCHC may be slightly increased (Figs. 8.19–8.25).

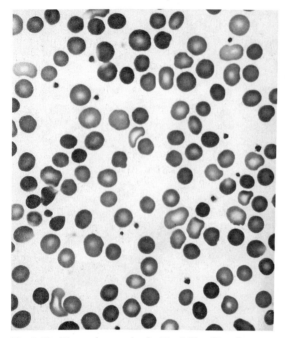

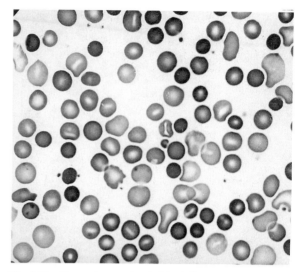

Fig. 8.21 Photomicrograph of a blood film. ABO haemolytic disease of the newborn. Spherocytosis is intense.

Fig. 8.19 Photomicrograph of a blood film. Hereditary spherocytosis. Shows a moderate degree of spherocytosis and anisocytosis. Note the round contour of the spherocytes.

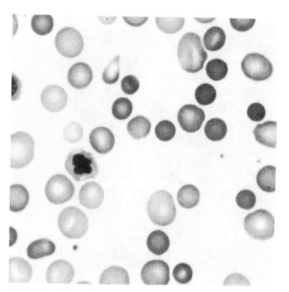

Fig. 8.22 Photomicrograph of a blood film. Auto-immune haemolytic anaemia. Shows a moderate degree of spherocytosis and anisocytosis.

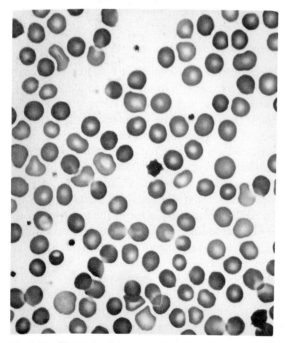

Fig. 8.20 Photomicrograph of a blood film. Hereditary spherocytosis. Clinically mild case; shows a lesser degree of spherocytosis than in Fig. 8.19.

rare and atypical hereditary haemolytic anaemias spherocytes may have an irregular contour (Fig. 8.25) and in haemolytic hereditary elliptocytosis any spherocytes present tend to be oval rather than round (Fig. 8.11). The blood film of a patient who has been transfused with stored blood may show a proportion of spherocytes.

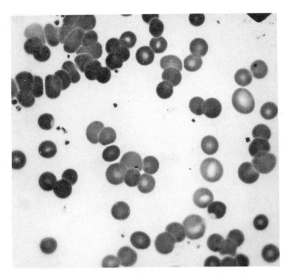

Fig. 8.23 Photomicrograph of a blood film. Auto-immune haemolytic anaemia, warm-antibody type. The majority of the cells are spherocytes.

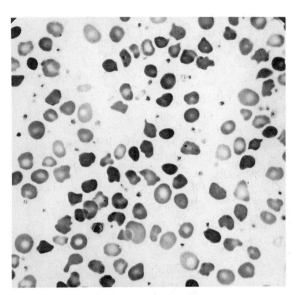

Fig. 8.25 Photomicrograph of a blood film. Atypical hereditary spherocytosis. Severe HS that did not respond fully to splenectomy. Densely-staining spherocytes with irregular contours are conspicuous in this film 23 years after splenectomy.

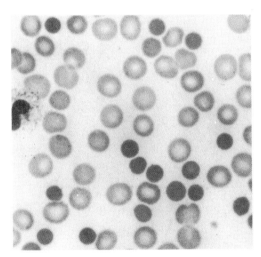

Fig. 8.24 Photomicrograph of a blood film. *Cl. welchi* septicaemia. Shows an extreme degree of spherocytosis; note the round contour of the spherocytes. A markedly dimorphic picture.

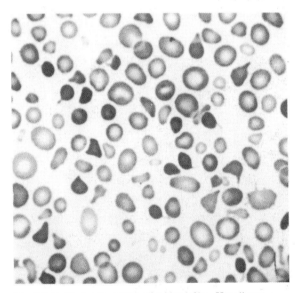

Fig. 8.26 Photomicrograph of a blood film. Hereditary haemolytic anaemia, a variant of hereditary ovalocytosis (pyropoikilocytosis). Shows spherocytes and numerous cell fragments, and a few ovalocytes.

Schistocytosis (fragmentation) (σχιστός, cleft)

Schistocytes, of varying shapes, are found in many blood diseases. Thus fragmentation occurs:

1. In certain genetically determined disorders, e.g. thalassaemias (Fig. 8.17) and hereditary elliptocytosis and allied disorders (Figs. 8.26 and 8.27).

2. In acquired disorders of red cell formation, e.g. megaloblastic (Fig. 8.7 and iron-deficiency anaemias (Fig. 8.14).

3. As the consequence of mechanical stresses, e.g. in the microangiopathic haemolytic anaemias

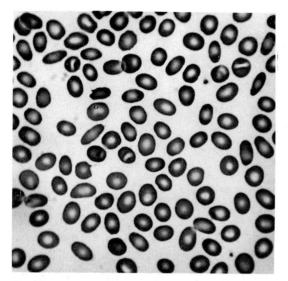

Fig. 8.27 Photomicrograph of a blood film. Mother of patient whose film is shown in Fig. 8.26. Many oval or elliptic cells are present.

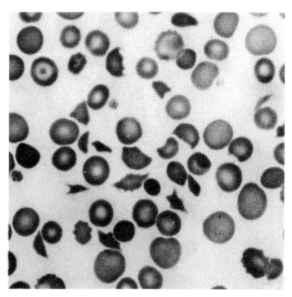

Fig. 8.29 Photomicrograph of a blood film. Microangiopathic haemolytic anaemia: haemolytic-uraemic syndrome. Shows spherocytosis and cell fragments and marked crenation.

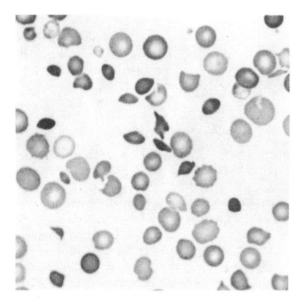

Fig. 8.28 Photomicrograph of a blood film. Microangiopathic haemolytic anaemia: renal cortical necrosis. Shows numerous small poikilocytes and cell fragments.

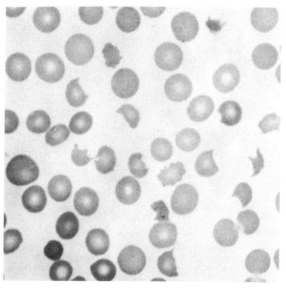

Fig. 8.30 Photomicrograph of a blood film. Microangiopathic haemolytic anaemia: disseminated carcinoma of breast. Shows many bizarre-shaped cells, crenation, cell fragments and 'burr' cells.

(Figs. 8.28–8.30) and cardiac haemolytic anaemias (Fig. 8.31).

4. As the result of direct thermal injury as in severe burns (Fig. 8.32).

In all conditions in which fragmentation is occurring three types of cell can be distinguished:

1. Small fragments of cells of varying shape, sometimes with sharp angles or spines (spurs), sometimes round in contour, usually staining deeply but occasionally palely as the result of loss of haemoglobin at the time of fragmentation.

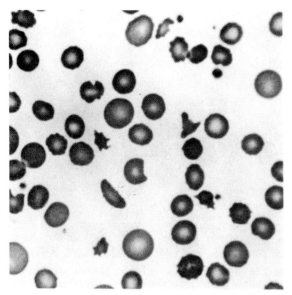

Fig. 8.31 Photomicrograph of a blood film. Post-cardiac surgery haemolytic anaemia. Shows numerous irregularly shaped cell fragments. Note presence of platelets.

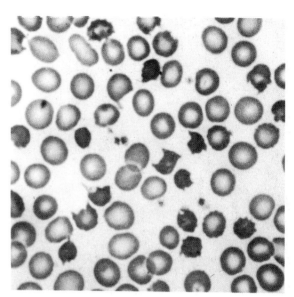

Fig. 8.33 Photomicrograph of a blood film. Haemolytic anaemia caused by an overdose of dapsone. Shows many irregularly-contracted cells.

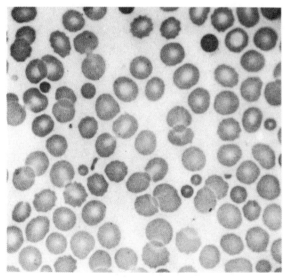

Fig. 8.32 Photomicrograph of a blood film. Severe burns. Shows many very small rounded cell fragments and a little crenation.

2. Larger cells, of irregular or mainly rounded contour from which fragments have been split off—these include 'helmet' cells.

3. Normal unfragmented adult red cells and reticulocytes.

Not infrequently, as for instance in the haemolytic-uraemic syndrome in children, the blood picture is made more bizarre by the superimposition of varying degrees of crenation (Fig. 8.29).

Irregularly-contracted red cells

Several types of irregularly-contracted cells can be distinguished. In drug- or chemical-induced haemolytic anaemias a proportion of the red cells are smaller than normal and unusually densely staining, i.e. they appear contracted, and their margins are slightly irregular and may be partly concave (Figs. 8.33, 8.34). These may be cells from which Heinz bodies have been extracted by the spleen. Similar cells may be seen in films of some unstable haemoglobinopathies before splenectomy, e.g. that due to the presence of Hb Köln (Fig. 8.35). Heinz bodies are not normally visible in Romanowsky-stained blood films but they may be seen in such films as pale purple-staining bodies in severe unstable haemoglobin haemolytic anaemias (Fig. 8.36). An extreme degree of irregular contraction is characteristic of severe favism, and it is typical to see that in some of the contracted cells the haemoglobin appears to have contracted away from the cell membrane (Fig. 8.37).

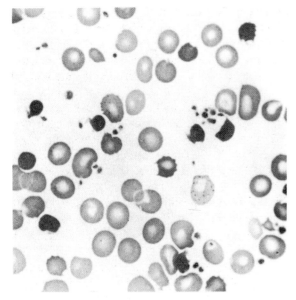

Fig. 8.34   Photomicrograph of a blood film. Haemolytic anaemia caused by an overdose of phenacetin. Shows many markedly and irregularly contracted cells; also punctate basophilia.

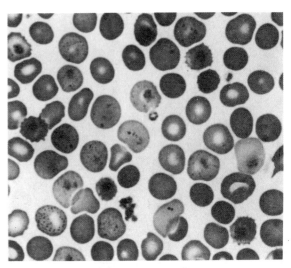

Fig. 8.36   Photomicrograph of a blood film. An unstable haemoglobin haemolytic anaemia (Hb Bristol). Shows contracted and crenated cells; also punctate basophilia and inclusions (Heinz bodies, punctate basophilia and Pappenheimer bodies).

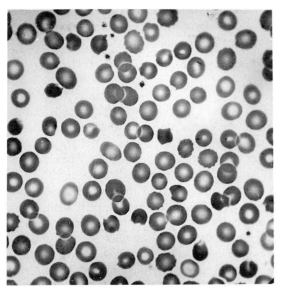

Fig. 8.35   Photomicrograph of a blood film. An unstable haemoglobin haemolytic anaemia (Hb Köln). Shows some moderately contracted cells with somewhat irregular contours.

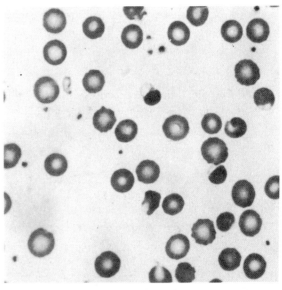

Fig. 8.37   Photomicrograph of a blood film. Favism. Shows numerous markedly contracted cells. Note condensation and contraction of haemoglobin from the cell membrane.

A type of irregular contraction of unknown origin has been described by the term pyknocytosis.[21] The pyknocytes closely resemble chemically damaged red cells. As already referred to (p. 88), a small number of pyknocytes may be found in the blood of infants in the first few weeks of life, especially in premature infants. The term 'infantile pyknocytosis' refers to a transient haemolytic anaemia of obscure origin affecting infants in which many pyknocytes are present (Fig. 8.38).[10,21]

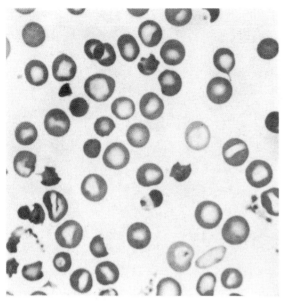

Fig. 8.38 Photomicrograph of a blood film. Infantile pyknocytosis. Shows irregularly-contracted cells similar to those seen in chemical- or drug-induced haemolytic anaemias (cf. Figs. 8.33 and 8.34).

MISCELLANEOUS CHANGES

Leptocytosis (λεπτός, thin)

This term has been used to describe unusually thin red cells, as in severe iron deficiency or thalassaemia in which the cells may stain as rings of haemoglobin with large almost unstained central areas (Figs. 8.14 and 8.17). The term *target cell* refers to a leptocyte in which there is a central round stained area in addition to a rim of haemoglobin. Target cells are thought to result from cells having a surface which is disproportionately large compared with their volume. They are seen in films in chronic liver diseases in which the cell membrane may be loaded with cholesterol (Fig. 8.39), and in varying numbers in iron-deficiency anaemia and in thalassaemia. They are often conspicuous in certain haemoglobinopathies, e.g. Hb CC disease (Fig. 8.40), Hb AC trait (Fig. 8.41), Hb SS disease (Figs. 8.42–8.44), Hb SC disease (Fig. 8.45), Hb S/β-thalassaemia, Hb EE disease (Fig. 8.46) and Hb AE trait (Fig. 8.47). In Hb-CC disease crystals of haemoglobin may be seen (Fig. 8.40).

Target cells appear after splenectomy (Fig. 8.48), even in otherwise healthy subjects whose spleens have been removed for traumatic rupture. Splenectomy in thalassaemia may result in an extreme degree of leptocytosis and target cell formation (Fig. 8.49).

Sickle cells (drepanocytes)

The varied film appearances in sickle-cell disease are illustrated in Figs. 8.42–8.44. In homozygous

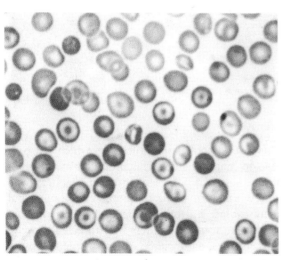

Fig. 8.39 Photomicrograph of a blood film. Chronic liver disease (obstructive jaundice). Shows many target cells.

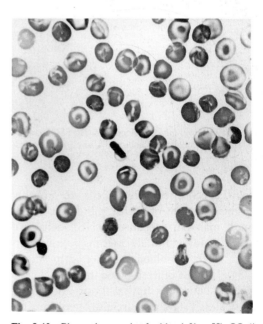

Fig. 8.40 Photomicrograph of a blood film. Hb CC disease. Shows many target cells and an extracellular crystal.

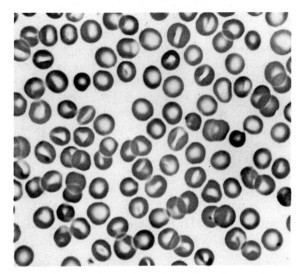

Fig. 8.41 Photomicrograph of a blood film. Hb AC trait.

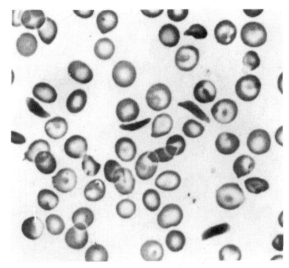

Fig. 8.43 Photomicrograph of a blood film. Hb SS disease. Shows sickled cells and target cells.

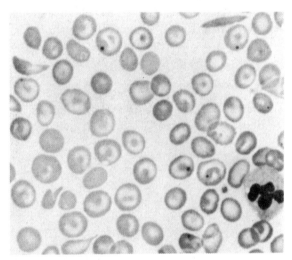

Fig. 8.42 Photomicrograph of a blood film. Hb SS disease. Shows a few sickled cells, target cells and Howell-Jolly bodies.

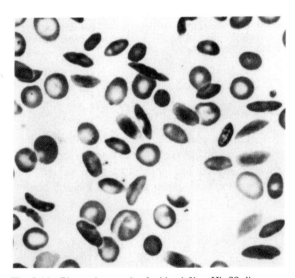

Fig. 8.44 Photomicrograph of a blood film. Hb SS disease. Shows numerous sickled cells.

sickle-cell (Hb-SS) disease sickle cells are probably always present in films of freshly withdrawn blood. Sometimes many irreversibly sickled cells are present (Fig. 8.44) and in all cases massive sickling takes place when the blood is subjected to anoxia (see p. 234). In films of fresh blood the sickled cells vary in shape between elliptical forms, oat-shaped cells and sickles. Target cells are also often a feature (Figs. 8.42, 8.43), and Howell-Jolly bodies are found when there is splenic atrophy.

Crenation

This term describes the process by which red cells develop many or numerous projections from their surface (Fig. 8.50). Described by Ponder[15] as disc-sphere transformation, crenation can result from many causes, e.g. by washing red cells free from plasma and suspending them in 9 g/l NaCl between glass surfaces, particularly at a raised pH, from the presence of traces of fatty substances on the slides on which films are made and from the presence of

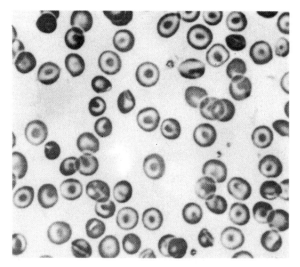

Fig. 8.45 Photomicrograph of a blood film. Hb SC disease. Shows numerous target cells.

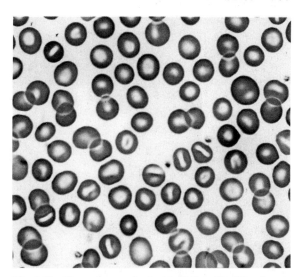

Fig. 8.47 Photomicrograph of a blood film. Hb AE trait.

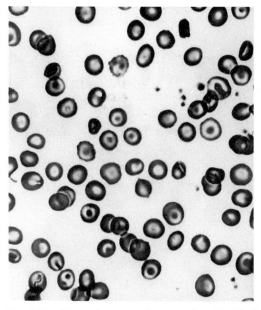

Fig. 8.46 Photomicrograph of a blood film. Hb EE disease.

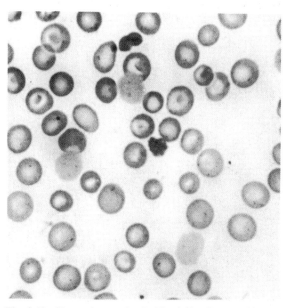

Fig. 8.48 Photomicrograph of a blood film. Pyruvate-kinase deficiency, after splenectomy. Shows macrocytosis, target cells and a markedly crenated cell.

traces of chemicals which at higher concentrations cause lysis. The end stages of crenation are the 'finely crenated sphere' and the 'spherical form' which closely resemble spherocytes (Fig. 8.51 and 8.52). The disc-sphere transformation may be reversible, e.g. that produced by washing cells free from plasma, and in this respect the contracted 'spherical form' (which has not lost surface) is quite distinct from the 'spherocyte' (which has lost surface), although they may closely resemble one another in stained films.

A few crenated cells may be seen in many blood films, even in those from healthy subjects. Crenation regularly develops if blood is allowed to stand overnight at 20°C before films are made (Fig. 8.50). It may be a marked feature, for obscure and probably diverse reasons, in freshly made blood films made from patients suffering from a variety of

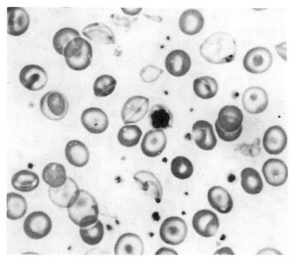

Fig. 8.49 Photomicrograph of a blood film. β-thalassaemia major, after splenectomy. Shows many target cells and cells grossly deficient in haemoglobin. The relatively deeply staining target cells are normal cells that have been transfused. Normoblasts are present.

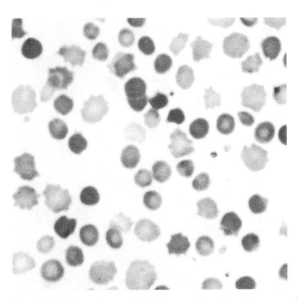

Fig. 8.51 Photomicrograph of a blood film. Hereditary spherocytosis. Shows marked spherocytosis and an unusual degree of crenation.

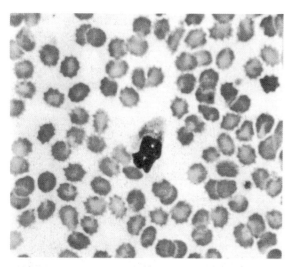

Fig. 8.50 Photomicrograph of a blood film. Normal blood after 18 h at *c* 20°C. Shows a marked degree of crenation.

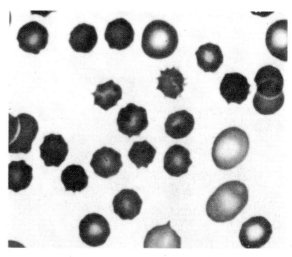

Fig. 8.52 Photomicrograph of a blood film. Acute renal failure following multiple bee stings. Shows crenation leading to finely-crenated spheres.

illnesses, e.g. uraemia. When crenation is superimposed on an underlying abnormality, the red cells may appear bizarre in the extreme (Fig. 8.29).

Acanthocytosis (ἄκανθα, spine)

The term acanthocytosis was introduced to describe an abnormality of the red cell associated with abnormal phospholipid metabolism (Fig. 8.53). [5,13,16] Characteristically, the majority of the red cells are coarsely crenated (acanthocytes), the size and number of the projections varying. Some cells have moderate numbers of small regularly arranged projections from their surface, others have smaller numbers of less regularly arranged finer projections with sharper points. Morphologically, rather similar

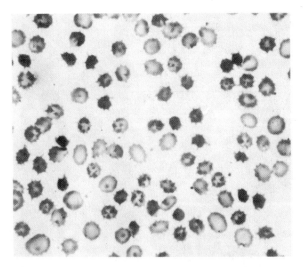

Fig. 8.53 Photomicrograph of a blood film. Acanthocytosis. Many cells show marked crenation and contraction.

lack of the Kell precursor (Kx) (Fig. 8.55).[24] The cause of these phenomena is obscure, but they may reflect an abnormality in the phospholipid content or phospholipid-cholesterol ratio of the red cell membrane.

In another type of ? acanthocytosis, a proportion of the red cells bear small numbers of irregularly situated but often quite large projections with rounded tips (Fig. 8.56). Although usually less than 10% of the cells are affected, the appearances are unusual and distinctive. The cause of the abnormality is obscure; the phenomenon is not rare and its relationship, if any, to other types of acanthocytosis has not been determined. The change has not yet been found to correlate with any particular type of illness, and in some instances the patients have not been anaemic.

irregularly crenated cells (? acanthocytes) are to be seen, often in quite large numbers, in blood films made from splenectomized patients (Fig. 8.54); and somewhat similar cells may be seen in the films of some patients with anaemia and chronic liver disease ('spur cell' anaemia).[18] Yet another cause of acanthocytosis is the McLeod phenotype, caused by

Burr Cells

The 'burr' abnormality was described by Schwartz and Motto[17] in the blood films of patients suffering from a variety of disorders, but particularly in uraemia. Burr cells are small cells or cell fragments bearing one or a few spines. They are probably

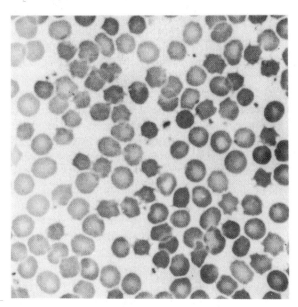

Fig. 8.54 Photomicrograph of a blood film. Hereditary spherocytosis. 11 yr after splenectomy. Shows spherocytosis and crenation (cf. Fig. 8.61 for other features of splenic atrophy or post-splenectomy blood films).

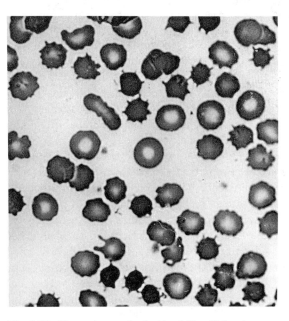

Fig. 8.55 Photomicrograph of a blood film. McLeod phenotype associated with chronic haemolytic anaemia. Acanthocytes are conspicuous.

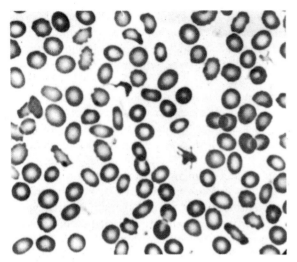

Fig. 8.56 Photomicrograph of a blood film. Acanthocytosis. Shows some bizarre-shaped acanthocytes and cell fragments; also moderate anisocytosis and ovalocytosis.

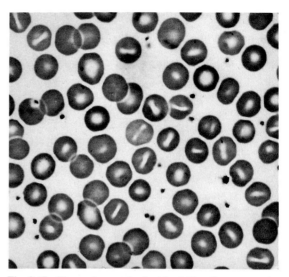

Fig. 8.57 Photomicrograph of a blood film. Stomatocytosis. Many of the cells have slit-like central unstained areas.

damaged or fragmented cells which have undergone a type of crenation (Figs. 8.29, 8.30).

Stomatocytosis (στόμα, mouth)

Stomatocytes are red cells in which the central biconcave area appears slit-like in dried films. The term was first used to describe the appearance of some of the cells in a rare type of haemolytic anaemia.[11] In 'wet' preparations, the stomatocyte is a cup-shaped red cell. The slit-like appearance of the cell's concavity, as seen in dried films, is thus to some extent an artefact. Subsequently, stomatocytes have been recognized in small numbers in many films and occasionally many or even the majority of the cells present are stomatocytes (Fig. 8.57). They have been reported in alcoholism.[3a] Their presence in large numbers has been attributed to a genetic factor, stomatocytes having been described as being particularly frequent in films of Australians of Mediterranean origin.[4,14] There is a suspicion that in some films the occurrence of stomatocytosis may be an artefact and it is known that the change can be produced by decreased pH and as the result of exposure to cationic detergent-like compounds and non-penetrating anions.[22] However, it remains to be explained, if the stomatocytic change is usually an artefact, why the change is seen in some films

and not in others and why some cells are affected and not others.

The advent of the scanning electron microscope, which has a resolving power at least ten times that of the light microscope, and has a great depth of focus and gives a three-dimensional view, has provided the stimulus and the means for a critical re-examination of red cell morphology.

Bessis and his co-workers have published excellent photographs of pathological red cells and have introduced a new nomenclature to describe what they have seen.[1,2,22] They use the term echinocyte (ἐχῖνοζ, sea urchin) for the crenated cell and clearly differentiate the echinocyte from the acanthocyte. (The normal cell is referred to as a discocyte.) Echinocytes (e.g. crenated red cells as produced by adding oleic acid or lysolecithin to plasma) have 10–30 evenly distributed spicules, while acanthocytes (in congenital abetalipoproteinaemia) have 5–10 spicules of varying length which are irregularly distributed. Acanthocytes can undergo crenation, the product being termed an 'acantho-echinocyte'. Bessis and his co-workers stressed how the echinocytic and stomatocytic change can be superimposed on other pathological forms. Thus, they illustrated 'sickle-stomatocytes' and 'stomato-acanthocytes'. They also discussed the difficult question of the in-vivo significance of crenation (echinocytic change) observed in vitro. It seems that neither echinocytosis nor acanthocytosis is necessarily associated with increased haemolysis. It cannot be concluded, either, that crenation is occurring in vivo, when the phenomenon is markedly evident in films made on glass slides. To ensure that cells are crenated in any blood sample as it is withdrawn, Brecher and Bessis recommended that the blood be examined immediately between plastic instead of glass cover-slips or slides, to avoid the known 'echinocytogenic' effect of glass surfaces, probably due to alkalinity.[2] Recently, marked echinocytosis has been reported in premature infants following exchange transfusion or transfusion of normal red cells.[6]

CHANGES ASSOCIATED WITH COMPENSATORY ERYTHROPOIESIS

Polychromasia ($\pi o\lambda \acute{v}\varsigma$, many)

This term suggests that the red cells are being stained many colours. In practice, it denotes that some of the red cells stain shades of bluish grey—these are the reticulocytes. Cells staining shades of blue, 'blue polychromasia', are unusually young reticulocytes. 'Blue polychromasia' is most often seen when there is extramedullary erythropoiesis, as, for instance, in myelosclerosis or carcinomatosis.

Punctate basophilia

'Classical' punctate basophilia is found, as a variant of diffuse basophilia, in many blood diseases, as well as in infections and intoxications such as lead poisoning. The granules of diffuse punctate basophilia are uniformly distributed in the cell (Figs. 8.58 and 8.59); they do not give a positive Perls's reaction for ionized iron in contrast to Pappenheimer bodies (see below) which do.

Erythroblastaemia

Erythroblasts may be found in the blood films of almost any patient with a severe anaemia; they are, however, very unusual in aplastic anaemia. They are more common in children than in adults and large numbers are a very characteristic finding in haemolytic disease of the newborn. Small numbers

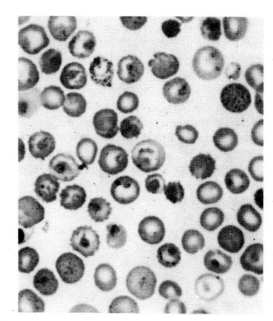

Fig. 8.58 Photomicrograph of a blood film. Unstable haemoglobinopathy (Hb Hammersmith); after splenectomy. There is a remarkable degree of punctate basophilia. Also shows Pappenheimer bodies and circular bodies corresponding to Heinz bodies.

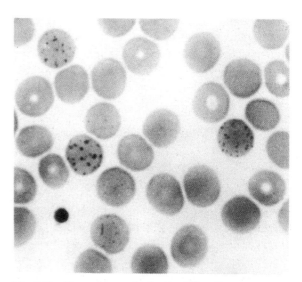

Fig. 8.59 Photomicrograph of a blood film. Punctate basophilia. Pyrimidine-5′-nucleotidase deficiency.

can be found in the cord blood of normal infants at birth and quite large numbers in that of premature infants.

When large numbers of erythroblasts are present, many of them are probably derived from extramedullary foci of erythropoiesis, e.g. in the liver and spleen. This seems likely to be true, for instance, in haemolytic disease of the newborn, leukaemia, myelosclerosis and carcinomatosis. In carcinomatosis the number of erythroblasts is often disproportionately high for the degree of anaemia, and a few immature granulocytes are usually present also (so-called leuco-erythroblastic anaemia).

Erythroblasts can usually be found in the peripheral blood after splenectomy and in the presence of

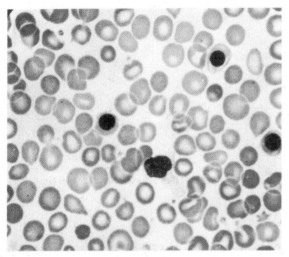

Fig. 8.60 Photomicrograph of a blood film. Myelosclerosis, after splenectomy. Shows three normoblasts and moderate anisocytosis and poikilocytosis; also a target cell and a cell fragment.

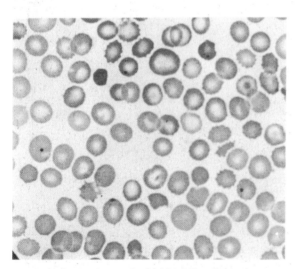

Fig. 8.61 Photomicrograph of a blood film. Steatorrhoea. Shows Howell-Jolly bodies, target cells and crenation, all consequences of splenic atrophy.

extramedullary erythropoiesis many may be present (Fig. 8.60). Large numbers are frequently seen in the blood films of Hb-SS disease patients in painful crises. Small numbers of erythroblasts are not uncommon in blood from patients suffering from cyanotic heart failure or septicaemias.

Howell-Jolly bodies

These are nuclear remnants and (usually singly) may be seen in a small percentage of red cells in pernicious anaemia. Cells containing them are regularly present after splenectomy and where there has been marked splenic atrophy. Usually only a few such cells are present, but they may be numerous in cases of steatorrhoea in which there is splenic atrophy and sometimes deficiency of folate (Fig. 8.61).

EFFECT OF SPLENECTOMY

Some of the changes have already been mentioned, namely, the occurrence of target cells, 'acanthocytes' (Figs. 8.48 and 8.54) and Howell-Jolly bodies. Pappenheimer bodies are also regularly found. These are granules, staining black with Romanowsky dyes; in size they are usually minute and usually are only present singly or in pairs. Not infrequently they may be found in the majority of circulating red cells (Fig. 8.62). They correspond to

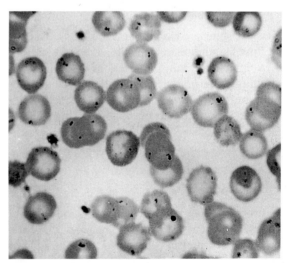

Fig. 8.62 Photomicrograph of a blood film. Pyruvate-kinase deficiency, after splenectomy. Shows many macrocytes, the majority containing Pappenheimer bodies; numerous platelets.

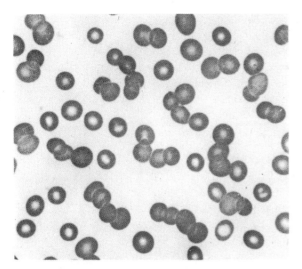

Fig. 8.63 Photomicrograph of a blood film. Shows rouleaux in a normal blood film (cf. Fig. 8.64).

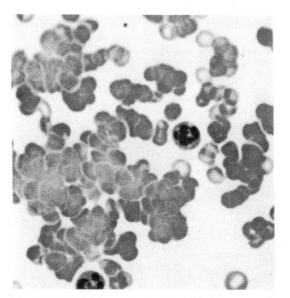

Fig. 8.64 Photomicrograph of a blood film. Shows massive auto-agglutination (cf. Fig. 8.63).

the siderotic granules of siderocytes and are never distributed uniformly throughout the cells as is classical punctate basophilia.

Rouleaux and auto-agglutination

The differences between rouleaux and auto-agglutination are described on p. 82 and there is usually no difficulty in determining which is which in stained films (cf. Figs. 8.63 and 8.64). However, in myelomatosis and in other conditions in which there is intense rouleaux formation the rouleaux may simulate auto-agglutination. Even so, if the film, apparently showing auto-agglutination, is carefully scanned, an area in which rouleaux can be clearly seen will almost certainly be found. Rouleaux occur to some extent in all films, and their presence adds point, as has been mentioned, to the importance of careful selection of the area of film to be examined.

SCANNING ELECTRON MICROSCOPY

The morphology of red cells, as illustrated in this chapter, may be distorted by spreading and drying films in the traditional way. A more authentic portrayal of red cell shape in vivo can be seen by scanning electron microscopy (Figs. 8.65–8.70). However, this specialized procedure is not practical as a routine.

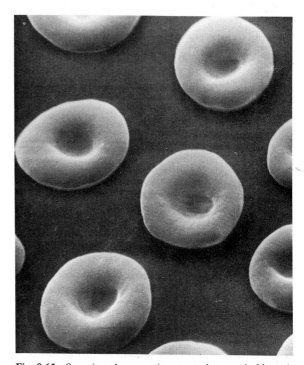

Fig. 8.65 Scanning electron microscope photograph. Normal red cells.

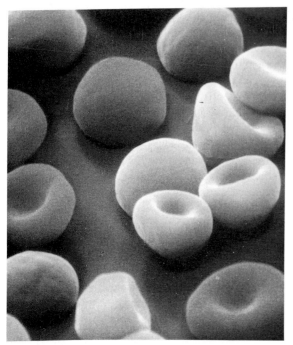

Fig. 8.66   Scanning electron microscope photograph. Hereditary spherocytosis. Note the round shape of spherocytes. Compare with Fig. 8.65; also see blood film appearances as shown in Fig. 8.19.

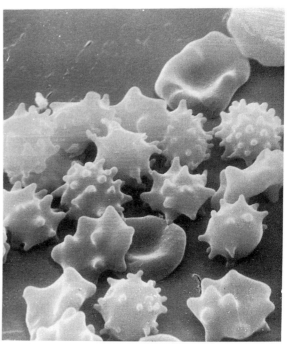

Fig. 8.68   Scanning electron microscope photograph. Acanthocytosis. Some cells also show crenation and contraction. Compare with Fig. 8.67; also see blood film appearances as shown in Fig. 8.53.

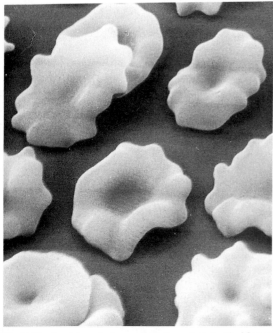

Fig. 8.67   Scanning electron microscope photograph. Normal blood after standing overnight. Note crenation.

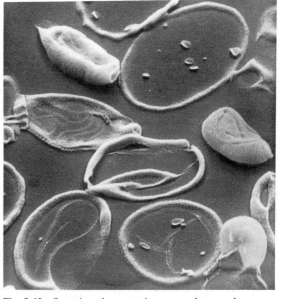

Fig. 8.69   Scanning electron microscope photograph. β-thalassaemia major, post-splenectomy. Shows cells grossly deficient in haemoglobin; there are also contracted cells and poikilocytes. In the hypochromic cells inclusions are seen, corresponding to Pappenheimer bodies.

MORPHOLOGY OF LEUCOCYTES

To describe adequately the normal morphology of the various types of leucocytes and the abnormalities met with in disease would require a lengthy text and many photomicrographs in colour. However, the recognition of leucocyte abnormalities and the appreciation of their significance are of great practical importance. Accordingly, the relatively common abnormalities will be referred to; less common abnormalities will not be described and for these readers are referred to an atlas where they are usually well illustrated.

NEUTROPHIL POLYMORPHONUCLEARS

The following are abnormalities to look for:

Granules

'Heavy', dark-staining, 'toxic' granules are characteristic of bacterial infections (Fig. 8.71), although with some Romanowsky stains normal granules are also darkly stained. Large reddish-staining granules are frequently seen in aplastic anaemia and also sometimes in myelosclerosis. In myeloid leukaemias, on the other hand, the granules often stain poorly and the recognition of 'agranular' neutrophils may help in diagnosis; sometimes only a proportion of the neutrophils is affected, and the cells with easily visible granules can then act as a standard against which the cells with poorly visible granules can be compared.

Large, dark-staining granules are a characteristic of the Alder abnormality (a genetic disorder). In this condition coarse azure granules may also be seen in lymphocytes and monocytes.

Vacuoles

These are not normally visible in the neutrophils in stained films of fresh blood viewed with the optical microscope. In bacterial infections they are, however, not uncommon, and they develop, along with other changes, in normal blood allowed to stand in vitro after withdrawal (see p. 4)

Döhle bodies

These are small round or oval patches up to 2–3 μm in size, usually in the periphery of the cytoplasm of neutrophils, which stain blue-grey with Romanowsky dyes. They are mostly seen in bacterial infections, and are not characteristic of

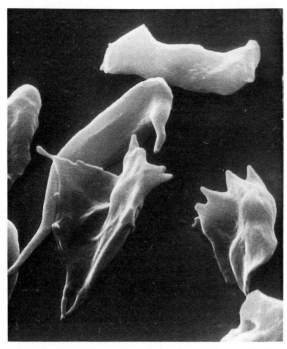

Fig. 8.70 Scanning electron microscope photograph. Hb SS disease. Shows sickled cells.

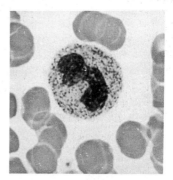

Fig. 8.71 Photomicrograph of a blood film. Severe infection. Shows neutrophil left shift and toxic granulation.

leukaemia. A similar structure occurs as a benign inherited anomaly, known as May-Hegglin anomaly.

Nuclei

Segmentation of the nucleus of neutrophils is a normal phenomenon which, it has been suggested, enables the cells to pass through small spaces in the course of leaving blood vessels more easily than they would be able to if their nucleus was in one large piece. A shift to the 'left' or 'right' of the segmentation of the nuclei of neutrophils in the peripheral blood has been noticed and studied for years and has been recorded quantitatively by various, mostly obsolete, indices. There is no doubt, however, but that recognition of a right shift can help in the diagnosis of a megaloblastic anaemia (Fig. 8.72). Uraemia is another cause of a right shift, and atypical hypersegmented neutrophils may sometimes be seen in leukaemia.

A shift to the left, with band and stab forms (Fig. 8.73) and perhaps a few myelocytes too is a common consequence of severe sepsis and is usually accompanied by 'toxic' granulation etc. More pronounced left shifts, e.g. with promyelocytes and a few blasts present, are more likely to denote leucoerythroblastic anaemia or leukaemia but such a picture can be seen in severe infections.

Abnormalities in nuclear shape, e.g. unusually elongated or bizarre-shaped lobes, are not uncommon in some leukaemias, and, at the opposite end

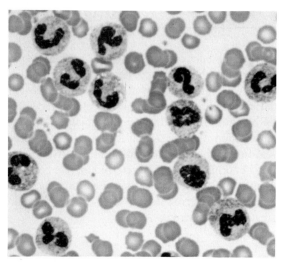

Fig. 8.73 Photomicrograph of a blood film. Infection. Shows left shift of neutrophils.

of the scale, Pelger-like nuclei may be encountered, too, in myeloid leukaemias. In such instances the nuclei are unusually densely staining and have rounded contours and there is a sharp distinction between acidophilic and basophilic chromatin. The majority of the cells will be unsegmented 'meta-myelocytes', and at the most the nucleus consists of two regular almost equal lobes. In some cases Pelger 'myelocytes' with small round nuclei may be present. Pelger cells, as seen in leukaemia, are morphologically very similar to the neutrophils of the benign inherited Pelger-Huet anomaly (Fig. 8.74).

Occasionally, unusually large neutrophils may be seen in films. Such cells often appear to contain about twice the normal amount of nuclear material; they are in fact probably tetraploid. Such cells are most frequent in leukaemia but small numbers may be found in a variety of benign conditions.

Small numbers of dead or dying polymorphonuclears may be found in blood films; they are to be seen in their largest numbers in severe sepsis or in blood which has been allowed to stand 18 h or more in vitro. The nuclei of such cells are densely staining, small and rounded off (see also p. 4).

An interesting phenomenon which has occasionally been observed is the adhesion of red cells to neutrophils (Fig. 8.75). At first sight, an immune

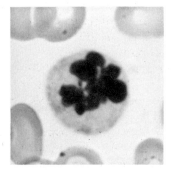

Fig. 8.72 Photomicrograph of a blood film. Pernicious anaemia. Shows a hypersegmented neutrophil.

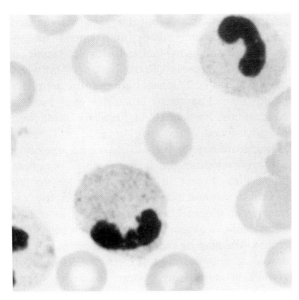

Fig. 8.74 Photomicrograph of a blood film. Pelger-Huet anomaly. Shows two 'Pelger' cells.

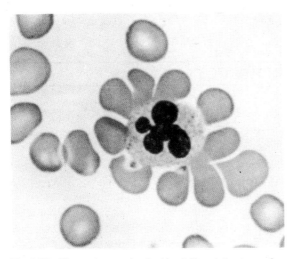

Fig. 8.75 Photomicrograph of a blood film. Adherence of red cells (and two platelets) to a neutrophil. Patient had acquired haemolytic anaemia, with negative direct antiglobulin test.

adherence phenomenon, the significance and mechanism of the occurrence is unknown.

LYMPHOCYTES

Normally, the majority of circulating lymphocytes are small cells with only a scanty rim of cytoplasm in which there are often a few scattered azurophil granules. About 10% of the lymphocytes in circulation are much larger cells with more abundant cytoplasm and a reduced nuclear:cytoplasmic ratio; the cytoplasm of these large lymphocytes frequently contains azurophil granules. In both small and large lymphocytes, the nucleus is relatively homogeneous. Prolymphocytes, as seen in prolymphocytic leukaemia, are relatively large cells in which several nucleoli are easily visible. Lymphoblasts, with relatively small amounts of cytoplasm, larger nuclei, less dense nuclear pattern and well-defined nucleoli, probably do not circulate in health, except possibly in small numbers in the blood of infants. In acute lymphoblastic leukaemia they may be the predominant cell type. Sometimes, the cells, although clearly blasts, are quite small (microblasts) and do not exceed mature lymphocytes in size.

In certain lymphomas, lymphocytes with clefts in their nuclei, giving rise sometimes to overlapping lobes, are not uncommon; usually these are small cells with little cytoplasm. (Lymphocytes with well marked lobes are likely to be artefacts developing in blood allowed to stand in vitro [see p. 4]). Plasmacytoid lymphocytes, with deeply basophilic cytoplasm, are not uncommon in infections, particularly in virus infections, e.g. in rubella, measles, influenza, hepatitis and cytomegalovirus infection; but cells identical with, or very closely similar to, marrow plasma cells are rare in the peripheral blood and their presence (if more than very occasional) may indicate underlying myelomatosis.

The lymphocytosis of infectious mononucleosis is rather characteristic. More abnormal cells are likely to be present than in other virus infections and the cells themselves, 'reactive lymphocytes', although rather variable in size and appearance, tend to be large and to have abundant, deeply basophilic cytoplasm.

Lymphocytes predominate in the blood films of infants and small children, and in such films large lymphocytes and reactive lymphocytes tend to be conspicuous.

A variety of lymphocyte types may be seen in chronic lymphocytic leukaemia (CLL). Usually the picture is relatively monotonous, the cells being superficially very similar and usually lacking the few azurophilic granules normally found in the cytoplasm of mature lymphocytes. On close scrutiny of CLL films a small proportion of larger, younger cells with one or two visible nucleoli may be seen as well as a few lymphoblasts with multiple nucleoli. In lymphomas, pathological cells, if present, vary in type and if there is lymphocytosis the blood lymphocyte picture is usually far less uniform than in CLL.

MONOCYTES

Monocytes are normally easy to distinguish from lymphocytes and neutrophil polymorphonuclears. In disease, however, this distinction may be less easy. Thus, it is sometimes difficult to separate clearly monocytes from lymphocytes in infectious mononucleosis and monocytes from neutrophils in sepsis and in some types of myeloid leukaemia. Leukaemic monocytes or 'monocytoid cells' tend to differ in subtle ways from their normal counterparts, but the diagnosis of leukaemia, fortunately, does not depend on the recognition of individual cells as leukaemic or normal, respectively. Rarely, monocytes which have acted as macrophages are seen in peripheral blood films. The classic circumstance is bacterial endocarditis, particularly if films are made from ear-prick blood.

Immature eosinophils, i.e. eosinophil myelocytes and promyelocytes, are seldom seen in peripheral blood films except in chronic granulocytic leukaemia. In non-leukaemic eosinophilias the vast majority of, if not all, the eosinophils are mature. In eosinophilic leukaemia, a varying number of the eosinophils may be partially or almost completely devoid of granules. The presence of such poorly granulated cells points toward leukaemia as the diagnosis but should not be taken as being absolute proof.

PLATELET MORPHOLOGY

It is possible, using EDTA as anticoagulant, to assess platelet numbers fairly accurately simply by inspection of stained films. In films of native blood, platelets clump and this assessment cannot be done with any pretence of accuracy—except in rare conditions such as Glanzmann's disease in which the platelets fail to clump. Platelets normally vary considerably in size and a small proportion of large platelets, up to 3—5 μm diameter, may be seen in health. More are present when platelets are being actively regenerated as after haemorrhage or in thrombocytopenic purpura. A higher proportion still of large platelets, and 'giant' platelets up to 7 μm in diameter, may be conspicuous features of thrombocythaemia or myelosclerosis (megakaryocytic myelosis) (Fig. 8.76) and in this group of disorders, megakaryocyte nuclei or fragments of nuclei may sometimes be found in peripheral blood films.

Although EDTA is a very convenient anticoagulant to use for routine platelet counts, occasionally

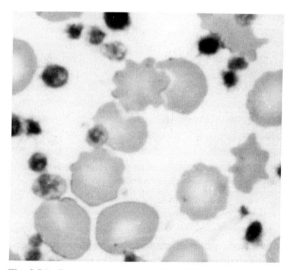

Fig. 8.76 Photomicrograph of a blood film. Essential thrombocythaemia. Shows platelet anisocytosis with some 'giant' platelets.

the presence of EDTA causes the platelets to clump and the count to be falsely low.[8] The mechanism of this phenomenon and its incidence is unknown. EDTA also affects the staining of platelets, some of which swell and stain relatively palely if EDTA-containing blood is allowed to stand at c 20°C for 2 h or more. Exceptionally, failure to stain develops much more rapidly.[20]

An interesting phenomenon which is occasionally seen is the adhesion of platelets to neutrophils (Fig. 8.77).[3,7,19] Its significance is uncertain for it has been observed in blood withdrawn from apparently healthy individuals. On the other hand, it has been seen in patients in whom platelet auto-antibodies have been demonstrated[23] and in other types of thrombocytopenia.[9] It is not seen in films made from uncoagulated blood.

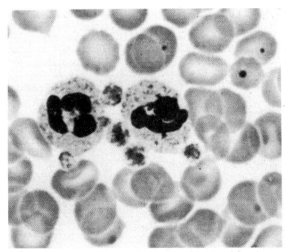

Fig. 8.77 Photomicrograph of a blood film. Idiopathic thrombocytopenic purpura after splenectomy. Shows adhesion of platelets to neutrophils; also Howell-Jolly bodies.

REFERENCES

[1] BESSIS, M. (1972). Red cell shapes. An illustrated classification and its rationale. *Nouvelle Revue Francaise d'Hématologie*, **12,** 721.

[2] BRECHER, G. and BESSIS, M. (1972). Present status of spiculated red cells and their relationship to the discocyte-echinocyte transformation: a critical review. *Blood*, **40,** 333.

[3] CROME, P. E. and BARKHAN, P. (1963). Platelet adherence to polymorphs. *British Medical Journal*, ii, 871.

[3a] DOUGLASS, C. and TWOMEY, J. (1970). Transient stomatocytosis with hemolysis: a previously unrecognized complication of alcoholism. *Annals of Internal Medicine*, **72,** 159.

[4] DUCROU, W. and KIMBER, R. J. (1969). Stomatocytes, haemolytic anaemia and abdominal pain in Mediterranean migrants: some examples of a new syndrome? *Medical Journal of Australia*, ii, 1087.

[5] ESTES, J. W., MORLEY, T. J., LEVINE, I. M. and EMMERSON, C. P. (1967). A new hereditary acanthocytosis syndrome. *American Journal of Medicine*, **42,** 868.

[6] FEO, C. J., TCHERNIA, G., SUBTIL, E. and LEBLOND, P. F. (1978). Observation of echinocytosis in eight patients: a phase contrast and SEM study. *British Journal of Haematology*, **40,** 519.

[7] FIELD, E. J. and MACLEOD, I. (1963). Platelet adherence to polymorphs. *British Medical Journal*, ii, 388.

[8] GOWLAND, E., KAY, H. E. M., SPILLMAN, J. C. and WILLIAMSON, J. R. (1969). Agglutination of platelets by a serum factor in the presence of EDTA. *Journal of Clinical Pathology*, **22,** 460.

[9] GREIPP, P. R. and GRALNICK, H. R. (1976). Platelet to leucocyte adherence phenomena associated with thrombocytopenia. *Blood*, **47,** 513.

[10] KEIMOWITZ, R. and DESFORGES, J. F. (1965). Infantile pyknocytosis. *New England Journal of Medicine*, **273,** 1152.

[11] LOCK, S. P., SEPHTON SMITH, R. and HARDISTY, R. M. (1961). Stomatocytosis: a hereditary red cell anomaly associated with haemolytic anaemia. *British Journal of Haematology*, **7,** 303.

[12] MARSH, G. W. (1966). Abnormal contraction, distortion and fragmentation in human red cells. London University MD Thesis.

[13] MIER, M., SCHWARTZ, S. O. and BOSHES, B. (1960). Acanthrocytosis [*sic*], pigmented degeneration of the retina and ataxic neuropathy: a genetically determined syndrome with associated metabolic disorder. *Blood*, **16,** 1586.

[14] NORMAN, J. G. (1969). Stomatocytosis in migrants of Mediterranean origin. *Medical Journal of Australian*, i, 315.

[15] PONDER, E. (1948). *Hemolysis and Related Phenomena*. Grune and Stratton, New York.

[16] SALT, H. B., WOLFE, O. H., LLOYD, J. K., FOSBROOKE, A. S., CAMERON, A. H. and HUBBLE, D. V. (1960). On having no beta-lipoprotein. A syndrome comprising a-beta-lipoprotinaemia, acanthocytosis, and steatorrhoea. *Lancet*, ii, 325.

[17] SCHWARTZ, S. O. and MOTTO, S. A. (1949). The diagnostic significance of 'Burr' red blood cells. *American Journal of Medical Sciences*, **218,** 563.

[18] SILBER, R., AMOROSI, E., LHOWE, J. and KAYDEN, H. J. (1966). Spur-shaped erythrocytes in Laennec's cirrhosis. *New England Journal of Medicine*, **275,** 639.

[19] SKINNIDER, L. F., MUSCLOW, C. E. and KAHN, W. (1978). Platelet satellitism—an ultrastructural study. *American Journal of Hematology*, **4,** 179.

[20] STAVEM, P. and BERG, K. (1973). A macromolecular serum component acting on platelets in the presence of EDTA—'Platelet stain preventing factor'. *Scandinavian Journal of Haematology*, **10,** 202.

[21] TUFFY, P., BROWN, A. K. and ZUELZER, W. W. (1959). Infantile pyknocytosis: a common erythrocyte abnormality of

the first trimester. *American Journal of Diseases of Children*, **98**, 227.

[22] WEED, R. I. and BESSIS, M. (1973). The discocyte-stomatocyte equilibrium of normal and pathologic red cells. *Blood*, **41**, 471.

[23] WHITE, L. A., BRUBAKER, L. H., ASTER, R. H., HENRY, P. H. and ADELSTEIN, E. H. (1978). Platelet satellitism and phagocytosis by neutrophils: association with antiplatelet antibodies and lymphoma. *American Journal of Hematology*, **4**, 313.

[24] WIMER, B. M., MARSH, W. L., TASWELL, H. F. and GALEY, W. R. (1977). Haematological changes associated with the McLeod phenotype of the Kell blood group system. *British Journal of Haematology*, **36**, 219.

9. Red cell cytochemistry

Cytochemical methods applied to erythroid cells are especially useful for demonstrating free iron and fetal haemoglobin. These and other applications are described in this chapter.

SIDEROCYTES AND SIDEROBLASTS

Siderocytes are red cells containing granules of non-haem iron; they were originally described by Grüneberg[13] in small numbers in the blood of normal rat, mouse and human embryos, and in large numbers in mice with a congenital anaemia. The granules are formed of a water-insoluble complex of ferric iron, lipid, protein and carbohydrate. This siderotic material (or haemosiderin) reacts with potassium ferrocyanide to form a blue coloured compound, ferriferrocyanide; this reaction is the basis of a positive Prussian blue (Perls's) test. The material also stains by Romanowsky dyes and then appears as basophilic granules which have been referred to as 'Pappenheimer bodies' (Fig. 9.1).[24] By contrast, ferritin, which is a water-soluble non-haem compound of iron with the protein apoferritin, is not detectable by Perls's reaction. Ferritin is normally present in all cells in the body whereas haemosiderin is mainly found in monocyte-macrophage cells in the bone marrow, liver (Kupffer cells) and spleen, except when the body is overloaded with iron as in haemochromatosis or transfusional haemosiderosis.

Iron is transported in plasma attached to a β-globulin, transferrin, and passes selectively to the bone marrow where, at the surface of the erythroblast, the iron is released and enters the cell. Most of the iron is rapidly converted to haem in the mitochondria. The non-haem residue is in the form of ferritin. Degradation of the ferritin turns some of it into haemosiderin which can be stained by Perls's reaction and visualized under the light microscope as golden-yellow refractile particles.

In health, siderotic granules can normally be seen in the cytoplasm of many of the normoblasts of human bone marrow and in marrow reticulocytes.[8,18] However, they are not normally seen in human peripheral-blood red cells. After splenectomy, on the other hand, siderocytes can always be found in the peripheral blood, often in large numbers. The reason for this is probably because reticulocytes, after delivery from the marrow, are normally sequestered for a time in the spleen and there complete haem synthesis and utilize, for this purpose, the iron stored in their cytoplasm

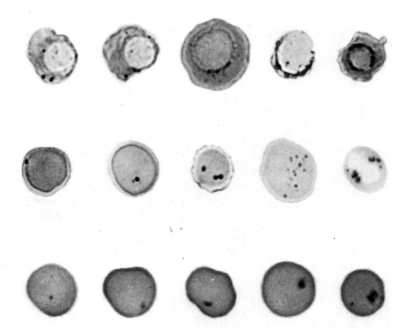

Fig. 9.1 Siderotic granules and 'Pappenheimer bodies'. Photomicrographs of normoblasts and red cells stained by the acid-ferrocyanide method to show siderotic granules (top two rows) and stained by Jenner-Giemsa's stain to demonstrate 'Pappenheimer bodies' (bottom row). × 1000.

within the siderotic granules. After splenectomy, this stage of reticulocyte ripening has to take place in the blood stream, with the result that even in an otherwise healthy person a small percentage of siderocytes can then be found in the peripheral blood.[7] The spleen is also probably able to remove large siderotic granules—as may be found in disease—from red cells by a process of pitting,[5] and in its absence such granules persist in the red cells throughout their life-span in the peripheral blood.

Method of staining siderotic granules

Air-dry films of peripheral blood or bone marrow and fix with methanol for 10–20 min. When dry, place the slides in a solution of 10 g/l potassium ferrocyanide in 0.1 mol/l HCl made by mixing equal volumes of 47 mmol/l (20 g/l) potassium ferrocyanide and 0.2 mol/l HCl immediately before use.

Leave the slides in the solution for about 10 min at c 20°C. Wash well in running tap water for 20 min, rinse thoroughly in distilled water and then counterstain with 1 g/l aqueous safranin or eosin for 10–15 s. Care must be taken to avoid contamination by iron which may have been present on the slides or in staining dishes. Prepare the glassware by soaking in 2 mol/l HCl before washing (see p. 540).

Prussian-blue staining can be applied to films which have previously been stained by Romanowsky dyes, even after years of storage. It is advisable to let the films stand in methanol overnight to remove most of the Romanowsky stain. Sundberg and Bromann described a technique whereby films were stained first by a Romanowsky dye (Wright's stain) and then over-stained by the acid-ferrocyanide method.[30] This can give beautiful pictures but the small blue-stained iron-containing granules tend to be masked in young erythroblasts by the general basophilia of the cell cytoplasm. Hayhoe and Quaglino described a method for combined PAS and iron staining.[14] A rapid method has been described for demonstrating siderotic granules by staining with 1% bromochlorphenol blue for 1 min.[19] Iron-containing granules stain dark purple.

Significance of siderocytes

Siderocytes contain one or two (rarely many) small iron-containing unevenly distributed granules which stain a Prussian-blue colour. In about 40% of polychromatic erythroblasts there are normally a few very small scattered siderotic granules.[18] They stain faintly and may be difficult to see by light microscopy. The percentage of erythroblasts recognizable as sideroblasts is increased in haemolytic anaemias and megaloblastic anaemias and in haemochromatosis and haemosiderosis, in proportion to the degree of saturation of transferrin, i.e. to the amount of iron available. A disproportionate increase in the percentage of erythroblasts that are sideroblasts occurs when the synthesis of Hb is impaired, in which case the granules in the sideroblasts are both more numerous and larger than normal. When there is a defect in haem synthesis, the granules are deposited in mitochondria and frequently appear to be arranged

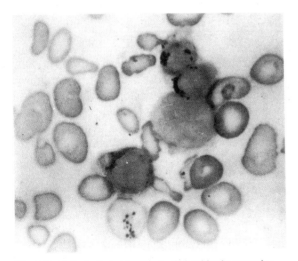

Fig. 9.2 Pathological sideroblasts. Sideroblastic anaemia (hereditary type). Three normoblasts are shown, in the cytoplasm of which is a massive accumulation of iron-containing granules. Perls's acid-ferrocyanide reaction. × 1000.

in a collar around the nucleus (Fig. 9.2) giving the 'ring sideroblasts' characteristic of sideroblastic anaemias. In contrast, the distribution of the granules within the cell tends to be normal in conditions in which globin synthesis alone is affected, e.g. in thalassaemia, or when there is iron overload.

There are several types of sideroblastic anaemia.[7,25] These include the primary acquired and congenital (hereditary) types. Pyridoxine (vitamin-B_6) deficiency also gives rise to a sideroblastic anaemia, and B_6-antagonists, e.g. drugs used in anti-tuberculosis therapy, produce the same effect. Secondary sideroblastic anaemia can also occur in alcoholism, lead poisoning and occasionally in rheumatoid arthritis and other 'medical' diseases. Ring sideroblasts are not uncommonly seen in primary haematological disorders, notably myelosclerosis, acute myeloid leukaemias and erythroleukaemia; they are also a feature of the myelodysplastic syndromes, and myelodysplastic marrows may contain 15% or more sideroblasts.[1]

In the primary acquired type, erythroblasts at all stages of maturity may be loaded with siderotic granules; whereas in some of the secondary sideroblastic anaemias and in the hereditary types the more mature cells seem most affected.

In addition to the siderotic granules within erythroblasts, haemosiderin can normally be seen in marrow films as accumulations of small granules, lying free or in phagocytes in marrow fragments.[27] The amount of haemosiderin will be markedly increased in patients with large iron stores, and reduced or absent in iron-deficiency anaemias (Fig. 9.3). In infections the iron stores may be increased, with much siderotic material in phagocytes but little or none visible in erythroblasts. Markedly excessive iron in phagocytes is also a feature of some dyserythropoietic anaemias. In practice, staining to demonstrate iron stores in marrow fragments and siderotic granules in erythroblasts is a simple and valuable diagnostic procedure and should be applied to marrow films as a routine.

There is no cytochemical method of demonstrating ferritin. Methods of assay are described in Chapter 25.

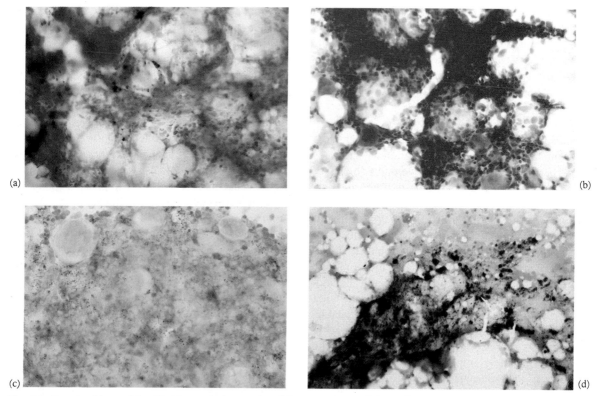

Fig. 9.3   Prussian blue staining (Perls's reaction) on aspirated bone marrow particles to demonstrate iron stores. (a) normal (b) absent (c) increased (d) grossly increased.

HAEMOGLOBIN DERIVATIVES

HEINZ BODIES IN RED CELLS

Heinz, in 1890, was the first to describe in detail inclusions in red cells developing as the result of the action of acetylphenylhydrazine on the blood.[16] Now it is known that 'Heinz' bodies can be produced by the action on red cells of a wide range of aromatic nitro- and amino-compounds, as well as by inorganic oxidizing agents such as potassium chlorate. They also occur when one or other of the globin chains of haemoglobin is unstable. In man, the finding of Heinz bodies is a sign of either chemical poisoning, drug intoxication, G6PD deficiency or the presence of an unstable haemoglobin, e.g. Hb Köln. When of chemical or drug origin, Heinz bodies are likely to be visible in red cells only if the patient has been splenectomized previously or when massive doses of the chemical or drug have

been taken. When due to an unstable haemoglobin they seem never to be visible in freshly withdrawn red cells except after splenectomy. They nevertheless develop in vitro when pre-splenectomy blood is incubated for 24–48 h.[6]

Heinz bodies are a late sign of oxidative damage, and represent an end-product of the degradation of Hb. Reviews dealing with Heinz bodies include those by Jacob[17] and by White.[37]

DEMONSTRATION OF HEINZ BODIES

Unstained preparations

Heinz bodies may be seen as refractile objects in dry unstained films, if the illumination is cut down by lowering the microscope condenser, and they can be seen by dark-ground illumination or phase-contrast microscopy. However, it is preferable to look for them in stained preparations (see below). In size they vary from 1 to 3 μm. One or more may be present in a single cell. They are usually close to the cell membrane, and in wet preparations may move around within the cells in a slow Brownian movement.

The degradation product of an unstable haemoglobin, e.g. Hb Köln, exhibits green fluorescence when excited by blue light at 370 nm in a fluorescent microscope.[9]

Stained preparations

Methyl violet stains the bodies excellently.

Dissolve c 0.5 g of methyl violet in 100 ml of 9 g/l NaCl and filter. Add 1 volume of blood (in any anticoagulant) to 4 volumes of the methyl violet solution and allow the suspension to stand for c 10 min at c 20°C. Then prepare films and allow them to dry or view the suspension of cells between slide and cover-glass. The Heinz bodies stain an intense purple (Figs. 9.4 and 9.5).

Heinz bodies also stain with other basic dyes. Brilliant green stains them well and none of the stain is taken up by the remainder of the red cell.[28] Rhodanile blue (5 g/l solution in 10 g/l NaCl) stains them rapidly,[29] i.e. within 2 min, at which time reticulocytes are only weakly stained. Compared with methyl violet, Heinz bodies stain less intensely with brilliant cresyl blue or New methylene blue. Nevertheless, they may be readily seen as pale blue bodies in a well-stained reticulocyte preparation, if the preparation is not counter-stained.

If permanent preparations are required, fix the vitally stained films by exposure to formalin vapour for 5–10 min. Then counterstain the fixed films with 1 g/l eosin or safranin, after thoroughly washing in water. If films are fixed in methanol, the bodies are decolourized.

In β-thalassaemia major, methyl violet staining of the bone marrow will demonstrate precipitated α-chains. These appear as large irregular inclusions in late normoblasts, usually single and closely adhering to the nucleus. If such patients are splenectomized, inclusions are also found in reticulocytes and mature red blood cells.

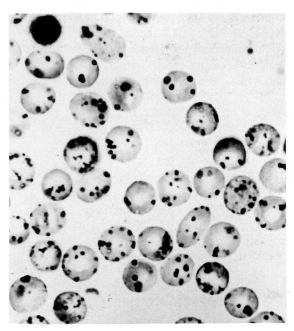

Fig. 9.5 G6PD deficiency. Blood exposed to acetyl phenylhydrazine. The majority of the cells contain several Heinz bodies. Stained supravitally by methyl violet. Reproduced by kind permission from E. Beutler, R. J. Dern and A. S. Alving (1955). The hemolytic effects of primaquine. VI. An in vitro test for sensitivity of erythrocytes to primaquine. *Journal of Laboratory and Clinical Medicine*, **45**, 40.

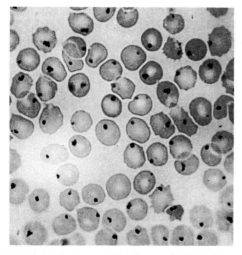

Fig. 9.4 Unstable haemoglobin disease. Hb Köln (after splenectomy). Many of the cells contain large Heinz bodies. Stained supravitally by methyl violet. × 700.

DEMONSTRATION OF HAEMOGLOBIN H

Patients with α-thalassaemia, who form Hb H (β_4), have red cells in which on exposure to brilliant cresyl blue, as in reticulocyte preparations, multiple blue-green spherical inclusions develop[12] (Fig. 9.6).

Method

Mix together in a small tube as for staining reticulocytes (p. 61) equal volumes of fresh blood and 10 g/l brilliant cresyl blue in iso-osmotic phosphate buffer pH 7.4 (p. 538). Leave the preparation at 37°C for 1–3 h before making films. Allow the films to dry and examine without counterstaining. Hb H precipitates as multiple pale-staining greenish-blue almost spherical bodies of varying size which can be clearly differentiated from the darker-staining reticulo-filamentous material of reticulocytes (Fig. 9.6 and Fig. 9.7).

The number of cells containing inclusions varies according to the type of α-thalassaemia. In α-thalassaemia-1 trait only 0.01–1% of the red cells contain inclusions, but this finding provides a significant clue to diagnosis. In Hb-H disease (α-thalassaemia-1/α-thalassaemia-2), as a rule at least 10% of the cells develop inclusions and, in some cases, the percentage is considerably greater.

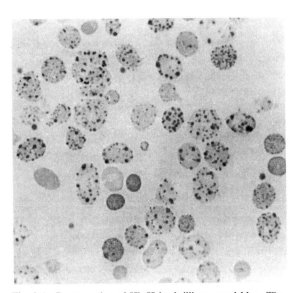

Fig. 9.6 Denaturation of Hb H by brilliant cresyl blue. The round bodies of varying size consist of precipitated Hb H. × 900.

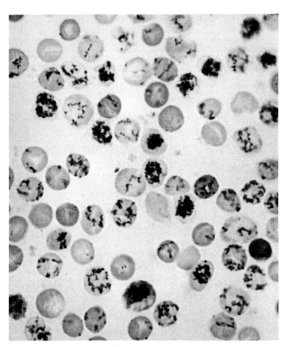

Fig. 9.7 Film of blood from patient with pyruvate kinase deficiency. Postsplenectomy. Almost every erythrocyte is a reticulocyte. Stained supravitally by brilliant cresyl blue. Compare with Fig. 9.6.

CARBOXYHAEMOGLOBIN

HbCO can be demonstrated in the red cells in a blood film. The method is a modification of the methaemoglobin (Hi) elution technique described below.[2,3] It is based on the fact that HbO_2 is oxidized by nitrite to Hi whereas HbCO is not. The method has, however, only limited practical value.

METHAEMOGLOBIN (Hi)

The peroxidatic capacity of Hi, but not of HbO_2 is reduced by cyanide. The peroxidatic activity prevents elution of haemoglobin by citric acid in the presence of hydrogen peroxide. Thus, normal red cells containing HbO_2 will remain intact and take up a counterstain whereas cells containing Hi will appear as ghosts when subjected to elution. Based on this principle, Kleihauer and Betke devised a simple method for demonstrating Hi in red cells in blood films.[20]

FETAL HAEMOGLOBIN

An acid-elution cytochemical method was introduced by Kleihauer et al in 1957.[21] It is a sensitive procedure which identifies individual cells containing Hb F even when few are present, and their detection in the maternal circulation has provided valuable information on the pathogenesis of haemolytic disease of the newborn.

The identification of cells containing Hb F depends upon the fact that they resist acid-elution to a greater extent than do normal cells; thus, in the technique described below, they appear as isolated darkly-stained cells amongst a background of palely-staining ghost-cells. The occasional cells which stain to an intermediate degree are less easy to evaluate; some may be reticulocytes as these also resist acid-elution to some extent. The following method in which elution is carried out at pH 1.5 is recommended.[22]

Reagents

Fixative. 80% ethanol.

Elution solution. Solution A: 7.5 g/l haematoxylin in 90% ethanol. Solution B: $FeCl_3$, 24 g; 2.5 mol/l HCl, 20 ml; doubly-distilled water to 1 litre.

For use, mix well 5 volumes of A and 1 volume of B. The pH is approximately 1.5. The solution can be used for c 4 weeks: if a precipitate forms, the solution should be filtered.

Counterstain. 1 g/l aqueous erythrosin or 2.5 g/l aqueous eosin.

Method

Prepare fresh air-dried films. Immediately after drying, fix the films for 5 min in 80% ethanol in a Coplin jar. Then rinse the slides rapidly in water and stand vertically on blotting paper for about 10 min to dry. Next, place the slides for 20 s in a Coplin jar containing the elution solution. Rinse in tap-water and allow them to dry in the air. Fetal cells stain red and adult ghost-cells stain pale pink (Fig. 9.8).

A number of modifications of the Kleihauer method have been proposed. In one, New methylene blue is incorporated in the buffer solution, the reaction time is prolonged and buffer is used for washing the films.[4] The advantage of this technique is that reticulocytes stain blue, whilst cells containing Hb F stain pink.

An immunofluorescent staining method has been developed based on the use of a specific antibody

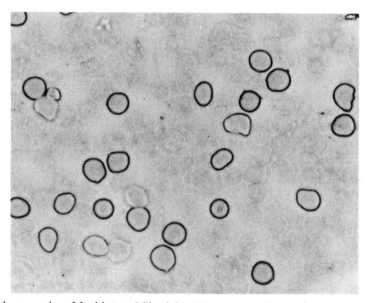

Fig. 9.8 Cytochemical demonstration of fetal haemoglobin. Acid elution method. The preparation consists of a mixture of cord blood and normal adult blood. The darkly staining cells are fetal cells. × 700.

against Hb F which does not react with Hb A.[33] By using a double-labelling procedure with rhodamine-labelled antibody against γ-globin and a fluorescein-labelled antibody against β-globin, it is possible to detect the presence of Hb F and Hb A in the same cell.[32]

A sensitive immunochemical method has been described for detecting maternal red cells in the fetal circulation;[36] the preparation is labelled sequentially with Rh immunoglobulin, rabbit anti-human IgG and goat anti-rabbit IgG conjugated to alkaline phosphatase, and is then stained as described on p. 148.

HAEMOGLOBIN S

Immunofluorescence with Hb-S antibody has been used for the identification of Hb S in red cells;[15,23] and by a double-labelling method similar to that described above it is possible to identify Hb S as well as another haemoglobin in individual cells.[15]

PERIODIC–ACID–SCHIFF (PAS) REACTION

The PAS reaction is used mainly for leucocyte cytochemistry. The method is described on p. 130. Mature red cells and the cytoplasm of normoblasts at any stage of development do not normally stain.

Erythroblasts may however react positively in disease. Deep diffuse staining has been observed in erythroleukaemia[26] and lesser degrees of staining may be seen in thalassaemia, iron-deficiency anaemia, cord-blood erythroblasts, sideroblastic anaemia, myelosclerosis, various types of leukaemia and in various types of haemolytic anaemia. Positive reactions have also been recorded in pernicious anaemia, aplastic anaemia, lead poisoning and polycythaemia vera. In acute myeloid leukaemia PAS-positive erythroid precursors have been associated with decreased remission rate.[31]

CYTOCHEMICAL TESTS FOR DEMONSTRATING DEFECTS OF RED CELL METABOLISM

Chemical tests for the recognition of defects of red cell metabolism are described in Chapter 14. Cytochemical methods have been developed by means of which some of these defects can be demonstrated in individual cells. Thus tests have been described for demonstrating red cells deficient in glucose-6-phosphate dehydrogenase (G6PD).[10,11,34] The principle on which the methods are based is that red cells are treated with sodium nitrite to convert their oxyhaemoglobin (HbO_2) to methaemoglobin (Hi). In the presence of G6PD, Hi reconverts to HbO_2, but in G6PD deficiency Hi persists. The blood is then incubated with a soluble tetrazolium compound (MTT) which will be reduced by HbO_2 (but not by Hi) to an insoluble formazan form.[20] Alternatively, the presence of Hi can be demonstrated by converting it to HiCN with potassium cyanide and then adding hydrogen peroxide which elutes HiCN but not HbO_2.[11] The cells are then stained, e.g. with eosin, and the HbO_2 containing cells can be readily distinguished from unstained ghosts, which had contained the Hi and which do not stain.

Attempts have been made to improve the reliability of the test for detecting heterozygotes, e.g. by controlled slight fixation of the red cells and accelerating the reaction with an exogenous electron carrier (1-methoxy phenazine methosulphate).[35] These cytochemical procedures are not more sensitive in the demonstration of G6PD deficiency than are the simple screening tests described on p. 204. They may, however, be useful when assessing G6PD activity in women, and may be the only way to detect deficiency in the hetero-zygous state. The method described below is satisfactory.

DEMONSTRATION OF G6PD DEFICIENCY

Reagents

Sodium Nitrite: 0.18 mol/l (12.5 g/l). The solution must be stored in a dark bottle and made up monthly.

Incubation Medium: 9 g/l NaCl, 4 ml; 50 g/l glucose, 1.0 ml; 0.3 mol/l phosphate buffer pH 7.0, 2.0 ml; 0.11 g/l Nile blue sulphate, 1.0 ml; water, 2.0 ml.

MTT Tetrazolium: 5 g/l of 3-(4,5-dimethylthiazolyl-1-2)-2,5-diphenyl tetrazolium bromide in 9 g/l NaCl.

Hypotonic Saline: 6 g/l NaCl.

Method[10]

Venous blood collected into ACD should be used. The test should be carried out within 8 h of collection and the blood should be kept at 4°C until it is tested. The blood is centrifuged at 4°C for 20 min at 1200–1500 g. The supernatant is discarded and 0.5 ml of packed red cells is added to a 15 ml glass centrifuge tube containing 9 ml of 9 g/l NaCl and 0.5 ml of sodium nitrite solution. The tube is incubated at 37°C for 20 min. After centrifuging at 4°C for 15 min at c 500 g, the supernatant fluid is discarded without disturbing the buffy coat and uppermost layer of red cells. The cells are washed three times in cold saline. After the last washing the buffy coat is removed, the packed cells are mixed well and 50 μl are transferred to a glass tube containing 1 ml of the incubation medium. The suspension is incubated undisturbed at 37°C for 30 min. Then 0.2 ml of MTT solution is added. The suspension is gently shaken and incubated at 37°C for 1 h. The cells are thoroughly resuspended. One drop is placed adjacent to one drop of hypotonic saline on a glass slide. The drops are thoroughly mixed, and covered with a cover-slip.

The red cells are examined with an oil-immersion objective and the presence of formazan granules is noted.

Interpretation

When G6PD activity is normal all the red cells are stained. In G6PD hemizygotes the majority of the red cells are unstained. In heterozygotes mosaicism is usually easily seen, a proportion of cells behaving as normal and the remainder being devoid or almost devoid of stainable material.

REFERENCES

[1] BENNETT, J. M. (1986). Classification of the myelodysplastic syndromes. *Clinics in Haematology*, **15**, 909.

[2] BETHLENFALVAY, N. C. (1971). Cytologic demonstration of carboxyhemoglobin: clinical and in vitro studies in man. *Journal of Laboratory and Clinical Medicine*, **77**, 543.

[3] BETKE, K. and KLEIHAUER, E. (1967). Cytological demonstration of carboxyhaemoglobin in human erythrocytes. *Nature* (London), **214**, 188.

[4] CLAYTON, E. M., FELHAUS, W. D. and PHYTHYON, J. M. (1963). The demonstration of fetal erythrocytes in the presence of adult red blood cells. *American Journal of Clinical Pathology*, **40**, 487.

[5] CROSBY, W. H. (1957). Siderocytes and the spleen. *Blood*, **12**, 165.

[6] DACIE, J. V., GRIMES, A. J., MEISLER, A. et al (1964). Hereditary Heinz-body anaemia. A report of studies on five patients with mild anaemia. *British Journal of Haematology*, **10**, 388.

[7] DACIE, J. V. and MOLLIN, D. L. (1966). Siderocytes, sideroblasts and sideroblastic anaemia. *Acta Medica Scandinavica*, **179**, Suppl, 445. p. 237.

[8] DOUGLAS, A. S. and DACIE, J. V. (1953). The incidence and significance of iron-containing granules in human erythrocytes and their precursors. *Journal of Clinical Pathology*, **6**, 307.

[9] EISENGER, J., FLORES. J., TYSON, J. A. and SHOHET, S. B., (1985). Fluorescent cytoplasm and Heinz bodies of hemoglobin Köln erythrocytes: evidence for intracellular heme catabolism. *Blood*, **65**, 886.

[10] FAIRBANKS, V. F. and LAMPE, L. T. (1968). A tetrazolium-linked cytochemical method for estimation of glucose-6-phosphate dehydrogenase activity in individual erythrocytes: applications in the study of heterozygotes for glucose-6-phosphate dehydrogenase deficiency. *Blood*, **31**, 589.

[11] GALL, J. C., BREWER, G. J. and DERN, R. J. (1965). Studies of glucose-6-phosphate dehydrogenase activity of individual erythrocytes: the methaemoglobin-elution test for identification of females heterozygous for G6PD deficiency. *American Journal of Human Genetics*, **17**, 359.

[12] GOUTTAS, A., FESSAS, Ph., TSEVRENIS, H. and XEFTERI, E. (1955). Description d'une nouvelle variété d'anémie hémolytique congénitale, *Sang*, **26**, 911.

[13] GRÜNEBERG, H. (1941). Siderocytes: a new kind of erythrocytes. *Nature* (London), **148**, 469.

[14] HAYHOE, F. G. J. and QUAGLINO, D. (1960). Refractory sideroblastic anaemia and erythraemic myelosis: possible relationship and cytochemical observations. *British Journal of Haematology*, **6**, 381.

[15] HEADINGS, V., BHATTACHARYA, S., SHUKLA, S. et al (1975). Identification of specific hemoglobins within individual erythrocytes. *Blood*, **45**, 263.

[16] HEINZ, R. (1890). Morphologische Veränderungen der rother Blutkörperchen durche Gifte. *Virchows Archiv*, **122**, 112.

[17] JACOB, H. S. (1970). Mechanisms of Heinz body formation and attachment to red cell membrane. *Seminars in Hematology*, **7**, 341.

[18] KAPLAN, E., ZUELZER, W. W. and MOURIQUAND, C. (1954). Sideroblasts. A study of stainable nonhemoglobin iron in marrow normoblasts. *Blood*, **9**, 203.

[19] KASS, L. and EICKHOLT, M. M. (1978). Rapid detection of ringed sideroblasts with bromchlorphenol blue. *American Journal of Clinical Pathology*, **70**, 738.

[20] KLEIHAUER, E. and BETKE, K. (1963). Elution procedure for the demonstration of methaemoglobin in red cells of human blood smears. *Nature* (London), **199**, 1196.

[21] KLEIHAUER, E. BRAUN, H. and BETKE, K. (1957). Demonstration von fetalem Hämoglobin in den Erythrocyten eines Blutausstrichs. *Klinische Wochenschrift*, **35**, 637.

[22] NIERHAUS, K. and BETKE, K. (1968). Eine vereinfachte Modifikation der säuren Elution für die cytologische Darstellung von fetalem Hämoglobin. *Klinische Wochenschrift*, **46**, 47.

[23] PAPAYANNOPOULOU, Th., McGUIRE, T. C., LIM, G., GARZEL, E., NUTE, P. E. and STAMATOYANNOPOULOS, G.(1976). Identification of haemoglobin S in red cells and normoblasts, using fluorescent anti-Hb antibodies. *British Journal of Haematology*, **34**, 25.

[24] PAPPENHEIMER, A. M., THOMPSON, K. P., PARKER, D. D. and SMITH, K. E. (1945). Anaemia associated with unidentified erythrocytic inclusions after splenectomy. *Quarterly Journal of Medicine*, **14**, 75.

[25] PIPPARD, M. J. and HOFFBRAND, A. V. (1989). Iron. In *Postgraduate Haematology*. Eds A. V. Hoffbrand and S. M. Lewis, 3rd edn., p. 26. Heinemann, Oxford.

[26] QUAGLINO, D. and HAYHOE, F. G. J. (1960). Periodic-acid-Schiff positivity in erythroblasts with special reference to Di Guglielmo's disease. *British Journal of Haematology*, **6**, 26.

[27] RATH, C. E. and FINCH, C. A. (1948). Sternal marrow hemosiderin: a method for the determination of available iron stores in man. *Journal of Laboratory and Clinical Medicine*, **33**, 81.

[28] SCHWAB, M. L. L. and LEWIS, A. E. (1969). An improved stain for Heinz bodies. *American Journal of Clinical Pathology*, **51**, 673.

[29] SIMPSON, C. F., CARLISLE, J. W. and MALLARD, L. (1970). Rhodanile blue: a rapid and selective stain for Heinz bodies. *Stain Technology*, **45**, 221.

[30] SUNDBERG, R. D. and BROMANN, H. (1955). The application of the Prussian blue stain to previously stained films of blood and bone marrow. *Blood*, **10**, 160.

[31] SWIRSKY, D. M., DeBASTOS, M., PARISH, S. E., REES, J. K. H. and HAYHOE, F. G. J. (1986). Features affecting outcome during remission induction of acute myeloid leukaemia in 619 adult patients. *British Journal of Haematology*, **64**, 435.

[32] THORPE, S. J. and HUEHNS, E.G. (1983). A new approach for the antenatal diagnosis of β-thalassaemia: a double labelling immunofluorescence microscopy technique. *British Journal of Haematology*, **53**, 103.

[33] TOMODA, Y. (1964). Demonstration of foetal erythrocytes by immunofluorescent staining. *Nature* (London), **202**, 910.

[34] TÖNZ, O. and ROSSI, E. (1964). Morphological demonstration of two red cell populations in human females heterozygous for glucose-6-phosphate dehydrogenase deficiency. *Nature* (London), **202**, 606.

[35] VAN NOORDEN, C. J. F. and VOGELS, I. M. C. (1985). A sensitive cytochemical staining method for glucose-6-phosphate dehydrogenase activity in individual erythrocytes. *British Journal of Haematology*, **60**, 57.

[36] WANG XIN-HUA and ZIPURSKY, A. (1987). Maternal erythrocytes in the fetal circulation: the immunocytochemical identification of minor populations of erythrocytes. *American Journal of Clinical Pathology*, **88**, 346.

[37] WHITE, J. M. (1976). The unstable haemoglobins. *British Medical Bulletin*, **32**, 219.

10. Leucocyte cytochemical and immunological techniques

(By D. Catovsky)

CYTOCHEMICAL TESTS

Cytochemical tests applied to haemopoietic cells allow the demonstration of specific enzymes or other substances in individual cells. They are particularly useful for the study of immature cells (e.g. blasts) and lymphocytes because conventional morphology, as seen in Romanowsky-stained films, is not sufficient to identify differentiation features. Most tests are applied to the diagnosis and classification of leukaemia:

1. In distinguishing the patterns of differentiation of early granulocytic and early monocytic cells in the acute leukaemias and in recognizing some types of acute lymphoblastic leukaemia (ALL).

2. In characterizing the cells in chronic lymphoid leukaemias, and, to some extent, in normal lymphocyte subsets.

3. In distinguishing leucocytoses and leukaemoid reactions from genuine myeloproliferative disorders.

4. In studying abnormalities and/or enzyme deficiencies of neutrophils, for example, in the myelodysplastic syndromes.[10]

In erythroid cells, free iron, haemoglobin derivatives and red cell enzymes can be demonstrated.

In special cases, methods of ultrastructural cytochemistry need to be applied, as the resolution of light microscopy may not suffice to demonstrate the localization of the reaction product. One such example is the platelet peroxidase reaction demonstrable in the endoplasmic reticulum and nuclear membrane of mature and immature cells of the megakaryocytic series.[2,14] A number of techniques for enzyme histochemistry can now also be applied to semi-thin sections of plastic-embedded bone-marrow trephine biopsies.[6]

THE MYELOPEROXIDASE REACTION

Myeloperoxidase is a lysosomal enzyme localized in the azurophil granules of neutrophils and monocytes.[3,66] Azurophil granules in granulocytic cells correspond to the relatively large electron-dense (primary) granules seen under the electron microscope.[3,67] The secondary (specific) granules are less electron dense and appear at the myelocyte stage.[3,14] In the monocytic series the azurophil granules are smaller[83] and are not the first to appear during maturation in these cells. Thus the designation primary for them is not appropriate. The lysosomal granules present in early monocytic cells (monoblasts) are very small and have acid phosphatase but lack peroxidase activity.[67]

Myeloperoxidase can also be demonstrated in the specific granules of eosinophils and basophils. In eosinophils the specific granules are not newly formed but derive from primary granules which are also myeloperoxidase positive. The eosinophil peroxidase has been shown by chemical, cytochemical and immunological methods to be different from that of neutrophils and probably to be under separate genetic control.[1] The enzyme in eosinophils is cyanide-resistant and, in neutrophils, cyanide-sensitive.[94]

Most of the early methods for the demonstration of peroxidase use benzidine and hydrogen peroxide. The method of Kaplow[52] described in previous editions of this book uses benzidine dihydrochloride, a less carcinogenic compound. As there are difficulties, in some countries, in the use of methods which include benzidine, alternative and probably safer substrates should be considered. These are 3-amino-9-ethyl carbozole, o-tolidine,[41] 2,7-fluorenediamine (FDA)[7,45] and 3,3'-diamino benzidine (DAB) tetrahydrochloride.[39] Some of them, like α-naphthol, are less sensitive than benzidine-based methods and therefore are of little value in the study of leukaemic cells.[48]

DAB is the substrate of choice for ultrastructural studies because its oxidized product is electron-dense and can be intensified by post-fixation with osmium tetroxide.[14] DAB is also frequently used to visualize the immunoperoxidase reaction.[14] Hanker et al[39] described a method using DAB that we have found reliable in the diagnosis of acute myeloid leukaemia (AML). This method, as well as one with the alternative substrate (FDA) described by Inagaki et al[45], will be described here.

METHOD WITH DAB

Fixative. A mixture of 1.25% glutaraldehyde and 1% formaldehyde in 0.1 mol/l phosphate buffer (pH 7.3). Mix 50 ml of a 25% solution of glutaraldehyde, 27.8 ml of a 36% solution of formaldehyde and add the buffer up to 1 litre.

Incubation mixture. DAB, 5 mg; tris-HCl buffer, 50 mmol/l, pH 7.6, 10 ml; H_2O_2, 30% (w/v), 0.1 ml. Add the reagents in this order and mix well after each addition. This medium should be prepared just before use.

Enhancer. Dissolve copper sulphate ($CuSO_4$), 0.5 g or copper nitrate ($Cu(NO_3)_2.3H_2O$), 0.5 g in 100 ml of tris-HCl buffer, 50 mmol/l, pH 7.6.

Counterstain. Dissolve 10 g of Giemsa's stain in 100 ml of 66 mmol/l phosphate buffer, pH 6.4.

Method

Fix peripheral-blood or bone-marrow films for 1 min and then rinse in 9 g/l NaCl (saline). Immerse the slides in the incubation mixture for 1 min in a Coplin jar at room temperature (20–25°C). Rinse briefly in tris-HCl buffer (three changes) and then immerse the slides in the reaction enhancer. Rinse in saline and keep in the saline until counterstained. Counterstain for 10 min, dry and mount in DPX (BDH Ltd.)

METHOD WITH 2,7-FDA[7,45]

Fixative. 10% formal-ethanol solution: 9 volumes of 95% ethanol and 1 volume of 40% formaldehyde.

Incubation mixture. Dissolve 40 mg of 2,7-FDA in 40 ml of tris-HCl buffer (pH 8.6) in order to obtain a saturated solution. Stir vigorously for 5 min at room temperature and then filter to remove excess of precipitated substrate. The solution (without H_2O_2) is stable for at least 6 weeks at room temperature. Add just before use 2 drops of 30% H_2O_2 to clear filtrate.

Giemsa counterstain. 10 g of Giemsa stain in 66 mmol/l phosphate buffer (as above).

Method

Fix films for 1 min and rinse in water. Transfer the slides to the incubation mixture in a Coplin jar. Incubate for 5 min at room temperature. Wash for a few seconds and counterstain with Giemsa for 15 min, dry and mount in DPX mountant*.

Technical considerations

Either reaction works well with films made from freshly withdrawn (uncoagulated) blood or bone marrow. Myeloperoxidase is not inhibited by heparin, oxalate or EDTA and films made from such blood may be stained adequately if the blood is not allowed to stand at *c* 20°C for more than 6 h. Once films are made they should be left to dry and then fixed; they may then be kept at 4°C for up to 1 week until the reaction is performed. The fixation procedure described above can be interchanged for both cytochemical reactions, and counterstaining may be modified according to individual needs. The methods described above were tested mainly on cells from cases of acute leukaemia.

Significance

Developing granulocytes always give positive reactions; the reaction is strong in promyelocytes and myelocytes but may be negative in very early myeloblasts. Almost all mature neutrophils give a positive reaction despite the fact that few azurophil granules are visible when the cells are stained with Romanowsky dyes. Eosinophils and basophils give positive reactions, as do promonocytes and monocytes. Monoblasts, lymphocytes and lymphoblasts fail to react.

The main value of the myeloperoxidase reaction is in the distinction between acute myeloid and acute lymphoblastic leukaemia (see below).[8,32,41,42] For practical purposes only immature cells that show myeloperoxidase activity can be confidently referred to as myeloblasts; if the reaction is negative they could be any other type of blast cell.

---

*BDH Ltd.

Auer rods nearly always react positively in leukaemic myeloblasts, and the reaction permits a better identification of these characteristic rods than the May-Grünwald-Giemsa stain. An interesting difference has been observed when using the above methods in AML cells. The method with DAB demonstrates a significantly higher percentage of positive rods than techniques with other substrates.[39] In particular, DAB allows the visualization of the so-called Phi bodies,[39] small fusiform-shaped rods, which appear to derive from catalase-containing granules, whilst Auer rods derive from primary granules. Thus the apparent greater sensitivity of the method with DAB in samples of AML may result from the known property of DAB to demonstrate catalase in microperoxisomes as well as myeloperoxidase activity. Phi bodies are not seen using the reaction with 2,7-FDA but Auer rods are easily seen (Fig. 10.1). The latter give a clear brown reaction product without crystals or precipitates, which facilitates the morphological recognition of the cells reacting positively.

SUDAN BLACK B STAINING

Sudan Black B was used by Sheehan[81] and later by others to stain the granules of neutrophils, many of which appear to contain phospholipids. The close parallelism observed between sudanophilia and myeloperoxidase activity relates to the fact that both cytochemical reactions are positive in the azurophil granules of neutrophils and monocytes and in the specific eosinophil granules. The biochemical basis for the sudanophilia in these cells is poorly understood.[41] One possible view is that Sudan Black B stains the lipid membrane of the granules which contain the enzyme myeloperoxidase. Another is that the dye stains through an enzymatic mechanism, perhaps linked to myeloperoxidase, and not just by physical solution in the lipids.[41] Both reactions are positive in mature and immature myeloid cells and thus are useful in the differential diagnosis and classification of the acute leukaemias.[32,41,42] The simplicity of the Sudan Black B reaction makes its use mandatory in routine haematology laboratories. The method of Sheehan and Storey[82] which has been in use, almost unchanged, for more than 40 years, is given below.

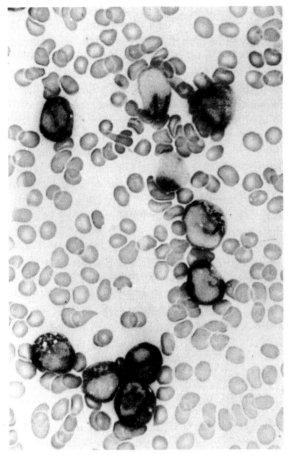

Fig. 10.1   Myeloperoxidase reaction (2,7-FDA method).
Bone-marrow cells from a case of acute myeloblastic
leukaemia with maturation (M2). The cells are
myeloperoxidase-positive. Note two blasts cells with positive
Auer rods.

Reagents

Fixatives. 40% formaldehyde.

Staining solution. This is a mixture of two
solutions, A and B.

(A) Sudan Black B. 0.3 g in 100 ml of absolute
ethanol. Shake well to dissolve the stain and filter to
remove particles.

(B) Buffer. 16 g of crystalline phenol in 30 ml of
absolute ethanol. Add the phenol-ethanol mixture
to 100 ml of water in which 0.3 g of disodium
hydrogen phosphate ($Na_2HPO_4.12H_2O$) has been
dissolved. Stir vigorously until all the phenol has
dissolved and filter. Add 30 ml (or 60 ml) of solution A to 20 ml (or 40 ml) of solution B and filter.
The mixture can be kept at 4°C for 2–3 months.

Counterstain.   May-Grünwald-Giemsa,   preferably, or safranin.

Method

Fix air-dried films of blood or bone marrow for 10
min in formalin vapour. This can be done by
soaking filter paper in formalin and placing inside a
37°C incubator.★ Wash gently in water for 5–10
min; longer periods (e.g. 1 h) may result in stronger
staining. Wash in 70% ethanol by waving the slides
in the alcohol in a Coplin jar for 3–5 min. Wash
with water for 2 min, dry, counterstain for 5 min
and mount.

The reaction product in the cytoplasm is black;
the nuclei stain blue (or red) depending on the
counterstain used.

NEUTROPHIL ALKALINE PHOSPHATASE (NAP)

Alkaline-phosphatase activity can be demostrated
cytochemically in the cytoplasm of mature neutrophils, typically in segmented forms and only rarely
in band forms. The enzyme is not demonstrable in
other blood leucocytes, but fibroblast-like reticulum
cells,[11] part of the bone-marrow stroma, react
strongly.

Recently, small amounts of NAP activity have
been demonstrated in the membrane of some
lymphoid cells[18] and shown histochemically in a
type of B-cell lymphoma.[62]

NAP was thought initially to be localized in the
specific (secondary) granules, by analogy with the
findings in rabbit neutrophils,[3] or in late-appearing
tertiary granules. Recent studies by Rustin et al[76]
have shown that NAP is associated with a membra-
nous component of the cytoplasm identified as an
irregularly-shaped tubular structure distinct from
primary or secondary granules or other cytoplasmic
organelles.

Early cytochemical methods for the demonstration of NAP were based upon the hydrolysis of the
substrate α-naphthyl phosphate at pH 9.0–10.0 and
the coupling of the liberated naphthol to a diazo-

★Alternatively, immerse the films for 5 min in a solution of 9
volumes of absolute ethanol and 1 volume of 40%
formaldehyde.

tized amine to form an insoluble coloured precipitate. The intensity of the precipitate is a rough measure of the enzyme content of individual neutrophils. Later methods have used substituted naphthols as substrates,[54] e.g. naphthol AS,[77] AS-BI or AS-MX[52] phosphate; they all give highly chromogenic and insoluble reaction products which are superior to those developed in previously decribed methods. We describe here below the method of Rutenburg et al[77] which is simple and highly reproducible and gives an easily recognizable blue reaction product. This method can also be applied to tissue sections. For the technical aspects of the preparation and storage of films and the effects of fixation on NAP activity, refer to the detailed review by Kaplow.[54]

Reagents

Fixative. Absolute methanol, 9 volumes; neutral formalin (40% formaldehyde), 1 volume. The mixture should be kept at − 20°C, or in the ice compartment of a refrigerator, and may be used for up to 2–3 weeks.

Stock substrate solution. Dissolve 30 mg of naphthol AS phosphate in 0.5 ml of N,N-dimethylformamide and add 0.3 mol/l tris buffer, pH 9 (p. 539) to make the volume up to 100 ml. This solution is stable for several months at 2–4°C, but its pH should be checked before use.

Diazonium salt. Fast Blue BB or BBN.

Counterstain. 1 g/l aqueous neutral red.

Control. Each batch of slides to be stained should include two controls, a normal blood film and a blood film giving a strong reaction, e.g. from a patient with a polymorphonuclear leucocytosis due to infection.

Method

Make films, if possible from freshly withdrawn blood (no anticoagulant). Films from blood collected into EDTA are less satisfactory, and if anticoagulated blood has to be used, films should be made as soon as possible, and in any case within 30 min of collection.

When made, fix the films without delay for 30 s in the formal-methanol fixative at 0–5°C. Then wash the slides in running tap-water for 10–15 s,

drain off excess water and allow to dry. If staining has to be delayed for more than 5–6 h, store the fixed films at − 20°C.

Prepare the incubation mixture by dissolving 10 mg of the diazonium salt in 10 ml of the stock substrate solution. Then filter this on to the slides and allow the reaction to continue for 15 min at *c* 20°C. Then rinse the slides in four changes of tap-water, allow them to dry and counterstain the films with neutral red for 6 min. After drying, place a drop of neutral mountant on the slide, and cover the film with a cover-slip.

Scoring results

Alkaline phosphatase activity is indicated by a precipitate of bright blue granules; the cell nuclei are stained red. Based on the intensity of staining and the number of blue granules in the cytoplasm of the neutrophils, individual cells can be rated as follows:

0: negative, no granules
1: positive but very few blue granules
2: positive with few to a moderate number of granules
3: strong positive with numerous granules
4: very strong positive with cytoplasm crowded with granules.

The score in an individual film consists of the sum of the scores of 100 consecutive neutrophils. As this mode of assessment is subjective, each laboratory should establish its own normal range.

Significance

The normal range of NAP is wide, 35–100 in our laboratory. In a few normal individuals occasional neutrophils score 3, none 4. The score is higher in women and children than in men, and in newborn infants the range is 150–300.

High scores are found in the neutrophilia of infections, in leukaemoid reactions, liver cirrhosis, Down's syndrome and polycythaemia vera. The enzyme seems to be influenced by oestrogens and corticosteroids, which may explain the gradual rise in score in pregnancy. High scores are found in active Hodgkin's disease but they are uncommon in non-Hodgkin's lymphomas; in Hodgkin's disease, however, the determination of NAP has no apparent advantage over simpler tests such as the ESR in the assessment of the activity of the disease.[68] Low scores are found in chronic granulocytic leukaemia in relapse and in myeloblastic leukaemias while the scores in lymphocytic leukaemias are normal or high. Intermediate scores, more often than not rather high, are found in monocytic and myelomonocytic leukaemias.

Low scores are found in paroxysmal nocturnal haemoglobinuria[58] and high scores in aplastic anaemia.[68] The development of PNH in a patient with aplastic anaemia is associated with a falling score.

The value of the NAP reaction in the differential diagnosis of the chronic myeloproliferative disorders is discussed later (see p. 139).

PERIODIC ACID-SCHIFF (PAS) REACTION

The PAS reaction depends on the liberation of carbohydrate radicals from combination with protein and their oxidation to aldehydes by the Schiff reagent. A positive reaction usually denotes the presence of glycogen. This can be confirmed by demonstrating that the positive reaction disappears when the film is treated with saliva or diastase before it is stained. Other PAS-positive material is unchanged by diastase digestion.

Developing granulocytes react positively at all stages of development. Mature polymorphonuclear neutrophils react most strongly (Fig. 10.2) and their cytoplasm contains large amounts of positively-staining material in the form of small granules. Myeloblasts and myelocytes contain fewer positively-staining granules but the cytoplasm stains diffusely pale pink. In eosinophils the background cytoplasm is PAS-positive but the large specific granules are PAS-negative.

Lymphocytes normally contain much less staining material than granulocytes, but a few fine or even coarse granules may often be demonstrated. Monocytes contain a small amount of fine, scattered, positively-staining material. The cytoplasm of normoblasts does not normally stain at any stage of development.

The PAS reaction of blood cells differs from the normal in disease and the findings have some diagnostic value.

Lymphocytes in the B-lymphoproliferative disorders (e.g. chronic lymphocytic leukaemia and prolymphocytic leukaemia) often contain an increased number of positively-staining granules (Fig. 10.2); in lymphoblasts, 'blocks' of staining material may be present.[32,41,42] This is the typical reaction in the common type of childhood lymphoblastic leukaemia (Fig. 10.3); in the less common T-cell variant the PAS reaction is, however, either weakly positive or negative.[20]

Erythroblasts may react positively in disease. Deep diffuse staining has been observed in erythroleukaemia[70] and in thalassaemia; and lesser degrees of staining may be seen in iron-deficiency anaemia, myelosclerosis, various types of leukaemia and in various types of haemolytic anaemia. Positive reactions have also been recorded in pernicious

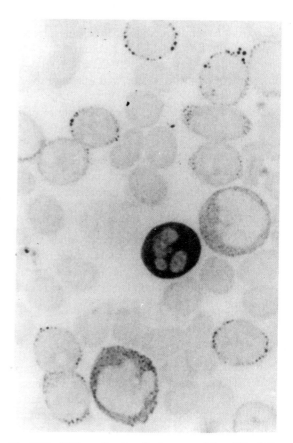

Fig. 10.2 PAS reaction in cells from a peripheral-blood film. Chronic lymphocytic leukaemia. Most of the lymphoid cells are PAS-positive with medium size granules; two large cells with fine granules are monocytes and in the centre there is a neutrophil showing a diffuse positive reaction.

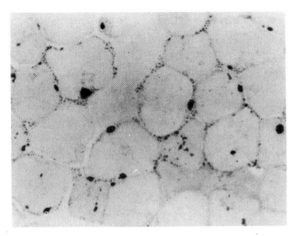

Fig. 10.3   PAS reaction in cells from cerebrospinal fluid.
Cytocentrifuge preparation; acute lymphoblastic leukaemia.
Most of the cells are PAS-positive with medium size granules
and single blocks.

anaemia, aplastic anaemia, lead poisoning and polycythaemia vera.

The reaction is best carried out on fresh blood or
bone-marrow films but old methanol-fixed films or
films stained by Romanowsky dyes months or years
before can be quite satisfactorily stained.

Reagents

Periodic acid (HIO$_4$.2H$_2$O), 10 g/l.

Schiff's reagent (leucobasic fuchsin). Basic
fuchsin, 1.0 g, dissolved in 400 ml of boiling water.
Cool the solution to 50°C and then filter. To the
filtrate add 1 ml of thionyl chloride (SOCl$_2$) and
allow the solution to stand in the dark for 12 h.
Then add 2.0 g of activated charcoal and after
shaking for 1 min filter the preparation. Store in the
dark at 0–4°C.

Rinsing solution. Sodium metabisulphite, 100 g/l,
6 ml; HCl, 1 mol/l, 5 ml; water to 100 ml.

Counterstain. Mayer's haemalum or Harris's
aqueous haematoxylin, 2.0 g; water to 100 ml.

Method

Fix the films in methanol for 5–15 min. Then wash
in running tap-water for 15 min. Expose the films
to digestion in diastase (1 g in 1 litre of 9 g/l NaCl)
for 1 h at room temperature. Thereafter, allow both
treated and untreated slides to stand in the periodic
acid solution for 10 min, then wash and immerse
them in Schiff's reagent for 30 min at room temperature in the dark. Rinse the slides three times in
the rinsing solution, then wash in distilled water for
5 min, counterstain with haematoxylin for 10 min
and then blue in tap-water for 5 min. Finally, dry in
the air and mount in a neutral mountant.

ACID PHOSPHATASE REACTION

There are several techniques for the demonstration
of acid phosphatase in leucocytes in films and tissue
sections. Some utilize the same reagents used for
the demonstration of NAP but at pH 5.0. For
example, the method of Li et al[60] uses naphthol
AS-BI phosphate and Fast Garnet GBC and gives a
highly chromogenic reaction product; it is easily
reproducible and suitable for demonstrating the
enzyme in the granulocytic series. For lymphocytes
and monocytes, a method using naphthol AS-BI
phosphate coupled with freshly hexazotized pararosanilin buffered to pH 5.0[33] may be better,
although its final reaction product is less distinctly
granular than when Fast Garnet GBC is used.[41]
Another good coupling agent is Fast red ITR salt.

Acid phosphatase activity is present in the lyso-
somes of many types of haemopoietic cell, i.e.
myelocytes, polymorphonuclear neutrophils, lymphocytes, plasma cells, megakaryocytes, platelets,
and all the cells of the mononuclear phagocyte
system (monoblasts, promonocytes, monocytes and
macrophages). It is one of the acid hydrolases that
can be demonstrated in lymphoid cells, and is of
diagnostic value in the differential diagnosis of
lymphoproliferative conditions (see below). Studies
in tissue sections have demonstrated a greater
enzyme content in T-cell-dependent areas than in
B-cell-dependent areas (e.g. germinal centres) of
lymphoid tissues from men and rodents. The activity of acid phosphatase increases after lymphocyte
transformation with phytohaemagglutinin and during the transition from monocyte to tissue macrophage. The technique of Goldberg and Barka[33]
has been shown, in our hands, to be reliable in
the study of lymphocytic and monocytic proliferations.[17,19,20] For hairy cell leukaemia (HCL)
the method of Li et al[60] has been recommended.[83]

Reagents

Fixative. Methanol, 10 ml; acetone, 60 ml; water, 30 ml; citric acid, 0.63 g. This solution should be adjusted to pH 5.4 with 1 mol/l NaOH and controlled weekly.

Stock solutions.

A. Buffer, pH 5.0. Sodium acetate, trihydrate, 19.5 g; sodium barbiturate, 29.5 g; water to 1 litre (Michaeli's veronal acetate buffer).

B. Substrate. Naphthol AS-BI phosphate dissolved in N, N dimethylformamide, 10 mg/ml (i.e. 25 mg in 2.5 ml).

C. Sodium nitrite ($NaNO_2$). 4% aqueous solution.

D. Pararosanilin chloride (Sigma). 2 g in 50 ml of 2 mol/l HCl. Heat gently, without boiling; cool down to room temperature and filter.

Solutions A, B and D can be stored at 4°C; solution C should be freshly made each time or can only be stored for up to 1 week at 4°C.

Working solution. Mix together 92.5 ml of solution A, 2.5 ml of solution B, 32.5 ml of water and 4 ml of hexazotized pararosanilin solution. Make the latter by mixing well 2 ml of solution C and 2 ml of solution D; allow to stand for 2 min before adding to the other constituents. Mix well and adjust the pH of the working solution to pH 5.0 with 1 mol/NaOH.

Counterstain. 1% methyl green in veronal acetate buffer, pH 4.0.

Mounting medium. Glycerol/gelatin. Add 15 g of gelatin to 100 ml of glycerol and 100 ml of water.

Method

Dry the films well before starting the reaction. (It is desirable to leave them for this purpose for at least 24 h at room temperature.) Fix the films for 10 min, then rinse the slides well in water. They can now be kept for 1–2 weeks at −20°C if required.

Incubate the slides for 1 h at 37°C in the working solution; rinse in tap-water, counterstain the films for 1 min, rinse in tap-water and mount whilst still wet. For this, the glycerol/gelatin mixture has to be in liquid phase; i.e. warmed to 37°C or higher.

The cytoplasmic reaction product is bright red; the nuclei stain pale green.

Test of tartrate resistance

This is often carried out in parallel with the above reaction or preferably the method using Fast Garnet GBC[60,83] for the study of hairy cells. Add 375 mg of crystalline L(+)-tartaric acid (Sigma) to 50 ml of the working solution; the final concentration is then 50 mmol/l. Then carry out the cytochemical reaction. Most positively-reacting leucocytes are tartrate-sensitive and fail to react in the presence of tartrate. The majority of hairy cells of HCL react equally positively in both solutions.[95]

Significance

The most common application of the acid phosphatase reaction is in the classification of lymphoproliferative disorders. Almost all acute and chronic T-cell lymphoproliferations are characterized by a strong acid phosphatase reaction. In T-ALL (Fig. 10.4)[17,20] the reaction is localized to an area of the cytoplasm which at ultrastructural level corresponds to the Golgi zone. In the chronic T-cell leukaemias the reaction is also positive but with variable consistency. For example, most cases of T-cell chronic lymphocytic leukaemia (CLL) but only two-thirds of those with T-cell prolymphocytic leukaemia (PLL) have cells which react strongly positively. The enzyme activity in these cases is tartrate-sensitive.

In normal T-cells, acid phosphatase activity is an early differentiation feature, e.g. the reaction is

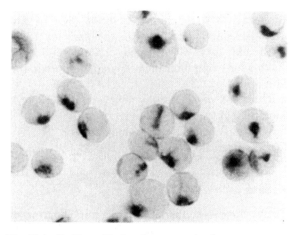

Fig. 10.4 Positive acid phosphatase-reaction in a peripheral-blood film. Acute lymphoblastic leukaemia of T-cell type.

positive in fetal thymocytes and it persists in some mature T-lymphocytes.[5] In the B-cell disorders the reaction is often weak or negative with the exception of HCL, the cells of which show a strong acid phosphatase activity[60] resistant to inhibition by tartrate in the majority of cases.[95] This enzyme corresponds to a unique isoenzyme 5 found predominantly in hairy cells.[95] Tartrate-resistant cells have not been found in the peripheral blood of normal individuals but a few such cells can be found in the normal bone marrow.[63] In B-cell PLL one-third of the cells show a positive acid phosphatase reaction if tested by the method of Goldberg and Barka[33] and some of these cells have been shown to be tartrate-resistant, as in HCL.[20]

In AML, blasts of the monocytic lineage react more strongly than those of the granulocytic lineage. The reaction in monoblasts is diffuse over the whole cytoplasm and can be seen at ultrastructural level to be localized in small lysosomal granules.[67] The reaction may be of value in the distinction of the various types of AML (see below).

ESTERASES

These are a group of hydrolases with a wide range of pH activity which vary in their localization in cells of different bone-marrow lineages. It is best to consider separately the results obtained with the various substrates used for their cytochemical demonstration. Those currently in use are: α-naphthol acetate, α-naphthol butyrate, naphthol AS (or AS-D) acetate and naphthol AS-D chloracetate.[91]

Li et al described nine esterase isoenzymes in leucocytes:[59] 1, 2, 7, 8 and 9 represent the 'specific' esterase of granulocytes which can be demonstrated by means of naphthol AS-D chloracetate; 3, 4, 5 and 6 represent the so-called 'non-specific' esterases which are sensitive to sodium fluoride (NaF) and are found in monocytes, megakaryocytes and platelets, and are demonstrated by α-naphthol esters (acetate and butyrate). Naphthol AS (or AS-D) reacts with most isoenzymes but is inhibited by NaF in its reaction with the non-specific esterases.

α-NAPHTHOL ACETATE ESTERASE (ANAE)

The cytochemical reaction for ANAE is of practical value because it gives distinct patterns in lympho-

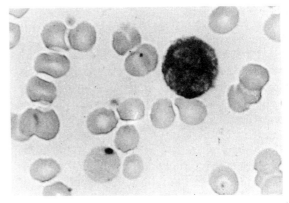

Fig. 10.5 Alpha-naphthyl acetate esterase reaction.
ANAE-positive reaction in normal cells. A lymphocyte (presumably T) has a characteristic single 'dot-like' reaction; a monocyte shows a strong diffuse reaction over the whole cytoplasm.

cytes (a dot-like reaction)[18,55] and in monocytes (a diffuse positive reaction)[19] as illustrated in Fig. 10.5. The localized reaction in lymphocytes is resistant to NaF,[19,28] whilst that in monocytes is NaF-sensitive. In normal blood there is a good correlation between the proportion of E-rosettes (a T-cell marker) and the percentage of ANAE-positive lymphocytes. The reaction in immature T-cells (thymocytes) is also localized, but it is weak and seen in only one-third of those cells. The dot-like reaction in peripheral-blood T-lymphocytes is seen mainly in the subset with Fc receptors for IgM, Tμ cells.[27] Results with the substrate α-naphthyl butyrate are, in general, very similar to those obtained with ANAE. Some authors have made a distinction between the ANAE reaction carried out at different pHs, acid or alkaline, the latter favouring the reaction in monocytes and the former being more specific for T-lymphocytes. The method of Yam et al[94] at pH 6.1 permits the adequate demonstration of the distinct reaction in both cell types.[18, 19]

Reagents

Fixative. Phosphate buffered acetone-formaldehyde. Acetone, 40 ml; 35% formaldehyde, 25 ml; Na_2HPO_4, 20 mg, and KH_2PO_4, 100 mg, in 30 ml of water. Filter the solution before use; it must be clear. It will keep at room temperature for 1 month.

Stock solutions.

A. α-Naphthyl acetate. 50 mg dissolved in 2.5 ml of 2-methoxyethanol.

B. Phosphate buffer. 0.1 mol/l, pH 7.6, 44.5 ml.

C. Hexazotized pararosanilin. 3 ml. This is prepared by mixing equal volumes of pararosanilin solution (solution D of the acid phosphatase reaction, see p. 132) and fresh 4% aqueous $NaNO_2$ for 1 min just before use.

Incubation mixture. Mix solutions A and B and add to them the freshly prepared solution C. Adjust the pH to 6.1 with 1 mol/l NaOH. Filter before use; the solution must be clear.

Counterstain and mounting medium. As for acid phosphatase (methyl green and glycerol/gelatin).

Method

Fix the films for 30 s, rinse the slides well in water and allow to dry. Incubate the slides for 45 min in the incubation mixture. After the incubation, wash the slides in tap-water and counterstain for 1 min and mount whilst still wet.

A positive reaction results in dark red granules; the nuclei stain pale green.

Inhibition with sodium fluoride (NaF)

Add 75 mg of NaF to 50 ml of the incubation mixture (concentration 1.5 mg/ml = 37.5 mmol/l).

Carry out the test simultaneously with the ANAE reaction to investigate the NaF sensitivity of a cell population. This may be necessary for the identification of monocytes within a mixture of mononuclear cells or to characterize a particular leukaemic cell type.

Significance[4,27,44,55,94]

The ANAE cytochemical reaction is often applied to the study of normal and leukaemic cell populations. In normal samples it helps to distinguish between T-lymphocytes and monocytes because of the different pattern of reaction and the different sensitivity to NaF (see above). In leukaemias and lymphoproliferative disorders it has three main applications:

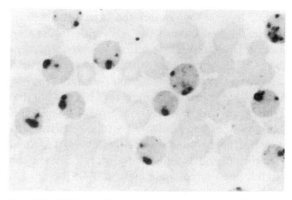

Fig. 10.6 Alpha-naphthyl acetate esterase reaction. Strong localized ANAE reaction in peripheral blood cells of a T-cell prolymphocytic leukaemia. (Photograph by courtesy of Dr. A. D. Crockard).

1. In AML it facilitates the diagnosis of monocytic leukaemia (FAB M5), the cells of which give a strong diffuse reaction sensitive to NaF. In erythroleukaemia (FAB M6) and megakaryoblastic leukaemia (FAB M7) the blast cells give a positive ANAE reaction localized to the Golgi zone and sensitive to NaF.[28] In contrast to M5, the reaction in M6 and M7 is not observed (or is very weak) when α-napthyl butyrate is used as substrate.[28]

2. In ALL, together with the acid phosphatase reaction, it helps to identify T-ALL.[4,44]

3. In the chronic B and T lymphoid leukaemias it helps to distinguish T-PLL (positive reaction) (Fig. 10.6) from B-PLL (negative reaction). The typical dot-like pattern of normal T-lymphocytes is not observed, however, in T-CLL. This probably relates to a similar finding in the cell subset that is the normal counterpart of the lymphocyte of T-CLL (T-lymphocytes[27] or large granular lymphocytes).

Erythroblasts are normally ANAE-negative. However, they can react positively in megaloblastic anaemia. Weak reactions have also been described in thalassaemia and sideroblastic anaemia.

NAPHTHOL AS (OR AS-D) ACETATE ESTERASE

Both substrates are commonly used: naphthol AS acetate (NASA) or naphthol AS-D acetate (NASDA) can demonstrate non-specific esterase activity in monocytic cells. They do not show, as does ANAE, a consistent localized reaction in T-lymphocytes. Fast Blue BB has been recommended as coupling agent.[83] The reaction with both substrates is carried out at pH 6.9.[94] At this pH, however, prolonged incubation can result in hydrolysis of the substrate by the chloracetate esterase of granulocytes,[59] thus making the reaction less specific for monocytes. Therefore, the simultaneous incubation with NaF is needed to improve the recognition of promonocytes and monocytes and to distinguish them from promyelocytes and myelocytes. NaF is less necessary with ANAE (or α-naphthol butyrate) because the reaction is strong in monocytic cells and is weak or negative in granulocytes. The reaction product with NASDA is often stronger than with NASA and diffuses less; it is thus the substrate of choice. The main value of the reaction is in differentiating between the myeloblastic types (M1 and M2) and the monocytic types (M5a and M5b) of AML.[8] In myelomonocytic leukaemia (M4), it helps in assessing the relative size of the monocytic component.

CHLORACETATE ESTERASE

The specific esterase present in granulocytes and mast cells is distinct from that in monocytes and megakaryocytes; it can be demonstrated by using naphthol AS-D chloracetate as substrate and Fast Garnet GBC,[62] Fast Red Violet or Fast Blue BB[41] as coupling agents. Recently a method with New fuchsin has been recommended by the International Committee for Standardization in Haematology.[83] The enzyme is optimally active at pH 7.0–7.6 and is not inhibited by NaF. The positive reaction is found in mature and immature granulocytes and, in general, the reactions parallel those of myeloperoxidase and Sudan Black B in the granulocytic lineage; Auer rods often react positively. Little or no enzyme activity is demonstrable in lymphocytes and monocytes.

One advantage of the chloracetate method is the possibility of demonstrating enzyme activity in paraffin-embedded histological sections of formalin-fixed material. It can be applied as well to material from other tissues, being particularly useful for the diagnosis of granulocytic sarcoma (chloroma).

The chloracetate esterase reaction has been widely used on haematological material in combination with ANAE or α-naphthol butyrate esterase in a single method—the so-called combined or dual esterase reaction.[41,94] The end-result is the demonstration, in the same preparation, of both types of esterase; they can be distinguished by the colour of the reaction products by using different coupling agents, e.g. blue when using Fast Blue BB for the chloracetate esterase and dark red using hexazotized pararosanilin for ANAE. This procedure simplifies the cytochemical characterization of leukaemic cells. In acute myelomonocytic leukaemia (M4) it helps to identify both the granulocytic and monocytic components.

OTHER ACID HYDROLASES

Two enzymes, β-glucuronidase[32] and β-glucosaminidase[27,71] have been shown by histochemical methods to be present in high concentrations in T-cell-dependent areas of lymphoid tissues and to be either absent or present in only small amounts in the B-cell-dependent areas. Both enzymes have now been shown to be useful markers of leukaemic T-lymphocytes. The reaction product in cells of chronic B-cell leukaemias is usually weak or negative.[27]

LYSOZYME ACTIVITY

A simple cyto-bacterial method for the demonstration of lysozyme (muramidase) activity based on the technique of Briggs et al,[15] as modified by Syrén and Raeste[86] was described in previous editions of this book. As the method is not often performed nowadays in the characterization of blast cells, we do not reproduce it here.

Normal blood monocytes and neutrophils always give a positive lysis test but lymphocytes do not. In normal bone marrow, lysozyme activity can be demonstrated in granulocytes as far back as the myelocyte stage. In acute leukaemia, myeloblasts and lymphoblasts are lysozyme-negative but promonocytes and monocytes, and sometimes monoblasts, give positive reactions.

Because lysozyme appears relatively late during monocyte maturation, at the promonocyte stage, this reaction is consistently positive in differentiated forms of monocytic leukaemia, i.e. in M4, M5b and CMML of the FAB classification,[8,11] but may be negative in the poorly differentiated type, i.e. M5a. In the former case, a high proportion of leukaemic monocytes (50–90%) are lysozyme-positive. In general, the number of lysozyme-positive cells in the circulation and the serum lysozyme concentration are closely correlated.[21]

PRACTICAL VALUE OF CYTOCHEMICAL REACTIONS

There are three major groups of malignancies of haemopoietic cells in which the cytochemical methods described above have been found to be useful for a correct diagnosis and classification:

1. The acute leukaemias, proliferations of immature haemopoietic precursors (blast cells).
2. The chronic myeloproliferative disorders, proliferations of differentiated cells of the myeloid lineage.
3. The chronic lymphoproliferative disorders, proliferations of mature-looking lymphoid cells.
4. The myelodysplastic syndromes,[10] a group of conditions distinct from, but possibly related to, the acute leukaemias should also be considered in the differential diagnosis.

Well-prepared peripheral-blood and bone-marrow films stained with May-Grünwald-Giemsa are the basis for any classification. The cytochemical tests provide clues regarding the type and direction of cellular differentiation and should be regarded as complementing and not substituting for the morphological analysis.

DIFFERENTIAL DIAGNOSIS OF THE ACUTE LEUKAEMIAS—THE FAB CLASSIFICATION[8–12]

Two main forms of acute leukaemia are recognized: myeloid (AML), more frequent in adults (>20 years), and lymphoblastic (ALL), predominantly found in children (<15 years).

AML

Seven types of AML can be identified by morphology with the help of cytochemistry. The main features of each type (M1–M7) are summarized in Table 10.1. Certain cytochemical reactions are essential in distinguishing AML from undifferentiated forms of ALL (e.g. L2). This is particularly so in cases where the cells are immature, e.g. in M1 (myeloblastic leukaemia without maturation) and M5a (monoblastic leukaemia, poorly differentiated). The peroxidase, Sudan Black B and chloracetate esterase reactions reveal granulocytic differentiation in the M1, M2, M3 and M4 types of AML whilst the non-specific esterases (NASDA and ANAE ± NaF), and the acid phosphatase and lysozyme reactions, demonstrate monocytic differentiation. In addition to the cytobacterial test referred to on p. 135, lysozyme can be investigated in samples of serum and urine by turbimetric methods.

Although most cases of hypergranular promyelocytic leukaemia (M3) can be diagnosed in May-Grünwald-Giemsa-stained films, an M3-variant characterized by having fewer azurophil granules may require for its identification a positive reaction with the cytochemical methods for granulocytic cells (Table 10.1). Because of their (typical) bilobed nuclei, cells of the M3-variant can sometimes be confused with atypical monocytes (as in M4 and M5 leukaemias). However, the non-specific esterase reactions are usually weak or negative in M3.

In erythroleukaemia (M6) the PAS reaction may be strongly positive, with a diffuse or granular pattern being found in erythroblasts and sometimes in erythrocytes, too; the ANAE reaction may also be positive in red-cell precursors,[75] and is often localized in the Golgi zone.[28]

A rare form of AML is acute megakaryoblastic leukaemia.[12,14] The blast cells appear undifferentiated, and may resemble lymphoblasts.[2] The cytochemical profile of these cells is similar to that of megakaryocytes: i.e. positive reactions with PAS, acid phosphatase and ANAE (NaF-sensitive as in monocytes). A specific test for megakaryoblasts, the

Table 10.1 Classification and cytochemistry of AML

Reaction	Myeloblastic@ M1	M2	Promyelocytic M3	Myelomonocytic M4	Monocytic M5	Erythroleukaemia M6	Megakaryoblastic[10] M7
May-Grünwald-Giemsa stain	Blasts with few or no granules (90%); Auer rods	Blasts (>30%) Maturation beyond promyelocytes. Abnormal neutrophils	Hypergranular promyelocytes; faggots. Bilobed nuclei. Hypogranular variant	Blasts (>30%). Evidence of granulocytic and monocytic differentiation	(a) Monoblasts; (b) Monoblasts, promonocytes & monocytes. (a) & (b) >80% monocytic cells.	Over 50% of erythroid cells, often bizarre. Myeloblasts with Auer rods. The % of blasts is >30% by excluding erythroid cells from the differential count.[11]	Blasts (>30%); often dry tap aspirate; bone marrow trephine biopsy required
Peroxidase Sudan Black B	+ or + + (>5% blasts)	+ +	+ + +	+ or + + (2 populations)	− or +	+ (blasts)	−
Esterases							
1. Chloroacetate	+	+ +	+ + +	+ or + +	− or ±	+	−
2. NASDA	+	+	+ +	+ or + + +*	+ + +*	+ +*	+ +* in Golgi zone
3. ANAE	−	±	±	+ or + + +*	+ + +	+* (erythroid precursors) in Golgi zone	+ +* in Golgi zone
Acid phosphatase	− or +	+	+ or + +	+ or + +	+ + +	±	+ +
Lysozyme	−	−	±	+ or + +	± or + + +	−	−
PAS	+ diffuse	+ diffuse	+ + diffuse	+ or + + variable	+ or + + granules	+ (erythroblasts)	+ or + +
Incidence	23%	30%	8%	16%	16%	6%	1%

*NaF sensitive. *Degree of reaction:* − negative; ± weak (few positive cells); + moderate to strong; + + moderate to strong; + + + most of the cells strongly positive. Cytochemical reactions that are useful for differential diagnosis are printed in bold type. @Cases of myeloblastic leukaemia may give negative cytochemical reactions with peroxidase, Sudan Black B, and also give negative esterase reactions. These forms of AML have been designated as M0*; the evidence for the myeloid nature is provided by the presence of myeloid antigens[29,38,79] and by myeloperoxidase activity demonstrated at ultrastructural level.[61]

so-called 'platelet peroxidase' reaction, can be demonstrated by electron microscopy in the nuclear membrane and endoplasmic reticulum of these cells although not in the Golgi apparatus.[2,14]

The enzyme content of mature neutrophils in AML, particularly in M2 and M6, can often be shown by negative cytochemical reactions to be deficient. The NAP score is often low in M2 (myeloblastic leukaemia with maturation),[50] especially in M2 cases with the chromosome translocation t (8;21). An interesting difference between the low NAP values seen in CGL and in M2 has been reported by Kamada et al[50]—namely, that if the leukaemic cells are suspended in liquid culture for 1 week the NAP score increases in CGL whilst it remains unchanged in M2. The peroxidase, Sudan Black B and chloracetate reactions may also be negative in variable proportions of neutrophils in AML, more frequently in M2 and M6.[22] In contrast, the neutrophils in AML and in M5 react positively in these reactions to about the same degree as do normal neutrophils.

ALL

Three morphological types have been described by the FAB group: L1, L2 and L3.[8,9] The differences in age incidence (L1 is more common in children and L2 more frequent in adults), the strong correlation of L3 with B-ALL (with monoclonal membrane immunoglobulins) and the difference in prognosis between L1 and L2 (worse in L2) within similar age-groups together suggest that the three morphological types may reflect true biological differences.

L1 lymphoblasts tend to be small and to have scanty cytoplasm; the nucleo-cytoplasmic (N:C) ratio is high in the majority and they have a small and not easily visible nucleolus; the nuclear membrane is often regular. L2 lymphoblasts, in contrast to L1, are larger, have more abundant cytoplasm (low N:C ratio) and have one or more prominent nucleoli; the nuclear outline is irregular in over 25% of cells. The differences between L1 and L2 can be more easily solved in borderline cases by the simple scoring system proposed by the FAB group.[9] L3 cells (or Burkitt type), because of their resemblance to cells of the endemic African lymphoma, are uniformly large, have finely stippled nuclear chromatin and, characteristically, a deep basophilic cytoplasm often associated with prominent vacuolation.[8]

Two cytochemical tests are useful in the study of ALL; the PAS and acid phosphatase reactions. They do not correlate with the L1, L2 or L3 morphological types but they do show some relationship to the immunological subtypes of ALL (Table 10.2). In cases in which the cells are undifferentiated (usually L2 blast cells in adult patients), it is important to exclude AML (usually M1 and M5a). For this, the peroxidase, Sudan Black B and NASDA reactions should be shown to be negative. The PAS reaction is often positive in ALL—at least, in a proportion of blasts, as shown by coarse granules or blocks of positively-reacting material (usually glycogen). This pattern of reaction, particularly with a negative background, is rarely seen in AML. It is more typical of the common form of childhood ALL which can be defined by immunological tests for the ALL antigen (glycoprotein [gp] 100). This was described initially by Greaves et al[36] as common-ALL. This form of ALL is now recognized by monoclonal antibodies (McAb) of the cluster of differentiation (CD10), i.e. CD10.[35,74]

Table 10.2 Cytochemistry and the immunological classification of ALL*

Method	Null-ALL	Common-ALL	T-ALL	B-ALL
Morphology	L1–L2	L1–L2	L1–L2	L3
PAS	– or + +	+ or + +	– or +	–
	coarse granules	coarse granules		
Acid phosphatase	– or +	– or +	+ + or + + +	–
Peroxidase } Sudan Black B }	–	–	–	–
Lysozyme	–	–	–	–

*For details of the membrane and enzyme markers in ALL, see Table 10.4.
Degree of reaction as in Table 10.1.

In T-ALL (positive T-cell markers), the PAS reaction is negative in two-thirds of cases; in B-ALL it is almost always negative. The differences shown by the PAS reaction probably reflect the different proliferation kinetics of the immunologically-defined subtypes of ALL. For example, in B-ALL (PAS-negative) a greater number of cells are in cycle; this is also reflected in the numerous mitotic figures seen in bone marrow with L3 morphology. The acid phosphatase test gives a consistently localized positive reaction in T-ALL and pre-T-ALL blast cells.[4,17,44]

Chronic myeloproliferative disorders

Low NAP scores are typical of untreated chronic granulocytic leukaemia (CGL) and high NAP scores are characteristic of polycythaemia vera, leucocytoses and leukaemoid reactions secondary to infection or neoplasia and of most cases of myelosclerosis. Normal scores are often found in secondary polycythaemia due to hypoxia, 'stress' or renal disorders. In CGL the low initial scores may change to normal or high in about one-third of patients during remission; scores become high during severe infections, after splenectomy and in up to 50% of cases undergoing blast-cell transformation.

The possibility of characterizing more precisely the type of blast cells seen during the transformation of CGL has improved significantly in recent years. The cytochemical methods applied to the study of AML may provide useful information. Often, however, CGL blasts are very undifferentiated by cytological and cytochemical criteria. Ultrastructural studies, e.g. the platelet-peroxidase reaction, may help in the diagnosis of megakaryoblastic transformation (15% of cases).[14] Nowadays a number of McAb against platelet glycoproteins can be used to demonstrate the megakaryoblastic nature of the blasts.[28,88] A 'lymphoid' transformation occurs in 20% of cases of CGL; most cytochemical tests are negative in this form, but the PAS reaction may show granular positivity. Lymphoblastic transformation can now be diagnosed by positive criteria by demonstrating the common ALL-antigen (CD 10),[35,46] and the enzyme terminal deoxynucleotidyl transferase (TdT).[13] A mixed population of blast cells is not rare during transformation of CGL; thus mixed lymphoid and myeloid blast crises have been documented.[19]

Myelodysplastic syndromes (MDS)

Precise diagnostic criteria for the MDS were recently proposed by the FAB group.[10] All of them are characterized by hypercellular bone marrows. Five conditions are included under the broad term MDS:

1. Refractory anaemia (RA), with erythroid hyperplasia and/or dyserythropoiesis.

2. RA with ring sideroblasts, also designated as acquired idiopathic sideroblastic anaemia (AISA), the main feature being the presence of ring sideroblasts in at least 15% of erythroblasts. (See p. 116 for staining techniques.)

3. RA with excess of blasts (RAEB) which shows dyspoiesis in the three bone-marrow cell lineages, dysgranulopoiesis being always conspicuous. The percentage of bone-marrow blasts is between 5 and 20%; these cells may have a few or no azurophil granules.

4. Chronic myelomonocytic leukaemia (CMML), with many features of RAEB plus a significant peripheral blood monocytosis (usually over $1 \times 10^9/l$).

5. RAEB in transformation, a group close to AML and defined by the presence of blasts in the peripheral blood (over 5%) and between 20 and 30% in the bone marrow.

In order to distinguish RAEB from AML with more than 50% erythroid cells in the bone marrow the FAB group recommended in those circumstances that erythroid cells be excluded from the differential count and then, if more than 30% of the residual bone marrow cells are blasts, the diagnosis is M6.

In addition to staining for iron, the other cytochemical methods used in AML may be useful for the study of the MDS. They may help to define the monocytic component in CMML or the type of blasts in RAEB and they are particularly useful in demonstrating dysgranulopoiesis, e.g. by the presence of neutrophils negative for peroxidase and/or Sudan Black B reactions or giving extremely low NAP scores.

MDS features can be demonstrated in patients presenting as de-novo AML. When there is evidence that the three bone marrow cell lines are dysplastic, the designation AML with trilineage myelodysplasia has been coined.[16] These patients remit less readily than those with primary AML without MDS changes, and may relapse with pure MDS and without blast cells.[16] Because these patients may have a preceding preleukaemic process and abnormal erythropoiesis they often present with more severe anaemia than other patients with AML without MDS.

CHARACTERIZATION OF CHRONIC LYMPHOPROLIFERATIVE DISORDERS[19,27]

Analysis using immunological membrane markers shows that the majority of lymphoproliferative disorders are of the B-cell type (Table 10.3). In the most common of these, chronic lymphocytic leukaemia (CLL), and in prolymphocytic leukaemia (PLL), the PAS reaction is often positive in a granular form.[20] This reaction is variable, often negative, in the chronic T-cell disorders.

The reactions for acid hydrolases (acid phosphatase, ANAE, β-glucuronidase and β-glucosaminidase) are positive in most T-cell disorders and negative in the B-cell types (Table 10.3). The non-specific esterase reaction can also help to diagnose the rare 'true' histiocytic lymphomas within the group of large-cell lymphomas, which are usually of B-cell type. True histiocytic lymphomas are tumours of monocytic lineage and show strong diffuse positivity with NASA, NASDA or ANAE, the reactions being NaF-sensitive. These cytochemical reactions are negative in the majority of B-cell lymphomas. Despite the characteristic cytochemical patterns set out in Table 10.3, the current trend is to classify the lymphoid malignancies on the basis of reactions to immunological reagents, chiefly McAb, which cover a wide range of differentiation antigens demonstrable in the B- and T-cell lineages. These reagents have the additional advantage that they detect antigens which characterize early or late stages of lymphoid maturation.

DEMONSTRATION OF DNA AND RNA

Methods for demonstrating DNA and RNA in haemopoietic cells were referred to briefly in the Sixth Edition of this book. As the methods are now seldom used, we are omitting any reference to them in this edition.

Table 10.3 Cytochemistry of chronic lymphoproliferative disorders and relation to membrane phenotype

Disease	Immunological subtype*	Relative incidence@	ANAE	Acid phosphatase	β-glucuronidase β-glucosaminidase
CLL‖	B	98%	−	−	−
	T	2%	− or ±	+ +	+ + +
PLL‖	B	70%	−	− or +	−
	T	30%	+ + +	± or + +	+ + +
Non-Hodgkin's	B	85%	−	− or +	−
lymphomas	T**	15%	+ +	+ or + + +	+ +
HCL@@	B	100%	− or +	+ +†	−

*B-cell markers: membrane bound and/or cytoplasmic monoclonal immunoglobulins; mouse RBC rosettes and B-cell lineage McAb, e.g. CD19, CD20.
T-cell markers: sheep RBC rosettes, heteroantisera and McAbs to T-cell antigens, e.g. CD2, CD3, CD4, CD8, etc.
@ Based on over 2000 cases studied in the MRC Leukaemia Unit Laboratories by D.C.
** Includes Sézary syndrome and adult T-cell lymphoma-leukaemia (HTLV-1 positive).
†Resistant to tartaric acid.
‖Chronic lymphocytic leukaemia.
‖Prolymphocytic leukaemia.
@@Hairy cell leukaemia.

CELL MARKERS

Cells can be identified, not only by their morphology and cytochemistry, but also by the presence of characteristic receptors and antigens on the cell membrane, immunoglobulin molecules on the membrane (SmIg) and/or in the cytoplasm (CyIg) and by enzymes such as terminal deoxynucleotidyl transferase (TdT) in the nucleus.[13] By this means it is possible to distinguish B- and T-lymphocytes and also subsets within the major types of lymphocytes. Market studies help in identifying the lineage of immature cells; they have also contributed to the study of early and late stages of lymphoid differentiation, and to the diagnosis and classification of the acute and chronic lymphoid leukaemias.

Separation of mononuclear (MN) cells

For most cell marker studies it is necessary to separate the MN cell fraction containing lymphocytes, monocytes, blasts and other mononuclear cells (according to the sample) and to exclude neutrophils, eosinophils, basophils and erythrocytes. Methods include density gradient centrifugation with Ficoll-Triosil, Hypaque or Lymphoprep.* The method with Lymphoprep is described below. When necessary, platelets can also be excluded by defibrinating the blood before separation.

Method

Dilute 10 ml of the anticoagulated (e.g. heparinized) blood with an equal volume of 9 g/l NaCl (saline). Add the diluted blood drop by drop to 7.5 ml of Lymphoprep and then centrifuge at 400 g for 30 min. The MN layer separates from the upper plasma layer and from the red cells and neutrophils (which settle to the bottom of the tube). After separation, take up the MN cell layer into another tube and wash three times with TC 199.

METHODOLOGY FOR THE STUDY OF CELL MARKERS

There are several ways of testing for cell markers:

*Nyegaard, Oslo

1. In suspensions of viable cells;
2. In cells on cytospin-made slides, or directly using blood or bone-marrow films;
3. In cells in frozen sections of bone marrow or other haemopoietic tissues (immunocytochemistry).

Tests on cell suspensions will only detect membrane antigens while tests on fixed cells will often detect cytoplasmic as well as membrane antigens. Some antigens are expressed first in the cytoplasm of early blasts, e.g. CD3 in early T-cells, CD22 in early B-cells and CD13 in early myeloid cells, and only later on the surface of the cell membrane. Thus tests for markers may be negative when tested on cell suspensions but positive on fixed cells.

Cells in suspension can be tested by rosetting methods or by staining directly (1 layer) or indirectly (2 or more layers) with antibodies labelled with fluorescent dyes (immunofluorescence, IF). IF labelling is detected using fluorescence microscopes equipped with ultraviolet light or in-flow cytometers, like FACS or EPICS, which are equipped with a laser source of illumination. Fixed cells can be studied also by direct or indirect IF, or more frequently by peroxidase or alkaline phosphatase labelled reagents.[30] The latter methods do not require special microscopy equipment and provide permanent preparations.

ROSETTE TESTS

These are based on the affinity of red cells (RBC) to bind specifically to membrane receptors. This binding can be demonstrated with the RBC of various species (sheep, mouse, ox, etc.) which form rosettes (Fig. 10.7) with various types of lymphocytes. There are two types of rosette, immune and spontaneous, depending on whether the RBC are or are not coated by Ig molecules.

Immune rosettes are used to demonstrate receptors for the Fc part of IgG (Fc γ) or IgM (Fc μ) in B-and-T-lymphocytes and can also be used to test McAb.[46] Human RBC (Rh positive) coated with anti-D can also be used to detect high affinity Fc receptors in monocytes.

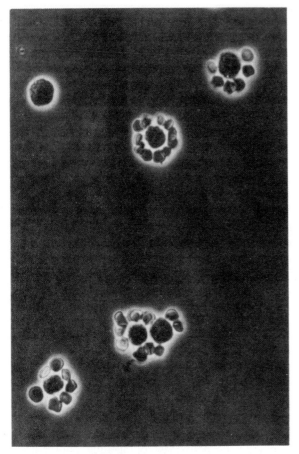

Fig. 10.7   E-rosette formation. Leukaemia T-cells from a case of T-PLL are seen forming rosettes with sheep RBC. Viewed under phase-contrast microscopy.

Spontaneous binding of sheep or mouse RBC has been used, respectively, as markers for T-lymphocytes[46,51,93] and for a subset of B-lymphocytes, chiefly those proliferating in B-CLL.[18,24,85]

SHEEP RED BLOOD CELLS (SRBC) ROSETTES (E-ROSETTES)[51,93]

This test is used as a marker of T-lymphocytes. Almost all peripheral-blood T-lymphocytes and most mature T-lymphocytes in other organs form E-rosettes. The receptor for SRBC appears early during T-cell maturation, and thus it is present also on immature T-cells, including most thymocytes. Because of this, it is usually considered a good marker for T-cell leukaemias, both acute (T-ALL)

and chronic (T-CLL, T-PLL, etc). The only exceptions are cases of pre-T-ALL, an immature variant constituting 25–30% of T-ALL cases (Table 10.4) in which some T-antigens are present but few or no E-rosettes are formed.[44] In the chronic T-cell lymphoproliferative disorders (Table 10.5) E-rosettes are, as a rule, demonstrable.

As the formation of E-rosettes requires active cell metabolism, viable cells are necessary. The sensitivity of the test can be increased by treating the SRBC with papain, neuraminidase[46] or the sulphydryl compound AET.[51] AET treatment results in the highest values for E-rosettes and it gives consistent reactions with strong rosettes which are resistant to disruption. An interesting property of E-rosettes is their temperature dependence. Mature T-lymphocytes form a maximum number of rosettes at 4°C and these dissociate at 37°C. Thymocytes, on the other hand, form rosettes at 4°C and 37°C. This property was used in the past for the diagnosis of T-ALL in which the proliferating cells have characteristics of thymic cells.

Because of difficulties in securing a regular supply of sheep RBC for testing, the receptor for E-rosettes is demonstrated with more consistent results by McAb of the CD2 group (OKT11, LEU5, RFT11, etc.) by indirect IF rather than by a rosetting technique. The rosetting test with sheep RBC has, however, the advantage that it can be read quickly.

Reagents

Sheep red cells. Wash SRBC three times in 9 g/l NaCl (saline); then treat with AET (see below). It is convenient to use formalized SRBC, obtainable from Tissue Culture Services Ltd (UK).

Lymphocytes. Fresh normal blood human lymphocytes (10×10^6/ml) in saline suspension.

Fetal calf serum (FCS). Absorb 4 volumes of FCS with 2 volumes of SRBC for 2 h at 37°C. Then centrifuge, transfer the supernatant serum to another tube and inactivate it for 30 min at 56°C. Store in 5–10 ml volumes at −20°C.

Method

Add to 0.1 ml of AET-treated SRBC (1% suspension in TC 199) 0.05 ml of absorbed, inactivated FCS and 0.05 ml of lymphocyte suspension.

Table 10.4   Immunological classification of ALL

Reactivity against	Marker*	Null	B-lineage**		B-ALL	T-lineage***	
			cALL	pre-B		pre-T	T-ALL
Precursor cells	HLA-Dr	+	+	+	+	− or ±	−
	TdT	+	+	+	− or ±	+	+
	CD34 (3C5)	+	+	+	−	−	−
B-cell antigens	CD19 (B4)	+	+	+	+	−	−
	CD22-Cyt	+	+	+	+	−	−
	CD10 (J5)	−	+	+	− to +	− to +	−
	Cyt μ chain	−	−	+	+	−	−
T-cell antigens	CD7(3A1)	−	−	−	−	+	+
	CD3-Cyt	−	−	−	−	+	+
	CD5 (UCHT2)	−	−	−	−	− to +	+
	E-rosettes	−	−	−	−	−	+
Incidence in children		10%	60%	15%	1%	4%	10%

*Given according to cluster of differentiation (CD) number with the McAbs used in our laboratory shown in brackets. The McAbs are listed according to the sequential order in which they are first expressed in cells of the B- and T-lineages.
**All cases show rearrangement of the Ig heavy chain gene.
***All cases show rearrangement of the T-cell receptor β and/or γ and/or δ chain genes
Cyt: Cytoplasmic; negative by membrane staining (in cell suspension).

Centrifuge at 150 *g* for 5 min and then allow the mixture to stand (without resuspension) at 4°C for 1 h. The mixture can stand overnight, if convenient.

Resuspend the cells gently and add 2 drops of 0.05% methylene blue. Fill a counting chamber and inspect 200 lymphocytes.

The E-rosette test is considered to be positive when three or more SRBC are bound to a lymphocyte (Fig. 10.7). With normal T-lymphocytes, six or more SRBC are usually bound. It is important to visualize a lymphocyte in the centre of a rosette and to distinguish between rosetting and agglutination of SRBC.

Table 10.5   Markers in mature T-cell leukaemias*

Marker (McAb)	T-CLL	T-PLL	ATLL	Sézary
CD2/E rosettes	+ +	+ +	+ +	+
CD3(OKT3)**	+ +	+ +	+ +	+ +
CD4(OKT6)	−	+ + to −	+ +	+ +
CD5(UCHT2)	−	+ +	+ +	+ +
CD7(3A1)	−	+ +	−	−
CD8(OKT8)	+ +	+ to −	−	−
CD11b(OKM1)	− to +	−	−	−
Leu7	− to +	−	−	−
CD16(Leu11)	− to +	−	−	−
CD25(anti-TAC)	−	−	+ +	− to +

*All cases TdT −, CD1a −; B-markers (−); HLA-Dr may be positive in some cases.
**Membrane and cytoplasm.

AET treatment of SRBC

AET. 2-aminoethyl*iso*thiouronium bromide. Dissolve 400 mg of AET in 10 ml of water and adjust the pH to 9.0 with 4 mol/l NaOH. The AET solution should be prepared immediately before use.

AET-treated SRBC. Add 1 volume of packed washed SRBC to 4 volumes of AET and incubate the mixture for 15 min at 37°C. Then wash the cells three times in saline and prepare finally a 1% suspension of the cells in TC 199 (e.g. 0.1 ml of washed packed SRBC in 10 ml of TC 199).

The AET-treated SRBC can be kept at 4°C for 5–7 days before use.

Mouse RBC (M) rosettes[18,24,85]

The principle of this test is similar to that of the E-rosette test. Mouse RBC are freshly drawn by cardiac puncture from a laboratory mouse, e.g. CBA strain. One ml of blood is added to 1 ml of 32 g/l trisodium citrate and 9 ml of saline. These cells have to be used within 3 days. The best results in B-CLL (Table 10.6) are obtained when lymphocytes of normal peripheral blood (5–10%) form M-rosettes. A high percentage of B-CLL cells (usually over 50%, up to 90%) react similarly. This finding is useful for distinguishing B-CLL from other B-cell lymphoproliferative disorders (Table 10.6) in which the percentages of M-rosettes are low or zero. For unknown reasons, even in B-CLL, the percentages of cells giving M-rosettes are lower in bone-marrow samples;[24] and the differences shown in Table 10.6 are only seen in peripheral blood samples. Despite the high specificity of M-rosettes for the diagnosis of B-CLL, the test is currently used less often than in the past because it is now possible to characterize the B-lymphocyte of B-CLL by means of several McAb, such as CD5 (+ reaction), FMC7 (− reaction), and by the intensity of the surface membrane immunoglobulin (SmIg) staining (± reaction) (Table 10.6).

IMMUNOFLUORESCENCE TESTS

In general, to detect cellular antigens, antibodies conjugated with fluorescein*iso*thiocyanate (FITC) or tetra-ethylrhodamine*iso*thiocyanate (TRITC) are used. For details of the methods used to demonstrate antigens in immature haemopoietic cells and some blast cells, e.g. the common-ALL antigen, see Greaves et al,[37] and Janossy.[46] A method for SmIg is described below. Most mature B-cells fluoresce with anti-SmIg sera (Table 10.6). In the B-lymphoproliferative disorders, the degree of positivity (intensity of immunofluorescence) can help to distinguish the various conditions.

While the presence of SmIg is looked for with viable cells in suspension, CyIg (cytoplasmic immunoglobulin) is looked for in cells fixed on a slide, usually prepared by means of a cytocentrifuge (Cytospin). A good fluorescent microscope equipped with incident illumination and an appropriate filter system is essential.

DEMONSTRATION OF SURFACE MEMBRANE IMMUNOGLOBULINS (SmIg) BY FLUORESCENT ANTIBODY STAINING

Reagents

Acetate buffered saline, pH 5.5.[46] Add 8.8 ml of 0.2 mol/l (12 ml/l) glacial acetic acid to 41.2 ml of 0.2 mol/l (16.4 g/l) anhydrous sodium acetate and make the volume up to 200 ml with water. To each 200 ml add 1.8 g of NaCl and 0.2 g of anhydrous $CaCl_2$. Store in 10-ml volumes at $-20°C$.

Phosphate buffered saline (PBS), pH 7.4. See p. 538.

Azide. 0.02% sodium azide in PBS. This solution will keep for up to 1 month at 4°C without loss of potency.

Fluorescent antibodies. Preferably, use $F(ab)_2$ reagents, i.e. antibodies which have been treated with papain to destroy the Fc region. Such treatment

Table 10.6 Markers in chronic B-cell leukaemias and lymphomas*

Markers	B-CLL	B-PLL	NHL*	HCL	PCL
M-rosettes	+ +	−	− to +	− to +	−
SmIg (intensity)	±	+ +	+ +	+ +	−
CyIg**	−	− to +	−	− to +	+ +
CD19/CD20 CD24/HLA-Dr***	+ +	+ +	+ +	+ +	−
CD5	+ +	− to +	− to +	−	−
CD10	−	−	+ to −	−	− to +
CD22/FMC7	− to +	+ +	+ +	+ +	−
CD25/CD11c	−	−	−	+ +	−
anti-HC2	−	−	−	+ +	−
CD38	−	−	−	−	+ +

*Non-Hodgkin lymphomas: included here are disorders which often evolve with a leukaemia phase: follicular lymphoma (FL), intermediate (mantle zone) NHL and splenic lymphoma with circulating villous lymphocytes (SLVL). In general all these have similar markers except that FL cells are usually CD5 −, CD10 + and intermediate lymphoma cells are CD5 +, CD10±.

**Tested by IF on fixed cells; when fixed cells are tested by IP or APAAP they will detect both membrane (SmIg) and cytoplasmic (CyIg) immunoglobulin molecules.

***Pan-B markers detected by different McAb, B4 (CD1), B1 (CD20), BA1 (CD24), anti-class II MHC antigens (HLA-Dr).

leaves the F(ab)$_2$ antigen-binding fragment intact. This is essential when using rabbit antisera, although it may not be necessary with goat or sheep immunoglobulins.[46]

Pipettes. Use Eppendorf-type pipettes (e.g. Oxford sampler system) and tips and plastic tubes throughout the test.

Method

Wash the separated lymphocytes in 9 g/l NaCl (saline), and resuspend in acetate buffered saline, e.g. 0.2 ml of cell suspension (containing 1–2 × 10^6 cells) in 2 ml of buffer. Incubate the mixture at 37°C for 15 min.

Wash the cells twice in PBS and then incubate the deposited cells in 5 ml of TC 199 at 37°C for 1 h to remove cytophilic antibodies.

Centrifuge the cells, remove the supernatant and resuspend the cells in 0.2 ml of the azide solution. (The cell concentration should be 10–15 × 10^6/ml.).

Add 0.2 ml of diluted (usually 1 in 20) anti-Ig fluorescent conjugated antiserum. Mix the cell suspension well and allow to stand at 4°C or (preferably) in crushed ice for 30 min. Then top up the tube containing the cell suspension with TC 199 and centrifuge for 5 min at 40 **g** (to remove unbound conjugates). Discard the supernatant and wash the deposited cells twice in PBS.

Remove the supernatant and add to the deposited cells 1 drop of a mixture of equal volumes of PBS and glycerol.* Resuspend the cells and place 1 drop on a slide; cover with a cover-slip and seal with nail varnish.

Examine under the fluorescent microscope.

TERMINAL TRANSFERASE (TdT)

This remarkable DNA polymerase can be demonstrated by a biochemical assay[26] but is usually now demonstrated by an immunofluorescence test.[13,46] Both these methods give similar results[13,25,26] but the demonstration of TdT in cell nuclei by immunofluorescence is to be preferred because of its speed, simplicity and sensitivity to low numbers of cells. As shown in Table 10.4, tests for TdT are positive in all types of ALL with the exception of the rare B-ALL. Thus, it is the method of choice to distinguish ALL from AML. However, it should be noted that 15–20% of cases of AML, particularly immature forms, may show TdT activity.[47,69] On the other hand, the common-ALL antigen is almost never demonstrable in AML. By combining both methods the majority of cases of ALL can now be diagnosed confidently. If the tests for the common ALL antigents and TdT are positive the likelihood of a case being AML is remote. In our experience two sorts of AML cases may show TdT activity: in mixed (biphenotypic) ALL/AML cases the test for TdT is positive in blasts and in 30–50% of AML cases of M1 (peroxidase positive) and MO (peroxidase negative) TdT activity persists in myeloblasts. Three other situations in which the TdT assay gives useful information are:

1. In blast crisis of CGL, in which the TdT test is almost always positive in the lymphoblastic type of transformation (20% of cases).

2. In T-lymphoblastic lymphoma, which is the only non-Hodgkin's lymphoma with positive TdT activity.[13,37]

3. In the chronic (mature) T-cell proliferations (Table 10.5), in which TdT activity is always absent, contrasting with the positive findings in acute (immature) T-cell proliferations (T-ALL, pre-T-ALL and T-lymphoblastic lymphoma).[23,37]

SLIDE ASSAY FOR TERMINAL DEOXYNUCLEOTIDYL TRANSFERASE (TdT)

Reagents

*Anti-TdT.*** For use, dilute 1 in 10 in phosphate buffered saline (PBS), pH 7.4 (p. 538).

Fluorescent-conjugated (FITC) goat anti-rabbit Ig serum. For use, dilute 1 in 10 in phosphate buffered saline. (Rhodamine-conjugated antibodies and porcine anti-rabbit Ig may be used instead of the goat antiserum.)

---

*To reduce fading during examination the following alternative mixture has been recommended.[49] Add 10 ml of PBS containing 10 mg of p-phenylenediamine to 90 ml of glycerol. Adjust the pH to 8.0 with 0.5 mol/l carbonate bicarbonate buffer, pH 9.0.
**This can be purchased from Bethesda Research Laboratories In. (USA) or Sera Lab (UK).

Mounting medium. Glycerol 48 ml, PBS 48 ml, formalin 4 ml.

Method

Make cytocentrifuge (Cytospin) preparations, using 250 µl of a 1 × 10⁶/ml cell suspension per slide. Centrifuge for 1 min at 300 rpm (*c* 7 *g*) and allow the film to dry in the air. Ring the deposited cells with a wax pencil.

Such slides may be stored at room temperature for up to a week but it is preferable to carry out the test as soon as possible.

Fix the film in methanol for 15 min at 4°C. Then wash in PBS for 10 min in a jar provided with a magnetic stirrer. Wipe off the excess PBS around the ring of cells and cover the ring with 10 µl of the diluted anti-TdT serum. Leave for 10 min at room temperature in a moist chamber.

Wash the slides in PBS for a further 15 min using a magnetic stirrer as before.

Wipe off the excess PBS around the ring of cells and cover the cells with 10 µl of the diluted fluorescent-conjugated anti-rabbit Ig serum. Allow to stand for 30 min at room temperature in a moist chamber.

Wash the slide in PBS for 15 min at room temperature, as before; then cover the ring of cells with a cover-glass, using as mountant the glycerol/PBS/formalin mixture.

Examine under the fluorescent microscope. A positive reaction is denoted by nuclear fluorescence. Using the appropriate filters, this will be bright yellow with fluorescein conjugation and bright red with rhodamine conjugation.

Controls

Negative. Carry out the test leaving out the anti-TdT and also on cells known not to react (e.g. B-CLL cells).

Positive. Use a common-ALL cell line (e.g. NALM-1) or cells from a patient with known common-ALL who is not in remission.

MONOCLONAL ANTIBODIES (McAbs)

A significant development in the last few years has been the possibility of producing antibodies of great purity by means of the hydridoma technology. The principles of their preparation have been reviewed by Janossy.[46] A great number of reagents reactive with antigens present on haemopoietic cells are now available. Their major applications have been in defining the stages of T- and B-cell differentiation, from early T- and B-cells to mature (peripheral-blood) lymphocytes. The order of appearance of antigens (on the cell membrane unless specified) in the T-cell lineage is as follows: CD3 (cytoplasm), CD7, CD5, CD2 (E-rosette receptor), CD1a (cortical thymocyte antigen), CD(T4), CD8(T8) and CD3 (membrane).[23,46,72] Equivalent findings in the B-cell lineage are as follows: CD19, CD24, CyIg (µ chain only), CD10, CD20, M-rosette receptor, SmIg (heavy and light chains) and FMC7.[35-37,46,64,74] When applied to the diagnosis of acute lymphoblastic leukaemia (ALL) of B- and T-cell lineage (Table 10.4), the combined findings with McAb characterize certain types of ALL and also indicate both the direction (B or T) and the stage of differentiation of the lymphoblasts. For example, the presence of the common-ALL antigen, a glycoprotein of 100 kD demonstrable by McAb of the CD10 group[35,46,74] is used to define common-ALL. On the other hand, the presence of the antigen demonstrable by CD1a (OKT6) characterizes cortical thymocytes and the cells of T-lymphoblastic lymphoma which arise from that particular stage of thymic maturation.

Recently it has been possible to develop McAb with specificity for myeloid cells which are useful for the study of early AML. Thus, early myeloid antigens are characterized by McAbs of the CD13[29,32,38] and CD33[29,32] groups (Table 10.7). In addition, McAb with specificity for platelet

Table 10.7 Cell markers in AML

McAb	M0*	M1	M2/M3	M4/M5	M6	M7
CD34(3C5)	+	+	± to −	± to −	−	±
CD13(MCS2)**	+	+	+	+	+	+
CD33(MY9)	±	+	+	+	±	+
CD11b(OKM1)	−	−	+	±	−	−
CD14(FMC17)	−	−	−	+	−	−
Glycoph/Gero	−	−	−	−	+	−
CDw41/42	−	−	−	−	−	+
TdT***	− to +	− to +	−	−	−	−

*Undifferentiated myeloblastic leukaemia with negative light microscopy cytochemistry for AML, absence of lymphoid antigens, and positive peroxidase by electron microscopy.
**More sensitive when tested on fixed cells (cytoplasmic expression).[29]
***Positive in up to 50% of M0 and M1 cases, and in less than 10% in other types (M2 to M7).[69]

glycoproteins[88] are used to characterize megakaryoblasts and other platelet-precursor cells.[28]

Instructions for using McAb are usually provided by the manufacturers. The antigens are demonstrated by indirect IF (fluorescence microscopy or flow cytometry) or by staining fixed cells by the immunoperoxidase (IP)[29] or alkaline phosphatase anti-alkaline phosphatase (APAAP)[30] methods. The APAAP method is suitable for use on blood and bone marrow films and allows good preservation of cell morphology. The IF methods are quicker and simpler and flow cytometry allows rapid and accurate counting of thousands of cells. The McAb, a mouse antibody of IgG or IgM class, is used as the first layer, the second layer is an FITC or TRIC conjugated anti-mouse Ig, prepared in goats or rabbits. The use of F(ab$_2$) fragments of antibody in the second layer is recommended in order to prevent non-specific binding of the Fc portion of the Ig molecule to high affinity Fc receptors. When testing myeloid cells it is also important to block non-specific binding of the Fc portion of the McAb (first layer) by pre-incubation of the cells in 0.5% of human AB serum.[29,61] The method we use for the demonstration of membrane antigens by IF with McAb is given below.

METHOD FOR TESTING McAb ON CELL SUSPENSIONS BY IF

1. Isolate mononuclear cells using Lymphoprep (see p. 141).
2. Wash twice in phosphate buffer saline (PBS) (p. 538) or Hanks solution.
3. Remove all supernatant.
4. Resuspend the cells in the buffer: PBS containing 0.2% sodium azide (azide) and 0.2% bovine serum albumin (BSA) or Hanks solution.
5. Place in small tube: 50 μl of cells (total 2×10^6); add first layer of McAb (the amount varies with each McAb)*
6. Keep for 30 min at 4°C or 10 min at room temperature (c 20°C).
7. Wash twice in PBS-azide-BSA (see 4 above).
8. Remove all supernatant.
9. Add 50 μl of PBS-azide-BSA and as second layer 50 μl of FITC F(ab$_2$) fragment of goat antimouse IgG.**
10. Keep for 30 min at 4°C or 10 min at c 20°C.
11. Wash twice in PBS-azide-BSA.
12. Remove all supernatant.
13. Add 1 drop of PBS/glycerol (50:50).
14. Mount on glass slide and cover with cover-slip.
15. Seal with nail varnish.

---

*McAb-Mouse Ig against specific antigenic determinants. The amount of McAb to be used will depend on the reagent tested.
**The reagent for the second layer is usually conjugated with fluorescein (FITC); rhodamine (TRITC) labelled antibodies may, however, also be used. The use of F(ab$_2$) fragments, as opposed to whole antibody molecules, is to prevent non-specific binding of the second layer to cells with high affinity Fc receptors (e.g. monocytes), thus resulting in a false positive test which could be detected by a positive control when the McAb (first layer) is omitted.

It is important to set up a control with the McAb and preferably also with mouse ascitic fluid (without antibody activity against human antigens) of the same Ig isotype as that of the McAb used.

TESTS ON FIXED CELLS

Ig, McAb and TdT can be stained for on fixed cells by immunocytochemical methods. Those most commonly used are the immunoperoxidase (IP) and the APAAP techniques.[30] They are more elaborate and slower than IF on cell suspensions but have, on the other hand, several practical advantages. Films (Cytospin or hand-spread) can be stored unfixed at −20°C (the slides being covered in foil) and the tests can be performed in batches immediately or days or even weeks after the sample is obtained, if that is required. They also provide permanent preparations and allow good comparison with the equivalent film stained with May-Grünwald-Giemsa. Thus with mixed preparations of cells, e.g. blasts and normal cells, it is possible to identify which cells are positive or negative.

IP is simpler than APAAP and is useful for the study of lymphoid cells (mature and immature) but it may present problems when studying bone-marrow samples that contain myeloid cells with endogenous peroxidase, which may give a false positive reaction unless precautions to inhibit its activity are taken. These measures often affect cell morphology and thus defeat one of the purposes of the test. The IP method can be carried out with directly labelled antibodies (e.g. anti-human Ig) or more often by indirect methods using two or three layers. The first layer is a McAB (mouse Ig); the second layer is an anti-mouse Ig antibody conjugated with horse radish peroxidase; a third layer, a complex of peroxidase anti-peroxidase which binds to the second layer, can be used to reinforce the reaction. The reaction is completed by testing for peroxidase using diaminobenzidine (DAB).

The APAAP method involves several steps but the end results are quite satisfactory for peripheral blood and bone-marrow films. The stages include: incubation with the McAb, incubation with a rabbit anti-mouse Ig, and incubation with immune complexes of alkaline phosphatase and anti-alkaline phosphatase (APAAP). The second and third steps can be repeated to reinforce the reaction.

THE IMMUNOLOGICAL CLASSIFICATION OF LEUKAEMIA

The use of immunological methods, in particular McAbs, has improved the possibility of classifying more objectively the acute leukaemias in which the cells are too poorly differentiated to be characterized by morphology and cytochemistry. It has also enabled the lymphoproliferative disorders to be classified more precisely because B- and T-cells and their subsets can be defined by marker studies.

ALL

The immunological classification of ALL is summarized in Table 10.4. It is important to remember that some antigens appear first in the cytoplasm (CD3 in T-blasts and CD22 in B-lineage blasts) and will not be detected when testing the cells in suspension. Similarly, in early myeloid cells CD13 is expressed first in the cytoplasm before the membrane.[29]

There are two major lineages in the lymphoid system and lymphoblastic leukaemias will therefore arise from early B- or T- precursor cells. Table 10.4 illustrates that only a few McAb react positively with the most immature lymphoblasts; with maturation, however, more McAbs react. Thus to demonstrate all cases of a particular lineage it is important to include in the battery of McAbs used those which will detect the most immature cells. In B-lineage ALL these are CD19 and CD22 (cytoplasmic), in T-lineage ALL they are CD7 and CD3 (cytoplasmic) and with myeloid cells CD13 (cytoplasmic) and CD33. The expression of the antigens reacting with the two anti-myeloid reagents often correlates with the expression of myeloperoxidase detectable at the ultrastructural level.[61] Several reagents are particularly needed in cases with mixed lymphoblastic and myeloblastic proliferations and in the so-called biphenotypic acute leukaemias in which antigens denoting one lineage are found in the cells of another. Both types of apparent lineage infidelity may represent the proliferation of multipotent stem cells[34] with potential for differentiation in several directions.

T-cell leukaemias (Tables 10.3 and 10.5)

Proliferating mature T-lymphocytes are always TdT and CD1a negative.[23] Cells with these characteristics are found in T-CLL (large granular lymphocytes), in T-PLL (prolymphocytes) and with so-called leukaemia-lymphoma syndromes like Sézary syndrome and adult leukaemia/lymphoma (ATLL), a disorder associated with the human retrovirus HTLV-1.[23] These disorders share common antigens (markers), but there are differences that can be exploited for differential diagnosis.

B-cell leukaemias (Table 10.6)

The malignant proliferations of mature (differentiated) B-lymphocytes are the chronic B-cell leukaemias: B-CLL, B-PLL and HCL and non-Hodgkin lymphomas (NHL) which often evolve with peripheral blood and/or bone marrow involvement (leukaemic phase). As stated above, the membrane phenotype of B-CLL is different from that of the other B-cell disorders and this facilitates the more precise characterization of this disease which is the most common form of leukaemia in adults over the age of 50 years.

AML (Table 10.7)

In recent years a number of McAb with specificity for myeloid cells have become available. When used in combination with some of the lymphoid markers (to exclude ALL), they show a pattern which may be characteristic of some types of AML and which may complement the FAB classification. For example antibodies to glycophorin A or the Gerbich blood group (McAb Ge) help to characterize the immature erythroblasts of M6; and McAbs against platelet glycoproteins[88] are useful for the diagnosis of M7 (megakaryoblastic) leukaemia and megakaryoblastic blast crisis in CGL. CD34 (McAb 3C5 or My10) reacts with early precursor cells, the antigen being expressed as in immature AML (MO, M1) and B-lineage but not T-lineage ALL.

In general, it is not necessary to apply all the tests suggested in Tables 10.4 to 10.7, but it is useful to select pairs of reagents which are useful for immature B-cells (CD19, CD10), T-cells (CD7, CD3 cyt.), mature T-cells (CD4, CD8), mature B-cells (SmIg, HLA-Dr) and, depending on the findings, to extend the number of tests as required, according to the diagnostic problem.

DEMONSTRATION OF CHROMOSOMES

The demonstration of human chromosome abnormalities has become a subject of increasing importance in clinical haematology. Description of how to obtain adequate mitosis and of the various methods of chromosome banding (Q: quinacrine mustard; G: Giemsa stain; R: reverse banding pattern) are beyond the scope of this book. Details can be found in the references at the end of this chapter.[78,87,92,96]

For analysis, chromosomes are usually studied in mitoses arrested at metaphase by the addition of colchicine, demecolcine or vinblastine. Bone-marrow aspirates provide the best material for study in cases of leukaemia; peripheral blood may be adequate when the leucocyte count is very high, particularly in CGL. Blood lymphocytes should be studied simultaneously to define the normal constitutional karyotype. This is done by short-term culture with the mitogen phytohaemagglutinin (PHA).

Since the discovery of the Philadelphia (Ph[1]) chromosome, due to the translocation of material from the long arm (q) of chromosome 22 (22q −) to the long arm of chromosomes 9 (9q +), numerous haemopoietic malignancies have been found to be associated with specific abnormalities. These are summarized in Table 10.8.

The abnormalities in a karyotype may be numerical, e.g. trisomy (an extra chromosome) or mono-

Table 10.8 Non-random,* acquired⁺ chromosome abnormalities in haemopoietic malignancies[32,79,80,89,92,96-98]

Disease	Abnormality
I. Acute leukaemia	
i) ALL	
B-lineage	t(9;22)**; t(4;11); 6q − ; t(1;19)
Burkitt type (L3, B-ALL)	t(8;14); t(2;8); t(8;22)
T-lineage	t or del (9); t(11;14) 6q −
ii) AML	+ 8
M2	t(8;21)
M3 and M3-variant	t(15;17)
M4***	Inv or del (16q)
M5	t or del (11q)
M2 with basophilia	t(6;9)
II. Chronic leukaemias/NHL	
i) Lymphoid	
B-CLL	+ 12
B-PLL	t(11;14)
Follicular NHL	t(14;18)
Mantle zone	+ 12; t(11;14)
T-PLL	inv (14q)
ii) CGL	t(9;22)
Blast crisis	iso(17); + 8; + 19
III. MDS/RAEB****	− 5,5q − , − 7,7q −

*Present in the majority of the abnormal metaphases.
+ Present in the leukaemic cell population but not in normal cells (e.g. T-lymphocytes, fibroblasts, etc.).
**Ph[1] + ALL.
***Myelomonocytic leukaemic with bone marrow eosinophilia (10%).
****Refractory anaemia with excess of blasts.

somy (only one chromosome of the pair), or structural. The modal number of chromosomes, 46 in man, may be less than 46 (hypodiploid) or more than 46 (hyperdiploid). For example, a hyperdiploid karyotype (47 chromosomes or more) is seen in 23% of children with ALL.[89,92] A modal chromosome number greater than 50 is associated with the best prognosis in childhood ALL.[89]

Marker chromosomes are structurally abnormal chromosomes in banded or unbanded karyotypes. When the banding pattern can be recognized it should be described by the standard nomenclature.[73] Non-random abnormalities refer to consistent changes seen in a particular cell population which are unlikely to have occurred by chance. A clone refers to a population of cells, presumably derived from a single progenitor cell, which is characterized by the same marker chromosome(s).

The karyotype of the bone-marrow cells of a particular leukaemia (e.g. AML) may show that all the metaphases are abnormal(AA), or that some are

normal and others abnormal (AN), or that all the metaphases are normal (NN). AA suggests that no normal cells are present and has usually a bad prognosis.[78,80] AN represents a mixture of normal and leukaemic cells; recent studies suggest that examination of mitotic figures after 24–48 h culture may yield more abnormal metaphases compared with direct preparations of the same material.[97] NN indicates that there are no gross abnormalities; this might mean that the method is insensitive or that only the karyotype of normal cells is being analysed rather than that of the leukaemic population.

The more sensitive techniques for the study of human chromosomes (long chromosomes, prometaphase banding) that are now becoming available may be expected to provide more information. For example, finely banded chromosome preparations can be obtained by high-resolution techniques, in particular those using culture techniques, and cell synchronization with amethopterin.

Abnormalities in the chronic lymphoid leukaemias can be obtained by stimulating the cells with specific (B or T) mitogens or non-specific mitogens (e.g. phorbolester TPA). Peripheral blood samples from patients with these leukaemias are usually sufficient to document abnormalities. In the acute leukaemias the material of choice is bone marrow.

NUCLEAR SEXING OF LEUCOCYTES

Sex chromosome anomalies are not uncommon and they can usually be identified readily by nuclear sexing. Buccal mucosa is the material usually examined but in experienced hands valuable information can also be gained by inspection of the neutrophil leucocytes. The feature to be identified is a nuclear appendage, the drumstick, which is present in a proportion of the neutrophils of normal females but not of normal males. The drumstick represents one X chromosome and is equivalent to the single Barr body which may be seen in normal (XX) female cell nuclei.

Method

Make blood films, stain them and cover with a cover-glass in the usual way. Then scan them systematically with an oil-immersion lens for drumsticks of the correct size and staining quality. The use of a micrometer ocular may be necessary to measure the drumsticks.

The drumsticks are pedunculated nuclear appendages, with a spherical or oval head of between 1.4 and 1.6 µm in diameter, formed of densely staining chromatin attached by a thread-like neck to the rest of the nucleus (Fig. 10.8). Very often a small space or chink can be seen in the chromatin of the head of the drumstick. These sex drumsticks have to be distinguished from non-specific nodules which may be of smaller or larger size, irregular in shape, and sometimes deficient in chromatin. Sessile chromatin sex nodules of the same size as drumsticks may also be seen; they stain densely and project by more than half their diameter beyond the nuclear membrane (Fig. 10.8). They also occur only in females, but they are less easily distinguished from other non-specific nodules and appendages which have no diagnostic significance.

As a screening test, scrutinize at least 50 neutrophils for drumsticks (and sessile nodules). In females, three or more definite sessile nodules and one or more drumsticks are usually seen in the first

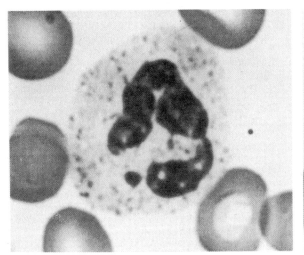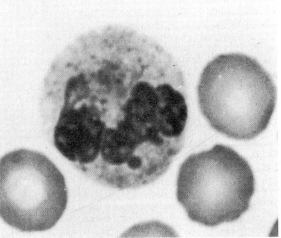

Fig. 10.8 Nuclear sexing of neutrophils. Photomicrographs of neutrophils showing female sex appendages. The left-hand cell has a 'drumstick'; the right-hand cell has a sessile nodule.

50 cells. On the other hand, in males no drumsticks and no definite sessile nodules should be seen. If there is any doubt, examine further cells, and if at least two definite drumsticks and accompanying sessile nodules are identified in the first 500 cells, it can reliably be assumed that the cells are chromatin-positive and the subject female (XX). Usually at least six definite drumsticks are found in

less than 200 neutrophils. If neither drumsticks nor sessile nodules are seen in the first 200 neutrophils, the cells can be regarded as chromatin-negative and the subject male (XY) or XO. When there is a shift to the left in the segmentation of the neutrophil nuclei it is more difficult to arrive at a clear-cut answer, and it may be necessary to examine many more cells.

REFERENCES

[1] ARCHER, G. T., AIR, G., JACKAS, M. and MORELL, D. B. (1965). Studies on rat eosinophil peroxidase. *Biochimica et Biophysica Acta*, **99**, 96.

[2] BAIN, B. J., CATOVSKY, D., O'BRIEN, M., PRENTICE, H. G., LAWLOR, E., KUMARAN, T.O., McCANN, S. R., MATUTES, E. and GALTON, D. A. G. (1981). Megakaryoblastic leukaemia presenting as acute myelofibrosis. A study of four cases with the platelet-peroxidase reaction. *Blood*, **58**, 206.

[3] BAINTON, D. F., ULLVOT, J. L. and FARQUHAR, M. G. (1971). The development of neutrophilic polymorphonuclear leukocytes in human bone marrow. *Journal of Experimental Medicine*, **134**, 907.

[4] BASSO, G., COCITO, M.G., POLETTI, A., MESSINA, C., COLLESELLI, P. and ZANESCO, L. (1980). Study of cytochemical markers ACP and ANAE in childhood lymphoma and leukaemia. *British Journal of Cancer*, **41**, 835.

[5] BASSO, G., COCITO, M. G., SEMENZATO, G., PEZZUTTO, A. and ZANESCO, L. (1980). Cytochemical study of thymocytes and T lymphocytes. *British Journal of Haematology*, **44**, 577.

[6] BECKSTEAD, J. H., HALVERSON, P. S., RIES, C. A. and BAINTON, D. F. (1981). Enzyme histochemistry and immuno histochemistry on biopsy specimens of pathologic human bone marrow. *Blood*, **57**, 1088.

[7] BENAVIDES, I. and CATOVSKY, D. (1978). Myeloperoxidase cytochemistry using 2,7-fluorenediamine. *Journal of Clinical Pathology*, **31**, 1114.

[8] BENNETT, J. M., CATOVSKY, D., DANIEL, M. T., FLANDRIN, G., GALTON, D. A. G., GRALNICK, H.R. and SULTAN, C. (1976). Proposals for the classification of the acute leukaemias. *British Journal of Haematology*, **33**, 451.

[9] BENNETT, J. M., CATOVSKY, D., DANIEL, M. T., FLANDRIN, G., GALTON, D. A. G., GRALNICK, H. R. and SULTAN, C. (1981). The morphological classification of acute lymphoblastic leukaemia—concordance among observers and clinical correlations. *British Journal of Haematology*, **47**, 553.

[10] BENNETT, J. M., CATOVSKY, D., DANIEL, M. T., FLANDRIN, G., GALTON, D. A. G., GRALNICK, H. R. and SULTAN, C. (1982). Proposals for the classification of the myelodysplastic syndromes. *British Journal of Haematology*, **51**, 189.

[11] BENNETT, J. M., CATOVSKY, D., DANIEL, M. T., FLANDRIN, G., GALTON, D. A. G., GRALNICK, H. R. and SULTAN, C.(1985). Proposed revised criteria for the classification of acute myeloid leukemia. *Annals of Internal Medicine*, **103**, 620.

[12] BENNETT, J. M., CATOVSKY, D., DANIEL, M. T., FLANDRIN, G., GALTON, D. A. G., GRALNICK, H. R. and SULTAN, C. (1985). Criteria for the diagnosis of acute leukemia of

megakaryocyte lineage (M7). A report of the French-American-British Cooperative Group. *Annals of Internal Medicine*, **103**, 460.

[13] BOLLUM, F. J. (1979). Terminal deoxynucleotidyl transferase as a hematopoietic cell marker. *Blood*, **54**, 1203.

[14] BRETON-GORIUS, J., GOURDIN, M. F. and REYES, F. (1981). Ultrastructure of the leukemic cell. In *The Leukemic Cell*. Ed. D. Catovsky, Chapter 4. Churchill Livingstone, Edinburgh.

[15] BRIGGS, R. S., PERILLIE, P. E. and FINCH, S. C. (1966). Lysozyme in bone marrow and peripheral blood cells. *Journal of Histochemistry and Cytochemistry*, **14**, 167.

[16] BRITO-BABAPULLE, F., CATOVSKY, D. and GALTON, D.A.G. (1987). Clinical and laboratory features of de novo acute myeloid leukaemia with trilineage myelodysplasia. *British Journal of Haematology*, **66**, 445.

[17] CATOVSKY, D., CHERCHI, M., GREAVES, M. F., PAIN, C., JANOSSY, G. and KAY, H. E. M. (1978). The acid phosphatase reaction in acute lymphoblastic leukaemia. *Lancet* i, 749.

[18] CATOVSKY, D., CHERCHI, M., OKOS, A., HEGDE, U. and GALTON, D.A.G. (1976). Mouse red cell rosettes in B-lymphoproliferative disorders. *British Journal of Haematology*, **33**, 173.

[19] CATOVSKY, D., CROCKARD A. D., MATUTES, E. and O'BRIEN, M. (1981). Cytochemistry of leukaemic cells. In *Histochemistry: the Widening Horizons*. Eds. P. J. Stoward and J. M. Polak, Chapter 6. John Wiley & Sons, Chichester.

[20] CATOVSKY, D., GALETTO, J., OKOS, A., MILLANI, E. and GALTON, D. A. G. (1974). Cytochemical profile of B and T leukaemic lymphocytes with special reference to acute lymphoblastic leukaemia. *Journal of Clinical Pathology*, **27**, 767.

[21] CATOVSKY, D. and GALTON, D. A. G. (1973). Lysozyme activity and nitroblue-tetrazolium reduction in leukaemic cells. *Journal of Clinical Pathology*, **26**, 60.

[22] CATOVSKY, D., GALTON, D. A. G. and ROBINSON, J. (1972). Myeloperoxidase-deficient neutrophils in acute myeloid leukaemia. *Scandinavian Journal of Haematology*, **9**, 142.

[23] CATOVSKY, D., LINCH, D. C. and BEVERLEY, P. C. L. (1982). T-cell disorders in haematological diseases. *Clinics in Haematology*, **11**, 661.

[24] CHERCHI, M. and CATOVSKY, D. (1980). Mouse RBC rosettes in chronic lymphocytic leukaemia—different expression in blood and tissues. *Clinical and Experimental Immunology*, **39**, 411.

[25] CIBULL, M. L., COLEMAN, M. S., NELSON, O., HUTTON, J. J., GORDON, D. and BOLLUM, F.J. (1982). Evaluation of methods of detecting terminal deoxynucleotidyl transferase

in human hematologic malignancies. *American Journal of Clinical Pathology*, **77**, 420.

[26] COLEMAN, M. S. and HUTTON, J. J. (1981). Terminal transferase. In *The Leukemic Cell*. Ed. D. Catovsky, p. 203. Churchill Livingstone, Edinburgh.

[27] CROCKARD, A. D., CHALMERS, D., MATUTES, E. and CATOVSKY, D. (1982). Cytochemistry of acid hydrolases in chronic B and T cell leukemias. *American Journal of Clinical Pathology*, **78**, 437.

[28] de OLIVEIRA, M.S.P., GREGORY, C., MATUTES, E., PARREIRA, A. and CATOVSKY, D. (1987). Cytochemical profile of megakaryoblastic leukaemia: a study with cytochemical methods, monoclonal antibodies, and ultrastructural cytochemistry. *Journal of Clinical Pathology*, **40**, 663.

[29] de OLIVEIRA, M. S. P., MATUTES, E., RANI, S., MORILLA, R. and CATOVSKY, D. (1988). Early expression of MCS2 (CD13) in the cytoplasm of blast cells from acute myeloid leukaemia. *Acta Haematologica* (Basel), **80**, 61.

[30] ERBER, W. N., MYNHEER, L. C. and MASON, D. Y. (1986). APAAP labelling of blood and bone-marrow samples for phenotyping leukaemia. *Lancet*, **i**, 761.

[31] FAIRBANKS, V. F. and LAMPE, L. T. (1968). A tetrazolium-linked cytochemical method for estimation of glucose-6-phosphate dehydrogenase activity in individual erythrocytes: applications in the study of heterozygotes for glucose-6-phosphate dehydrogenase deficiency. *Blood*, **31**, 589.

[32] FIRST MIC COOPERATIVE STUDY GROUP (1986). Morphologic, immunologic and cytogenetic (MIC) working classification of acute lymphoblastic leukemias. *Cancer Genetics and Cytogenetics*, **23**, 189.

[33] GOLDBERG, A. F. and BARKA, T. (1962). Acid phosphatase activity in human blood cells. *Nature* (London), **195**, 297.

[34] GREAVES, M. F., CHAN, L. C., FURLEY, A. J. W., WATT, S. M. and MOLGAARD, H. V. (1986). Lineage promiscuity in hemopoietic differentiation and leukemia. *Blood*, **67**, 1.

[35] GREAVES, M. F., HARIRI, G., NEWMAN, R. A., SUTHERLAND, D. R., RITTER, M. A., and RITZ, J. (1983). Selective expression of the common acute lymphoblastic leukemia (gp 100) antigen on immature lymphoid cells and their malignant counterparts. *Blood*, **61**, 628.

[36] GREAVES, M. F., JANOSSY, G., PETO, J. and KAY. H. (1981). Immunologically defined subclasses of acute lymphoblastic leukaemia in children: their relationship to presentation features and prognosis. *British Journal of Haematology*, **48**, 179.

[37] GREAVES, M. F., RAO, J., HARIRI, G. VERBI, W., CATOVSRY, D., RUNG, P. and GOLDSTEIN, G. (1981). Phenotypic heterogeneity and cellular origins of T cell malignancies. *Leukemia Research*, **5**, 281.

[38] GRIFFIN, J. D., LINCH, D., SABBATH, K., LARCOM, P. and SCHLOSSMAN. S. F. (1984). A monoclonal antibody reactive with normal and leukaemic human myeloid progenitor cells. *Leukemia Research*, **8**, 521.

[39] HANKER, J. S., AMBROSE, W. W., JAMES, C. J. MANDELKORN, J., YATES, P. E., GALL, S. A., BOSSEN, E. H. FAY, J. W., LAZLO, J. and MOORE, J. O. (1979). Facilitated light microscopic cytochemical diagnosis of acute myelogenous leukemia. *Cancer Research*, **39**, 1635.

[40] HAYHOE, F. G. J. and QUAGLINO, D. (1960). Refractory sideroblastic anaemia and erythraemic myelosis: possible relationship and cytochemical observations. *British Journal of Haematology*, **6**, 381.

[41] HAYHOE, F. G. J. and QUAGLINO, D. (1980). *Haematological Cytochemistry*. Churchill Livingstone,Edinburgh.

[42] HAYHOE, F. G. J., QUAGLINO, D. and DOLL, R. (1964). *The Cytology and Cytochemistry of Acute Leukaemias: A study of 140 Cases*. Her Majesty's Stationery Office, London.

[43] HAYHOE, F. G. J., QUAGLINO, D. and FLEMANS, R. J. (1960). Consecutive use of Romanowsky and periodic-acid-Schiff techniques in the study of blood and bone-marrow cells. *British Journal of Haematology*, **6**, 23.

[44] HUHN, D., THIEL, E., RODT, H. and ANDREEWA, P. (1981). Cytochemistry and membrane markers in acute lymphatic leukaemia (ALL). *Scandinavian Journal of Haematology*, **26**, 311.

[45] INAGAKI, A., UNO, S., YONEDA, M. and OHKAWA, K. (1976). 2,7-fluorenediamine and 2,5-fluorenediamine as peroxidase reagents for blood smears. *Journal of Laboratory and Clinical Medicine*, **88**, 334.

[46] JANOSSY, G. (1981). Membrane markers in leukemia. In *The Leukaemic Cell*. Ed. D. Catovsky, Chapter 5. Churchill Livingstone, Edinburgh.

[47] JANOSSY, G., HOFFBRAND, A. V., GREAVES, M. F., GANESHAGURU, K., PAIN, C., BRADSTOCK, K. F., PRENTICE, W. G., RAY, H. E. M. and LISTER, T. A. (1980). Terminal transferase enzyme assay and immunological membrane markers in the diagnosis of leukaemia—a multiparameter analysis of 300 cases. *British Journal of Haematology*, **44**, 221.

[48] JOHAIS, T., DANIEL, M. T. and FLANDRIN, G. (1981). Valeur comparée des réactions à la benzidine et à l'α-naphtol pour la mise en évidence de l'activité peroxydase dans les cellules leucémiques. *Pathologie Biologie*, **29**, 189.

[49] JOHNSON, G. D. and NOQUEIRA ARAUJO, G .M. de C. (1981). A simple method of reducing the fading of immunofluorescence during microscopy. *Journal of Immunological Methods*, **43**, 349.

[50] KAMADA, N., DOHY, H., OKADA, K. OGUMA, N., KURAMOTO, A., TANARA, A. and UCHINO, H. (1981). In vivo and in vitro activity of neutrophil alkaline phosphatase in acute myelocytic leukemia with 8;21 translocation. *Blood*, **58**, 1213.

[51] KAPLAN, M. E. and CLARK, C. J. (1974). An improved rosetting assay for detection of human T-lymphocytes. *Journal of Immunological Methods*, **5**, 131.

[52] KAPLOW, L. S. (1963). Cytochemistry of leukocyte alkaline phosphatase. Use of complex naphthol AS phosphates in azo dye-coupling technics. *American Journal of Clinical Pathology*, **39**, 439.

[53] KAPLOW, L. S. (1965). Simplified myeloperoxidase stain using benzidine dihydrochloride. *Blood*, **26**, 215.

[54] KAPLOW, L. S. (1968). Leukocyte alkaline phosphatase cytochemistry: applications and methods. *Annals of New York Academy of Sciences*, **155**, 911.

[55] KULENKAMPFF, J., JANOSSY, G. and GREAVES, M. F. (1977). Acid esterase in human lymphoid cells and leukaemic blasts: marker for T lymphocytes. *British Journal of Haematology*, **36**, 235.

[56] KUNG, P. C., GOLDSTEIN, G., REINHERZ, E. L. and SCHLOSSMAN, S. F. (1979). Monoclonal antibodies defining distinctive human T cell surface antigens. *Science*, **206**, 347.

[57] LENNOX, B. and DAVIDSON, W. M. (1964). Nuclear sexing. *Association of Clinical Pathologists Broadsheet No. 47*.

[58] LEWIS, S. M. and DACIE, J. V. (1965). Neutrophil (leucocyte) alkaline phosphatase in paroxysmal nocturnal haemoglobinuria. *British Journal of Haematology*, **11**, 549.

[59] LI, C. Y., LAM, K. W. and YAM, L. T. (1973). Esterases in human leukocytes. *Journal of Histochemistry and Cytochemistry*, **21**, 1.

[60] LI, C. Y., YAM, L. T. and LAM, K. W. (1970). Acid phosphatase isoenzyme in human leukocytes in normal and pathologic conditions. *Journal of Histochemistry and Cytochemistry*, **8**, 473.

[61] MATUTES, E., de OLIVEIRA, M. P., FORONI, L., MORILLA, R. and CATOVSKY, D. (1988). The role of ultrastructural cytochemistry and monoclonal antibodies in clarifying the nature of undifferentiated cells in acute leukaemia. *British Journal of Haematology*, **69**, 205.

[62] MOLONEY, W. C., MCPHERSON, K. and FLIEGELMAN, L. (1960). Esterase activity in leukocytes demonstrated by the use of napthol AS-D chloracetate substrate. *Journal of Histochemistry and Cytochemistry*, **8**, 200.

[63] MOVER, S., LI, C. Y. and YAM, L. T. (1972). Semiquantitative evaluation of tartrate-resistant acid phosphatase activity in human blood cells. *Journal of Laboratory and Clinical Medicine*, **80**, 711.

[64] NADLER, L. M., KORSMEYER, S. J., ANDERSON, K. C., BOYD, A. W., SLAUGHENHOUPT, B., PARK, E., JENSEN, J., CORAL, F., MAYER, B. J., SALLAN, S. E., RITZ, J. and SCHLOSSMAN, S. F. (1984). B cell origin of non T cell acute lymphoblastic leukemia: a model for discrete stages of neoplastic and normal pre B-cell differentiation. *Journal of Clinical Investigation*, **74**, 332.

[65] NANBA, K., JAFFE, E. S., BRAYLAN, R. C., SOBAN, E. J. and BERARD, C. W. (1977). Alkaline phosphatase-positive malignant lymphoma—a subtype of B-cell lymphoma. *American Journal of Pathology*, **68**, 535.

[66] NICHOLS, B. A., BAINTON, D. F. and FARQUHAR, M. G. (1971). Differentiation of monocytes—origin, nature and fate of their azurophil granules. *Journal of Cell Biology*, **50**, 498.

[67] O'BRIEN, M., CATOVSKY, D. and COSTELLO, C. (1980). Ultrastructural cytochemistry of leukaemic cells: characterization of the early small granules of monoblasts. *British Journal of Haematology*, **45**, 201.

[68] OKUN, D. B. and TANAKA, K. R. (1978). Leukocyte alkaline phosphatase. *American Journal of Hematology*, **4**, 293.

[69] PARREIRA, A., de OLIVEIRA, M. S. P., MATUTES, E., FORONI, L., MORILLA, R. and CATOVSKY, D. (1988). Terminal deoxynucleotidyl transferase positive acute myeloid leukaemia: an association with immature myeloblastic leukaemia. *British Journal of Haematology*, **69**, 219.

[70] QUAGLINO, D. and HAYHOE, F. G. J. (1960). Periodic-acid-Schiff positivity in erythroblasts with special reference to Di Guglielmo's disease. *British Journal of Haematology*, **6**, 26.

[71] REED, C. E. and BENNETT, J. M. (1975). N-Acetyl-β-glucosaminidase activity in normal and malignant leukocytes. *Journal of Histochemistry and Cytochemistry*, **23**, 752.

[72] REINHERZ, E. L., KUNG, P. C., GOLDSTEIN, G., LEVEY, R. H. and SCHLOSSMAN, S. F. (1980). Discrete stages of human intrathymic differentiation: analysis of normal thymocytes and leukemia lymphocytes of T cell lineage. *Proceedings of the National Academy of Sciences*, USA, **77**, 1588.

[73] Report of the Standing Committee on Human Cytogenetic Nomenclature (1978). An international system for human cytogenetic nomenclature: ISCN, 1978. *Cytogenetics and Cell Genetics*, **21**, 309.

[74] RITZ, J., PESANDO, J. M., NOTIS-MCCONARTY, J., LAZARUS, H. and SCHLOSSMAN, S. F. (1980). A monoclonal antibody to human acute lymphocytic leukaemia. *Nature* (London), **283**, 583.

[75] ROZENSZAJN, L., LEIBOVICH, M., SHOHAM, D. and EPSTEIN, J. (1968). The esterase activity in megaloblasts, leukaemic and normal haemopoietic cells. *British Journal of Haematology*, **14**, 605.

[76] RUSTIN, G. J. S., WILSON, P. D. and PETERS, T. J. (1979). Studies on the subcellular localisation of human neutrophil alkaline phosphatase. *Journal of Cell Science*, **36**, 401.

[77] RUTENBURG, A. B., ROSALES, C. L. and BENNETT, J. M. (1965). An improved histochemical method for the demonstration of leukocyte alkaline phosphatase activity: clinical application. *Journal of Laboratory and Clinical Medicine*, **65**, 698.

[78] SANDBERG, A. A. (1980). *Chromosomes in Human Cancer and Leukemia.* Elsevier, New York.

[79] Second MIC Cooperative Study Group (1988). Morphologic, immunologic and cytogenetic (MIC) working classification of the acute myeloid leukaemias. *British Journal of Haematology*, **68**, 487.

[80] Second International Workshop on Chromosomes in Leukemia—1979 (1980). Cytogenetic, morphologic and clinical correlations in acute non-lymphocytic leukaemia with t(8q – ;21q +), *Cancer Genetics and Cytogenetics*, **2**, 99.

[81] SHEEHAN, H. L. (1939). The staining of leucocyte granules by Sudan Black B. *Journal of Pathology and Bacteriology*, **49**, 580.

[82] SHEEHAN, H. L. and STOREY, G. W. (1947). An improved method of staining leucocyte granules with Sudan Black B. *Journal of Pathology and Bacteriology*, **59**, 336.

[83] SHIBATA, A., BENNETT, J. M., CASTOLDI, G. L., CATOVSKY, D., FLANDRIN, C., JAFFE, E. S., KATAYAMA, I., NANBA, K, SCHMALZL, F., YAM, L. T. and LEWIS, S. M. [International Committee for Standardization in Haematology (ICSH)] (1985). Recommended methods for cytological procedures in haematology. *Clinical and Laboratory Haematology*, **7**, 55.

[84] SIMPSON, C. F., CARLISLE, J. W. and MALLARD, L. (1970). Rhodanile blue: a rapid and selective stain for Heinz bodies. *Stain Technology*, **45**, 221.

[85] STATHOPOULOS, G. and ELLIOTT, E. V. (1974). Formation of mouse or sheep red-blood-cell rosettes by lymphocytes from normal and leukaemic individuals. *Lancet*, **i**, 600.

[86] SYRÉN, E and RAESTE, A.-M. (1971). Identification of blood monocytes by demonstration of lysozyme and peroxidase activity. *Acta Haematologica* (Basel), **45**, 29.

[87] TESTA, J. R. and ROWLEY, J. D. (1981). Chromosomes in leukaemia and lymphoma with special emphasis on methodology. In *The Leukaemic Cell.* Ed. D. Catovsky, Chapter 6. Churchill Livingstone, Edinburgh.

[88] TETTEROO, P. A. T., LANSDORP, P. M., LEEKSMA, O. C. and von dem BORNE, A. E. G. Kr. (1983). Monoclonal antibodies against human platelet glycoprotein IIIa. *British Journal of Haematology*, **55**, 509.

[89] Third International Workshop on Chromosomes in Leukemia—1980 (1981). *Cancer Genetics and Cytogenetics*, **4**, 95.

[90] UNGERLEIDER, R. S. (Ed.) (1981). Conference on Cell Markers in Acute Leukemia. *Cancer Research*, **41**, 4749.

[91] WACHSTEIN, M. and WOLF, G. (1958). The histochemical demonstration of esterase activity in human blood and bone marrow smears. *Journal of Histochemistry and Cytochemistry*, **6**, 457.

[92] WILLIAMS, D. L., HARRIS, A., WILLIAMS, K. J., BROSIUS, M. J. and LEMONDS, W. (1984). A direct bone marrow chromosome technique for acute lymphoblastic leukemia. *Cancer Genetics and Cytogenetics,* **13,** 239.

[93] WYBRAN, J., CHANTLER, S. and FUDENBERG, H. H. (1973). Isolation of normal T-cells in chronic lymphatic leukaemia. *Lancet,* **i,** 126.

[94] YAM, L. T., LI, C. Y. and CROSBY, W. H. (1971). Cytochemical identification of monocytes and granulocytes. *American Journal of Clinical Pathology,* **55,** 283.

[95] YAM, L. T., LI, C. Y. and LAM, K. W. (1971). Tartrate-resistant acid phosphatase isoenzyme in the reticulum cells of leukemic reticuloendotheliosis. *New England Journal of Medicine,* **284,** 357.

[96] YUNIS, J. J. (1981). Chromosomes and cancer: new nomenclature and future directions. *Human Pathology,* **12,** 494.

[97] YUNIS, J. J. (1981). New chromosome techniques in the study of human neoplasia. *Human Pathology,* **12,** 540.

[98] YUNIS, J. J., OKEN, M. M., KAPLAN, M. E., ENSRUD, K. M., HOWE, R. R. and THEOLOGIDES, A. (1982). Distinctive chromosomal abnormalities in histologic subtypes of non-Hodgkin's lymphoma. *New England Journal of Medicine,* **307,** 1231.

11. Bone-marrow biopsy

Biopsy of bone marrow is an indispensible adjunct to the study of diseases of the blood and may be the only way in which a correct diagnosis can be made. Marrow can be obtained by needle aspiration, percutaneous trephine biopsy or surgical biopsy. *Needle biopsy* is simple, safe and relatively painless, and it can be repeated many times and performed on out-patients. It seems to be safe in almost all circumstances, even in thrombocytopenic purpura. However, it should never be attempted when there is a major disorder of coagulation as in haemophilia without appropriate cover and checking by coagulation factor assay. *Trephine biopsy*, using a 'microtrephine', is a little less simple, but it too can be performed on out-patients.

The disadvantage of aspiration biopsy is that the arrangement of the cells in the marrow and the relationship between one cell and another are more or less destroyed by the process of aspiration, and in fibrotic marrows little but blood may be aspirated. On the other hand, when marrow is aspirated, individual cells are perfectly preserved in well made films and, after staining, subtle differences between cells can be recognized usually to a far greater degree than is possible with sectioned material. If present, particles of aspirated marrow can be concentrated and subsequently sectioned and this allows the structure of small pieces of marrow to be studied. The great value of microtrephine biopsy is that it can provide a perfect view of the structure of relatively large pieces of marrow—that is, if the material obtained by the biopsy has been skilfully processed. At the same time morphological features of individual cells may be identified by making an imprint or a smear from the material obtained.

Microtrephines of 2 mm bore or less can be inserted into the sternum, vertebral spines or iliac crest; the larger trephines should only be inserted into the iliac crest. Studies on large numbers of cases have demonstrated that, whereas microtrephine-biopsy specimens are superior to films of aspirated material in some circumstances, e.g. for diagnosing marrow involvement by lymphoma or non-haematological neoplastic diseases, the simple procedure of aspiration marrow biopsy seldom fails to provide important information in patients who have a blood disease.[11,20,42] Both techniques have an important and complementary role in their investigation.

NEEDLE (ASPIRATION) BIOPSY OF THE BONE MARROW

Satisfactory samples of bone marrow can be aspirated from the sternum, iliac crest or anterior or posterior iliac spines and from the spinous processes of the lumbar vertebrae, and in children aged <2 yr from the upper end of the tibia. The iliac spines have the advantage that if no material is aspirated a microtrephine biopsy can be performed immediately. These sites may, however, be difficult in obese subjects, and puncture of the sternum is still frequently undertaken.

Puncture of the sternum

The usual site for puncture is the manubrium or the first or second pieces of the body of the sternum. The manubrium is formed of rather denser bone than the body of the sternum, and, in elderly subjects at least, it tends to contain more fatty marrow than is found elsewhere in the sternum.[12] It is also sometimes less easy to be certain that the needle point has reached the cavity of the bone. However, completely satisfactory samples are obtained more often than not from the manubrium. If serial punctures are being performed, a different site should be selected for each, in order to avoid marrow possibly disorganized by haemorrhage resulting from previous punctures.

Only needles designed for the purpose should be used. They should be stout and made of hard stainless steel, about 7–8 cm in length, with a well-fitting stilette, and must be provided with an adjustable guard. The point of the needle and the edge of the bevel must be kept well sharpened. The most commonly used ones are the Salah and the Klima needles (Fig. 11.1). The patient lies on his back in a semi-recumbent position and the skin covering the upper part of the sternum is cleaned with 70% alcohol (e.g. ethanol) or 0.5% chlorhexidine (5% diluted 1 in 10 in ethanol). If hairy, the site must be shaved. The skin, subcutaneous tissue and periosteum overlying the site selected for the puncture are carefully infiltrated with a local anaesthetic such as 2% lignocaine.

If the manubrium is selected, the site of the puncture should be about 1 cm above the sterno-manubrial angle and slightly to one side of the

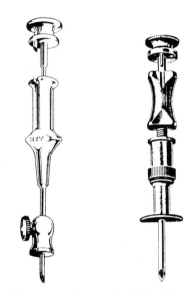

Fig. 11.1   Marrow-puncture needles. Salah (left) and Klima (right). (reduced × 3/4.

mid-line; if the body of the bone is to be punctured, this should be done opposite the second or third intercostal spaces slightly to one side of the mid-line.

Puncture the skin and pierce the subcutaneous tissues. When the needle-point reaches the periosteum, adjust the guard on the needle to allow it to penetrate for about 5 mm further, and fix the guard tightly in position. Then push the needle with a boring motion into the cavity of the bone. The amount of force required varies, but may need to be considerable. It is usually easy to appreciate when the cavity of the bone has been entered. Then remove the stilette and with a well fitting 2 or 5 ml syringe suck up not more than 0.3 ml of marrow contents. —bone marrow diluted with a variable amount of blood. As a rule, material can be sucked into the syringe without difficulty; occasionally it may be necessary to re-insert the stilette and to push the needle in a little further and to suck again.

Make films from some of the aspirated material without delay (see p. 160). The remainder of the material may then be delivered into a suitable fixative for the preparation of histological sections (see p. 160). Fix some of the films in absolute methanol as soon as they are dry for subsequent staining by a Romanowsky method or by PAS or for iron. Further films should be fixed in formal-ethanol if other cytochemical staining is to be carried out (p. 126). If there has been a 'dry tap', insert the stilette into the needle and push any material in the lumen of the needle on to a slide; in lymphomas and carcinomas, especially, sufficient material may be obtained to make a diagnosis.[14]

Puncture of the ilium

The iliac crest is another site from which active marrow may be withdrawn. Pass the needle perpendicularly into the cavity of the ilium at a point just posterior to the anterior superior iliac spine or 2 cm posterior and 2 cm inferior to the anterior superior iliac spine. As with spinous-process puncture the bone is often appreciably harder to pierce than is the sternum. The anterior superior iliac spine can also be punctured. It may be easier to locate in very obese individuals and the bone overlying it is said to be thinner than that of the iliac crest.[32]

The posterior iliac spine overlies a large marrow-containing area and relatively large volumes of marrow can be aspirated from this site.[8] An advantage of puncturing the ilium is that the patient can lie on his side and cannot see what is happening, and several attempts at puncture and aspiration can be made, if necessary, in the same anaesthetized area. Posterior iliac puncture can be carried out with the patient lying prone or on his side.

Puncture of spinous processes

Good samples of marrow may be obtained from adults by puncturing the spines of lumbar vertebrae.[35] Puncture is not difficult since the bones lie superficially, but rather more pressure is required than for sternal puncture.

Pass the needle into the spine of a lumbar vertebra slightly lateral to the mid-line in a direction at right angles to the skin surface, with the patient either sitting up or lying on his side as for a lumbar puncture. With this technique, too, the patient cannot see what is happening.

Comparison of the different sites for needle puncture

There is considerable variation in the composition of cellular marrow withdrawn from adjacent or different sites. Aspiration from only one site may give misleading information;[25] especially is this true in aplastic anaemia as the marrow may be affected patchily.[16,34] In general, however, the overall cellularity and type of maturity of haemopoiesis and the balance between erythropoiesis and leucopoiesis are similar.[3,15] In practice, it is a distinct advantage to have a choice of several sites for puncture, particularly when puncture at one site results in a 'dry tap' or when blood alone is withdrawn. Aspiration at a different site may yield cellular marrow or strengthen suspicion of a widespread change affecting the bone marrow, such as fibrosis or hypoplasia. In aplastic anaemia several punctures may be necessary in order to arrive at the diagnosis.

Which site is used is a matter of personal preference. The sternum is probably the easiest bone to puncture and on the whole seems to yield the most cellular marrow samples.[3] Sternal puncture, however, has the disadvantage that the patient is aware of what is happening and is often not unreasonably apprehensive.

The actual risks of sternal puncture, in particular of perforating the sternum, are extremely small in adults. Care and the use of a guarded needle should reduce the incidence to zero. In children aged <12 yr the risks are greater and a site for puncture other than sternum should be chosen (see below).

NEEDLE BIOPSY OF THE BONE MARROW IN CHILDREN

In very young children, from birth to 2 yr, the medial aspect of the upper end of the tibia just below the level of the tibial tubercle may be punctured and active marrow withdrawn. In older children the tibial cortical bone is usually too dense and the marrow within is normally less active. Iliac puncture, particularly in the region of the posterior crest, is then the method of choice. Sternal puncture, although possible, is not free from danger for the bone is thin and the marrow cavities are small. The dimensions of the marrow cavities in the sternum of children were given by Diwany.[13]

ASPIRATION OF BONE MARROW FOR TRANSPLANTATION

Bone-marrow grafting has led to the introduction of techniques suitable for obtaining large volumes (1 litre or more) of bone marrow from a donor. The method in general use is the multiple puncture technique which was described by Thomas and Storb.[49] They devised a special needle with a 45° bevel to avoid plugging of the lumen during aspiration, but ordinary marrow puncture needles (p. 158) can be used satisfactorily.

Aspiration of bone marrow in laboratory animals

Several procedures have been suggested for obtaining marrow from small animals without having to kill them. In one method a dental drill is used and bone marrow is aspirated through the hole thus made, by means of a pipette[53] or a fine needle attached to a syringe.[40] Archer et al have designed a needle which, attached to an ordinary 5 ml syringe, can be used to puncture the femur: marrow can be aspirated readily and repeatedly.[1]

EXAMINATION OF ASPIRATED BONE MARROW

Quite large volumes of marrow (plus blood) can be aspirated, but the more material aspirated the greater is the proportion of contaminating blood. There is, as already stated, little if any advantage in aspirating more than 0.3 ml of marrow fluid. The material aspirated can be dealt with in at least four ways: films can be made of the material as aspirated; films can be made after it has been concentrated; 'particle smears' can be made, and histological sections can be cut.

Bone-marrow films

Careful preparation is essential and it is desirable, if possible, to concentrate the marrow cells at the expense of the blood in which they are diluted.

The following simple manoeuvre is generally satisfactory. Deliver single drops of aspirate onto slides about 1 cm from one end and then quickly suck off most of the blood with a fine Pasteur pipette applied to the edge of each drop. Alterna-tively, place the slides on a slope to allow the blood to drain away. The irregularly shaped marrow fragments tend to adhere to the slide and most of them will be left behind. Then make films, 3–5 cm in length, of the marrow fragments and the remaining blood using a smooth-edged glass spreader of not more than 2 cm in width (Fig. 11.2). The marrow fragments are dragged behind the spreader and leave a trail of cells behind them. (It is in these cellular trials that differential counts should be made, commencing from the marrow fragment and working back towards the head of the film; in this way smaller numbers of cells from the peripheral blood become incorporated in a differential count.)

The preparation can be considered satisfactory only when marrow particles as well as free marrow cells can be seen in stained films, as is usual with the above technique. No attempt should be made to squash the marrow particles. Their structure—whether hypocellular or hypercellular—can be readily appreciated without recourse to squashing.

Fix the films of bone marrow and stain them with Romanowsky dyes as for peripheral blood films (p. 76). However, a longer fixation time (at least 20 min in methanol) is essential for high quality staining. Films should be stained by Perls's method as a routine to demonstrate iron (see p. 116).

Some workers add the aspirated marrow routinely to an anticoagulant, e.g. dried EDTA, in a tube and prepare films on return to the laboratory. While this is convenient, it is all too easy to use an excess of anticoagulant. When films of marrow containing a gross excess of anticoagulant are spread (as when a few drops of marrow are added to a tube containing sufficient EDTA to prevent the clotting of 5 ml of

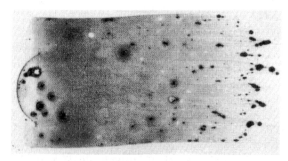

Fig. 11.2   Film of aspirated bone marrow. The marrow particles are easily visible, mostly at the tail of the film (× 1.5).

blood) masses of pink-staining amorphous material may be seen and some of the erythroblasts and reticulocytes may clump together.

Concentration of bone marrow by centrifugation

Centrifugation can be used to concentrate the marrow cells and to assess the relative proportions of marrow cells, peripheral blood and fat in aspirated material. While concentration of poorly cellular samples is useful, it is unnecessary when the aspirated material is of average or increased cellularity. Volumetric data, too, are of little value in individual patients because of the wide range of values encountered even in health.

Methods for separation of marrow cells are described on p. 83.

'Particle smears'

Some workers deliberately isolate aspirated marrow particles and make 'smears' of them on slides or between two cover-slips using slight pressure.[44] While this technique undoubtedly gives preparations of authentic marrow cells, squashing and smearing out of the particle causes disruption and distortion of cells, and the resultant thick preparations are difficult to stain really well. The authors feel that this technique has no advantages over the method described on p. 160.

Imprints

One or two glass slides are gently touched in several places by the exposed marrow at the surface of the biopsy. These imprints are allowed to dry; the slides are then fixed and stained in the same manner as films. When there is a dry tap on aspiration the biopsy core should be gently rolled on a slide before putting it into fixative (see below). The slide should then be fixed and stained as before.

Preparation of films of post-mortem bone marrow

Films made of bone marrow obtained post mortem are seldom satisfactory. When the marrow is spread in the ordinary way the majority of the cells tend to break up and appear as smears. Berenbaum described how the blood cells are much better preserved if the marrow is suspended in albumin before the films are made.[5] He recommended that a small piece of marrow be suspended in 1–2 ml of 5% bovine albumin (1 volume 30% albumin, 5 volumes 9 g/l NaCl). The suspension is then centrifuged and the deposited marrow cells are resuspended in a volume of supernatant approximately equal to, or slightly less than, that of the deposit. Films are made of this suspension in the usual way. Berenbaum also pointed out that the addition of albumin to blood so as to give a 5% concentration improves the preservation of lymphocytes in cases of lymphocytic leukaemia in which many 'smear cells' are often seen in films of peripheral blood prepared in the ordinary way.

The rate and pattern of cellular autolysis during the first 15 h after death has been studied and the differences between the changes of post-mortem autolysis and those which occur in life as a result of blood diseases have been defined.[26]

QUANTITATIVE CELL COUNTS ON ASPIRATED BONE MARROW

A number of values for the cell content of aspirated normal bone marrow have been given in the literature.[41,51] The percentage marrow that is cellular rather than fatty in the sternum of healthy adults was given by Berman and Axelrod as 48–79%.[7] But quantitation of the cell content of aspirated marrow is not reliable in view of the tendency of the marrow to be aspirated in the form of particles of varying size as well as free cells and the uncontrollable factor of dilution with peripheral blood, which according to some authors may amount to 40–100% in 0.25–0.5 ml bone-marrow samples.[6]

For the above reasons quantitative cell counts on aspirated marrow seem hardly worth carrying out; instead, the degree of cellularity can be assessed within broad limits as increased, normal or reduced by inspection of a stained film containing marrow particles, and for practical purposes this is all that is usually necessary. As a rough guide, if less than 25% of the particle is occupied by haemopoietic cells it is probably hypocellular, and if more than 75–80% it is hypercellular.

Less subjective quantitative measurement can be obtained by 'point counting' of sections;[24,29] a normal range of 30–80% has been reported in the anterior iliac crest.[24]

Physiological variation in the cell content has to be taken into account. The cellularity of the marrow is affected by age. In adults, a smaller proportion of the marrow cavity is occupied by haemopoietic marrow than in children and the proporation of fat cells to cellular marrow is increased. In one study, by means of point counting of sections from the iliac crest, the range of cellularity in children under 10 years was reported as 59–95% with a mean of 79%; at 30 years the mean was 50%, and at 70 years it was 30% with a range of 11–47%.[24] The decrease in cellularity in elderly subjects is even more marked in the manubrium sterni. The marrow undergoes slight to moderate hyperplasia in pregnancy.[36]

DIFFERENTIAL CELL COUNTS ON ASPIRATED BONE MARROW; THE 'MYELOGRAM'

Many workers perform differential counts on marrow films and by presenting the data in the form of a myelogram express the incidence of the various cell types as percentages. Such figures are not as accurate as they might appear. Films made from aspirated material inevitably include cells from the peripheral blood as well as from the bone marrow, and the variable dilution with blood involves an error for which no compensation is possible. In addition, the more fixed and primitive cells may resist aspiration or, if aspirated, tend to remain embedded in marrow fragments. Megakaryocytes in particular are most irregularly distributed and tend to be carried to the tail of the film.

Ideally, differential counts should be performed on sectioned material. However, difficulties in identification make this impractical, although methacrylate embedding offers a better opportunity for correctly identifying cells. Fadem and Yalow recommended that differential counts be done on preparations made by the particle-smear technique.[15] As mentioned on p. 160, a fairly reliable method is to count the cells in the trails of cells left behind the marrow particles as they are carried to the tail during spreading.

Because of the naturally variegated pattern of the bone marrow and the irregular distribution of the marrow cells when spread in films, differential cell counts on marrow aspirated from normal subjects are likely to vary widely in health—so widely that minor degrees of deviation from the normal occurring in disease are difficult to establish. Lymph follicles occur in the bone marrow as a normal constituent, and chance aspiration at the site of such a follicle would result in a film with an unusually high proportion of lymphocytes. Follicles have been reported to occur especially in infants, although in one large study they were reported to be quite rare in children and more common in middle-aged and elderly people.[37]

The normal values given in Table 11.1 can be taken only as an approximate guide. Glaser et al gave figures for the cellular composition of the bone marrow in normal infants, children and young adults, based on 151 samples.[21] Variation is marked in the first year, particularly so in the first month. The percentage of erythroblasts falls from birth, and at 2–3 weeks they constitute only c 10% of the nucleated cells. Myeloid cells (granulocyte precursors) increase during the first two weeks of life, following which a sharp fall occurs at about the third week, but by the end of the first month c 60% of the cells are myeloid. Lymphocytes constitute up to 40% of the nucleated cells in the marrow of small infants; the mean value at 2 yr is c 20%, falling to c 15% during the rest of childhood. The percentage of plasma cells is especially low from infancy up to the age of 5 yr.[48]

The hyperplasia which occurs in pregnancy affects both erythropoiesis and granulopoiesis, the latter proportionately less, though with some increase in the relative proportion of immature cells.[36] The hyperplasia is maximal in the third trimester; a return to normal begins in the puerperium but is not completed until at least 6 weeks post partum.

Ratios

Ratios based on a count of 200–500 cells provide useful qualitative information without recourse to more time-consuming differential counts.

The myeloid:erythroid ratio has been widely used. Leucocytes of all types and stages of maturation are lumped together. The very wide normal

Table 11.1 Normal ranges for differential counts on aspirated bone marrow

Reticulum cells	0.1–2%
Myeloblasts	0.1–3.5%
Promyelocytes	0.5–5%
Myelocytes	
neutrophil	5–20%
eosinophil	0.1–3%
basophil	0–0.5%
Metamyelocytes	10–30%
Polymorphonuclears	
neutrophil	7–25%
eosinophil	0.2–3%
basophil	0–0.5%
Lymphocytes	5–20%
Monocytes	0–0.2%
Megakaryocytes	0.1–0.5%
Plasma cells	0.1–3.5%
Proerythroblasts	0.5–5%
Normoblasts★	
polychromatic	2–20%
pyknotic★★	2–10%

★ or erythroblasts
★★The term 'pyknotic' is preferred to 'orthochromatic' as a description of the most mature normoblasts. Cells with fully ripened cytoplasm (orthochromatic in the strict sense) are rarely found in normal bone marrow.

range, 2.5–15:1, reflects the variegated pattern of normal marrow.

As an alternative, the leuco-erythrogenetic ratio can be calculated; for this mature leucocytes are excluded. The normal ratio has been reported as 0.56–2.67:1.[43]

The myeloid:lymphoid ratio varies widely, 1–17:1, and the lymphoid:erythroid ratio is similarly a wide one, 0.2–4.0:1.[18]

REPORTING ON BONE-MARROW FILMS

The first thing to do is to look with the naked eye at a selection of slides and to choose from them several of the best spread films containing easily visible marrow particles. The particles should then be examined with a low-power (16 mm) objective with particular reference to their cellularity, and an estimate of whether the marrow is hypoplastic, normoplastic or hyperplastic can usually be made without much difficulty, if sufficient particles are available for study (Fig. 11.3). The next step is to select for detailed examination—still using the 16 mm objective—a highly cellular area of the film where the nucleated cells are well stained and well

spread. Areas such as these can usually be found towards the tails of films in the vicinity of marrow particles. The cells in these cellular areas should be examined first with a higher power (e.g. 4 mm) objective and subsequently, if necessary, with the 2 mm oil-immersion objective. Megakaryocytes should be looked for at this stage of the examination; they are most often found towards the tail of the film.

Systematic examination, backed by a knowledge of the patient's peripheral blood count and his history, will usually enable a diagnosis to be made without recourse to a differential count. A detailed 'myelogram' is, in fact, not often required in clinical practice. A description of the general cellularity of the marrow and the type of erythropoiesis (e.g. whether normoblastic, megaloblastic or dyserythropoietic) and of the general maturity of the erythropoietic and leucopoietic cells, and perhaps an estimate of the myeloid:erythroid ratio, are all that are usually needed when reporting on bone-marrow films for diagnostic purposes.

This is not to say that detailed differential counts are never useful and need never be done. Thus, changes in the proportion of primitive to maturing

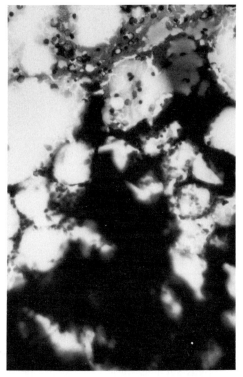

(a)

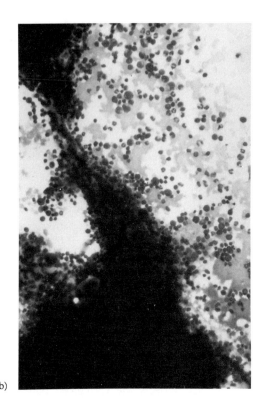

(b)

Fig. 11.3 Films of aspirated marrow. Photomicrographs of particles illustrating cellularity. a. normal, b. hypercellular, c. hypocellular.

myeloid cells reflect response to treatment in leukaemia or recovery from agranulocytosis, and the actual percentage of blast cells may be of significance in the differentiation of refractory anaemias and myelodysplasia.

The proportion of lymphoid cells is an important indicator of prognosis in chronic lymphocytic leukaemia.[46] On the other hand, time is often much better spent in examining a series of slides than in performing a detailed differential count as a routine on the first few hundred cells looked at in the marrow film of each patient. A wide search may, for instance, in a case of obscure anaemia, settle the diagnosis by revealing isolated groups of metastatic carcinoma cells. In addition, a film should always be stained and examined for iron.

Other features of possible diagnostic value include the presence of erythrophagocytosis, abnormal numbers of phagocytic reticulum cells, excess plasma cells, non-haemopoietic cells and degenerate or necrotic cells. Bone-marrow necrosis is a not

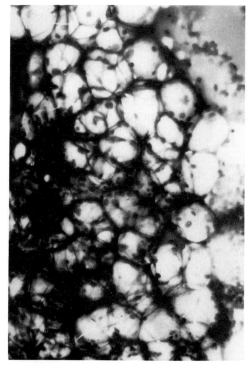

(c)

ROYAL POSTGRADUATE MEDICAL SCHOOL
HAMMERSMITH HOSPITAL

CASE No

DATE OF BIRTH

HAEMATOLOGY
BONE MARROW REPORT

SURNAME

SEX

FIRST NAMES

WARD

CONSULTANT

BM

LAB. No.

DISEASE CLASSIFICATION

NAME

DATE TAKEN

LAB. No.   BM

Site(s)

Aspiration

Consistency of Bone

Cellularity

Erythropoiesis

Leucopoiesis

Megakaryocytes

Plasma Cells

Reticulum Cells

Abnormal Cells

Iron

Mitoses

Myeloid-Erythroid Ratio
   (Normal Range   2.5-15 : 1)

CONCLUSION

Signature

Date

Fig. 11.4   Report form for bone-marrow films. In use at the Royal Postgraduate Medical School.

uncommon complication of sickle-cell disease; it also occurs occasionally in lymphomas, lymphoblastic and chronic lymphocytic leukaemia, myeloproliferative diseases and metastatic carcinoma as well as in septicaemia, tuberculosis and anorexia nervosa.[9,30,38,47,52]

In marrow necrosis cells stain irregularly, with blurred outlines, cytoplasmic shrinkage and nuclear pyknosis. In anorexia there is also gelatinous transformation of ground substance of the marrow.[47]

It is helpful in reporting on bone-marrow films to have a printed form on which the report and conclusion can be set out in an ordered fashion (Fig. 11.4).

PREPARATION OF SECTIONS OF ASPIRATED BONE MARROW

Sections give a better picture of the marrow architecture than can be deduced from films. In a good preparation the relationship between cellular marrow and fat spaces is preserved, hypoplasia or hyperplasia can be recognized, and tumour cells and granulomata can be seen. However, for cytological detail sectioned material is usually less satisfactory, especially when it has had to be decalcified and is paraffin embedded. The subtle differences between cells such as normoblasts and megaloblasts, which are usually easy to appreciate in well stained films, are difficult to recognize in sections and it may sometimes be difficult even to differentiate erythroblasts from leucocytes with complete certainty.

The fragments obtained by aspirating bone marrow are small, rarely greater than 1 mm in size, and a careful technique in handling them is required. They are usually free from bone and the marrow architecture is well preserved, but their usefulness is limited because their small size makes it uncertain how representative of the bone marrow they are. A more serious disadvantage of the aspiration technique is that fragments are often not obtained by suction in just those patients—with perhaps marrow hypoplasia, myelosclerosis or invasion by tumour—in whom histological evidence of any marrow abnormality is particularly required. In these patients trephine biopsy may be necessary.

A number of methods of dealing with aspirated fragments have been published which differ in the

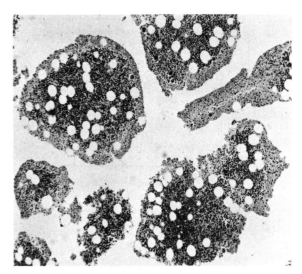

Fig 11.5   Section of aspirated bone-marrow particles. Method of Raman[45] × 60.

details of handling and concentrating the fragments, fixation and embedding.[11,45] The following method gives adequate concentration of the marrow particles and is simple to carry out (Fig. 11.5). Fixation is good and sections may be successfully stained by Romanowsky dyes as well as by other methods.

Preparation of sections of aspirated bone-marrow particles[45]

Fixative

Absolute ethanol is diluted with an equal volume of 15% formalin (150 ml/l of 40% formaldehyde). The sp gr of the mixture is 0.93, almost exactly the same as that of human fat. When a marrow aspirate is added to this fixative, the blood remains in suspension while the marrow particles rapidly sediment. Even fatty marrow settles down in a few seconds.

Method

Add 0.25 ml of bone-marrow aspirate to 20 ml of the fixative in a stoppered container and mix thoroughly. Allow it to fix overnight at room temperature.

The following morning resuspend the sediment by inversion. With a Pasteur pipette provided with a teat, pick out the coarser marrow fragments after they have re-settled to the bottom of the bottle, which usually takes only a few seconds. Then transfer them to a round-bottomed test-tube, provided with a rubber bung, containing 70% (v/v) ethanol. Leave for at least 15 min, then dehydrate with two changes of absolute ethanol, leaving the particles for 1 h in each. Then drain off the ethanol and replace with toluene. After 1 h decant off the toluene and replace it by a toluene-paraffin wax mixture and then by two changes of paraffin wax. Free the block by breaking the tube when the wax has cooled and hardened. The marrow fragments will have settled as a small mass at the bottom of the block and little or no trimming will be required. Cut sections of 4–5 µm thickness, the thinner the better.

PRECUTANEOUS TREPHINE BIOPSY OF THE BONE MARROW

Several types of trephines have been used. Türkel and Bethell described a microtrephine of about 2 mm bore which could be passed through a hollow introducing needle only slightly larger than a marrow aspirating needle.[50] No skin incision was necessary and the instrument could be safely used on the sternum and the procedure carried out in the ward. However, the cylinders of bone and underlying marrow obtained with the Türkel and Bethell trephine were small, and they were apt to break up while being prepared for sectioning. Needles of the Vim-Silverman type[10] are suitable for use in posterior iliac-crest punctures; but they yield smaller specimens of marrow than most other needles. However, the specimens are as a rule free from bone dust.

A disadvantage of most marrow trephines is that not infrequently the specimen is crushed and its

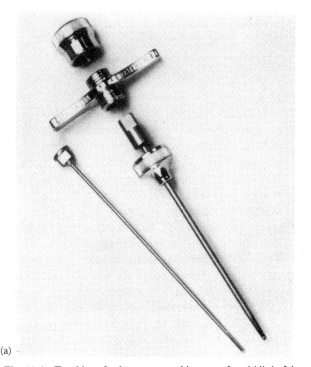

(a)

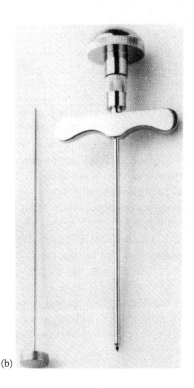

(b)

Fig. 11.6 Trephines for bone-marrow biopsy. a. Jamshidi, b. Islam.

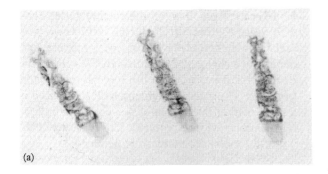

(a)

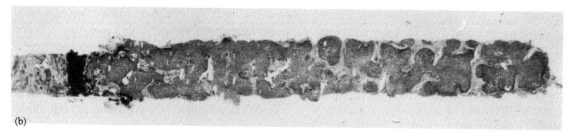

(b)

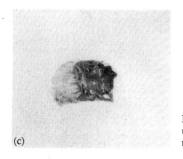

(c)

Fig. 11.7 Biopsy specimens of human bone marrow from iliac crest. Obtained using a. Jamshidi trephine ($\times 3$), b. Islam trephine ($\times 5$) and c. Sacker-Nordin trephine ($\times 3$).

architecture altered. The Jamshidi needle[*][28] which has a tapering end was designed to overcome this problem. The trephine should be inserted by to-and-fro rotation through approximately 90°. It should not be continuously rotated as this tends to distort and twist the core of marrow. Sometimes, however, the sample fractures while being extracted from the needle and in other cases the specimen does not detach readily from its base and efforts to detach it by movement of the needle result in it being crushed. These disadvantages have been overcome by having a core-securing device, as in the Islam trephine.[**][27a] This makes it possible to obtain a long uniform core of marrow-containing bone without the marrow architecture being distorted (Figs.

11.6 and 11.7). A modified version of the Islam trephine has multiple holes in the distal portion of the shaft in addition to the opening at the tip, in order to overcome sampling error when the marrow is not uniformly involved in a pathological lesion.[27b]

A larger trephine is sometimes of value as it may provide sufficient material for an accurate diagnosis when the result of a smaller and perhaps less representative biopsy is inconclusive. Trephines have been developed which have bores of 4 – 5 mm.[31,54] They can safely be used on the iliac crest, under local anaesthesia, but as a small skin incision is necessary the biopsy should be performed in the operating theatre where full aseptic precautions can be taken. Full-scale bone biopsy involving, for instance, removal of a piece of rib ('surgical biopsy') is nowadays seldom carried out.

[*] A. R. Horwell Ltd., London NW6 2BP.
[**] Downs Surgical Ltd., Mitcham, Surrey.

PREPARATION OF SECTIONS OF BONE MARROW OBTAINED BY TREPHINE BIOPSY

Fix the specimen in 10% formal saline, buffered to pH 7.0, or preferably in Helly's fluid (potassium dichromate 2.5 g, mercuric chloride 5 g, formalin [40% formaldehyde] 5 ml, water 100 ml) for 12–48 h. Then wash in running water overnight before decalcifying, dehydrating and embedding in paraffin wax by the usual histological procedures. Then cut and stain 4–5 μm thick sections. The relatively thick sections prepared in this way, together with cell shrinkage and the distortion produced by decalcification, make if difficult to interpret cellular detail. Almost all these disadvantages can be overcome by methyl methacrylate ('plastic') embedding.[19] In this process the undecalcified biopsy specimen is fixed in the usual way. It is then embedded in glycol or methyl methacrylate. Sections 1–2 μm thick can then be obtained using a tungsten carbide knife and a purpose-built expensive microtome, e.g. Reichert-Jung Autocut.[19,23] Not only does this provide clearer detail of cell morphology but cell and tissue relationships are maintained and the embedding procedure is less damaging to the tissue than paraffin embedding. Aspirated marrow can also be processed in this way after special fixation to separate the marrow particles from blood and precipitated protein.[22]

Before staining plastic-embedded sections, the methyl methacrylate must be dissolved from the sections by passing them sequentially through benzol or acetone, methanol, methanol-ammonia solution and water.[19]

Sections of marrow should be stained as a routine by haematoxylin and eosin (H & E) and by a

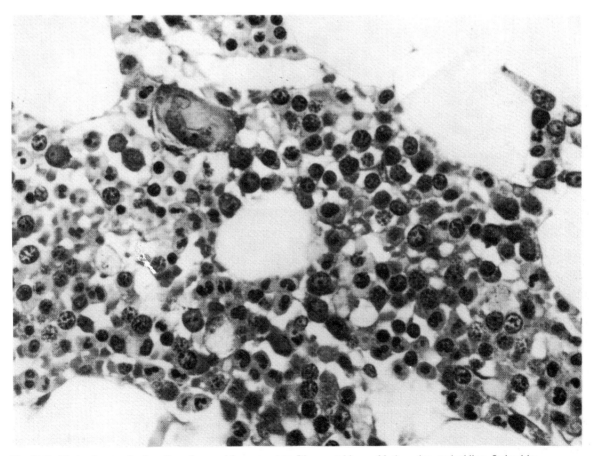

Fig. 11.8 Photomicrograph of section of normal bone marrow. Iliac crest biopsy. Methacrylate embedding. Stained by May-Grünwald-Giemsa. × 300.

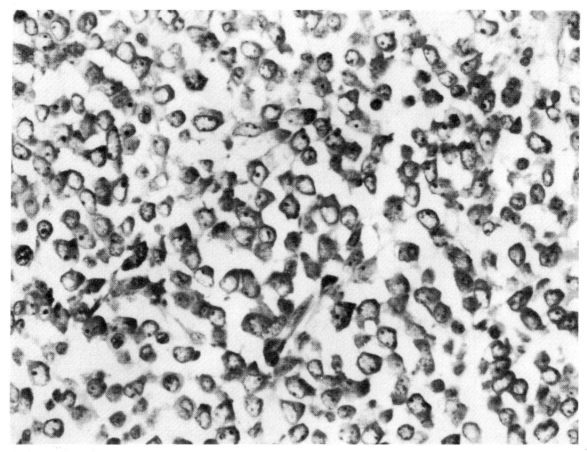

Fig. 11.9 Photomicrograph of section of bone marrow. Iliac crest biopsy. Methacrylate embedding. Myeloblastic leukaemia. Stained by May-Grünwald-Giemsa. × 300.

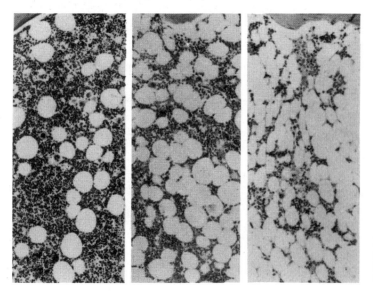

Fig. 11.10 Biopsy specimens of normal bone marrow. Photomicrographs of sections of iliac-crest bone marrow illustrating range of cellularity in health. × 100.

reticulin impregnation method. It is worthwhile also to stain sections by a Romanowsky stain, and for iron by Perls's reaction. H & E staining is excellent for demonstrating the cellularity and pattern of the marrow and for revealing pathological changes such as fibrosis or the presence of granulomata or carcinoma. Haemopoietic cells, on the hand, may be more easily identified in a Romanowsky-stained preparation (Figs. 11.8 and 11.9). In Fig. 11.10 is shown the extent to which the cellularity of the marrow varies in health. Sections can also be stained for various cytochemical reaction; however, specimens which have been embedded in plastic are unsuitable for immunohistology.[2]

Silver impregnation stains the glycoprotein matrix which is associated with connective tissue. The boen marrow always contains a small amount of this material which is referred to as 'reticulin' and which is actually collagen.[4] The reticulin content of normal iliac bone marrow is shown in Fig. 11.11.

The term myelofibrosis strictly refers to an increase in fine fibres and myelosclerosis to the condition when there is an increase in coarse fibres (Fig. 11.11). The latter type predominates in chronic ('idiopathic') myelofibrosis/myelosclerosis. Increased reticulin also occurs in other myeloproliferative disorders, particularly in cases associated with proliferation of megakaryocytes and in lymphoproliferative disorders, secondary carcinoma with marrow infiltration, osseous disorders such as hyperparathyroidism and Paget's disease, and in inflammatory reactions.[17,33,39]

Staining of sections of bone marrow by May-Grünwald-Giemsa

The many techniques which have been recommended for staining sectioned bone marrow by Romanowsky dyes are evidence of the real difficulty in obtaining good results. The following method is fairly satisfactory. It may be applied to aspirated marrow fragments, trephine or post-mortem material.

Place the cut sections which have been processed, as described on p. 169, in Lugol's iodine for 2 min. Then wash in several changes of water and finally rinse in water buffered to pH 6.8. Stain the sections for 1 h in May-Grünwald's stain diluted with an equal volume of buffered water. Then stain for a further 2 h in a fresh solution of Giemsa's stain diluted with 19 volumes of buffered water. The sections become grossly over-stained and deep blue in colour. Rinse in buffered water (pH 6.8) before differentiation.

Differentiate the sections by covering with a small volume of glycerin-ether, freshly diluted with four volumes of absolute ethanol. Differentiation takes place quickly and is usually adequate in a few

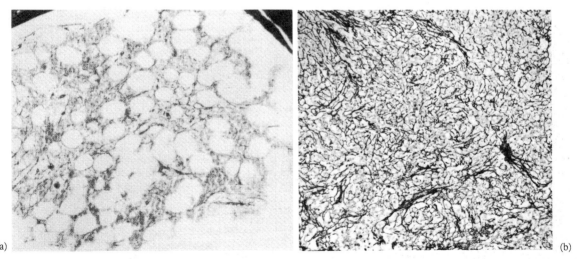

(a)   (b)

Fig. 11.11 Photomicrographs of sections of bone marrow. Iliac crest biopsy. Stained for reticulin by silver impregnation method. a. normal; b. myelofibrosis. × 100.

seconds. Next dehydrate the sections by a rapid dip in absolute ethanol, clear them in xylol and finally mount them in a xylol-miscible mounting medium (e.g. Diatex, R. A. Lamb). The use of glycerin-ether helps to prevent 'blueing' of the section during dehydration.

In a successfully stained section the cytoplasm of primitive cells should be blue, that of myelocytes and segmented neutrophils pale pink, the eosinophil granules should be bright red and the cytoplasm of the red cells orange. Neutrophil granules are not as a rule easily seen.

REFERENCES

[1] ARCHER, R. K., RILEY, J. and GWILLIAM, R. V. E. (1981). Aspiration of bone marrow from laboratory rats. *British Journal of Haematology*, **48**, 165.

[2] BARTL, R., FRISCH, B., BUCHENRIEBER, B. et al (1984). Multiparameter studies on 650 bone marrow biopsy cores. *Bibliotheca Haematologica*, **50**, 1.

[3] BENNIKE, T., GORMSEN, H. and MØLLER, B. (1956). Comparative studies of bone marrow punctures of the sternum, the iliac crest and the spinous process. *Acta Medica Scandinavica*, **155**, 377.

[4] BENTLEY, S.A., ALABASTER, O. and FOIDART, J. M. (1981). Collagen heterogeneity in normal human bone marrow. *British Journal of Haematology*, **48**, 287.

[5] BERENBAUM, M. C. (1956). The use of bovine albumin in the preparation of marrow and blood films. *Journal of Clinical Pathology*, **9**, 381.

[6] BERLIN, N. I., HENNESSY, T. G. and GARTLAND, J. (1950). Sternal marrow puncture: the dilution with peripheral blood as determined by P^{32} labelled red cells. *Journal of Laboratory and Clinical Medicine*, **36**, 23.

[7] BERMAN, L. and AXELROD, A. R. (1950). Fat, total cell and megakaryocyte content of sections of aspirated marrow of normal persons. *American Journal of Clinical Pathology*, **20**, 686.

[8] BERMAN, H. R. and KELLY, K. H. (1956). Multiple marrow aspiration in man from the posterior ilium. *Blood*, **11**, 370.

[9] CONRAD, M. E. and CARPENTER, J. T. (1979). Bone marrow necrosis. *American Journal of Haematology*, **7**, 181.

[10] CONRAD, M. E. and CROSBY, W. H. (1961). Bone marrow biopsy: modification of the Vim-Silverman needle. *Journal of Laboratory and Clinical Medicine*, **57**, 642.

[11] DEE, J. W., VALDIVIESO, M. and DREWINKO, B. (1976). Comparison of the efficacies of closed trephine needle biopsy, aspirated paraffin-embedded clot section and smear preparation in the diagnosis of bone-marrow involvement by lymphoma. *American Journal of Clinical Pathology* **65**, 183.

[12] DENST, J. and MULLIGAN, R. M. (1950). The distribution of bone marrow in the human sternum. *American Journal of Clinical Pathology*, **20**, 610.

[13] DIWANY, M. (1940). Sternal marrow puncture in children. *Archives of Disease in Childhood*, **15**, 159.

[14] ENGESET, A., NESHEIM, A. and SOKOLOWSKI, J. (1979). Incidence of 'dry tap' on bone marrow aspirations in lymphomas and carcinomas. Diagnostic value of the small material in the needle. *Scandinavian Journal of Haematology*, **22**, 417.

[15] FADEM, R. S. and YALOW, R. (1951). Uniformity of cell counts in smears of bone marrow particles. *American Journal of Clinical Pathology*, **27**, 541.

[16] FERRANT, A. (1980). Selective hypoplasia of pelvic bone marrow. *Scandinavian Jounal of Haematology*, **25**, 12.

[17] FRISCH B. and BARTL, R. (1985). Histology of myelofibrosis and osteomyelosclerosis. In *Myelofibrosis: Pathophysiology and Clinical Management*. Ed. S. M. Lewis, p. 51–86. Marcel Dekker, New York.

[18] FRISCH B. and LEWIS, S. M. (1974). The bone marrow in aplastic anaemia: diagnostic and prognostic features. *Journal of Clinical Pathology*, **27**, 231.

[19] FRISCH B., LEWIS, S. M. BURKHARDT, R. and BARTL, R. (1985). *Biopsy Pathology of Bone and Bone Marrow*. Chapman and Hall, London.

[20] GARRETT, T. J., GEE, T. S., LIEBERMAN, P. H. and McKENZIE, S. (1976). The role of bone marrow aspiration and biopsy in detecting marrow involvement by nonhematogenic malignancies. *Cancer*, **38**, 240.

[21] GLASER, K., LIMARZI, L. R. and PONCHER, H. G. (1950). Cellular composition of the bone marrow in normal infants and children. *Pediatrics*, **6**, 789.

[22] GREEN, G. H. (1970). A simple method for histological examination of bone marrow particles using hydroxyethyl methacrylate embedding. *Journal of Clinical Pathology*, **23**, 640.

[23] GREEN, G. H. and KURREIN, F. (1981). Glycol methacrylate embedding in general histopathology. *ACP Broadsheet No. 97*, Association of Clinical Pathologists, London.

[24] HARTSOCK, R. J., SMITH, E. B. and PETTY, C. S. (1965). Normal variations with aging of the amount of hematopoietic tissue in bone marrow from the anterior iliac crest. *American Journal of Clinical Pathology*, **43**, 326.

[25] HASHIMOTO, M. (1960). The distribution of active marrow in the bones of normal adults. *Kyushu Journal of Medical Science*, **11**, 103.

[26] HOFFMAN, S. B., MORROW, G. W. Jnr, PEASE, G. L. and STROEBEL, C. F. (1964). Rate of cellular autolysis in postmortem bone marrow. *American Journal of Clinical Patholgy*, **41**, 281.

[27] ISLAM, A. (1981). A new bone marrow biopsy needle with core securing device. *Journal of Clinical Pathology*, **35**, 359.

[27b] ISLAM, A. (1983). A new bone marrow aspiration needle to overcome the sampling errors inherent in the technique of bone marrow aspiration. *Journal of Clinical Pathology*, **36**, 954.

[28] JAMSHIDI, K. and SWAIM, W. R. (1971). Bone marrow biopsy with unaltered architecture: a new biopsy device. *Journal of Laboratory and Clinical Medicine*, **77**, 335.

[29] KERNDRUP, G., PALLESEN, G., MELSEN, F. and MOSEKILDE, L. (1980). Histological determination of bone marrow cellularity in iliac crest biopsies. *Scandinavian Journal of Haematology*, **24**, 110.

[30] KIRALY, J. F. and WHEBY, M. S. (1976). Bone marrow necrosis. *American Journal of Medicine*, **60**, 361.

[31] LANDYS, K. (1980). A new trephine for closed bone marrow biopsy. *Acta Haematologica*, **64**, 216.

[32] LEFFLER, R. J. (1957). Aspiration of bone marrow from the anterior superior iliac spine. *Journal of Laboratory and Clinical Medicine*, **50**, 482.

[33] LENNERT, K., NAGAI, K. and SCHWARZE, E.-W. (1975). Patho-anatomic features of the bone marrow. *Clinics in Haematology*, **4**, 331.

[34] LEWIS, S. M. (1965). Course and prognosis in aplastic anaemia. *British Medical Journal*, **i,** 1027.

[35] LOGE, J. P. (1948). Spinous process puncture. A simple clinical approach for obtaining bone marrow. *Blood*, **3**, 198.

[36] LOWENSTEIN, L. and BRAMLAGE, C. A. (1957). The bone marrow in pregnancy and the puerperium, *Blood*, **12**, 261.

[37] MAEDA, K., HYUN, B. H. and REBUCK, J. W. (1977). Lymphoid follicles in bone marrow aspirates. *American Journal of Clinical Pathology*, **67**, 41.

[38] MACFARLANE, S. D. and TAURO, G. P. (1986). Acute lymphocytic leukaemia in children presenting with bone marrow necrosis. *American Journal of Hematology*, **22**, 341.

[39] MCCARTHY, D. M. (1985) Fibrosis of the bone marrow; content and causes. *British Journal of Haematology*, **59**, 1.

[40] MCFADZEAN, A. J. S. (1948). Marrow biopsy in laboratory animals. *Journal of Pathology and Bacteriology*, **60**, 332.

[41] OSGOOD, E. E. and SEAMAN, A. J. (1944). The cellular composition of normal bone marrow as obtained by sternal puncture. *Physiological Reviews*, **24**, 46.

[42] PASQUALE, D. and CHIKKAPPA, G. (1981). Comparative evaluation of bone marrow aspirate particle smears, biopsy imprints, and biopsy sections. *American Journal of Hematology*, **22**, 381.

[43] PONTONI, L. (1936). Su alcuni rapporti citologici ricavati dal mielogramma; metodica e valutazione fisopatognostica generale. *Haematologica*, **17**, 833.

[44] PROPP, S. (1951). An improved technic of bone marrow aspiration, *Blood*, **6**, 585.

[45] RAMAN, K. (1955). A method of sectioning aspirated bone-marrow. *Journal of Clinical Pathology*, **8**, 265.

[46] ROZMAN, C., MONTSERRAT, E., RODRÍGUEZ-FERNÁNDEZ, J. M. et al (1984). Bone marrow histologic pattern— the best single prognostic parameter in chronic lymphocytic leukemia; a multivariate survival analysis of 329 cases. *Blood*, **64**, 642.

[47] SMITH, R. R. L. and SPIVAK, J. L. (1985). Marrow cell necrosis in anorexia nervosa and involuntary starvation. *British Journal of Haematology*, **60**, 525.

[48] STEINER, M. L. and PEARSON, H. A. (1966). Bone marrow plasmacyte values in childhood. *Journal of Pediatrics*, **68**, 562.

[49] THOMAS, E. D. and STORB, R. (1970). Technique for human marrow grafting. *Blood*, **36**, 507.

[50] TÜRKEL, H. and BETHELL, F. H. (1943). Biopsy of bone marrow performed by a new and simple instrument. *Journal of Laboratory and Clinical Medicine*, **28**, 1246.

[51] VAUGHAN, S. L. and BROCKMYRE, F. (1947). Normal bone marrow as obtained by sternal puncture. *Blood*, Special Issue, No. 1, p. 54.

[52] VESTERBY, A. and JENSEN, O. M. (1985). Aseptic bone/bone marrow necrosis in leukaemia. *Scandinavian Journal of Haematology*, **35**, 354.

[53] VIGRAM, M. (1947). A method of bone marrow biopsy from the rat. *Journal of Laboratory and Clinical Medicine*, **32**, 102.

[54] WILLIAMS, J. A. and NICHOLSON, G. I. (1963). A modified bone-biopsy drill for outpatient use. *Lancet*, **i**, 1408.

12. Diagnosis of blood disorders

The diagnosis of a blood disorder depends on a consideration of both clinical and laboratory evidence: neither is sufficient on its own. The clinical evidence includes the history of the patient's present illness and past history, his or her age, sex and occupation, family history and racial origin, and the result of a physical examination. Consideration of the clinical evidence in any detail is beyond the scope of this book, and it will not be discussed further; its appreciation is, however, an essential facet in the solving of any patient's problem. The laboratory evidence is derived from two kinds of test: those that are generally termed haematological—with which this book is concerned—and non-haematological tests, e.g. biochemical tests, radiological examination, etc., a consideration of which is again beyond the scope of this book. The results of such non-haematological tests are, however, not infrequently of critical significance in arriving at a diagnosis, as when, for instance, a patient is found to have a high blood urea or a paraprotein in his or her serum.

There are three ways in which the results of the haematological tests that are described in this book may be useful in diagnosis. These are:

1. Screening a blood sample for an abnormality.
2. Making a tentative diagnosis of a blood disorder.
3. Investigating in detail a patient in whom a tentative diagnosis of a particular blood disorder has been made.

SCREENING FOR AN ABNORMALITY

The choice of screening tests depends on what facilities are available, especially whether an automated counting system is used. In the absence of an electronic counter, measurement of PCV, estimation of haemoglobin and inspection of a stained film may be all that is practicable as a minimum 'screening' procedure. The measurement of PCV and haemoglobin estimation provide a check on one measurement against the other and the MCHC, if subnormal, gives a presumptive indication of iron deficiency. If a leucocyte or platelet abnormality is suspected, total counts of these should be undertaken.

In assessing whether the haemoglobin, PCV, leucocyte or platelet count of an individual is normal or abnormal, the results have to be considered in relation to the range of values generally considered to be normal. In this respect the patient's age and sex are important as well as the altitude at which he or she lives. Diurnal variation and the possible effects of exercise and of the patient's posture when the sample was taken, and its source, are additional factors that may influence the results. These questions have been considered in some detail in Chapter 2 (see p. 9).

The availability of an electronic counter allows blood-count data to be obtained quickly and with considerable accuracy. In particular, the figures obtainable for red cell count, MCV and MCH are far more reliable and consequently more valuable than those obtained by visual counting. However, in

175

relation to screening for an abnormality the main value of automated equipment lies in the speed with which blood-count data can be obtained.

Irrespective of the degree to which automated procedures can be used in blood counting, it is highly desirable to make and examine blood films. It is ideal, although not always practical, to make films from every sample of blood submitted to the laboratory even if the PCV or Hb is normal. Inspection of a film may reveal signs of an unsuspected blood disease, for example, compensated haemolytic anaemia or chronic lymphocytic leukaemia, which might not be revealed by quantitative counts, as well as interesting abnormalities such as hereditary elliptocytosis or the Pelger-Hüet leucocyte abnormality, and the presence in the film of excessive rouleaux may draw attention to a protein abnormality.

Ideally, all blood films—and not necessarily only those showing a definite abnormality—should be filed away and kept for as long as possible. From time to time it will be important to have available a film made many years previously. Re-examination may show, for instance, the early stages of an abnormality which had been missed, but had become more obvious later, or that the earlier film was normal. Each type of information may be important in a particular case.

DIAGNOSIS OF THE TYPE OF BLOOD DISORDER

When a patient's blood has been shown to be abnormal as the result of a screening procedure, it is necessary to make an accurate diagnosis. Sometimes this can be arrived at simply from knowledge of the patient's clinical history and the results of a physical examination and by examination of a well stained and well spread blood film, supplemented by a reticulocyte count and the quantitative cell count data already available. In other cases, no certain diagnosis is possible without bone-marrow aspiration or microtrephine biopsy. Other simple tests that may be helpful in appropriate cases include measurement of the ESR and the direct antiglobulin test. Only occasionally when, for example, a patient has a haemolytic anaemia, haemoglobinopathy or haemorrhagic disorder, have more complicated laboratory tests to be undertaken before even a tentative diagnosis can be made.

FURTHER HAEMATOLOGICAL INVESTIGATION OF A PATIENT AFTER A TENTATIVE DIAGNOSIS HAS BEEN MADE

The patient is investigated further usually for one of two reasons:

1. The diagnosis is not in doubt but further studies are required to elucidate the cause and mechanism of the patient's blood disorder or to classify it more precisely.

2. The diagnosis is not yet clear and further investigations are required in order to arrive (if possible) at the correct diagnosis.

The choice of tests and procedures to be undertaken depends upon the results of the preliminary tests already carried out and the facilities and time available. Recommended procedures for the further investigation of the more important types of blood disorder are given below. The more valuable and informative procedures are given first; the less important or more complicated tests, only applicable in certain circumstances, follow.

Hypochromic anaemias

Chemical tests for occult gastro-intestinal bleeding; bone-marrow aspiration (including staining for iron), if not already undertaken; measurement of serum ferritin, serum iron and total iron-binding capacity; tests for malabsorption syndrome; tests for absorption of iron; measurement of blood loss using ^{51}Cr. If thalassaemia or a haemoglobinopathy is suspected: haemoglobin electrophoresis; Hb-F and Hb-A_2 estimation; tests for an unstable haemoglobin; family studies; globin chain synthesis; globin chain molecular-genetic analysis.

Megaloblastic anaemias

See Chapter 25.

'Secondary anaemias'

These include too wide a range of blood disorders and mechanisms of anaemia to be summarized here.

The haematologist should direct his or her efforts towards explaining the patient's anaemia, which may be dyshaemopoietic, haemolytic and/or due to blood loss, and excluding a 'primary' blood disease or replacement of normal haemopoietic marrow by tumour. When an anaemia remains unexplained, blood volume measurements may show that it is a 'pseudoanaemia'.

Aplastic anaemia

Bone-marrow aspiration or microtrephine biopsy, possibly in more than one site, if not already undertaken; acidified-serum test for PNH; test for haemosiderin in urine deposit; neutrophil alkaline phosphatase, ^{59}Fe (and ^{52}Fe scan if available) to study red cell production; red cell survival study using ^{51}Cr, including measurement of blood loss in the faeces. Ascertainment of tissue (HLA) group in relation of possible bone-marrow transplanation.

Haemolytic anaemias

See Chapters 13–16 and 29.

Haemorrhagic disorders

See Chapters 17–20.

Leucopenia

Bone-marrow aspiration, if not already undertaken; serial observations on peripheral leucocyte count to test for cyclical neutropenia; tests for leucocyte antibodies (see Chapter 27).

Acute leukaemia

Bone-marrow aspiration, if not already undertaken, including PAS staining and staining for iron; alkaline-phosphatase reaction of neutrophils; myeloperoxidase reaction of neutrophils and precursor cells; other cytochemical and enzyme tests and immunological studies on cells from blood and marrow to identify cell type (see Chapter 10); serum-protein estimation; serum-B_{12} estimation; tests for abnormal haemoglobins, e.g. Hb H; chromosome studies.

Chronic granulocytic leukaemia

Bone-marrow aspiration, alkaline phosphatase reaction of neutrophils; chromosome studies.

Chronic lymphocytic leukaemia

Bone-marrow aspiration, cytochemical and enzyme tests and immunological studies (see Chapter 10); serum-protein estimation; lymph-node biopsy (aspiration and/or surgical).

Myelomatosis

Bone-marrow aspiration; serum-protein and serum Ca estimation; tests for Bence-Jones and other urine proteins; tests of renal functions; X-ray examination of skeleton.

Polycythaemia

Blood-volume estimation; bone-marrow aspiration or microtrephine biopsy; alkaline-phosphatase reaction of neutrophils; estimation of serum uric acid; renal function tests and pyelogram; measurement of oxygen saturation and oxygen dissociation; spleen scan and measurement of red cell pool; identification of an abnormal haemoglobin; erythropoietin assay.

Myelosclerosis (Myelofibrosis)

Bone-marrow trephine; estimation of serum folic acid and uric acid; alkaline-phosphatase reaction of neutrophils; use of ^{59}Fe (or ^{52}Fe) to demonstrate extramedullary erythropoiesis and ^{51}Cr to demonstrate rate and site of red cell destruction; spleen scan and measurement of red cell pool.

Pancytopenia and splenomegaly

Bone-marrow aspiration; lymph-node biopsy (if lymph nodes enlarged); liver biopsy; ^{51}Cr to study red cell survival and sites of haemolysis; ^{59}Fe (or ^{52}Fe) to demonstrate extramedullary haemopoiesis; spleen scan; measurement of splenic red cell pool.

13. Laboratory methods used in the investigation of the haemolytic anaemias

Normally, effete red cells undergo lysis at the end of their life-span of 100–120 days within cells of the reticulo-endothelial (RE) system in the spleen and elsewhere (extravascular haemolysis) and haemoglobin is not liberated into the plasma in appreciable amounts. In a haemolytic anaemia the red cell life-span is, by definition, shortened (accelerated haemolysis). In some types of haemolytic anaemia the increased haemolysis is predominantly extravascular and the plasma haemoglobin concentration is barely raised: in other disorders a major degree of haemolysis takes place within the blood stream (intravascular haemolysis): the plasma haemoglobin rises substantially, and in some cases the amount of haemoglobin so liberated may be sufficient to lead to haemoglobin being excreted in the urine (haemoglobinuria).

The clinical and laboratory phenomena of increased haemolysis reflect the nature of the haemolytic mechanism, where the haemolysis is taking place and the response of the bone marrow to the anaemia resulting from the increased haemolysis, namely, erythroid hyperplasia and reticulocytosis.

INVESTIGATION OF HAEMOLYTIC ANAEMIA: A SUMMARY

The two pathways by which haemoglobin derived from effete red cells is metabolized are illustrated in Figure 13.1.

The investigation of patients suspected of suffering from a haemolytic anaemia comprises several distinct stages: recognizing the existence of increased haemolysis; determining the type of haemolytic mechanism; making the precise diagnosis; and, if facilities are available, carrying out tests of scientific rather than of immediate diagnostic or prognostic value. In practice, the procedures are often telescoped, for the diagnosis in some instances may be obvious to the experienced observer from a glance down the microscope at the patient's blood film.

The following practical scheme of investigation is recommended. The tests are arranged 1, 2, 3 and 4 in order of importance and practicability.

Is there evidence of increased haemolysis?

1. Hb estimation; reticulocyte count; inspection of a stained blood film for presence of spherocytes, elliptocytes, irregularly-contracted cells, schistocytes or auto-agglutination (see Chapter 8).

2. Osmotic-fragility test or glycerol lysis test; serum bilirubin estimation.

3. Measurement of life-span of patient's red cells

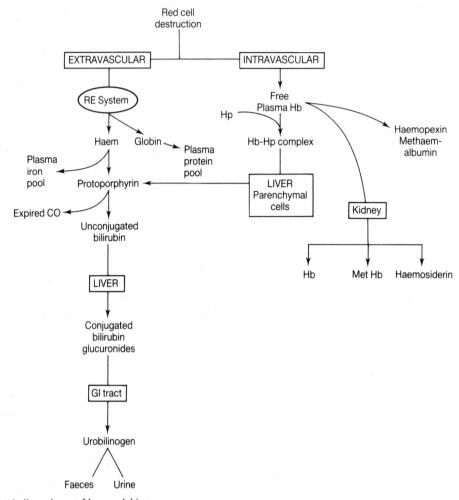

Fig. 13.1 Catabolic pathway of haemoglobin.

(^{51}Cr method); demonstration of haptoglobins; test for increased urinary urobilinogen excretion.

4. Measurement of faecal urobilinogen.

What is the type of haemolytic mechanism?

1. Direct antiglobulin test (DAT) with broad spectrum serum.

2. Test for haemosiderin and Hb in urine; estimation of plasma Hb; Schumm's test.

What is the precise diagnosis?

Which test should be done depends upon the results of the tests which have already been carried out. Not all are appropriate in every case.

1. If a hereditary haemolytic anaemia is suspected:

Osmotic-fragility determination after 24 h incubation at 37°C; autohaemolysis test ± the addition of glucose; screening test for red cell G6PD deficiency; red cell pyruvate kinase assay; assay of other red cell enzymes involved in glycolysis; estimation of red cell glutathione.

Electrophoresis for abnormal haemoglobins; estimation of Hb A$_2$; estimation of Hb F; tests for sickling; tests for heat-labile Hb (Hb Köln, etc.).

2. If an auto-immune acquired haemolytic anaemia is suspected:

Direct antiglobulin test using anti-Ig and anti-complement (C) sera; tests for auto-antibodies in the patient's serum; titration of cold agglutinins; Donath-Landsteiner test; electrophoresis of serum proteins.

3. If the haemolytic anaemia is suspected of being drug-induced:

Screening test for red cell G6PD; glutathione stability test; staining for Heinz bodies; identification of methaemoglobin (Hi) and sulphaemoglobin (SHb); tests for drug-dependent antibodies.

4. In all instances of haemolytic anaemia of obscure type (and in all cases of aplastic anaemia):

Acidified serum test (Ham's test) for paroxysmal nocturnal haemoglobinuria (PNH); sucrose lysis test etc.

Tests primarily of scientific interest

1. Red cell glucose consumption; red cell lactate production.
2. Elution of auto-antibodies and determination of antibody specificity (of practical but not diagnostic importance); tests for agglutination and/or lysis of enzyme-treated cells by auto-antibodies; tests for lysis of normal cells by auto-antibodies; demonstration of thermal range of auto-antibodies.
3. Determination of sites of haemolysis by surface counting (may be of practical importance if splenectomy is contemplated).

In this and subsequent chapters, descriptions will be given of most of the tests which have been referred to. This chapter will include tests of general importance in providing evidence of increased haemolysis. The investigation of hereditary haemolytic anaemias is described in Chapter 14, haemoglobinopathies in Chapter 15, PNH in Chapter 16 and autoimmune acquired haemolytic anaemias in Chapter 29. Some relevant tests, which are normally carried out in clinical chemistry laboratories, will not be described in detail. Instead, recommended methods are referred to.

ESTIMATION OF PLASMA HAEMOGLOBIN

The technique described below is adapted from Crosby and Furth's[8] modification of Wu's original peroxidase method.[37] The catalytic action of haem-containing proteins brings about the oxidation of benzidine by hydrogen peroxide to give a green colour which changes to blue and finally to reddish violet. The intensity of reaction may be compared in a photoelectric colorimeter or spectrophotometer with that produced by solutions of known Hb content. Methaemalbumin and Hb are measured together. Tetramethyl benzidine has been recommended as a non-carcinogenic analogue of benzidine;[19] it should, however, be handled with care. When the plasma Hb concentration is >50 mg/l it can be measured by means of a spectrophotometer at 540 nm by a modification of the whole-blood haemiglobincyanide method.[21]

Sample collection

Every effort must be made to prevent haemolysis during the collection and manipulation of the blood. A clean venepuncture is essential; a relatively wide-bore needle should be used and the syringe, first rinsed with sterile 9 g/l NaCl (saline), should fill spontaneously with blood. When the required amount of blood has been withdrawn, the needle should be detached and 9 volumes of blood added to 1 volume of 32 g/l sodium citrate. All glassware must be scrupulously clean.

In order to reduce haemolysis to a minimum, Hanks and his colleagues recommended that blood should be collected through a wide-bore needle direct into a siliconized centrifuge tube containing heparin.[14] The blood is then lightly centrifuged and the supernatant recentrifuged after being transferred to a clean tube. With this technique, the upper limit for plasma Hb in health was found to be as low as 6 mg/l.

PEROXIDASE METHOD[29]

Reagents

Benzidine reagent. Dissolve 1 g of 3,3′, 5,5′ tetramethyl benzidine in 90 ml of glacial acetic acid and make up to 100 ml with water. The solution will keep for several weeks in a dark bottle at 4°C.

Hydrogen peroxide. Dilute 1 volume of 3% ('10 vols') H_2O_2 with 2 volumes of water before use.

Acetic acid. 100 g/l glacial acetic acid.

Standard. A blood sample of known Hb content is diluted with water to a final concentration of 200 mg/l. It is convenient to use a HiCN standard solution (p. 38) as the source of Hb.

Method

Add 20 μl of plasma to 1 ml of the benzidine reagent in a large glass tube. At the same time set up a control tube, in which 20 μl of water are substituted for the plasma, and a standard tube, containing 20 μl of the Hb standard. Add 1 ml of the H_2O_2 solution to each tube and mix the contents well.

Allow the mixture to stand at *c* 20°C for 20 min and then add 10 volumes of the acetic acid solution to each tube and, after mixing, allow the tubes to stand for a further 10 min. Compare the coloured solutions at 600 nm or in a photoelectric colorimeter provided with an orange (e.g. Ilford 607) filter, using the colour developed by the control tube as a blank. If the Hb content of the plasma to be tested is abnormally high, the plasma should be diluted with saline until it is just visibly tinged red.

Normal range

10–40 mg/l;[7] up to 6 mg/l.[14]

Significance of raised plasma-haemoglobin concentrations

Haemoglobin liberated from the vascular or extravascular breakdown of red cells interacts with the plasma haptoglobins to form a haemoglobin-haptoglobin complex[18] which is subsequently removed from the circulation by, and degraded in, RE cells. Hb in excess of the capacity of the haptoglobins to bind it, is partly cleared in the urine in an uncomplexed form, resulting in haemoglobinuria, and partly degraded in the plasma into haem and globin. The haem complexes with albumin forming methaemalbumin (see p. 184) and with haemopexin (see p. 186); the globin

competes with Hb to form a complex with haptoglobin. In effect, the plasma-haemoglobin level is significantly raised in haemolytic anaemias when haemolysis is sufficiently severe for the available haptoglobin to be fully bound. The highest levels are found when haemolysis takes place predominantly in the blood stream (intravascular haemolysis). Thus marked haemoglobinaemia, with or without haemoglobinuria, may be found in paroxysmal nocturnal haemoglobinuria, paroxysmal cold haemoglobinburia, the cold-haemagglutinin syndrome, blackwater fever, and in march haemoglobinuria and in other mechanical haemolytic anaemias, e.g. that after cardiac surgery. In warm-type auto-immune haemolytic anaemias, sickle-cell anaemia and severe Mediterranean anaemia, the plasma-haemoglobin level may be slightly or moderately raised, but in hereditary spherocytosis, in which haemolysis occurs predominately in the spleen, the levels are normal or only very slightly raised.

It cannot be over-emphasized that the presence of excess Hb in the plasma is a reliable sign in intravascular haemolysis only if the observer can be sure that the lysis has not been caused during or after the withdrawal of the blood. Chaplin et al reported 5–30-fold rises above their upper normal level of 6 mg/l as the result of violent exercise,[5] and similar rises have been recorded by Vanzetti and Valente,[35] although others have failed to detect lysis after prolonged exercise, e.g. in long-distance runners.[2]

ESTIMATION OF SERUM HAPTOGLOBINS

Haptoglobin is a glycoprotein consisting of two pairs of α-chains and two pairs of β-chains. Free haemoglobin readily dissociates into dimers of α and β chains; the α chains bind avidly with the β chains of haptoglobin in plasma or serum to form a complex which can be differentiated from free haemoglobin by column chromatographic separation on Sephadex[25] or by its altered rate of migration on electrophoresis. For electrophoretic separation, paper,[18] cellulose acetate,[3,32] starch gel[28] and acrylamide gel[12] have been used. The method described below uses cellulose-acetate electrophoresis.

ELECTROPHORETIC METHOD

Principle. A known amount of haemoglobin is added to serum. The Hb-haptoglobin complex is separated by electrophoresis on cellulose acetate, and the relative amounts of bound and free Hb are estimated by scanning the electrophoresis strips after staining. The concentration of haptoglobin can then be expressed as mg Hb-binding capacity per litre serum.

Reagents

Buffer (pH 7.0, ionic strength 0.05) Na_2HPO_4. H_2O 7.1 g/l, 2 volumes; $NaH_2PO_4.H_2O$ 6.9 g/l, 1 volume. Store at 4°C.

Haemolysate. Prepare as described on p. 231. Adjust the Hb concentration to 35–40 g/l with water. This solution is stable at 4°C for several weeks.

Stain. Dissolve 0.5 g of o-dianisidine (3,3'-dimethoxybenzidine) in 70 ml of 95% ethanol; prior to use add together 10 ml of acetate buffer, pH 4.7 (sodium acetate 2.92 g, glacial acetic acid 1 ml, water to 1 litre), 2.5 ml of 3% (10 vol) H_2O_2 and water to 100 ml.

Clearing solution. Glacial acetic acid 25 ml, 95% ethanol 75 ml.

Acetic acid rinse. Glacial acetic acid, 50 ml/l.

Method

Serum is obtained from blood allowed to clot undisturbed at 37°C. As soon as the clot starts to retract, remove the serum by pipette and centrifuge it to rid it of suspended red cells. The serum may be stored at −20°C until used.

Mix well 1 volume of haemolysate with 9 volumes of serum. Allow to stand for 10 min at room temperature.

Impregnate cellulose acetate membrane filter-strips (12 × 2.5 cm) in buffer solution and blot to remove all obvious surface fluid. Apply 0.75 µl samples of the serum haemolysate mixture across the strips as thin transverse lines, and electrophorese at 0.5 mA/cm width. Good separation patterns about 5–7 cm in length should be obtained in 30 min (Fig. 13.2).

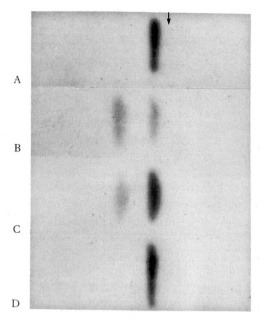

Fig. 13.2 Demonstration of serum haptoglobins.
Electrophoresis on paper.
A. Aqueous solution of haemoglobin (0.4 g/l) run as a reference. The band appears in the β globulin position.
B. Normal serum with added haemoglobin. Bands appear in both the β globulin position (Hb) and in the α_2 globulin position (Hb-haptoglobin complex).
C. Slightly reduced haptoglobulin with added haemoglobin. The β globulin band is denser than that of the α_2 globulin band (cf. B).
D. Serum from a case of haemolytic anaemia with added haemoglobin. Haptoglobins are absent and the haemoglobin appears only in the β globulin position. The line of origin is indicated by the arrow.

After electrophoresis is completed, immerse the membranes in freshly prepared o-dianisidine stain for 10 min. Then rinse with water and immerse in 50 ml/l acetic acid for 5 min. Remove the membranes and place in 95% ethanol for exactly 1 min. Transfer the membranes to a tray containing freshly prepared clearing solution and immerse for exactly 30 s. While still in the solution, position the membranes over a glass plate placed in the tray. Remove the glass plate with the membranes on it, drain the excess solution from the membranes, transfer the glass plate to a ventilated oven pre-heated to 100°C, and allow the membranes to dry for 10 min.

After the plate has cooled, scan the membranes by a densitometer at 450 nm with a 0.3 mm slit width.

Calculation

Calculate the density of the haptoglobin band as a fraction of the total Hb in the electrophoretic strip:

Haptoglobin (g/l) = haptoglobin fraction × Hb conc (g/l).

Another method for the estimation of haptoglobins is based on radial immunodiffusion in a plate of agarose gel containing a monospecific equine or goat antiserum to human haptoglobin. The test sample and a series of reference samples of known haptoglobin concentration are dispensed into wells in the plate and left for 18 h. Precipitation rings form by the reaction of haptoglobin with the antibody; the diameter of each ring is proportional to the concentration of haptoglobin in the sample. A calibration graph is prepared from the reference samples. The reagents for this procedure are available in a test kit (Endoplate Haptoglobin Test Kit, Kallestad Laboratories). Technical instructions are provided with the kit.

Significance of haptoglobin levels

In normal sera, haptoglobins are present in sufficient amounts to bind 0.3–2.0 g of Hb/l. The mean has been given as 1.1 g.[24] However, it is possible that the haptoglobin level depends to some extent on the haptoglobin group, and that the levels are higher in men than in women.[24]

Haptoglobins begin to be depleted when the daily Hb turnover exceeds about twice the normal.[3] This occurs irrespective of whether the haemolysis is predominantly extravascular or intravascular; but rapid depletion, often with the formation of methaemalbumin, occurs as a result of small degrees of intravascular haemolysis, even when the daily total Hb turnover is not increased appreciably above normal. Low concentrations of haptoglobins, in the absence of increased haemolysis, may be found in hepatocellular disease, and are characteristic of congenital ahaptoglobinaemia. Low concentrations may also be found in megaloblastic anaemias, probably because of increased haemolysis, and following haemorrhage into tissues.

The haptoglobin-haemoglobin complex is cleared by the RE system, mainly in the liver. The rate of removal is influenced by the concentration of free haemoglobin in the plasma: at levels below 10 g/l the clearance $T_{1/2}$ is 20 min; at higher concentrations clearance is considerably slower.

Increased haptoglobin concentrations may be found in pregnancy, chronic infections, malignancy, tissue damage, Hodgkin's disease, rheumatoid arthritis, systemic lupus erythematosus, biliary obstruction and as a consequence of steroid therapy or the use of oral contraceptives. Under these circumstances a normal haptoglobin concentration does not exclude increased haemolysis.

EXAMINATION OF PLASMA (OR SERUM) FOR METHAEMALBUMIN

A simple but not very sensitive method is to examine the plasma using a hand spectroscope.

Free the plasma from suspended cells and platelets by centrifuging at 1200–1500 *g* for 15–30 min. Then view it in bright daylight with a hand spectroscope using the greatest possible depth of plasma consistent with visibility. Methaemalbumin gives a rather weak band in the red (at 624 nm) (Fig. 13.3). As HbO_2 is usually present as well, its characteristic bands in the yellow-green may also be visible. The position of the methaemalbumin absorption band in the red can be readily differentiated from that of methaemoglobin (Hi) by means of a reversion spectroscope.

Presumptive evidence of the presence of small quantities of methaemalbumin, giving an absorption band too weak to recognize, can be obtained by extracting the pigment by ether and then converting it to an ammonium haemochromogen which gives a more intense band in the green (Schumm's test).

SCHUMM'S TEST

Method

Cover the plasma (or serum) with a layer of ether. Add a one-tenth volume of saturated yellow ammonium sulphide and mix it with the plasma. Then view it with a hand spectroscope. If methaemalbumin is present, a relatively intense narrow absorption band will be seen in the green (at 558 nm) (Fig. 13.3).

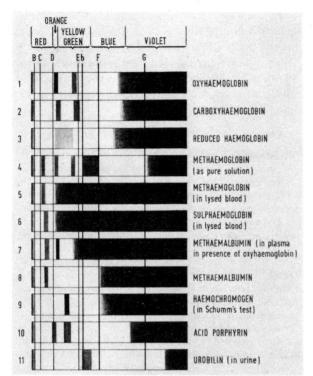

Fig. 13.3 Absorption spectra of derivatives of human haemoglobin. The absorption bands are shown in relation to the Fraunhofer lines, the positions of which are as follows: B at 686.7 nm, C at 656.3 nm, D at 589 nm, E at 527 nm, b at 518.4 nm, F at 486.1 nm and G at 430.8 nm.

Significance of methaemalbuminaemia

Methaemalbumin is found in the plasma when haptoglobins are absent in haemolytic anaemias in which lysis is predominantly intravascular. It was first observed by Fairley and Bromfield in blackwater fever.[11] It is a haem-albumin compound formed subsequent to the degradation of Hb liberated into plasma. In contrast to haptoglobin-bound Hb and haemopexin-bound haem, the haem-albumin complex is thought to remain in circulation until the haem is transferred from albumin to the more highly avid haemopexin.[23]

QUANTITATIVE ESTIMATION OF METHAEMALBUMIN BY A SPECTROPHOTOMETRIC METHOD

To 2 ml of plasma (or serum) add 1 ml of iso-osmotic phosphate buffer, pH 7.4. Centrifuge the mixture for 30 min at 1200–1500 g and measure its absorbence in a spectrophotometer at 569 nm. Add c 5 mg of solid sodium dithionite to the supernatant diluted plasma. Shake the tube gently to dissolve the dithionite and leave for 5 min to allow complete reduction of the methaemalbumin. Remeasure the absorbence. The difference between the two readings represents the absorbence due to methaemalbumin; its concentration can be read off from a calibration graph.

The calibration graph is constructed as follows: solutions containing 10–100 mg/l methaemalbumin are obtained by dissolving appropriate amounts of haemin (e.g. BDH Ltd, Sigma) in a minimum volume of 40 g/l human serum albumin. The absorbence of each solution is measured in a spectrophotometer at 569 nm, and a graph drawn from the figures obtained.

DEMONSTRATION OF HAEMOSIDERIN IN URINE

Method

Centrifuge 10 ml of urine at 1200 g for 10–15 min. Transfer the deposit to a slide, spread out to occupy an area of 1–2 cm and allow to dry in the air. Fix by placing the slide in methanol for 10–20 min and then stain by the method used to stain blood films for siderocytes (p. 116). Haemosiderin, if present, appears in the form of isolated or grouped blue-staining granules, usually from 1 to 3 μm in size (Fig. 13.4). If haemosiderin is present in small amounts, and especially if distributed irregularly on the slide, or if the findings are difficult to interpret, the test should be repeated on a fresh sample of urine collected into an iron-free container and centrifuged in an iron-free tube. (For the preparation of iron-free glassware, see p. 540.)

Significance of haemosiderinuria[9]

Haemosiderinuria is a sequel to the presence of Hb in the glomerular filtrate. It is a valuable sign of chronic intravascular haemolysis, for the urine will be found to contain iron-containing granules even if there is no haemoglobinuria at the time. However, haemosiderinuria is not found in the urine at the

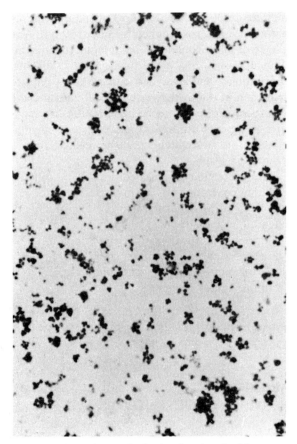

Fig. 13.4 Photomicrograph of urine deposit stained by Perls's reaction. Numerous granules of haemosiderin are present × 1200.

onset of a haemolytic attack even if this is accompanied by haemoglobinaemia and haemoglobinuria, as the haemoglobin has first to be absorbed by the cells of the renal tubules. The intracellular breakdown of Hb liberates iron which is then re-excreted. Haemosiderinuria may persist for several weeks after a haemolytic episode.

DEMONSTRATION OF SERUM HAEMOPEXIN

Haem derived from Hb, which fails to bind to haptoglobins, complexes with either albumin or haemopexin. The latter has a much higher affinity, and when complexed the haem is eliminated from the circulation, e.g. by the liver Kupffer cells.

Haemopexin is a haem-binding serum glycoprotein of molecular weight 70 000. In normal adults of both sexes its concentration is 0.5–1 g/l;[23] in newborn infants there is much less, c 0.3 g/l, but adult levels are reached by the end of the first year of life. In severe intravascular haemolysis haemopexin levels are low or zero when haptoglobins are depleted. With less severe haemolysis, although haptoglobins are likely to be reduced or absent, haemopexin may be normal or only slightly lowered, and it has been suggested that the haemopexin level gives a more reliable measure of haemolysis than does the haptoglobin level. Haem binds in a 1:1 molar ratio to haemopexin; 6 μg/ml of free haem is required to deplete the normal binding levels of haemopexin. Haemopexin seems to be disproportionately low in thalassaemia major,[23] and low levels may be found in certain pathological conditions other than haemolytic disease, namely, renal and liver diseases. The concentration is raised in diabetes mellitus, infections and carcinoma.[23]

Haemopexin can be measured by starch-gel electrophoresis[16] or immunochemically by radial immunodiffusion.[15]

CHEMICAL TESTS OF HAEMOGLOBIN CATABOLISM

Measurement of serum bilirubin, urinary urobilin and faecal urobilinogen can provide important information in the investigation of haemolytic anaemias. As these tests come within the province of the clinical chemist, they are, nowadays, seldom performed in a haematological laboratory. Accordingly, the principles of the tests and their interpretation will be described, but for details of the techniques readers are referred to text books of

clinical chemistry, e.g. *Microanalysis in Medical Biochemistry* by Wootton and Freeman.[36]

SERUM BILIRUBIN

Bilirubin is present in serum in two forms: as unconjugated prehepatic bilirubin and bilirubin conjugated to glucuronic acid. Normally, the serum-bilirubin concentration is <17 μmol/l (10 mg/l), and is mostly unconjugated.

In haemolytic anaemias the serum bilirubin usually lies between 17 and 50 μmol/l (10–30 mg/l) and most is unconjugated. Sometimes the level may be normal, despite a considerable increase in haemolysis. Levels >85 μmol/l (50 mg/l) and/or a large proportion of conjugated bilirubin suggest liver disease. Tisdale et al, who reported on the concentration of direct-reacting (conjugated) pigment in haemolytic jaundice, concluded that some of this type of bilirubin may often be regurgitated into the blood stream from the bile when the excretion of pigment is high, even in the absence of overt liver disease.[31]

In haemolytic disease of the newborn (HDN) the bilirubin level is an important factor in determining whether an exchange transfusion should be carried out, as high values of unconjugated bilirubin are toxic to the brain and can lead to kernicterus. In normal newborn infants the level may often reach 85 μmol/l, whilst in HDN infants levels of 350 μmol/l are not uncommon and need to be urgently lowered by exchange transfusion.

Moderately raised serum-bilirubin levels are frequently found in dyshaemopoietic anaemias, e.g. pernicious anaemia, where there is ineffective erythropoiesis. Although part of the bilirubin comes from red cells which have circulated, a major proportion is derived from red cell precursors in the bone marrow which have failed to complete maturation.

Total bilirubin can be measured by direct spectrophotometry at 460 nm in which the colour of serum is compared with a permanent yellow glass standard.★ Erroneous high results result from the presence of free haemoglobin or lipochromic pigments. In these circumstances bilirubin is more reliably measured by its reaction with aqueous diazotized sulphanilic acid. A red colour is produced which is compared in a photoelectric colorimeter with that of a freshly prepared standard or read in a spectrophotometer at 600 nm. Only conjugated bilirubin reacts directly with this aqueous reagent; unconjugated bilirubin, which is bound to albumin, requires the addition of ethanol to free it from albumin to enable it to react or the

action of an accelerator such as methanol or caffeine. The method of Michaelson et al[20] in which caffeine benzoate is used as the accelerator is said to have advantages.[36]

Bilirubin is destroyed by exposure to direct sunlight or any other source of ultraviolet light, including fluorescent lighting. Solutions are stable for 1–2 days if kept at 4°C in the dark.

UROBILIN AND UROBILINOGEN

Urobilin and its reduced form urobilinogen are formed by bacterial action on bile pigments in the intestine. The excretion of faecal urobilinogen is increased in patients with a haemolytic anaemia. Estimations are best expressed as mg of urobilinogen per 100 g of circulating Hb. In health this amounts to 18–35 μmol (11–21 mg) per day.[36]

The estimation of faecal urobilinogen is, however, a crude and often unsatisfactory method of assessing rates of haemolysis, and minor degrees are more reliably demonstrated by red cell life-span studies. Urobilinogen excretion is also increased in dyshaemopoietic anaemias such as pernicious anaemia because of ineffective erythropoiesis.

The amount of urobilinogen in the urine is a still less reliable index of haemolysis, for excessive urobilinuria can be a consequence of liver dysfunction as well as of increased red cell destruction.

For estimation in the faeces the bile-derived pigments (stercobilin) are reduced to urobilinogen which is extracted with water. The solution is then treated with Ehrlich's dimethylaminobenzaldehyde reagent to produce a pink colour which can be compared with either a natural or an artificial standard in a quantitative assay.[36]

QUALITATIVE TEST FOR UROBILINOGEN AND UROBILIN IN URINE[36]

Schlesinger's zinc test

To 5 ml of urine, add 2 drops of 0.5 mol/l iodine to convert urobilinogen to urobilin. After mixing and standing for 1–2 min, add 5 ml of a 100 g/l suspension of zinc acetate in ethanol and centrifuge the mixture. A green fluorescence becomes apparent in the clear supernatant if urobilin or urobilinogen is present.

★AO Bilirubinometer (British American Optical Co.)

If a spectroscope is available the fluid may be examined for the broad absorption band (due to urobilin) at the green-blue junction (Fig. 13.3).

Urobilinogen can also be detected in freshly voided urine by a commercially available reagent strip (Urobilistix, Ames Co.); the reagent is 4-dimethylaminobenzaldehyde which produces a brown colour in the presence of urobilinogen.

PORPHYRINS

Deranged haem synthesis results in alteration in the quantities of porphyrin synthesized and excreted by the body. The three porphyrins of clinical importance in man are: protoporphyrin, uroporphyrin and coproporphyrin together with their precursor δ-aminolaevulinic acid. Protoporphyrin is widely distributed in the body, and, in addition to its main role as a precursor of haem in Hb and myoglobin, it is a precusor of cytochromes and catalase. Uroporphyrin and coproporphyrin, which are precursors of protoporphyrin, are normally excreted in small amounts in urine and faeces, and red cells, too, normally contain a small amount of free protoporphyrin and coproporphyrin (Fig. 13.5).

ESTIMATION OF REDCELL PORPHYRINS

Principle. Porphyrins are extracted from washed red cells by a mixture of ethyl acetate and acetic acid. The preparation is treated with ether. Coproporphyrin is extracted from the ethereal solution by 0.1 mol/l HCl and protoporphyrin by 1.5 mol/l HCl. The porphyrin concentration in each extract is determined by a spectrophotometric method. Details of the procedure are given by Moore.[22]

DEMONSTRATION OF PORPHOBILINOGEN IN URINE

Principle. Ehrlich's dimethylaminobenzaldehyde reagent reacts with porphobilinogen to produce a pink aldehyde compound which can be differentiated from that produced by urobilinogen by the fact that the porphobilinogen compound is insoluble in chloroform.

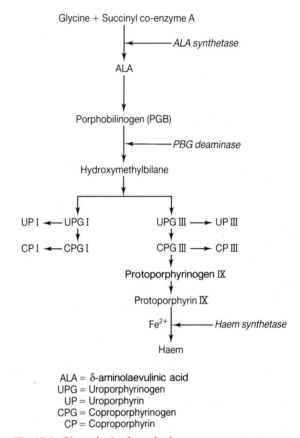

ALA = δ-aminolaevulinic acid
UPG = Uroporphyrinogen
UP = Uroporphyrin
CPG = Coproporphyrinogen
CP = Coproporphyrin

Fig. 13.5   Biosynthesis of porphyrin.

Ehrlich's reagent. Dissolve 0.7 g of *p*-dimethylaminobenzaldehyde in a mixture of 150 ml of 10 N (360 g/l) HCl and 100 ml of water.

Method

The test is best carried out on a freshly passed specimen of urine. Mix a few ml of urine and an equal volume of Ehrlich's reagent in a large test-tube. Add 2 volumes of a saturated solution of sodium acetate. The urine should then have a pH of about 5.0, giving a red reaction with Congo red indicator paper.

If a pink colour develops in the solution, add a few ml of chloroform and shake the mixture thoroughly to extract the pigment. The colour due to urobilinogen or indole will be extracted by the chloroform; whereas that due to porphobilinogen will not, and remains in the supernatant aqueous fraction. When present, the concentration of porphobilinogen in the urine may be estimated quantitatively by a spectrophotometric method at 555 nm.[22]

Aminolaevulinic acid (ALA)

When ALA is present in the urine it can be concentrated with acetyl acetone. It then reacts with Ehrlich's reagent in the same way as porphobilinogen to give a red solution with an absorbence maximum at 553 nm. It can be separated from porphobilinogen by ion exchange resins and estimated quantitatively by a spectrophotometric method.[22]

DEMONSTRATION OF PORPHYRINS IN URINE

Principle. Porphyrins exhibit pink-red fluorescence when viewed by UV light (at 405 nm). Uroporphyrin can be distinguished from coproporphyrin by the different solubilities of the two substances in acid solution.

Method

Mix 25 ml of urine with 10 ml of glacial acetic acid in a separating funnel and extract twice with 50 ml volumes of ether. Set the aqueous fraction (Fraction 1) aside. Wash the ether extracts in a separating funnel with 10 ml of 1.6 mol/l HCl and collect the HCl fraction (Fraction 2). View both fractions in UV light (at 405 nm) for pink-red fluorescence. Its presence in Fraction 1 indicates uroporphyrin; in Fraction 2, coproporphyrin. The presence of the porphyrins should be confirmed spectroscopically (see below).

If uroporphyrin has been demonstrated, the reaction can be intensified by the following procedure. Adjust the pH of Fraction 1 to 3.0–3.2 with 0.1 mol/l HCl and extract the fraction twice with 50 ml volumes of ethyl acetate. Combine the extracts and extract three times with 2 ml volumes of 3 mol/l HCl. View the acid extracts for pink-red fluorescence in UV light and spectroscopically for acid porphyrin bands.

SPECTROSCOPIC EXAMINATION OF URINE FOR PORPHYRINS

This is carried out on extracts, made as described above, or on urine which is acidified with a few drops of 10 N HCl. If porphyrins are present, a narrow band will appear in the orange at 596 nm and a broader band in the green at 552 nm (Fig. 13.3).

Qualitative tests are adequate for screening purposes. Accurate determinations require spectrophotometry or fluorimetry.[22]

Significance of porphyrins in blood and urine

Normal red cells contain <650 nmol/l of protoporphyrin and <64 nmol/l of coproporphyrin.[22] Increased amounts are present during the first few months of life. At all ages there is an increase in red cell protoporphyrin in iron-deficiency anaemia or latent iron deficiency, in lead poisoning, thalassaemia, some cases of sideroblastic anaemia and the anaemia of chronic infection.

Normally, a small amount of coproporphyrin is excreted in the urine (<430 nmol/day). This is demonstrable by the qualitative test described above, the intensity of pink-red fluorescence being proportional to the concentration of coproporphyrin. The excretion of coproporphyrin is increased when erythropoiesis is hyperactive, e.g. in haemolytic anaemias, polycythaemia and in pernicious anaemia, sideroblastic anaemias, etc. It is exceptionally high in lead poisoning and it is also high in liver disease; renal impairment results in diminished excretion.

Table 13.1 Distribution of porphyrins in red cells, urine and faeces in different forms of porphyria

	Red cells	Urine	Faeces
Congenital erythropoietic porphyria	UP I CP I	UP I CP I	UP I CP I
Hereditary coproporphyria		CP III	CP III
Erythropoietic protoporphyria	PP		PP
Acute intermittent porphyria		PBG ALA	
Variegate porphyria		PBG* ALA*	CP III PP
Acquired porphyria		UP I CP III	

* Mainly during acute attacks
UP = Uroporphyrin
CP = Coproporphyrin
PP = Protoporphyrin
ALA = δ aminolaevulinic acid
PBG = Porphobilinogen

Normally, porphobilinogen cannot be demonstrated in urine, and only traces of uroporphyrin (<50 nmol/day[22]) not detectable by the qualitative test described above, are present. Aminolaevulinic acid excretion is <40 μmol/day;[22] it is increased in lead poisoning.

The increase in urinary coproporphyrin excretion occurring in the above conditions is known as 'porphyrinuria'. There is no increase in uroporphyrin excretion. The porphyrias, on the other hand, are a group of disorders associated with abnormal porphyrin metabolism. There are several forms of porphyria, each with a different clinical and biochemical manifestation.[13] Two are of haematological importance, namely, congenital erythropoietic porphyria and erythropoietic protoporphyria. In the former, uroporphyrin and coproporphyrin are present in red cells and urine in increased amounts; in the latter, increased protoporphyrin is found in the red cells, but the urine is normal. In erythropoietic porphyria haemolytic anaemia may occur. The patterns of excretion of porphyrin and precursors in the different types of porphyria are shown in Table 13.1.

RECOGNITION AND MEASUREMENT OF ABNORMAL HAEMOGLOBIN PIGMENTS

Methaemoglobin (Hi), sulphaemoglobin (SHb) and carboxyhaemoglobin (HbCO) are of clinical importance, and each has a characteristic absorption spectrum demonstrable by simple spectroscopy or, more definitely, by spectrophotometry. If the absorbence of a dilute solution of blood (e.g. 1 in 200) is measured at wavelengths between 400 and 700 nm, characteristic absorption spectra are obtained (Fig. 13.6). In practice, the abnormal substance represents usually only a fraction of the total Hb (except in coal-gas poisoning), and its identification and accurate measurement may be difficult. Hi can be measured more accurately than SHb.

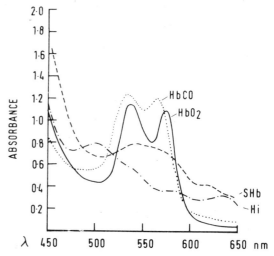

Fig. 13.6 Absorption spectra of various haemoglobin pigments. HbCO = carboxyhaemoglobin; HbO$_2$ = oxyhaemoglobin; SHb = sulphaemoglobin; Hi = methaemoglobin.

SPECTROSCOPIC EXAMINATION OF BLOOD FOR METHAEMOGLOBIN AND SULPHAEMOGLOBIN

Method

Dilute blood 1 in 5 or 1 in 10 with water and then centrifuge. Examine the clear solution, if possible in daylight, using a hand spectroscope. It is important that the greatest possible depth or concentration of solution consistent with visibility should be examined and that a careful search should be made (with varying depths or concentrations of solution) for absorption bands in the red part of the spectrum at 620–630 nm. If bands are seen in the red, add a drop of yellow ammonium sulphide to the solution. A band due to Hi, but not that due to SHb, will disappear. For comparison, lysed blood may be treated with a few drops of potassium ferricyanide (50 g/l) solution which will cause the formation of Hi. SHb may be prepared by adding to 10 ml of a 1 in 100 dilution of blood 0.1 ml of a 1 g/l solution of phenylhydrazine hydrochloride and a drop of water which has been previously saturated with hydrogen sulphide. The spectra of the unknown and the known pigments may then be compared in a reversion spectroscope. The absorption band in the red due to Hi is at 630 nm (cf. methaemalbumin at 624 nm) (Fig. 13.3).

Hi and SHb are formed intracellularly; they are not found in plasma except under very exceptional circumstances, e.g. when their formation is associated with intravascular haemolysis.

MEASUREMENT OF METHAEMOGLOBIN IN BLOOD

Principle. Hi has a maximum absorption at 630 nm. When cyanide is added this absorption band disappears and the resulting change in absorbence is directly proportional to the concentration of Hi. Total Hb in the sample is then measured after complete conversion to HiCN by the addition of ferricyanide-cyanide reagent. The conversion will measure HbO_2 and Hi but not SHb. Thus, the presence of a large amount of SHb will result in an erroneously low measurement of total Hb.

The method described below is based on that of Evelyn and Malloy.[10] Turbidity of the haemolysate can be overcome by the addition of a non-ionic detergent such as Nonidet P40[34] (see p. 38).

Reagents

Phosphate buffer. 0.1 mol/l, pH 6.8.
Potassium cyanide. 50 g/l.
Potassium ferricyanide. 50 g/l.
Non-ionic detergent (see p. 38). 10 ml/l.

Method

Lyse 0.2 ml of blood in a solution containing 4 ml of buffer and 6 ml of detergent solution. Divide the lysate into two equal volumes (A and B). Measure the absorbence of A in a spectrophotometer at 630 nm (D_1). Add 1 drop of KCN solution and measure the absorbence again, after mixing (D_2). Add 1 drop of potassium ferricyanide solution to B, and after 5 min, measure the absorbence at the same wavelength (D_3). Then add 1 drop of KCN solution to B and after mixing make a final reading (D_4). All the measurements are made against a blank containing buffer and detergent in the same proportion as present in the sample.

Calculation

$$\text{Methaemoglobin (\%)} = \frac{D_1 - D_2}{D_3 - D_4} \times 100.$$

The test should be carried out within 1 h of collecting the blood. After dilution, the buffered lysate can be stored for up to 24 h at 2–4°C without significant auto-oxidation of Hb to Hi.

SCREENING METHOD FOR DETERMINATION OF SULPHAEMOGLOBIN IN BLOOD

Principle. An absorbence reading at 620 nm measures the sum of the absorbence of HbO_2 and SHb in any blood sample. In contrast to HbO_2, the absorption band due to SHb is unchanged by the addition of cyanide. The residual absorbence, as read at 620 nm, is therefore proportional to the concentration of SHb.

The absorbence of the HbO_2 alone at 620 nm can only be inferred from a reading at 578 nm, and a conversion factor[34], A^{578}/A^{620}, has to be determined experimentally for each instrument on a series of normal blood samples. The absorbence of SHb is obtained by subtracting the absorbence of the HbO_2 from that of the total Hb. This provides an approximation only, but it may be regarded as adequate for clinical purposes in the absence of a more reliable method.

Method

Mix 0.1 ml of blood with 10 ml of a 20 ml/l solution of a non-ionic detergent (Sterox SE or Nonidet P40). Record the absorbence (A) at 620 nm (total Hb). Add 1 drop of 50 g/l KCN and after standing for 5 min, record A at 620 nm and at 578 nm.

Calculation

$$\text{Sulphaemoglobin (SHb) (\%)} = 2 \times \frac{A^{620} \text{SHb}}{A^{620} \text{HbO}_2}$$

where

$$A^{620}\text{HbO}_2 = \frac{\text{Absorbence read at 578 nm}}{\text{Conversion factor}}$$

and $A^{620}\text{SHb} = A^{620}$ total Hb $- A^{620}\text{HbO}_2$.

Significance of methaemoglobin and sulphaemoglobin in blood

Hi is present in small amounts in normal blood, and constitutes 1–2% of the total Hb. Its concentration is very slightly higher in infants, especially in premature infants, than in older children and adults.[17] Excessive formation of Hi occurs as the result of oxidation of Hb by drugs and chemicals such as phenacetin, sulphonamides, aniline dyes, nitrates and nitrites, etc.

The Hi produced by drugs is chemically normal and the pigment can be reconverted to HbO_2 by reducing agents such as methylene blue.

Other (rare) types of methaemoglobinaemia are caused by inherited deficiency of the enzyme NADH-methaemoglobin reductase and by inherited haemoglobin abnormalities (types of Hb M). The absorption spectra of the Hb Ms differ from that of normal Hi and they react slowly and incompletely with cyanide; their concentration cannot be estimated by the method of Evelyn and Malloy.[10]

Methaemoglobinaemia leads to cyanosis which becomes obvious with as little as 15 g Hi per litre, i.e. c 10%.

SHb is usually formed at the same time as Hi; it represents a further and irreversible stage in Hb degradation. It is present as a rule at a much lower concentration than is Hi.

DEMONSTRATION OF CARBOXYHAEMOGLOBIN

Principle. HbO_2, but not HbCO, is reduced by sodium dithionite and the percentage of HbCO in a mixture can be determined by reference to a calibration graph.

Calibration graph

Dilute 0.1 ml of normal blood in 20 ml of 0.4 ml/l ammonia and divide into two parts. To each add 20 mg of sodium dithionite. Then bubble pure CO into one for 2 min, so as to provide a 100% solution of HbCO.

Add various volumes of the HbCO solution to the reduced Hb solution to provide a range of concentrations of HbCO. Within 10 min of adding the dithionite, measure the absorbence of each solution at 538 nm and 578 nm. Plot the quotient A^{538}/A^{578} on arithmetical graph paper against the % HbCO in each solution.

Method[33,34]

Dilute 0.1 ml of blood in 20 ml of 0.4 ml/l ammonia and add 20 mg of sodium dithionite. Measure the absorbence in a spectrophotometer at 538 nm and 578 nm within 10 min. Calculate the quotient A^{538}/A^{578} and read the % HbCO in the blood from the calibration curve[34] or calculate it from the equation:[33]

$$\% \text{ HbCO} = \left\{ 2.44 \times \frac{A^{538}}{A^{578}} \right\} - 2.68$$

Significance of carboxyhaemoglobin in circulating blood

Carbon monoxide has an affinity for Hb c 200 times that of oxygen. This means that even low concentrations of CO rapidly lead to the formation of HbCO. Less than 1% of HbCO is present in normal blood and up to 10% in smokers.[26,27] A high concentration in blood causes tissue anoxia and may lead to death. Recovery can take place, as HbCO dissociates in time in the presence of high concentrations of oxygen.

IDENTIFICATION OF MYOGLOBIN IN URINE

Myoglobin is the principal protein in muscle, and may be released into the circulation when there is cardiac or skeletal muscle damage. Some may be excreted in the urine where its concentration can be measured by a sensitive and specific radio-immune assay.[30] As the absorption spectra of myoglobin and Hb are similar, although not identical, it is not possible to distinguish them readily by spectroscopy or even by spectrophotometry. But they can be separated by column chromatography.[4] The following is a simple screening test for identifying the presence of myoglobin in urine; it is based on the fact that Hb and myoglobin are precipitated in urine at different degrees of ammonium sulphate saturation. First, it is necessary to demonstrate by precipitation with sulphosalicyclic acid that the pigment in the urine is a protein.

Method[1]

Add 3 ml of a 30 g/l solution of sulphosalicylic acid to 1 ml of urine. Mix well and filter. If the pigment is a protein, it will be precipitated. (If the filtrate retains the abnormal colour, this must be due to a non-protein pigment, perhaps a porphyrin). If the pigment has been shown to be protein, add 2.8 g of ammonium sulphate to 5 ml of urine (= 80% saturation). Shake the mixture to dissolve the ammonium sulphate, then filter or centrifuge. In myoglobinuria the filtrate will be abnormally coloured; in haemoglobinuria the filtrate will be of normal colour and the precipitate coloured.

REFERENCES

[1] BLODHEIM, S. H., MARGOLIASH, E. and SHAFRIR, E. (1958). A simple test for myohemoglobinuria (myoglobinuria). *Journal of American Medical Association*, **167**, 453.

[2] BROTHERHOOD, J., BROZOVIC, B. and PUGH, L. G. C. (1975). Haematological status of middle- and long-distance runners. *Clinical Science and Molecular Medicine*, **48**, 139.

[3] BRUS, I. and LEWIS, S. M. (1959). The haptoglobin content of serum in haemolytic anaemia. *British Journal of Haematology*, **5**, 348.

[4] CAMERON, B. F., AZZAM, S. A., KOTITE, L. and AWAD, E. S. (1965). Determination of myoglobin and hemoglobin. *Journal of Laboratory and Clinical Medicine*, **65**, 883.

[5] CHAPLIN, H. Jnr, CASSELL, M. and HANKS G. E. (1961). The stability of the plasma hemoglobin level in the normal human subject. *Journal of Laboratory and Clinical Medicine*, **57**, 612.

[6] CHONG, G. C. and OWEN, J. A. (1967). Determination of methaemalbumin in plasma. *Journal of Clinical Pathology*, **20**, 211.

[7] CROSBY, W. H. and DAMESHEK, W. (1951). The significance of hemoglobinemia and associated hemosiderinuria, with particular reference to various types of hemolytic anemia. *Journal of Laboratory and Clinical Medicine*, **38**, 829.

[8] CROSBY, W. H. and FURTH, F. W. (1956). A modification of the benzidine method for measurement of hemoglobin in plasma and urine. *Blood*, **11**, 380.

[9] DACIE, J. (1985). *The Haemolytic Anaemias: Volume I: The Hereditary Haemolytic Anaemias*, 3rd edn p. 45. Churchill Livingstone, Edinburgh.

[10] EVELYN, K. A. and MALLOY, H. T. (1938). Microdetermination of oxyhemoglobin, methemoglobin and sulfhemoglobin in a single sample of blood. *Journal of Biological Chemistry*, **126**, 655.

[11] FAIRLEY, N. H. and BROMFIELD, R. J. (1934). Laboratory studies in malaria and blackwater fever. Part III. A new blood pigment in blackwater fever and other biochemical observations. *Transactions of the Royal Society of Tropical Medicine and Hygiene*, **28**, 307.

[12] FERRIS, T. G., EASERLING, R. E., NELSON, K. J. and BUDD, R. E. (1966). Determination of serum-hemoglobin binding capacity and haptoglobin-type by acrylamide gel electrophoresis. *American Journal of Clinical Pathology*, **46**, 385.

[13] GOLDBERG, A., MOORE, M. R., McCOLL, K. E. L. and BRODIE, M. J. (1987). Porphyrin metabolism and the porphyrias. In: *Oxford Textbook of Medicine*, 2nd edn. Eds D. J. Weatherall, J. G. G. Ledingham and D. A, Warrell, p. 9. 136. Oxford University Press, Oxford.

[14] HANKS, G. E., CASSELL, M., RAV, R. N. and CHAPLIN, H. Jnr (1960). Further modifications of the benzidine method for measurement of hemoglobin in plasma: definition of a new range of normal values. *Journal of Laboratory and Clinical Medicine*, **56**, 486.

[15] HANSTEIN, A. and MULLER-EBERHARD, U. (1968). Concentration of serum hemopexin in healthy children and adults and in those with a variety of hematological disorders. *Journal of Laboratory and Clinical Medicine*, **71**, 232.

[16] HEIDE, K., HAUPT, H., STÖRIKO, K. and SCHULTZE, H. E. (1964). On the heme-binding capacity of hemopexin. *Clinica Chimica Acta*, **10**, 460.

[17] KRAVITZ, H., ELEGANT, L. D., KAISER, E. and KAGAN, B. M. (1956). Methemoglobin values in premature and mature infants and children. *American Journal of Diseases of Children*, **91**, 1.

[18] LAURELL, C. B. and NYMAN, N. (1957). Studies on the serum haptoglobin level in hemoglobinemia and its influence on renal excretion of hemoglobin. *Blood*, **12**, 493.

[19] LIJANA, R. C. and WILLIAMS, M. C. (1979). Tetramethyl benzidine—a substitute for benzidine in hemoglobin analysis. *Journal of Laboratory and Clinical Medicine*, **94**, 266.

[20] MICHAELSSON, M., NOSSLIN, B. and SJÖLIN, S. (1965). Plasma bilirubin determination in the new born infant. A methodological study with special reference to the influence of haemolysis. *Paediatrica*, **35**, 925.

[21] MOORE, G. L., LEDFORD, M. E. and MERYDITH, A. (1981). A micromodification of the Drabkin hemoglobin assay for measuring plasma hemoglobin in the range of 5 to 2000 mg/dl. *Biochemical Medicine*, **26**, 167.

[22] MOORE, M. R. (1983). Laboratory investigation of disturbances of porphyrin metabolism. *Association of Clinical Pathologists, Broadsheet No. 109*. British Medical Association, London.

[23] MULLER-EBERHARD, U. (1970). Hemopexin. *New England Journal of Medicine*, **283**, 1090.

[24] NYMAN, M. (1959). Serum haptoglobin: methodological and clinical studies. *Scandinavian Journal of Clinical and Laboratory Investigation*, **11**, Suppl 39.

[25] RATCLIFF, A. P. and HARDWICKE, J. (1964). Estimation of serum haemoglobin-binding capacity (haptoglobin) on Sephadex G 100. *Journal of Clinical Pathology*, **17**, 676.

[26] RUSSELL, M. A. H., WILSON, C., COLE, P. V. and IDLE, M. (1973). Comparison of increases in carboxyhaemoglobin after smoking 'extra mild' and 'non mild' cigarettes. *Lancet*, **ii**, 687.

[27] SHIELDS, C. E. (1971). Elevated carbon monoxide level from smoking in blood donors. *Transfusion* (Philadelphia), **11**, 89.

[28] SMITHIES, O. (1959). An improved procedure for starch-gel electrophoresis: further variations in the serum proteins of normal individuals. *Biochemical Journal*, **71**, 585.

[29] STANDEFER, J. C. and VANDERJOGT, D. (1977). Use of tetramethyl benzidine in plasma hemoglobin assay. *Clinical Chemistry*, **23**, 749.

[30] STONE, M. J., WILLERSON, J. T. and WATERMAN, M. R. (1982). Radioimmunoassay of myoglobin. *Methods in Enzymology*, **84**, 172.

[31] TISDALE, W. A., KLATSKIN, G. and KINSELLA, E. D. (1959). The significance of the direct-reacting fraction of serum bilirubin in hemolytic jaundice. *American Journal of Medicine*, **26**, 214.

[32] VALERI, C. R., BOND, J. C., FLOWER, K. and SOBUCKI, J. (1965). Quantitation of serum hemoglobin-binding capacity using cellulose acetate membrane electrophoresis. *Clinical Chemistry*, **11**, 581.

[33] VAN ASSENDELFT, O. W. (1970). *Spectrophotometry of Haemoglobin Derivatives*. Royal VanGorcum Ltd, Assen, The Netherlands.

[34] VAN KAMPEN, E. J. and ZIJLSTRA, W. G. (1965). Determination of hemoglobin and its derivates. *Advances in Clinical Chemistry*, **8**, 141.

[35] VANZETTI, G. and VALENTE, D. (1965). A sensitive method for the determination of hemoglobin in plasma. *Clinica Chimica Acta*, **11**, 442.

[36] WOOTTON, I, D. P. and FREEMAN, H. (1982). *Micro-Analysis in Medical Biochemistry*, 6th edn. Churchill Livingstone, Edinburgh.

[37] WU, H. (1923). Studies on hemoglobin: ultra-method for determination of hemoglobin as peroxidase. *Biochemical Journal*, **2**, 189.

14. Investigation of the hereditary haemolytic anaemias: membrane and enzyme abnormalities

(Written in collaboration with L. Luzzatto)

The various initial steps to be taken in the investigation of a patient suspected of having a haemolytic anaemia are outlined in Chapter 13 and the changes in red cell morphology which may be found in haemolytic anaemias are illustrated in Chapter 8. In this chapter are descibed procedures useful in the investigation of patients thought to have haemolytic anaemias based on defects within the red cell membrane or defective enzymes important in red cell metabolism.

The technical expertise required to identify precisely the defect in a particular instance of hereditary haemolytic anaemia is beyond the scope of most haematological laboratories. The precise identification of an enzyme defect, for example, depends upon the isolation and purification of the enzyme and the characterization of its kinetic and structural uniqueness. In a service laboratory it is sufficient to identify the general nature of the defect, whether it be in the membrane or the metabolic pathways of the red cell. With metabolic defects an attempt should be made, where possible, to pin-point the enzyme involved. Most of the enzyme assays have been standardized by the International Committee for Standardization in Haematology (ISCH). A number of commercial kits are also available for the assay of various enzymes and for 2,3-diphosphoglycerate (DPG). In the first part of this chapter are described screening test for spherocytosis, including hereditary spherocytosis (HS), and glucose 6-phosphate dehydrogenase (G6PD) deficiency. In the later sections specific enzyme assays are described and the measurement of DPG and reduced glutathione (GSH).

OSMOTIC FRAGILITY, AS MEASURED BY LYSIS IN HYPOTONIC SALINE

Principle. The method to be described is based upon that of Parpart and co-workers.[37]

Small volumes of blood are mixed with a large excess of buffered saline solutions of varying concentration. The fraction of red cells lysed at each saline concentration is determined colorimetrically. The test is normally carried out at room temperature (15–25°C).

Reagents

Prepare a stock solution of buffered sodium chloride (AR), osmotically equivalent to 100 g/l (1.71 mol/l) NaCl, as follows: dissolve NaCl, 90 g; Na_2HPO_4, 13.65 g* and $NaH_2PO_4.2H_2O$, 2.34 g in water and adjust the final volume to 1 litre. This solution will keep for months in a well stoppered bottle.

In preparing hypotonic solutions for use it is convenient to make first a 10 g/l solution from the 100 g/l NaCl stock solution by dilution with water. Dilutions equivalent to 9.0, 7.5, 6.5, 6.0, 5.5, 5.0, 4.0, 3.5, 3.0, 2.0 and 1.0 g/l are convenient concentrations. Intermediate concentrations such as 4.75 and 5.25 g/l are useful in critical work and an additional 12.0 g/l dilution should be used for incubated samples.

It is convenient to make up 50 ml of each dilution. The solutions keep well at 4°C if sterile, but they should be inspected for moulds each time they are used and discarded if moulds develop.

Method

Heparinized venous blood or defibrinated blood may be used: oxalated or citrated blood is not suitable because of the additional salts added to it. The test should be carried out within 2 h of collection with blood stored at room temperature or within 6 h if the blood has been kept at 4°C.

1. Deliver 5.0 ml of each of the 11 saline solutions into 1 × 12 cm test-tubes. Add 5.0 ml of water to tube 12.

2. Add to each tube 50 µl of well mixed blood,

---

*or $Na_2.2H_2O$, 17.115 g.

and mix immediately by inverting the tubes several times avoiding foam.

3. Incubate the suspensions for 30 min at room temperature. Mix again, and then centrifuge for 5 min at 1200 *g*.

4. Remove the supernatants and estimate the amount of lysis in each using a spectrophotometer at a wavelength setting of 540 nm or a photoelectric colorimeter provided with a yellow-green (e.g. Ilford 625) filter. Use as a blank the supernatant from tube 1 (osmotically equivalent to 9 g/l NaCl).

5. Assign a value of 100% lysis to the reading with the supernatant of tube 12 (water) and express the readings from the other tubes as percent of the value of tube 12. Plot the results against the NaCl concentration (Fig. 14.1).

Notes

1. The measurement of osmotic fragility (OF) is a simple procedure which requires a minimum of equipment. It will yield gratifying results if carried out carefully.

2. The blood must be delivered into the 12 tubes with great care. The critical point is not that the amount be exactly 50 µl, but rather that the amount

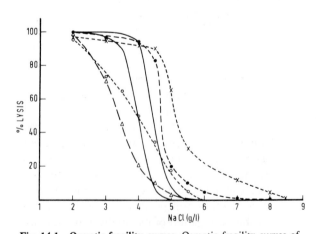

Fig. 14.1   Osmotic-fragility curves. Osmotic fragility curves of patients suffering from: (a) sickle cell anaemia △-----△, (b) β-thalassaemia major ○-----○, (c) hereditary spherocytosis ●----●, (d) 'idiopathic' warm auto-immune haemolytic anaemia X-----X. The normal range is indicated by the unbroken lines.

added to each tube must be the same. Two methods are recommended:

(a) Using an automatic pipette (e.g. a Pipetman with a yellow tip). After aspirating the blood gently, the outside should be wiped with tissue paper taking care not to suck out any blood from the inside of the tip by capillary action. The blood is then delivered into the saline solution and the pipette rinsed in and out several times until no blood is visible inside its tip.

The tip has to be changed before moving on to the next tube.

(b) Using a Pasteur pipette with a perfectly flat end, 1 mm in diameter. About 1 ml of blood should be sucked up, avoiding any bubbles, and the outside of the pipette wiped. With the pipette held vertically above tube 1, a single drop (about 50 µl) is delivered without the blood touching the wall of the tube. Further single drops are then delivered into the remaining 11 tubes.

Method (b) appears to be primitive, but with practice it is perfectly satisfactory; it is also more economical and much faster than method (a). With either method, the best way to test its accuracy is to do a preliminary test by delivering the blood into several tubes all containing the same saline solution (e.g. either 3.0 or 1.0 g/l). The readings with the supernatants should be all within 5% of each other.

3. If the amount of blood available is limited (e.g. from babies), and the spectrophotometer takes 1 ml cuvettes, the volumes can be scaled down to 1 ml of saline solution and 10 µl of blood. However, to deliver reproducibly 10 µl of blood is not easy. With method (b) a Pasteur pipette or capillary pipette with a much smaller diameter, calibrated to give 10 µl drops of blood would have to be used. It is then more difficult to maintain accuracy. Method (a) may be preferable in this case.

4. With the method using 50 µl of blood and with non-anaemic blood the reading for 100% lysis will be about 0.7. With a modern spectrophotometer any figure between 0.5 and 1.5 is acceptable. If the value is below 0.5, the test should be repeated using more blood or less saline (the reverse if the reading is above 1.5). With photoelectric colorimeters values above 0.5 are often not very accurate.

· 5. When transferring the supernatant from a tube to the spectrophotometer cuvette care has to be

taken not to disturb the pellet. If it is well packed, the supernatant can be simply poured from the tube into the cuvette; with a spectrophotometer provided with an automatic suction device, this is usually satisfactory. Alternatively, a Pasteur pipette should be used (fitted with a little plastic tubing at the end in order not to scratch the cuvette).

6. Even when a normal range has been established, it is essential always to run a normal control sample along with that of the patients to be tested in order to check, for example, the saline solutions.

The sigmoid shape of the normal osmotic fragility curve indicates that normal red cells vary in their resistance to hypotonic solutions. Indeed, this resistance varies gradually (osmotically) as a function of red cell age, with the youngest cells being the most resistant and the oldest cells the most fragile. The reason for this is that old cells have a higher sodium content and a decreased capacity to pump out sodium.

OSMOTIC FRAGILITY AFTER INCUBATING THE BLOOD AT 37°C FOR 24 HOURS

Method

Defibrinated blood should be used, care being taken to ensure that sterility is maintained.

Incubate 1 ml or 2 ml volumes of blood in sterile 5 ml screw-capped bottles. It is advisable to set up the samples in duplicate in case one bottle has become infected, as indicated by gross lysis and change in colour.

After 24 h, pool the contents of the duplicate bottles after thoroughly mixing the sedimented red cells in the overlying serum and estimate the fragility as previously described.

As the fragility may be markedly increased (Fig. 14.2), set up additional hypotonic solutions containing 7.0 g/l and 8.0 g/l NaCl. In addition, use a solution equivalent to 12.0 g/l NaCl, for sometimes, as in hereditary spherocytosis (HS), lysis may take place in 9.0 g/l NaCl. In this case use the supernatant of the tube containing 12.0 g/l NaCl as the blank in the colorimetric estimation.

The incubation fragility test is conveniently combined with the estimation of the amount of spontaneous autohaemolysis (see p. 202).

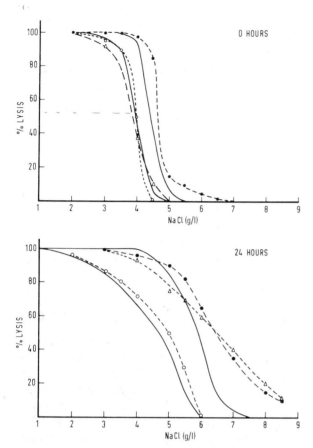

Fig. 14.2 Osmotic-fragility curves before and after incubating blood at 37°C for 24 hours. From patients suffering from: (a) hereditary spherocytosis ●-----●, (b) pyruvate-kinase deficiency △-----△ and (c) hereditary non-spherocytic haemolytic anaemia of undiagnosed type ○-----○. The normal range is indicated by the unbroken lines.

Factors affecting osmotic-fragility tests

In carrying out osmotic-fragility tests by any method three variables capable of markedly affecting the results must be controlled, quite apart from the accuracy with which the saline solutions have been made up. These are:

1. The relative volumes of blood and saline.
2. The final pH of the blood in saline suspension.
3. The temperature at which the tests are carried out.

A proportion of 1 volume of blood to 100 volumes of saline is chosen because the concentration of blood is so small that the effect of the plasma on the final tonicity of the suspension is negligible. When weak suspensions of blood in saline are used it is necessary to control the pH of the hypotonic solutions and it is for this reason that phosphate buffer is added to the saline. Even so, small differences will be found between the fragility of venous blood and maximally aerated (i.e. oxygenated) blood. For the most accurate results it is recommended that the blood should be mixed until bright red. Finally, it is ideal for tests to be carried out always at the same temperature, although for most purposes room temperature is sufficiently constant.

The extent of the effect of pH and temperature on osmotic fragility was well illustrated in the paper of Parpart and co-workers.[37] The effect of pH is more important: a shift of 0.1 of a pH unit is equivalent to altering the saline concentration by 0.1 g/l, the fragility of the red cells being increased by a fall in pH. A rise in temperature decreases the fragility, a rise of 5°C being equivalent to an increase in saline concentration of about 0.1 g/l.

Lysis is virtually complete at the end of 30 min at 20°C and the hypotonic solutions may be centrifuged at the end of this time.

Further details of the factors which affect and control haemolysis of red cells in hypotonic solutions were given by Murphy.[36]

Recording the results of osmotic-fragility tests

In the past, osmotic fragility most often has been expressed in terms of the highest concentration of saline at which lysis is just detectable (initial lysis or minimum resistance) and the highest concentration of saline in which lysis appears to be complete (complete lysis or maximum resistance). It is however, useful also to record the concentration of saline causing 50% lysis, i.e. the median corpuscular fragility (MCF), and to inspect the entire fragility curve (Fig. 14.1). The findings in health are summarized in Table 14.1.

Alternative methods of recording osmotic fragility

Two simple alternative methods of recording the results quantitatively are available: the data may be plotted on probability paper or increment-haemolysis curves can be drawn (see below). Both

Tables 14.1 Osmotic fragility in health (at 20°C and pH 7.4)

	Fresh blood (g/l NaCl)	Blood incubated for 24 h at 37°C (g/l NaCl)
Initial lysis	5.0	7.0
Complete lysis	3.0	2.0
MCF (50% lysis)	4.0–4.45	4.65–5.9

methods emphasize heterogeneity of the cell population with respect to osmotic fragility. If the observed amounts of lysis of normal blood are plotted on the probability scale against concentrations of saline, an almost straight line can be drawn through the points, there being skewness only where lysis is becoming almost complete. This method enables the MCF to be read off with ease.

In disease, tailed curves result in varying degrees of skewness at the other end of the probability plot as well. In order to obtain increment-haemolysis curves, the differences in lysis between adjacent tubes are plotted against the corresponding saline concentrations. Definitely bimodal curves may be obtained during recovery from a haemolytic episode.[42]

Use of the Fragiligraph *

Because the osmotic-fragility test is somewhat laborious, the development of an automated method was welcome. Danon[17] designed a dedicated instrument based on turbidimetry, the Fragiligraph, which records the changes in light scattering that take place when a very diluted red cell suspension in saline is dialysed against water. The resulting curve depicts the time-course of lysis as the medium in which the red cells are suspended gradually becomes more hypotonic as the salt is dialysed out. The curve looks similar to a standard OF curve, but it is actually different because the scale of the ordinate is logarithmic and because the curve reflects a kinetic element. The instrument also records the changes in salt concentration, and the MCF, and the saline concentration causing 10% lysis and 90% lysis can be measured accurately. The procedure has to be calibrated for each set of tests, and in practice the saving in time is considerable

* Kalmedic Instruments Inc, 969 Park Avenue, New York 10028.

only if many tests are to be carried out. Partly for this reason the instrument has not become popular in the diagnostic laboratory, although it can be useful for research purposes.[31] Like the orthodox osmotic-fragility curve, the Fragiligraph gives a visual image of the spread of osmotic fragility within the red cell population. For instance, the curve will be skewed or even bimodal when both high resistance and low resistance red cells co-exist.

Interpretation of results

The osmotic fragility of freshly taken red cells reflects their ability to take up a certain amount of water before lysing. This is determined by their volume to surface area ratio. The ability of the normal red cell to withstand hypotonicity results from its biconcave shape which allows the cell to increase its volume by about 70% before the surface membrane is stretched: once this limit is reached lysis occurs.[27] Spherocytes have an increased volume to surface area ratio; their ability to take in water before stretching the surface membrane is thus more limited than normal and they are therefore particularly susceptible to osmotic lysis. The increase in osmotic fragility is a property of the spheroidal shape of the cell and is independent of the cause of the spherocytosis. Characteristically, osmotic fragility curves from patients with HS who have not been splenectomized show a 'tail' of very fragile cells (Fig. 14.3). When plotted on probability paper the graph indicates two populations of cells, the very fragile and the normal or slightly fragile. After splenectomy the red cells are more homogeneous, the osmotic-fragility curve indicating a more continuous spectrum of cells, from fragile to normal.

Decreased osmotic fragility indicates the presence of unusually flattened red cells (leptocytes) in which the volume to surface area ratio is decreased. Such a change occurs in iron-deficiency anaemia and thalassaemia in which the red cells with a low MCH and MCV are unusually resistant to osmotic lysis (Fig. 14.1). Reticulocytes and red cells from splenectomized patients also tend to have a greater amount of membrane compared with normal cells and are osmotically resistant. In liver disease, target

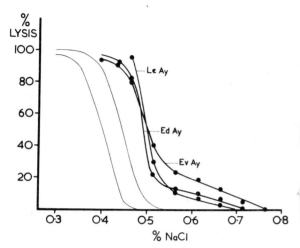

Fig. 14.3 Osmotic-fragility curves of three HS patients belonging to the same family [brother, sister and uncle (Le Ay)]. The area between the thin lines represents the normal range.

cells may be produced by passive accumulation of lipid and these cells, too, are resistant to osmotic lysis.[15]

The osmotic fragility of red cells after incubation for 24 h at 37°C is also a reflection of their volume to surface area ratio but the factors which alter this ratio are more complicated than in fresh red cells. The increased osmotic fragility of normal red cells which occurs after incubation (Fig. 14.2) is mainly caused by swelling of the cells associated with an accumulation of sodium which exceeds loss of potassium. Such cation exchange is determined by the membrane properties of the red cell which control the passive flux of ions and the metabolic competence of the cell which determines the active pumping of cations against concentration gradients. During incubation for 24 h the metabolism of the red cell becomes stressed and the pumping mechanisms tend to fail, one factor being a relative lack of glucose in the medium.

The osmotic fragility of red cells which have an abnormal membrane, such as those of HS and hereditary elliptocytosis (HE), increases abnormally after incubation (Fig. 14.2). The results with red cells with a glycolytic deficiency, such as those of pyruvate kinase (PK) deficiency, are variable. In severe deficiencies, osmotic fragility may increase substantially (Fig. 14.2) but in other cases the fragility may decrease due to a greater loss of

potassium than gain of sodium. In thalassaemia major and minor, osmotic fragility is frequently markedly reduced after incubation, again due to a marked loss of potassium.[24] A similar, though usually less marked, change is seen in iron-deficiency anaemia.

To summarize, measurement of red cell osmotic fragility provides a useful indication as to whether a patient's red cells are normal, for an abnormal result invariably indicates abnormality. The reverse is, however, not true, i.e. a result that is within the normal range does not mean that the red cells are normal. The findings in some important haemolytic anaemias are summarized in Table 14.2.

GLYCEROL LYSIS-TIME TESTS

The osmotic-fragility test is somewhat cumbersome and requires 2 ml or more of whole blood. It is thus not suitable for use in newborn babies nor as a population screening test. In 1974 Gottfried and Robertson[22] introduced a glycerol lysis-time (GLT) test, a one-tube test, to measure the time taken for 50% haemolysis of a blood sample in a buffered hypotonic saline-glycerol mixture. The original method had greater sensitivity in the osmotic resistant range but could also identify most patients with HS by a shorter GLT_{50}. Better identification of HS blood from normal was obtained by 24 h incubation of samples and by modifying the glycerol reagent.[21] Zanella and colleagues modified the original test further by decreasing the pH.[49] There is some loss of specificity for HS with the acidified compared with the original method but in practice this loss is unimportant.

ACIDIFIED GLYCEROL LYSIS-TIME TEST[49]

Reagents

Phosphate buffered saline (PBS). Add 9 volumes of 9.0 g/l (154 mmol/l) NaCl to 1 volume of 100 mmol/l phosphate buffer (2 volumes of Na_2HPO_4, 14.9 g/l added to 1 volume of KH_2PO_4, 13.61 g/l). Adjust the pH to 6.85 ± 0.05 at room temperature (15–25°C). This adjustment must be accurate.

AUTOHAEMOLYSIS (SPONTANEOUS HAEMOLYSIS DEVELOPING IN BLOOD INCUBATED AT 37°C FOR 48 HOURS)

thod

e sterile defibrinated blood and deliver four 1 ml 2 ml samples into sterile 5 ml screw-capped ttles.

Add to two of the bottles 50 or 100 µl of sterile 00 g/l glucose solution so as to provide a concenration of glucose in the blood of at least 30 mmol/l. Place the series of bottles in the incubator at 37°C.

After 24 h invert the bottles gently six times to mix the contents.

After incubating for 48 h, pool the contents of each pair of bottles. Remove a sample for the estimation of the PCV and centrifuge the remainder to obtain the supernatant serum.

Estimate the spontaneous lysis by means of a colorimeter or in a spectrophotometer at 625 nm. As a rule it is convenient to make a 1 in 10 dilution of the incubated serum in cyanide-ferricyanide (Drabkin's) solution, unless there is marked haemolysis when a 1 in 25 or 1 in 50 dilution is more suitable. A corresponding dilution of the pre-incubation serum is used as a blank and a 1 in 100 or 1 in 200 dilution of the whole blood in Drabkin's solution indicates the total amount of Hb present and serves as a standard.

Calculate the percentage lysis, allowing for the change in PCV resulting from the incubation as follows:[41]

$$\text{Lysis (\%)} = \frac{R_t}{R_o} \times \frac{D_o}{D_t} \times (1 - PCV_t) \times 100,$$

where, R_o = reading in colorimeter of diluted whole blood; R_t = reading in colorimeter of diluted serum at 48 h; PCV_t = packed cell volume at time T; D_o = dilution of whole blood (e.g. 1 in 200 = 0.005), and D_t = dilution of serum (e.g. 1 in 10 = 0.1).

The reading at time T is multiplied by $(1 - PCV_t)$ so as to give the concentration which would be found if the liberated haemoglobin was dissolved in whole blood, i.e. in both plasma and red cell compartments, not in the plasma compartment alone.

Normal range of autohaemolysis[23]

Lysis at 48 h. Without added glucose 0.2–4.0%; with added glucose 0–0.5%.

The results obtained are sensitive to slight differences in technique and each laboratory should use a carefully standardized procedure and establish its own normal range. It is more accurate (although more time consuming) to measure lysis by a chemical method rather than by a direct photometric method, particularly if the amount of liberated haemoglobin is small.[23]

Significance of increased autohaemolysis

Little or no lysis takes place when normal blood is incubated for 24 h under sterile conditions and the amount present after 48 h is small.[41] If glucose is added so that it is present throughout the incubation the development of lysis is markedly slowed. The amount of autohaemolysis which occurs after 48 h with and without glucose is determined by the properties of the membrane and the metabolic competence of the red cell. In membrane disorders such as HS the rate of glucose consumption is increased to compensate for an increased cation leak through the membrane. During the 48 h incubation glucose is therefore used up relatively rapidly so that energy production fails more quickly than normal unless glucose is added. This is one factor which contributes to the increased rate of autohaemolysis in HS. Usually, but not always, the addition of glucose to the blood decreases the rate of autohaemolysis in HS in about the same proportion as with normal blood (Fig. 14.4). This was referred to as Type-1 autohaemolysis.[41] When th utilization of glucose via the glycolytic pathway impaired, as in PK deficiency, the rate of au haemolysis at 48 h is usually increased and gluc fails to correct or may even aggravate lysis (Ty autohaemolysis, Fig. 14.5). A similar result m seen in severe HS (Type B), but in the absen spherocytosis failure of glucose to diminish haemolysis is a strong indication of a gly block. Blood from patients with G6PD de

Tables 14.2 Osmotic fragility in haemolytic anaemias: a summary

Condition	Notes
A. Associated with increased OF	
Hereditary spherocytosis (HS)	Entire curve may be 'shifted to the right', or most of it ma normal range, but with a 'tail' of fragile cells. Curve within i 10–20% of cases. After incubation for 24 h abnormalities usuall but still some 'false-negative'. Splenectomy does not affect MC the tail of fragile cells.
Hereditary elliptocytosis (HE)	As in HS, but in general changes less marked. Abnormal OF usua with severity of haemolysis, i.e. OF is normal in non-haemolytic
Other inherited membrane abnormalities	Results variable; with milder disorders curve more likely to be abn incubation for 24 h.
Auto-immune haemolytic anaemia	Tail of fragile cells roughly proportional to number of spherocytes; re: normal (or even left-shifted on account of high reticulocytosis)
B. Associated with decreased OF	
Thalassaemia	MCF decreased in all forms of thalassaemia, except in some α-thal zygotes; usually the entire curve is left-shifted.
Enzyme abnormalities	OF usually normal (anaemia originally referred to as hereditary spherocytic), but tail of highly resistant cells may be seen on account of reticulocytosis. After incubation for 24 h there may be a tail of fragile ce

Glycerol reagent (300 mmol/l). Add 23 ml of glycerol (27.65 g AR grade) to 300 ml of PBS and bring the final volume of 1 litre with water.

Method

Add 20 µl of whole blood, anticoagulated with EDTA, to 5.0 ml of PBS, pH 6.85. Mix the suspension carefully.

Transfer 1.0 ml to a standard 4 ml cuvette of a spectrophotometer equipped with a linear-logarithmic recorder. Fix the wavelength at 625 nm and start the recorder. Add 2.0 ml of the glycerol reagent rapidly to the cuvette with a 2.0 ml syringe pipette.

The rate of haemolysis is measured by the rate of fall of turbidity of the reaction mixture. The results are expressed as the time required for the optical density to fall to half the initial value ($AGLT_{50}$). The test can also be carried out using a colorimeter and stop-watch.

Results

Normal blood takes more than 1800 s (30 min) to reach the $AGLT_{50}$. The time taken is similar for blood from normal adults, newborn infants an cord samples. In patients with HS the range of the $AGLT_{50}$ is 25–150 s. A short $AGLT_{50}$ may also be found in chronic renal failure, chronic leukaemias, auto-immune haemolytic anaemia and in some pregnant women.

Significance of the AGLT

The glycerol in the hypotonic PBS slows the rate of entry of water molecules into the red cells so that the time taken for lysis may be conveniently measured. The same principles apply as with the osmotic-fragility test. Cells with a high volume to surface area ratio resist swelling for a shorter time than normal cells. This applies to all spherocytes, whether the spherocytosis is caused by HS or other mechanisms. The test is particularly useful in screening family members of patients with HS where morphological changes are too small to indicate clearly whether the disorder is present or not.

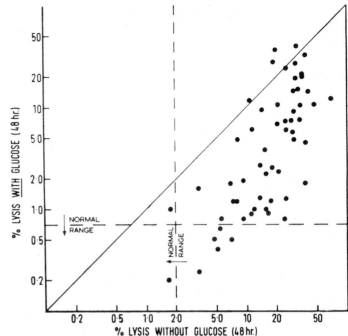

Fig. 14.4 Autohaemolysis after 48 hours' incubation at 37°C of sterile defibrinated blood derived from 57 patients suffering from hereditary spherocytosis, with and without the addition of glucose. Points lying near or on the diagonal line indicate that glucose had little or no effect on the rate of haemolysis (a Type-B result). (Reproduced from *The Hereditary Haemolytic Anaemias* by J. V. Dacie, Davidson Lecture, 1967. Publication No. 34 of the Royal College of Physicians of Edinburgh).

or other disorders of the pentose phosphate pathway may undergo a slight increase in autohaemolysis (without additional glucose) which is corrected by the addition of glucose. Commonly the result is normal but examination of the incubated blood may show an increase in methaemoglobin (Hi) (see

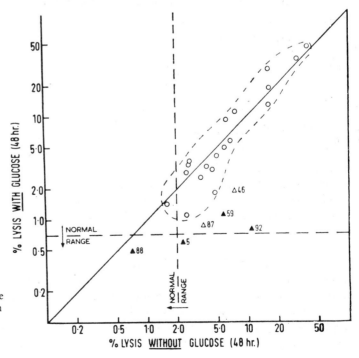

Fig. 14.5 Autohaemolysis after 48 hours' incubation at 37°C of sterile defibrinated blood derived from 19 patients suffering from pyruvate-kinase deficiency with and without the addition of glucose (hollow circles). Data from six other patients suffering from other types of hereditary non-spherocytic haemolytic anaemia have been added for comparison. Points lying near or on the diagonal line indicate that glucose had little or no effect on haemolysis. (For reference see Fig. 14.4)

below). Not all glycolytic enzyme deficiencies give a Type 2 reaction so that a Type 1 result does not exclude the possibility of such a defect.

In the acquired haemolytic anaemias the results of the autohaemolysis test are variable and generally not very helpful in diagnosis. In the auto-immune haemolytic anaemias lysis may be increased in the absence of additional glucose but the effect of added glucose is unpredictable. In paroxysmal nocturnal haemoglobinuria (PNH) the autohaemolysis of aerated defibrinated blood is usually normal.

Autohaemolysis may be increased in haemolytic anaemias caused by oxidant drugs or when there are defects in the reducing power of the red cell. Heinz bodies and/or Hi will be detectable at the end of incubation. Normally, red cells produce less than 4% Hi after 48 h incubation and Heinz bodies are not seen. Red cells containing an unstable haemoglobin also contain Heinz bodies at the end of the incubation period and increased amounts of Hi.

The nucleosides adenosine, guanosine and inosine, like glucose, diminish the rate of autohaemolysis when added to blood. Remarkably, adenosine triphosphate (ATP) strikingly retards haemolysis in PK deficiency, although glucose itself is ineffective.[18] ATP does not pass the red cell membrane.

The autohaemolysis test lacks specificity. This has drawn much criticism upon the test, including the suggestion that it has no place in the screening of blood for inherited defects.[6] The best way to detect metabolic defects in red cells is undoubtedly to measure glucose consumption, lactate production and the contribution to metabolism of the pentose phosphate pathway. These measurements are, unfortunately, difficult and are likely to be undertaken only by specialized laboratories. The autohaemolysis test does provide some information about the metabolic competence of the red cells and helps to distinguish membrane defects from enzyme defects if the results of the tests are taken together with other observations such as morphology, inheritance and presence or absence of associated clinical disorders. The autohaemolysis test will undoubtedly be abandoned as soon as a more suitable screening test becomes available.

DETECTION OF ENZYME DEFICIENCIES IN HEREDITARY HAEMOLYTIC ANAEMIAS

It should be possible for most haematological laboratories to identify the commoner enzyme deficiencies, i.e. of G6PD and PK, and to indicate where the probable defect lies in the rarer disorders. Detailed investigation of the aberrant enzymes and of the metabolism of the abnormal cells is probably best done in specialized laboratories. Comprehensive accounts of methods available for studying red cell metabolism are to be found in *Biochemical Methods in Red Cell Genetics* by Yunis (1969),[48] *Red Cell Metabolism, a Manual of Biochemical Methods,* 2nd edition by Beutler (1975)[5] and the ICSH recommendations.[9]

There are two stages in the diagnosis of red cell enzyme defects: first, screening procedures and, secondly, specific enzyme assays. The simple non-specific screening procedures such as the osmotic-fragility and autohaemolysis tests, which have already been described, may indicate the presence of a metabolic disorder and simple biochemical tests are available to show whether the disorder is in the pentose phosphate or the Embden-Meyerhof pathways; these intermediate stages of glycolysis are illustrated in Fig. 14.6.

SCREENING TESTS FOR G6PD DEFICIENCY AND OTHER DEFECTS OF THE PENTOSE PHOSPHATE PATHWAY

Many variants of the red cell enzyme, G6PD, have been detected and the methods used to identify variants have been standardized.[46] Inheritance is sex-linked as the enzyme is controlled by one gene locus in the X chromosome. Variants which have deficient activity produce one of several types of clinical disorder. The two most common variants

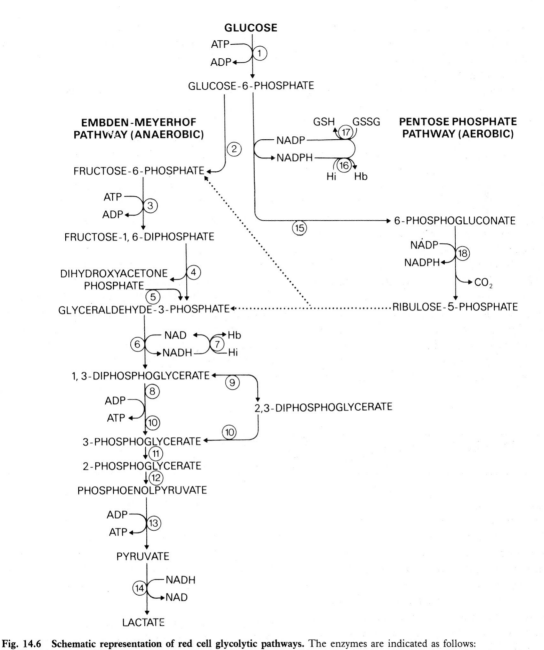

Fig. 14.6 Schematic representation of red cell glycolytic pathways. The enzymes are indicated as follows:
(1) Hexokinase; (2) Glucosephosphate isomerase; (3) Phosphofructokinase; (4) Aldolase; (5) Triose phosphate isomerase;
(8) Phosphoglycerate kinase; (9) Diphosphoglyceromutase; (10) Diphosphoglycerate phosphatase (11) Phosphoglyceromutase;
(12) Enolase; (13) Pyruvate kinase; (14) Lactate dehydrogenase; (15) Glucose-6-phosphate dehydrogenase;
(16) NADPH-methaemoglobin reductase; (17) Glutathione reductase; (18) 6-Phosphogluconate dehydrogenase. For explanation of abbreviations, see p. 223.

are the Mediterranean type which has very low activity and which may lead to favism, i.e. acute intravascular haemolysis following the ingestion of broad beans, and the A – type found in black populations in West Africa and the USA which leads to primaquine sensitivity. Both groups are susceptible to haemolysis produced by oxidant drugs and infections.

Much less frequently a chronic, non-spherocytic haemolytic anaemia is produced by rare variants of the enzyme. Severe neonatal jaundice with anaemia occurs in about 5% of patients who have major deficiencies of enzyme activity.

G6PD deficiency in hemizygous (male) or homozygous (female) individuals may be readily detected by screening tests but it is more difficult to detect heterozygous (female) carriers. Other defects of the pentose phosphate pathway (see p. 205) also lead to deficiency in the reducing power of the red cell. The clinical syndromes associated with these defects include intravascular haemolysis, with or without methaemoglobinaemia, in response to oxidative drugs.

G6PD catalyses the oxidation of glucose-6-phosphate (G6P) to 6-phosphogluconate (6PG) with the simultaneous reduction of nicotine adenine dinucleotide phosphate (NADP) to reduced NADP (NADPH):

$$G6P + NADP \underset{G6PD}{\overset{}{\rightleftharpoons}} 6PG + NADPH.$$

In a second, consecutive, oxidative reaction 6PG is converted to 6-phosphogluconolactone, with reduction of a further molecule of NADP to NADPH. The lactone then undergoes decarboxylation to ribulose 5-phosphate through a reaction catalysed by a specific lactonase, but which can also take place spontaneously. Thus the overall reaction catalysed by 6PG dehydrogenase (6PGD), can be written as:

$$6PG + NADP \underset{6PGD}{\overset{}{\longrightarrow}} Ru5P + CO_2 + NADPH.$$

The release of CO_2 drives the reaction to the right so that in practice the pathway is not reversible.

NADPH is an important reducing compound for the conversion of oxidized glutathione (GSSG) to glutathione (GSH) (see Fig. 14.6) and, under conditions of stress, the reconversion of Hi to Hb. Screening tests for G6PD deficiency depend upon the inability of cells from deficient subjects to convert an oxidized substrate to a reduced state. The substrates used may be the natural one of the enzyme, NADP, or other naturally occurring substrates linked by secondary reactions to the enzyme, for example GSSG or Hi or artificial dyes.

Which screening test is used in any particular laboratory will depend upon a number of factors such as cost, time required, temperature and humidity and availability of reagents. Two specific tests are described here.

FLUORESCENT SCREENING TEST FOR G6PD DEFICIENCY

The method is that of Beutler and Mitchell[11] modified on the recommendation of the ICSH.[9]

Principle. NADPH, generated by G6PD present in a lysate of blood cells, fluoresces under long-wave UV light.

Reagents

D-*Glucose-6-phosphate,* 10 mmol/l. Dissolve 305 mg of the disodium salt, or an equivalent amount of the potassium salt, in 100 ml of water.

NADP+, 7.5 mmol/l. Dissolve 60 mg of NADP+, disodium salt, in 10 ml of water.

Saponin. 750 mmol/l (10 g/l).

Tris-HCl buffer, pH 7.8. see p. 539.

Oxidized glutathione (GSSG), 8 mmol/l. Dissolve 49 mg of GSSG in 10 ml of water.

Mix the reagents in the following proportion: 2 volumes of G6P; 1 volume of NADP+; 2 volumes of saponin; 3 volumes of buffer; 1 volume of GSSG; 2 volumes of water.

The combined reagent is stable at $-20°C$ for 2 or more years and for 2 months at least if kept at $4°C$. Azide may be added to prevent growth of contaminants without loss of activity. 100 µl volumes of the reagent may be placed in appropriate small tubes and kept at $-20°C$ ready to use.

Method

Add 10 µl of whole blood, either anticoagulated (EDTA or heparin) or added before clotting, to 100 µl of the reagent mixture and keep at room temperature (15–25°C).

Apply 10 µl of the reaction mixture on to a Whatman No. 1 filter paper at the beginning of the reaction and after 5–10 min. A shorter interval may be appropriate at a high ambient temperature (c 25–30°C). Examine the spots under UV light. Always set up samples of normal blood and known G6PD-deficiency blood in parallel.

If the samples are to be collected away from the laboratory, place about 10 μl of blood on Whatman No.1 filter paper and allow it to dry. Cut out the disc of dried blood in the laboratory and add it to the reaction mixture.

The test can be carried out on blood stored in ACD (provided it is sterile) for up to 21 days at 4°C and for about 5 days at 25°C.

Interpretation

Fluorescence is produced by NADPH formed from NADP$^+$ in the presence of G6PD. Some of the NADPH produced is oxidized by GSSG, but this reaction, catalysed by glutathione reductase, is normally slower than the rate of NADPH production. Red cells with less than 20% of normal G6PD activity do not cause fluorescence.

Like all screening tests, this method is useful when large numbers of samples are to be tested but the result must be interpreted with caution in an individual patient. The main causes of erroneous inferences are as follows:

1. *False-normal.* If there is reticulocytosis, a vivid fluorescence may be seen with a genetically G6PD-deficient blood sample, because young red cells have more G6PD activity.

2. *False-deficient.* If the patient is anaemic, very little fluorescence may be seen despite the G6PD being genetically normal, simply because there are relatively few red cells in the 10 μl of blood used. Although it is possible to correct for either or both of these contingencies, it is best, if in doubt, to proceed directly to a quantitative enzyme assay (see below).

The test is meant to give only a + or − (normal or deficient) result, by comparison with the controls, and it does not make sense to grade by the eye the intensity of fluorescence. If a control G6PD-deficient sample is not available, the appearance of the 'zero time' spot can be used for reference. The threshold for a 'deficient' result can be worked out by making dilutions of a normal blood sample in saline, and is best set by regarding as deficient the fluorescence obtained when G6PD activity is 20% of normal or less (corresponding to a 1 in 5 dilution of normal blood). This means that very mildly deficient variants, and a substantial proportion of

heterozygotes (see p. 209), will be missed. However, clinically important haemolysis is unlikely to occur in subjects who have more than 20% G6PD activity, and therefore this seems an appropriate (though arbitrary) threshold for a diagnostic laboratory. Because the test depends on visual inspection, it is best to select the time of incubation in relation to ambient temperature in preliminary trials. NADPH production is a cumulative process. Therefore, given enough time, a G6PD-deficient sample will fluoresce! The time allowed for the reaction should be one at which the contrast in fluorescence between a G6PD-normal and a G6PD-deficient sample is maximal.

METHAEMOGLOBIN REDUCTION TEST

The method was developed by Brewer et al in 1962.[13]

Principle. Sodium nitrite converts Hb to Hi. When no methylene blue is added methaemoglobin persists, but incubation of the samples with methylene blue allows stimulation of the pentose phosphate pathway in subjects with normal G6PD levels. The Hi is reduced during the incubation period. In G6PD-deficient subjects the block in the pentose phosphate pathway prevents this reduction.

Reagents

Sodium nitrite. 180 mmol/l.

Dextrose. 280 mmol/l. Dissolve 5 g of AR dextrose and 1.25 g of $NaNO_2$ in 100 ml of water.

Methylene blue. 0.4 mmol/l. Dissolve 150 mg of methylthionine chloride (methylene blue chloride, Sigma) in 1 litre of water.

Nile blue sulphate. 22 mg in 100 ml of water. This may be used as an alternative to methylene blue. It is the better reagent if the test is to be combined with the Hi elution test (see p. 209).

The reagents may be used in a variety of ways to suit the convenience of the laboratory. A batch of tubes may be prepared in advance of use by mixing equal volumes of the reagents (sodium nitrite with methylene blue or Nile blue sulphate) and pipetting 0.2 ml of the combined reagent into individual glass tubes. Glass tubes must be used because plastic may adsorb some reagents. The contents of the tubes are allowed to evaporate to dryness at room temperature (15–25° C) or in an oven at a temperature not exceeding 37°C. The tubes must then be tightly stoppered. The reagent will keep for 6 months at room temperature. The reagents may, however, be used fresh, without drying.

Method

Use anticoagulated blood (EDTA, heparin or ACD) and test the samples preferably within 1 h of collection. Blood in ACD, however, can be stored for up to 1 week. With blood from severely anaemic patients adjust the PCV to 0.40 ± 0.05.

Add 2 ml of blood to the tube containing 0.2 ml of the combined reagent either freshly prepared or dried. Close the tube with a stopper and gently mix the contents by inverting it 15 times.

Prepare control tubes by adding 2 ml of blood to a similar tube without reagents (normal reference tube) and to a tube containing 0.1 ml of sodium nitrite-dextrose mixture without methylene blue ('deficient' reference tube).

Incubate the samples at 37°C for 3 h.

After the incubation, pipette 0.1 ml volumes from the test sample, the normal reference tube and the deficient reference tube into 10 ml of water in separate, clear glass test-tubes of identical diameter. Mix the contents gently. Compare the colours in the different tubes (see below).

Interpretation

Normal blood yields a colour similar to that in the normal reference tube—a clear red. Blood from deficient subjects gives a brown colour similar to that in the deficient reference tube. Heterozygotes give intermediate reactions.

The advantages of this method include the fact that it is extremely cheap, and that the only equipment required is a water-bath. In addition, the test can be complemented by cytochemical analysis which lends itself to detecting G6PD deficiency in patients with reticulocytosis and in heterozygotes.

The only disadvantage is the time taken to perform the test.

JACOB AND JANDL'S ASCORBATE-CYANIDE SCREENING TEST[28]

Principle. When sodium cyanide and sodium ascorbate are added to a sample of blood, catalase is inhibited by the cyanide and H_2O_2 is generated through a reaction that takes place between ascorbate and oxyHb (HbO_2). The H_2O_2 cannot be removed by catalase as this is inhibited by the cyanide. The H_2O_2 so generated will convert HbO_2 to hemichromes and Hi unless it is reduced by glutathione peroxidase. This reaction requires GSH as the proton donor. If the supply of GSH is impaired because of G6PD deficiency, Hi and hemichromes accumulate and the sample of blood will turn brown.

Reagents

Ascorbate. Dispense 10 mg of sodium ascorbate and 5 mg of glucose into a number of small tubes, which are then stoppered. They may be stored indefinitely at – 20°C.

Sodium cyanide. Dissolve 500 mg of NaCN in 50 ml of water and add 20 ml of iso-osmotic phosphate buffer, pH 7.4. Neutralize the solution (to pH 7.0) with 2 mol/l HCl and make up the volume to 100 ml with water. This solution is stable indefinitely at 20°C.

The neutralization should be carried out in a fume cupboard, and to avoid liberation of hydrocyanic acid gas the pH must not be allowed to fall below 7.0.

Cyanide solutions must *never* be pipetted by mouth. (Indeed, nowadays nothing should be pipetted by mouth.)

Method

Heparinized or EDTA, but not oxalated, whole blood is suitable.

First aerate to a bright red colour by inverting the container so that blood and air mix. Then add 2 ml to a tube containing ascorbate and glucose and add 2 drops of cyanide solution.

Incubate the mixture without a stopper in a water-bath at 37°C, and shake occasionally.

Mix the suspension thoroughly after 2 h and again at 3–4 h, noting its colour on each occasion.

The change in colour is not very great and the detection of the end-point of the test requires experience. The change is best appreciated by gently shaking the tubes and observing the colour of the film of blood on the side of the tubes. Normal blood remains red. Blood deficient in reducing power takes on a brownish hue.

As controls, samples of normal blood and known G6PD-deficient blood should be set up in parallel with the test sample(s).

Results and interpretation

G6PD-deficient blood becomes brown within 1–2 h while normal blood darkens slowly over several hours. Heterozygotes with intermediate levels of G6PD activity may (or may not) become brown within 2 h.

The ascorbate-cyanide test is not specific for G6PD deficiency. Thus positive reactions are also obtained in GSH deficiency, glutathione reductase (GR) deficiency, glutathione peroxidase (GPx) deficiency or a deficiency in one of the enzymes required for glutathione synthesis. Because all these enzyme defects are exceedingly rare, the method can be regarded as a screening test for G6PD deficiency.

False-positive results in newborn infants may be due to their relative deficiency of GPx.[30]

DETECTION OF HETEROZYGOTES FOR G6PD DEFICIENCY

Females heterozygous for G6PD deficiency have two populations of cells, one with normal G6PD activity and the other deficient. This is the result of inactivation of one of the two X chromosomes in individual cells early in the development of the embryo. All progeny cells (i.e. somatic cells) in females will have the characteristics of only the active X chromosome.[33] The total G6PD activity of blood in the female will depend on the proportion of normal to deficient cells. In most cases the activity will be between 20 and 80% of the normal. However, a few heterozygotes (about 1%) may have almost only normal or almost only G6PD-deficient cells.

Screening tests for G6PD deficiency fail to demonstrate most heterozygotes. The deficient red cells may, however, be identified in blood films by a cytochemical elution procedure based on the methaemoglobin reduction test[20] (see also p. 122.).

METHAEMOGLOBIN ELUTION TEST

Principle. HbO_2 cannot be eluted from red cells in the presence of H_2O_2 presumably because of its peroxidase activity. HiCN has no peroxidase activity and is eluted. This property has been adapted for use in a differential staining technique so that individual cells retaining HbO_2 in the methaemoglobin elution test are stained and Hi-containing cells appear as ghosts.[20]

Reagents

Potassium cyanide. 400 mmol/l. Dissolve 260 mg of KCN in 10 ml of water. Under no circumstances should this solution be pipetted by mouth.

Elution fluid. Mix 80 ml of ethanol (96% v/v, 16 ml of 200 mmol/l citric acid (3.84 g in 100 ml of water) and 5 ml of H_2O_2 (30% v/v). The solution is only active for 1 day.

Staining fluid. Haematoxylin, 7.5 g/l in 96% (v/v) ethanol.

Counterstain. Aqueous erythrosin, 1 g/l or aqueous eosin, 20 g/l.

Method

Use the incubated samples from the reduction test (see p. 207). For preference use samples incubated with Nile blue sulphate rather than methylene blue. Ideally the samples should be oxygenated during incubation by bubbling 95% O_2 – 5% CO_2 mixtures through them continously. However, it is equally adequate to blow air gently through the samples with a pipette from time to time.

After 2–3 h add 20 µl of KCN solution to 1 ml of the incubated mixture and mix gently. Make blood films on clean, dry glass slides.

Dry the films quickly in air. Immerse the slides in the elution fluid and agitate them up and down for 1 min.

Wash the slides first in methanol and then in water for 3 s each.

Stain the films for 2 min with haematoxylin, rinse in tap water, then counterstain with the erythrosin for 2 min.

Rinse the slides in tap water and allow to dry in the air.

Examine the films under the microscope and count the proportion of stained (HbO$_2$) cells to ghosts (Hi cells).

Interpretation and comments

In females heterozygous for G6PD deficiency the proportion of G6PD-deficient (ghost) cells varies from case to case: while usually 40–60% of the cells are deficient, the proportion may be much less and in extreme cases even only as few as 2–3% are deficient. Apparently normal subjects may, in a few instances, have a small residue of Hi-containing cells after the Hi reduction test, but this rarely exceeds 5% of the cells. Nearly all heterozygotes can be reliably detected if Nile blue sulphate is used and there is good oxygenation of the samples in the initial incubation. Nile blue sulphate increases the sensitivity of the test because the reduced form of the dye, which is produced in any normal cells that are present, diffuses less readily out of these cells than reduced methylene blue. An artefactual reduction of Hi in G6PD deficient cells from inward diffusion of an extrinsic reducing compound is thus less likely.

RED CELL ENZYME ASSAYS

As is illustrated in Figure 14.6, a large number of enzymes play a part in the metabolism of glucose in the red cell, and genetically-determined variants of almost all the enzymes are known to occur. This means that in investigating a patient suspected of suffering from a hereditary enzyme-deficiency haemolytic anaemia, multiple enzyme assays may be needed to identify the defect. In practice, however, G6PD deficiency and pyruvate kinase (PK) deficiency should be excluded first, because of the relative frequency (common in the case of G6PD, not rare in the case of PK) with which variants of these enzymes are associated with deficiency and increased haemolysis.

Many methods are available for assaying each enzyme, and for this reason the *International Committee for Standardization in Haematology* has produced simplified methods suitable for diagnostic purposes.[8] These methods are not necessarily the most appropriate for detailed study of the kinetic properties of the variant enzymes but they are relatively simple to set up and allow comparison of results between different laboratories.

GENERAL POINTS OF TECHNIQUE

Collection of blood samples

Blood samples may be anticoagulated with heparin (10 iu/ml blood), EDTA (1 mg/ml blood) or acid-citrate-dextrose (for formulae and volumes see p. 535). In any of these anticoagulants all normal enzymes are stable for 6 days at 4°C and 24 h at 25°C. However, enzymes variants in samples from patients may be less stable. Therefore, we recommend that ACD is used as anticoagulant and that the samples are tested promptly. Ideally, samples of blood should be transferred to central laboratories in tubes surrounded by wet ice (4°C). Frozen samples are unsuitable because the cells are lysed by freezing. Further details of enzyme stability were given by Beutler.[5] Approximately 1 ml of blood is required for each enzyme assay.

Separation of red cells from blood samples

Leucocytes and platelets generally have higher enzyme activities than red cells. Moreover, with abnormalities causing enzyme deficiency, the decrease in enzyme activity may be much less pronounced in leucocytes and platelets than in red cells, as for example in PK deficiency. It is, therefore, necessary to prepare red cells as free from contamination as possible. Various methods are suitable (see ICSH[8]); two are described below.

Washing the red cells

Centrifuge the anticoagulated blood at 1200–1500 g for 5 min and remove the plasma together with the buffy coat layer.

Resuspend the cells in 9 g/l NaCl (saline) and repeat the procedure three times. This will remove about 80–90% of the leucocytes.

This simple method is adequate in most instances when more complicated manoeuvres are impracticable, but it has the disadvantage that some of the reticulocytes and young red cells are lost together with the buffy coat. In addition, the remaining leucocytes may still be sufficient to cause misleading results, for instance in PK deficiency. Therefore, ideally the method below should be adopted.

Filtration through microcrystalline cellulose mixtures

Preparation of column:

Mix thoroughly together in ice-cold saline equal parts by weight of microcrystalline cellulose* (mean size 50 μm) and α-cellulose* just before use. The slurry produced should be just thin enough to pour easily.

Pour 4–5 ml of the slurry into a 5 ml plastic syringe clamped in the vertical position.

Place a pea-sized piece of cotton wool over the outlet of the syringe. When the slurry has settled there should be a bed of the microcrystalline cellulose α-cellulose mixture about 1.5 cm deep. The column should be made freshly for each batch of enzyme assays and used promptly.

Addition of blood

Add the washed cells to the column up to 2 ml at a time and wash the red cells through with c 1 ml of saline for each 1 ml of blood. At the end of this filtration pass a further 7 ml of saline through the column with gentle stirring. By this method about 99% of the leucocytes and about 90% of the platelets are removed. About 97% of the red cells are recovered and reticulocytes are not removed selectively.

---

* Sigma Chemical Co

Wash the cells collected from the column twice in 10 volumes of ice-cold saline and finally resuspend them in the saline to give a 50% suspension.

Determine the red cell count and haemoglobin in a sample of the suspension.

The 2 ml column can separate 18 ml of ACD, 15 ml of heparinized or 8 ml of EDTA blood. Defibrinated blood, which does not contain platelets, can also be used.

Preparation of haemolysate

Mix 1 volume of the washed or filtered suspension with 9 volumes of lysing solution consisting of 2.7 mmol/l EDTA, pH 7.0 and 0.7 mmol/l 2-mercaptoethanol (100 mg of EDTA disodium salt and 5 μl of 2-mercaptoethanol in 100 ml of water); adjust the pH to 7.0 with HCl or NaOH.

Ensure complete lysis by freeze-thawing. Rapid freezing is achieved using a dry-ice acetone bath or methanol which has been cooled to –20°C. Thawing is achieved in a water-bath at 25°C or simply in water at room temperature. Usually the haemolysate is ready for use without further centrifugation, but a 1-min spin in a microfuge is preferable in order to remove any turbidity. Dilutions, when necessary, are carried out in the lysing solution. The haemolysate should be prepared freshly for each batch of enzyme assays. Most enzymes in haemolysates are stable for 8 h at 4°C, but it is best to carry out assays immediately. The storing of frozen cells or haemolysates is not recommended; it is much better to store whole blood in ACD.

Control samples

Control samples should always be assayed at the same time as the test samples even when a normal range for the various enzymes has been established.

Take the control samples of blood at the same time as the test samples and treat them in the same way. When receiving samples from outside sources, always ask for a normal 'shipment control' to be included.

Reaction buffer

The ICSH recommendation is for a tris-HCl/ EDTA buffer which is appropriate for all the common enzyme assays. The buffer consists of 1 mmol/l tris-HCl and 5 mmol/l Na$_2$EDTA, the pH being adjusted to 8.0 with HCl.

Dissolve 15.75 g of tris-HCl and 186 mg of Na$_2$EDTA in water; adjust the pH to 8.0 with 1 mol/l HCl and bring the volume to 100 ml at 25°C.

Only two assays will be described in detail—those for G6PD and PK. However, the principles of these assays apply to all other enzyme assays. The assays are carried out in a spectrophotometer at a wavelength of 340 nm unless otherwise indicated. A final reaction mixture of 1.0 ml (or 3.0 ml) is suitable, the quantities given in the text being for 1.0 ml reaction mixtures unless otherwise stated. All dilutions of auxiliary enzymes are made in the lysing solution and all working materials should be kept in an ice-bath until ready for use. The assays are carried out at a controlled temperature, 30°C being the most appropriate. Cuvettes loaded with the assay reagents should be pre-incubated at this temperature for 10 min before starting the reaction. In most cases the reaction is started by the addition of substrate. Nowadays many spectrophotometers have a built-in or attached recorder, by which the absorbence changes can be conveniently measured. If no recorder is available, visual readings should be made every 60 s. In any case, the reaction should be followed for 5 to 10 min, and it is essential to ensure that during this time the change in absorbence is linear with time.

G6PD ASSAY

The reactions involving G6PD have already been described (p. 206). The activity of the enzyme is assayed by following the rate of production of NADPH which, unlike NADP, has a peak of ultraviolet light absorption at 340 nm.

Method

Assay conditions. The assays are carried out at 30°C, the cuvettes containing the first five reagents being incubated for 10 min before starting the reaction by adding the substrate, as shown in Table 14.3.

The change in absorbence following the addition of the substrate is measured over the first 5 min of

Table 14.3   G6PD assay

Reaction		Blank
Tris HCL EDTA buffer, pH 8.0	100 μl	100 μl
MgCl$_2$, 100 mmol/l	100 μl	100 μl
NADP, 10 mmol/l	20 μl	20 μl
1 in 20 haemolysate	20 μl	20 μl
Lysing solution	660 μl	760 μl
Start reaction by adding: G6P, 6 mmol/l	100 μl	...

the reaction. The value of the blank is subtracted from the test reaction, either automatically or by calculation.

In the 6th edition of this book (p.166) the recommended method for G6PD measurement included an assay for G6PD + 6PGD activity, with G6PD activity being calculated by subtraction. Although this assay can be regarded as more accurate for certain research purposes, it is not necessary for diagnostic purposes. Indeed, in G6PD deficiency it tends to introduce an error greater than the one it is meant to correct for.

Calculation of enzyme activity

The activities of the enzymes in the haemolysate are calculated from the initial rate of change of NADPH accumulation:

G6PD activity in the lysate (in mol/ml)

$$= \triangle A/min \times \frac{10^3}{6.22},$$

where 6.22 is the mmol extinction coefficient of NADPH at 340 nm and 10^3 is the factor appropriate for the dilutions in the reaction mixture. Results are expressed per 10^{10} red cells, per ml red cells or per g haemoglobin by reference to the respective values obtained with the washed red cell suspension. However, the ICSH recommendation is to express values per g haemoglobin, and it is ideal to determine the haemoglobin concentration of the haemolysate directly. When doing this, use a haemolysate to Drabkin solution ratio of 1:25.

G6PD is very stable and with most variants venous blood may be stored in ACD for up to 3 weeks at 4°C without loss of activity.

Some enzyme-deficient variants lose activity more rapidly, and this will cause deficiency to appear more severe than it is. Therefore, for diagnostic purposes a delay in assaying well-conserved samples should not be a deterrent.

Normal values

The normal range for G6PD activity should be determined in each laboratory. If the ICSH method is used, values should not differ widely from those given by that panel. Results are expressed in enzyme units (eu) which are the μmoles of substrate converted per min. These values are 8.34 ± 1.59 eu/g haemoglobin at 30°C.

Interpretation of results

In assessing the clinical relevance of a G6PD assay three important facts must be born in mind.

1. As already stated (p. 209) the gene for G6PD is on the X-chromosome, and therefore males, having only one G6PD gene, can be only either normal or deficient hemizygotes. By contrast, females, who have two allelic genes, can be either normal homozygotes or heterozygotes with 'intermediate' enzyme activity or deficient homozygotes.

2. Red cells are likely to haemolyse on account of G6PD deficiency only if they have less than about 20% of the normal enzyme activity.

3. G6PD activity falls off markedly as red cells age. Therefore, whenever a blood sample has a young red cell population G6PD activity will be higher than normal, sometimes to the extent that a genetically deficient sample may yield a value within the normal range. This will be usually but not always associated with a high reticulocytosis.

In practice, the following notes may be useful.

1. In males, diagnosis does not present difficulties in most cases, because the demarcation between normal and deficient subjects is sharp. There are very few acquired situations in which G6PD activity is decreased (one is pure red cell aplasia where there is reticulocytopenia); whereas an increased G6PD activity is found in all acute and chronic haemolytic states. Therefore a G6PD value below a well-established normal range always indicates G6PD deficiency. A value in the low-normal range in the face of reticulocytosis should also raise the suspicion of G6PD deficiency, because with reticulocytosis G6PD activity should be *higher* than normal. In such suspicious cases G6PD deficiency can be confirmed by repeating the assay when the reticulocytosis has subsided, or by assaying older red cells after fractionation by density, or by family studies.

2. In females, all the same criteria apply, with the added consideration that heterozygosity can *never* be rigorously ruled out by a G6PD assay: for this purpose, the cytochemical test described on p. 209 is more useful than a spectrophotometric assay, and a counsel of perfection is to use the two in conjunction with each other and with family studies. However, in most cases, a normal value in a female means that she is a normal homozygote, and a value below 10% of normal means that she is a deficient homozygote (see Table 14.4): but a few heterozygotes may fall in either of these ranges, because of the 'extreme phenotypes' that can be associated with an unbalanced ratio of the mosaicism consequent on X-chromosome inactivation. Any value between 10 and 90% of normal usually means a heterozygote, except for the complicating effect of reticulocytosis. As far as the clinical significance of heterozygosity for G6PD deficiency is concerned, it is important to remember that, because of mosaicism, a fraction of red cells in heterozygotes (on the average, 50%) are as enzyme-deficient as in a hemizygous male, and therefore susceptible to haemolysis. The severity of potential clinical complications is roughly proportional to the fraction of deficient red cells. Therefore, within the heterozygote range, the actual value of the assay (or the proportion of deficient red cells estimated by the cytochemical test) correlates with the risk of haemolysis.

Tables 14.4 G6PD in various clinical situations (Activity in enzyme units (eu) per g haemoglobin)

Male genotypes Female genotypes	Gd$^+$ GD$^+$GD$^+$	GD$^-$ Gd$^-$Gd$^-$	Gd$^+$Gd$^-$
In health	7–10	<2	2–7
In increased haemolysis unrelated to G6PD deficiency	15	4	4–9
During recovery from G6PD-related anaemia	...	6.5	6–10

The values quoted are examples.

IDENTIFICATION OF G6PD VARIANTS

There are many variants of G6PD in different populations with enzyme activities, ranging from nearly zero to 400–500% of normal activity (see full details in ref. 32). Classification and provisional identification of variants are based on their physico-chemical and enzymic characteristics. Criteria were laid down by a WHO scientific group in 1967[46] for the minimum requirements for identification of such variants and these recommendations have been revised recently.[47] The tests are carried out on male hemizygotes and are:

Red cell G6PD activity
Electrophoretic migration
Michaelis constant (K_m) for G6PD
Relative rate of utilization of 2-deoxyG6P (2dG6P)
Thermal stability.

Recently the full amino-acid sequence of G6PD has been established and definitive identification can be made by sequence analysis at the DNA level.[45] The provisional data have been confirmed in general but with some exceptions.[7]

PYRUVATE KINASE ASSAY

Many variants of PK have deficient enzyme activity in vivo.[34,35] In most cases deficient activity can be identified by simple enzyme assay. However, PK activity is subject in red cells to regulation by a number of effector molecules. With some PK variants the maximum velocity (V_{max}) of the enzyme is normal or nearly so, but at the low substrate concentrations found in vivo PK activity may be sufficiently low to cause haemolysis, either because affinity for the substrates, phosphoenolpyruvate (PEP) and ADP, is low or because binding of the important allosteric ligand, fructose-1,6-diphosphate, is altered. Some of these unusual variants can be identified by carrying out the enzyme assay not only under standard conditions but also at low substrate concentrations. Functional PK deficiency can also be identified by finding high concentrations of the substrates immediately above the block in the glycolytic pathway, particularly DPG.[26] (For measurement of DPG, see p. 217.)

Method

The preparation of haemolysate, buffer and lysing solution are exactly the same as for the G6PD assay. In the PK assay it is particularly important to remove as many contaminating leucocytes and platelets as possible because these cells may be unaffected by a deficiency affecting the red cells and contain high activities of PK. The principle of the assay is as follows:

$$PEP + ADP \xrightleftharpoons{PK} pyruvate + ATP.$$

The pyruvate so formed is reduced to lactate in a reaction catalysed by lactate dehydrogenase with the conversion of NADH to NAD:

$$pyruvate + NADH \xrightleftharpoons{LDH} lactate + NAD.$$

In order to ensure that this secondary reaction is not rate-limiting, LDH is added in excess to the reaction mixture and the PK activity is measured by the rate of fall of absorbence at 340 nm.

The reaction conditions are established in a 1 ml cuvette at 30°C by adding all the reagents except the substrate PEP to the cuvette and incubating them at 30°C for 10 min before starting the reaction by the addition of the PEP. In the following listing of reagents the amounts to be added for substrate conditions are shown in parenthesis.

Reagents

	Assay	Blank
Buffer. 1 mol/l tris-HCl with 5 mmol/l Na$_2$EDTA	100 µl	100 µl
KCl. 1 mmol/l	100 µl	100 µl
NADH. 10 mmol/l	20µl	20µl
ADP, neutralized. 15 mmol/l (6 mmol/l)	100 µl	...
LDH. 600 u/ml	10µl	10µl
1 in 20 haemolysate (p. 211)	20µl	20µl
Water	450 µl	550 µl
PEP. 50 mmol/l (2.5 mmol/l)	100 µl	100 µl

The change in absorbence (A) is measured over the first 5 min and the activity of the enzyme in μmoles NADH reduced/min/ml haemolysate is calculated as follows:

$$\frac{\Delta A/min}{6.22} \times 10,$$

where 6.22 is the mmol extinction coefficient of NADH at 340 nm.

Express results as for G6PD

Normal values

As with all enzyme assays, a normal range should be determined for each laboratory. Values should, however, not be widely different between laboratories if the ICSH methods are used. The normal range of PK activity at 30°C is 12 ± 2 eu/g Hb. At a low substrate concentration the normal activity is 15 ± 3% of that at the high substrate concentration.

Interpretation of results

PK, like G6PD, is a red cell age-dependent enzyme. But unlike G6PD deficiency, PK deficiency is usually associated with chronic haemolysis. Therefore, patients in whom PK deficiency is suspected almost invariably have a reticulocytosis, and if their PK level is below the normal range they can be considered to be PK-deficient. Thus, once the technique and normal values are well established in a laboratory, and provided shipment controls are always included, the main problem is of underdiagnosis rather than of overdiagnosis of PK deficiency. One way to pick up abnormal variants has been included in the method recommended, i.e. the use of low substrate concentrations. Even so, PK deficiency may be missed because high reticulocytosis may increase PK activity quite markedly. This means that a PK activity in the normal range in the presence of a high reticulocytosis is highly suspicious of inherited PK deficiency (because with reticulocytosis the activity ought to be *higher* than normal). In such cases the importance of family studies cannot be overemphasized. Heterozygotes have about 50% of the normal PK activity, sometimes less; but they do not suffer from haemolysis. Therefore, the heterozygous parents of a patient may well have a red cell PK activity lower than that of their homozygous PK-deficient offspring. This finding may clinch the diagnosis.

ESTIMATION OF REDUCED GLUTATHIONE (GSH)[10]

Principle. The method described is based on the development of a yellow colour when 5,5′-dithiobis (2-nitrobenzoic acid) (Ellman's reagent, DTNB) is added to sulphydryl compounds. The colour which develops is fairly stable for about 10 min and the reaction is little affected by variation in temperature.

The reaction is read at 412 nm. GSH in red cells is relatively stable and venous blood samples anticoagulated with ACD maintain GSH levels for up to 3 weeks at 4°C. GSH is slowly oxidized in solution, so only fresh lysates should be used for the assay.

Reagents

Lysing solution. Disodium EDTA, 1g/l.
Precipitating reagent. Metaphosphoric acid (sticks), 1.67 g; disodium EDTA 0.1g; NaCl 30g; water to 100ml.

Solution is more rapid if the reagents are added to boiling water and the volume made up after cooling.

This solution is stable for at least 3 weeks at 4°C. If any NaCl remains undissolved the clear supernatant should be used.

Disodium hydrogen phosphate. 3 mmol/l: $Na_2HPO_4.12H_2O$, 107.5 g/l, or $Na_2HPO_4.2HO$, 53.4 g/l or anhydrous Na_2HPO_4, 42.6 g/l.

DTNB reagent. Dissolve 20 mg of DTNB in 100 ml of buffer, pH 8.0. Sodium citrate, 100 mmol/l (10 g/l) or tris/HCl, are suitable buffers.

The solution is stable for up to 3 months at 4°C.

Glutathione standards. When standard curves are constructed, suitable dilutions are made from a 1.62 mmol/l (50 mg/dl) stock solution of GSH.

The stock solution should be made freshly with degassed (boiled) water or saline for each run as GSH oxidizes slowly in solution.

Method

Add 0.2 ml of well mixed, anticoagulated blood, of which the PCV, red cell count and haemoglobin have been determined, to 1.8 ml of lysing solution and allow to stand at room temperature for 5 min for lysis to be completed.

Add 3 ml of precipitating solution, mix the solution well and allow to stand for a further 5 min.

After remixing, filter through a single thickness Whatman No.42 filter paper.

Add 1 ml of clear filtrate to 4 ml of freshly made Na_2HPO_4 solution. Record the absorbence at 412 nm (A_1). Then add 0.5 ml of the DTNB reagent.

The colour develops rapidly and remains stable for about 10 min. Read its devlopment at 412 nm in a spectrophotometer (A_2).

A reagent blank is made using saline or plasma instead of whole blood.

Standard curves. If assays are carried out frequently, it is not necessary to construct standard curves for each batch. They are, however, essential initially to calibrate the apparatus used and should be done regularly to check the suitability of the reagents. Suitable dilutions of GSH are achieved by substituting 5, 10, 20 and 40 µl of the 1.62 mmol/l stock solution, made up to 0.2 ml with lysing solution, for the blood in the reaction.

Calculation

Determination of extinction coefficient (E). The molar extinction coefficient of the chromphore at 412 nm is 13 600. This only applies when a narrow band wave length is available. When a broader wave band is used, the extinction coefficient is lower.

The system may be calibrated by comparing the extinction absorbence in the test system (D_2) with that obtained in a spectrophotometer with a narrow band at 412 nm (D_1). The derived correction factor, E_1, is given by D_1/D_2 and is constant for the test system.

Calculation of GSH concentration

The amount of GSH in the cuvette sample (GSH_c) is given by:

$$\Delta A^{412} \times \frac{E_1}{E} \times 5.5 \; \mu mol.$$

The concentration of GSH in the whole blood sample is:

$$\frac{GSH_c \times 5}{0.2} \mu mol/ml.$$

The unit is often expressed in terms of mg/dl of red cells. The molecular weight of GSH is 307. Thus, GSH in mg/dl packed red cells is given by:

$$GSH_c \times \frac{5}{0.2} \times \frac{1}{PCV} \times 307 \times 100.$$

Normal range

The normal range may be expressed in a number of ways, e.g. 6.57 ± 1.04 µmol/g Hb or 223 ± 35 µmol/dl packed red cells or 69 ± 11 mg/dl packed cells.

THE GLUTATHIONE STABILITY TEST

Principle. In normal subjects incubation of red cells with the oxidizing drug acetylphenylhydrazine has little effect on the GSH content, since its oxidation is reversed by glutathione reductase, which in turn relies on G6PD for a supply of NADPH. Therefore, in G6PD deficient subjects the stability of GSH is significantly lowered.

Reagents

Acetylphenylhydrazine. Dissolve 100 mg in 1 ml of acetone.

Transfer 0.05 ml volumes (containing 5 mg of acetylphenylhydrazine) by pipette to the bottom of 12×75 mm tubes.

Dry the contents of the tubes in an incubator at 37°C, stopper with rubber bungs and store in the dark until used.

Method

Venous blood, anticoagulated with EDTA, heparin or ACD may be used; it may be freshly collected or previously stored at 4°C for up to 1 week.

Add 1 ml to a tube containing acetylphenyl-hydrazine and place a further 1 ml in a similar tube not containing the chemical. Invert the tubes several times and then incubate them at 37°C.

After 1 h mix the contents of the tubes once more and incubate the tubes for a further 1 h. At the end of this time determine and compare the GSH concentration in the test sample and in the control sample.

Interpretation

In normal adult subjects red cell GSH is lowered by not more than 20% by incubation with acetyl-phenylhydrazine. In G6PD-deficient subjects it is lowered by more than this: in heterozygotes (females) the fall may amount to about 50% whilst in hemizygotes (males) the fall is often much greater and almost all may be lost.

GSH and GSH stability in infants

During the first few days after birth the red cells have a normal or high content of GSH. On the addition of acetylphenylhydrazine the GSH is unstable in both normal and G6PD-deficient infants. In normal infants, however, the instability can be corrected by the addition of glucose and by the time the normal infant is 3–4 days old the cells behave like adult cells.[30,50]

2, 3-DIPHOSPHOGLYCERATE (DPG)

The importance of the high concentration of DPG in the red cells of man was recognized at about the same time by Chanutin and Curnish[14] and Benesch and Benesch.[4] DPG binds to a specific site in the β-chain of haemoglobin and it decreases its oxygen affinity by shifting the balance of the so-called T and R conformations of the molecule. The higher the concentration of DPG the greater the partial pressure of oxygen (pO_2) needed to produce the same oxygen saturation of haemoglobin. This is reflected in a DPG-dependent shift in the oxygen dissociation curve.

Measurement of the concentration of DPG in red cells may also be useful in identifying the probable site of an enzyme deficiency in the metabolic pathway. In general, enzyme defects cause an increase in the concentration of metabolic intermediates above the level of the block and a decrease in concentration below the block. Thus DPG is increased in PK deficiency and decreased in hexokinase deficiency. In most other disorders of the glycolytic-pathway, however, the DPG concentration is normal, because increased activity through the pentose phosphate pathway allows a normal flux of metabolites through the triose part of the glycolytic pathway.

MEASUREMENT OF RED CELL DPG

Various methods have been used to assay DPG. Krimsky[29] used the catalytic properties of DPG in the conversion of 3-phosphoglycerate (3PG) to 2-phosphoglycerate (2PG) by phosphoglycerate mutase (PGM). At very low concentrations of DPG the rate of conversion is proportional to the concentration of DPG. This method is elegant and extremely sensitive but too cumbersome for routine use. Rose and Liebowitz[39] found that glycolate-2-phosphate increased the 2,3DPG phosphatase activity of phosphoglycerate mutase (PGM) and a quantitative assay of the substrate, DPG, was evolved on this basis.

Principle. DPG is hydrolysed to 3PG by the phosphatase activity of PGM stimulated by glycolate-2-phosphate. This reaction is linked to the conversion of NADH to NAD by glyceraldehyde-

3-phosphate dehydrogenase (Ga3PD) and phosphoglycerate kinase (PGK):

$$2,3DPG \xrightarrow[\text{(glycolate-2-phosphate)}]{\text{2,3DPG phosphatase}} 3PG + Pi;$$

$$3PG + ATP \xrightarrow{PGK} 1,3DPG + ADP;$$

$$1,3DPG + NADH \xrightarrow{Ga3PD} Ga3P + Pi + NAD^+.$$

The fall in absorbence at 340 nm, as NADH is oxidized, is measured.

Method

Freshly drawn blood in EDTA or heparin may be used. If there is an unavoidable delay in starting the assay, blood (4 volumes) should be added to CPD anticoagulant (1 volume) and stored at 4°C. A control blood sample should be taken at the same time.

DPG levels are stable for 48 h if the blood is stored in this way. The haemoglobin, red cell count and PCV should be measured on part of the sample. It is not necessary to remove leucocytes or platelets.

Deproteinization. Add 1 ml of blood to 3 ml of ice-cold 80 g/l trichloracetic acid (TCA) in a 10 ml conical centrifuge tube.

Shake the tube vigorously, preferably on an automatic rotor mixer and then allow to stand for 5–10 min for complete deproteinization. The shaking is important, otherwise some of the precipitated protein will remain on the surface of the mixture.

Centrifuge at about 1200 *g* for 5–10 min at 4°C to obtain a clear supernatant. The DPG in the supernatant is stable for 2–3 weeks when stored at 4°C, and indefinitely if frozen.

Reagents

Triethanolamine buffer. 0.2 mol/l, pH 7.6.
Dissolve 9.3 g of triethanolamine hydrochloride in *c* 200 ml of water; then add 5.0 g of disodium EDTA and 2.5 g of $MgSO_4.7_2O$. Adjust the pH to 7.6 with 2 mol/l KOH (*c* 15 ml) and make up the volume to 250 ml with water.

ATP, sodium salt. 20 mg/ml. Dissolved in buffer, this is stable for several months when frozen.

NADH, sodium salt. 10 mg/ml. This is relatively unstable and should be made freshly each day.

Glyceraldehyde-3-phosphate dehydrogenase. Crystalline suspension from rabbit muscle in ammonium sulphate (Sigma).

Phosphoglycerate kinase. Crystalline suspension from yeast in ammonium sulphate.

Phosphoglycerate mutase. Crystalline suspension from rabbit muscle in ammonium sulphate.

Glycolate-2-phosphate. 2-Phosphoglycolic acid (Sigma), 10 mg/ml. This is stable for several months when frozen.

Reaction

Deliver the reagents into a silica or high quality glass cuvette, with a 1 cm light path. The following quantities are for a 4 ml cuvette:

	Test	Blank
Triethanolamine buffer	2.50 ml	2.50 ml
ATP	100 μl	100 μl
NADH	100 μ	100 μl
Deproteinized extract	250 μl	—
Ga-3-PD	20 μl	20 μl
PGK	10 μl	10 μl
PGM	20 μl	20 μl
Water	—	250 μl
	3.00 ml	3.00 ml

Warm the mixtures at 25°C for 5 min and record the absorbence of both test and blank mixtures at 340 nm. Then start the reaction by the addition of 100 μl of glycolate-2-phosphate.

Remeasure the absorbence (in 15 min) of the test and blank mixtures after completion of the reaction.

Make further measurements after a further 5 min to make sure the reaction is complete.

Only one blank is required for each batch of test samples.

Calculation

DPG (μmol/ml blood)

$$= (\Delta A \text{ test} - \Delta A \text{ blank}) \times \frac{3.10}{6.22} \times 16$$

$$= (\Delta A \text{ test} - \Delta A \text{ blank}) \times 8 = D,$$

where 3.10 = the volume of reaction mixture, 6.22 = mmolar extinction coefficient of NADH at

340 nm and 16 = dilution of original blood sample (1 ml in 3.0 ml of TCA, 0.25 ml added to cuvette).

The results of DPG assays are best expressed in terms of haemoglobin content or red cell volume. Thus, if the result of the above calculation is represented by D, then:

$$D \times \frac{1000}{(Hb)} = DPG \text{ in } \mu mol/g \text{ Hb or}$$

$$D \times \frac{1000}{(Hb)} \times \frac{64}{1000} = DPG \text{ in } \mu mol/\mu mol \text{ Hb}$$

and

$$D \times \frac{1}{PCV}$$

$$= DPG \text{ in } \mu mol/ml \text{ (packed) red cells,}$$

where (Hb) = haemoglobin in g/l of whole blood and 64 is the mol wt of haemoglobin $\times 10^{-3}$.

The molar ratio of DPG to haemoglobin in normal blood is about 0.75:1.

Normal range

3.5–5.0 μmol/ml packed red cells or 8.5–15.9 μmol/g haemoglobin.

Each laboratory should determine its own normal range.

Significance of DPG concentration

An increase in DPG concentration is found in most conditions in which the arterial blood is undersaturated with oxygen, as in congenital heart and chronic lung diseases; in most acquired anaemias; at high altitudes; in alkalosis, and in hyperphospha-taemia. Decreased DPG levels occur in hypophosphataemic states and in acidosis.

Acidosis, which shifts the oxygen dissociation curve to the right, causes a fall in DPG, so that the oxygen dissociation curve of whole blood from patients with chronic acidosis (such as patients in diabetic coma or pre-coma) may have nearly normal dissociation curves. A rapid correction of the acidosis will lead to a major shift of the curve to the left, that is to a marked increase in the affinity of haemoglobin for oxygen, which may lead to tissue hypoxia. Caution should therefore be exercised in correcting acidosis.

From the diagnostic point of view, the main importance of DPG determination is (1) in haemolytic anaemias and (2) in the interpretation of changes in the oxygen affinity of blood.

1. As already mentioned, increased or decreased DPG may be associated with glycolytic enzyme defects, and increased DPG (up to 2–3 times normal) is particularly characteristic of most patients with PK deficiency. Although this finding certainly cannot be regarded as diagnostic, a normal or low DPG makes PK deficiency most unlikely.

2. Whenever a shift in the oxygen dissociation curve is observed, and an abnormal haemoglobin with altered oxygen affinity is suspected, determination of DPG is essential. Indeed, there is a simple correlation between DPG level and p_{50}, from which it is possible to work out whether any change in p_{50} is explained by an altered level of DPG.[19]

DPG levels are generally slightly lower than normal in HS and this probably accounts for the slight erythrocytosis which is sometimes seen after splenectomy.

THE OXYGEN DISSOCIATION CURVE

The oxygen dissociation curve is the expression of the relationship between the partial pressure of oxygen and the saturation of haemoglobin with oxygen. Details of this relationship and the physiological importance of changes in this relationship were worked out in detail at the beginning of this century by the great physiologists Hüfner, Bohr, Barcroft, Henderson and many others. Their work was summarized by Peters and Van Slyke in *Quantitative Clinical Chemistry, Volume 1.*[38] The relevant chapters of this book have been reprinted and it would be difficult to better their description of the importance of the oxygen dissociation curve:

The physiological value of haemoglobin as an oxygen carrier lies in the fact that its affinity for oxygen is so nicely balanced that in the lungs haemoglobin becomes 95–96% oxygenated, while in the tissues and capillaries it can give up as much of the gas as is demanded. If the affinity were much less, complete oxygenation in the lungs could not be approached: if it were greater, the tissues would have difficulty in removing from the blood the oxygen they need. Because the affinity is adjusted as it is, both oxyhaemoglobin and reduced haemoglobin exist in all parts of the circulation but in greatly varied proportions.

MEASURING THE OXYGEN DISSOCIATION CURVE

Determination of the oxygen dissociation curve depends upon two measurements: the partial pressure of oxygen (pO_2) with which the blood is equilibrated, and the proportion of haemoglobin which is saturated with oxygen. Methods for determining the dissociation curve fall into three main groups:

1. The pO_2 is set by the experimental conditions and the percent saturation of haemoglobin is measured.

2. The percentage saturation is predetermined by mixing known proportions of oxygenated and deoxygenated blood and the pO_2 is measured.

3. The change in oxygen content of the blood is plotted continuously against pO_2 during oxygenation or deoxygenation and the percent saturation calculated.

The multiplicity of methods available for measuring the oxygen dissociation curve suggests that no method is ideal. The advantages and disadvantages of the various techniques have been reviewed.[3,43] The standard method with which new methods are compared is the gasometric method of Van Slyke and Neill.[44] This method is slow and demands considerable expertise and is not suitable for most haematological laboratories. The method described below[40] is based on similar principles to that of Van Slyke and Neill but employs spectrophotometric measurement of reduced oxyhaemoglobin rather than direct gasometric measurement. The method

may be used for suspensions of red cells as well as dilute haemoglobin solutions.

Method

Principle. Oxygen at known pO_2 is added step-wise to a tonometer which contains a dilute suspension of red cells in which the haemoglobin is completely deoxygenated. The haemoglobin in the cells is equilibrated with the gas and the percent saturation is measured spectrophotometrically after each addition. Because the haemoglobin concentration is low there is a negligible shift in the pO_2 in the gas phase after equilibration.

Apparatus

Tonometer-Cuvette. This is not available commercially but can be made in a glass-blowing workshop.*

A tonometer, 5 cm high by 5 cm maximum diameter, is made from Pyrex glass. To one end is fused a high vacuum stopcock[†] with a single side arm at right angles to the main axis of the apparatus. Small scratches should be made around the entry hole so that air can be admitted slowly. To the other end of the tonometer is fused, via a graded seal, a silica cuvette, 1 cm in light path and 4 ml in volume. Silica cuvettes should be used since the fusion process will distort ordinary glass cuvettes. The joints should be made to withstand pressures of at least 100 kPa (1 atmosphere). The whole apparatus (Fig. 14.7) should be no more than 20 cm high. The total volume of the tonometer and additions is measured. The stopcock is greased with silicone grease, taking care that none gets into the apparatus.

Spectrophotometer. Double-beam spectrophotometer with modified cuvette housing (e.g. Pye-Unicam, S.P.8000).

High Vacuum pump.

Gas burette. Made from a graduated 3 ml pipette.

---

*As designed by Professor E. R. Huehns and colleagues at University College Hospital, London.
[†]Quickfit, high vacuum stopcock TH6 (Baird and Tatlock (London) Ltd), suitably modified, is appropriate.

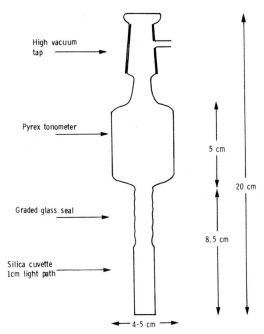

Fig. 14.7 Apparatus used in determination of oxygen dissociation curve.

High vacuum tap

Pyrex tonometer

Graded glass seal

Silica cuvette 1cm light path

5 cm

20 cm

8.5 cm

4-5 cm

Reagents

Stock phosphate buffer, pH 7.43. 80 ml of 150 mmol/l Na_2HPO_4 and 20 ml of 150 mmol/l NaH_2PO_4.

Working buffer. Add 1 volume of stock buffer to 4 volumes of 154 mmol/l (9 g/l) NaCl. The pH must be 7.43 ± 0.01.

Other phosphate buffers of suitable pH may be prepared for studying the Bohr effect.

Method

Weigh the freshly greased tonometer. Dilute 2–4 drops of heparinized blood in about 10 ml of working buffer and place in the tonometer which is then evacuated via the side arm of the stopcock using a high vacuum pump.

Close the stopcock and disconnect the tonometer from the pump and then rotate it horizontally in a water-bath at 37°C for 3 min. This allows equilibration between the gases in the blood and buffer and the vacuum. Repeat the evacuation and equilibration twice more to ensure complete deoxygenation of the haemoglobin.

After a further equilibration, dry the cuvette, wipe it clean and place it in the appropriate part of the spectrophotometer.

After 30 s, to allow movement of red cells to stop, record the absorbence between 500 and 600 nm as a continuous spectrum. Then remove the tonometer from the spectrophotometer, dry the interior of the side arm, and attach the side arm to the gas burette.

Let a known volume of air (about 2 ml) into the tonometer through the side arm, the exact amount of air being measured by movement of the mercury bubble and recorded. Again equilibrate the Hb with the gas in the tonometer by rotating the apparatus at 37°C for 3 min.

Measure the absorbence over the same range once more after 30 s.

Add further volumes of air in the same way and repeat the process after each additon. In this way a family of curves is built up until finally the stopcock is opened to the air and the haemoglobin becomes fully saturated.

Read the absorbence at 540, 560 and 576 nm from the tracings.

Finally weigh the tonometer and its contents.

Calculation

$$pO_2 \text{ (mmHg)} = \frac{\left(P - \dfrac{H \times SVP}{100}\right) \times 0.21}{V - v} \times A,$$

where P = atmospheric pressure in mm Hg[*]; H = relative humidity in percent; SVP = saturated vapour pressure at room temperature in mm Hg; 0.21 = fraction of O_2 in air; V = volume of tonometer in ml; v = volume of contents in ml, and A = volume of air added in ml.

$$V = W_2 - W_1,$$

where W_2 = weight of tonometer + contents and W_1 is weight of tonometer alone, assuming sp gr 1.0 for the blood/buffer suspension.

% saturation of Hb

$$= \frac{(A_{540} - A_{540}^{deoxy}) + (A_{560}^{deoxy})}{(A_{540}^{oxy} - A_{540}^{deoxy}) + (A_{560}^{deoxy} - A_{560}^{oxy})} \times 100$$

---

[*] × 0.133 kPa.

or

% saturation of Hb

$$= \frac{(A_{576} - A_{576}^{deoxy}) + (A_{560}^{deoxy} - A_{560})}{(A_{576}^{oxy} - A_{576}^{deoxy}) + (A_{560}^{deoxy} - A_{560}^{oxy})} \times 100$$

where A_{540}, A_{560} and A_{576} are the absorbences of the partially saturated Hb at the appropriate wavelength and A^{deoxy} and A^{oxy} indicate the absorbence of the totally desaturated and totally oxygenated samples, respectively. The results are then plotted as a graph to obtain the full dissociation curve.

Assessment of the method

The method has the advantages that the curve can be determined on a small sample of blood and that it is relatively quick (about 45 min for a complete curve) and fairly simple. It is, too, a reasonably inexpensive method, providing the spectrophotometer can be used for other purposes. The method is particularly suitable for determining the 'n' value of a haemoglobin and calculating the Bohr effect. Its major disadvantage is that dilute suspensions of blood do not behave like whole blood and that the curve determined in this way gives no indication of what is happening in vivo to the $p_{50}O_2$. For these reasons it is useful for diagnostic work in identifying abnormal haemoglobins but it is not useful for research work which requires a knowledge of shifts in the oxygen affinity of blood in vivo.

Interpretation

Fig. 14.8 shows the sigmoid nature of the oxygen dissociation curve of Hb A and the effect of hydrogen ions on the position of the curve. A shift of the curve to the right indicates decreased affinity of the haemoglobin for oxygen and hence an increased tendency to give up oxygen to the tissues: a shift to the left indicates increased affinity and so an increased tendency for haemoglobin to take up and retain oxygen. Hydrogen ions, DPG and some other organic phosphates such as ATP shift the curve to the right. The amount by which the curve is shifted may be expressed by the $p_{50}O_2$, i.e. the partial pressure of oxygen at which the haemoglobin is 50% saturated.

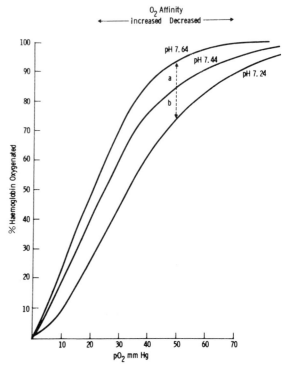

Fig. 14.8   The effect of pH upon the oxygen dissociation curve.

The oxygen affinity, as represented by the $p_{50}O_2$, is related to compensation in haemolytic anaemias.[2] 1 g of haemoglobin can carry about 1.34 ml of O_2. Fig. 14.9 shows the O_2 dissociation curves of Hb A and Hb S plotted according to the volume of oxygen contained in 1 litre of blood when the haemoglobin concentrations are 146 g/l and 80 g/l, respectively. The $p_{50}O_2$ of Hb A is given as 26.5 mm Hg (3.5 kPa) and Hb S as 36.5 mm Hg (4.8 kPa). It will be seen that in the change from arterial to venous saturation the same volume of oxygen is given up despite the difference in haemoglobin concentration. Patients with a high $p_{50}O_2$ achieve a stable haemoglobin at a lower level than normal and this should be taken into account when planning transfusion for these patients.

The Bohr effect

Bohr et al described the effect of CO_2 on the oxygen dissociation curve.[12] An increase in CO_2 concentration produces a shift to the right, i.e. a decrease in oxygen affinity. It was soon realised that this effect was mainly due to changes in pH, although CO_2 itself has some

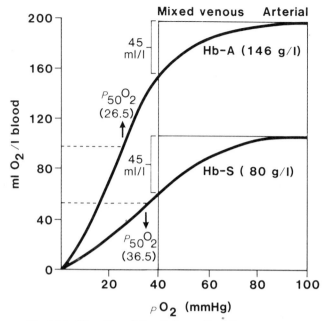

Fig. 14.9 The effect of O_2 affinity on O_2 delivery to tissues.

Hill's constant

Hill thought that there was a constant ('n') which represented the number of molecules of oxygen which would combine with 1 molecule of haemoglobin.[25] Experiment showed that the value was 2.6 rather than the expected 4. The explanation for this lies in the effect of binding 1 molecule of oxygen by haemoglobin on the affinity for binding further oxygen molecules by haemoglobin, the so-called allosteric effect of haem-haem interaction: 'n' is a measure of this effect and the calculation of the 'n' value helps in identifying abnormal haemoglobins,[1] the molecular abnormality of which leads to abnormal haem-haem interaction.

direct effect. The Bohr effect is given a numerical value, $\Delta \log p_{50}O_2/\Delta pH$, where $\Delta \log p_{50}O_2$ is the change in $p_{50}O_2$ produced by a change in pH (ΔpH). The normal value of the Bohr effect at physiological pH and temperature is about 0.45.

Abbreviations used in this chapter

ADP, AMP, ATP	Adenosine di-, mono- or triphosphate
ALD	Aldolase
DHAP	Dihydroxyacetone phosphate
1,3DPG	1,3-Diphosphoglycerate
DPG	2,3-Diphosphoglycerate
DPGM	Diphosphoglycerate mutase
2,3DPGPase	2,3-Diphosphoglycerate phosphatase
DTNB	5,5'-Dithiobis (2-nitrobenzoic acid) (Ellman's reagent)
En	Enolase
F1,6P	Fructose-1,6-diphosphate
F6P	Fructose-6-phosphate
Ga3P	Glyceraldehyde-3-phosphate
Ga3PD	Glyceraldehyde-3-phosphate dehydrogenase
G6P	Glucose-6-phosphate
2DG6P	2-Deoxyglucose-6-phosphate
G6PD	Glucose-6-phosphate dehydrogenase
GPI	Glucose phosphate isomerase
GPx	Glutathione peroxidase
GR	Glutathione reductase
GSH	Reduced glutathione
GSSG	Oxidized glutathione
Hx	Hexokinase
LAC	Lactate
LDH	Lactate dehydrogenase
NAD, NADH	Nicotine adenine dinucleotide,
NADP, NADPH	Nicotine adenine dinucleotide phosphate
Pi	Inorganic phosphate
PEP	Phosphoenolpyruvate
PFK	Phosphofructokinase
6PG	6-Phosphogluconate
6PGD	6-Phosphogluconate dehydrogenase
3PG, 2PG	3-(or 2-) Phosphoglycerate
PGK	Phosphoglycerate kinase
PGM	Phosphoglyceromutase
PK	Pyruvate kinase
Ru5P	Ribulose-5-phosphate
TPI	Triose phosphate isomerase

REFERENCES

[1] BELLINGHAM, A. J. (1972). The physiological significance of the Hill parameter 'n'. *Scandinavian Journal of Haematology*, **9**, 552.

[2] BELLINGHAM, A. J. and HUEHNS, E. R. (1968). Compensation in haemolytic anaemias caused by abnormal haemoglobins. *Nature* (London), **218**, 924.

[3] BELLINGHAM, A. J. and LENFANT, C. (1971). Hb affinity for O_2 determined by O_2-Hb dissociation analyser and mixing technique. *Journal of Applied Physiology*, **30**, 903.

[4] BENESCH, R. and BENESCH, R. E. (1967). The effect of organic phosphates from the human erythrocyte on the allosteric properties of haemoglobin. *Biochemical and Biophysical Research Communications*, **26**, 162.

[5] BEUTLER, E. (1975). *Red cell Metabolism. A Manual of Biochemical Methods* 2nd edn. Grune and Stratton, New York.

[6] BEUTLER, E. (1978). Why has the autohemolysis test not gone the way of the cephalin floculation test? *Blood*, **51**, 109.

[7] BEUTLER, E. (1989). Glucose-6-phosphate dehydrogenase: new perspectives. *Blood*, **73**, 1397.

[8] BEUTLER, E., BLUME, K. G., KAPLAN, J. C., LÖHR, G. W., RAMOT, B. and VALENTINE, W. N. (1977). International Committee for Standardization in Haematology. Recommended methods for red-cell enzyme analysis. *British Journal of Haematology*, **35**, 331.

[9] BEUTLER, E., BLUME, K. G., KAPLAN, J. C., LÖHR, G. W., RAMOT, B. and VALENTINE, W. N. (1979). International Committee for Standardization in Haematology. Recommended screening test for glucose-6-phosphate dehydrogenase (G-6-PD) deficiency. *British Journal of Haematology*, **43**, 465.

[10] BEUTLER, E., DURON, O. and KELLY, B. (1963). Improved method for the determination of blood glutathione. *Journal of Laboratory and Clinical Medicine*, **61**, 882.

[11] BEUTLER, E. and MITCHELL, M. (1968). Special modification of the fluorescent screening method for glucose-6-phosphate dehydrogenase deficiency. *Blood*, **32**, 816.

[12] BOHR, C., HASSELBACH, K. and KROGH, A. (1904). Ueber einen in biologischer Beziehung wichtigen Einfluss, den die Kohlensäurespannung des Blutes auf dessen Sauerstoffbindungübt. *Skandinavisches Archiv für Physiologie*, **16**, 402.

[13] BREWER, G. J., TARLOV, A. R. and ALVING, A. S. (1962). The methemoglobin reduction test for primaquine-type sensitivity of erythrocytes. A simplified procedure for detecting a specific hypersusceptibility to drug hemolysis. *Journal of the American Medical Association*, **180**, 386.

[14] CHANUTIN, A. and CURNISH, R. R. (1967). Effect of organic and inorganic phosphates on the oxygen equilibrium of human erythrocytes. *Archives of Biochemistry and Biophysics*, **121**, 96.

[15] COOPER, R. A. (1970). Lipids of human red cell membrane: normal composition and variability in disease. *Seminars in Hematology*, **7**, 296.

[16] DACIE, J. (1985). *The Haemolytic Anaemias, Vol.1. The Hereditary Haemolytic Anaemias, Part 1*, p. 146. Churchill Livingstone, Edinburgh.

[17] DANON, D. (1963). A rapid micromethod for recording red cell osmotic fragility by continuous decrease of salt concentration. *Journal of Clinical Pathology*, **16**, 377.

[18] DE GRUCHY, G. C, SANTAMARIA, J. N., PARSONS, I. C. and CRAWFORD, H. (1960). Nonspherocytic congenital hemolytic anemia. *Blood*, **16**, 1271.

[19] DUHM, J. (1971). Effects of 2,3-diphosphoglycerate and other organic phosphate compounds on oxygen affinity and intracellular pH of human erythrocytes. *Pflügers Archiv für die gesampte Physiologie des Menschen und der Tiere*, **326**, 341.

[20] GALL, J. C., BREWER, G. J. and DERN, R. J. (1965). Studies of glucose-6-phosphate dehydrogenase activity of individual erythrocytes: the methemoglobin-elution test for identification of females heterozygous for G6PD deficiency. *American Journal of Human Genetics*, **17**, 359.

[21] GOTTFRIED, E. L. and ROBERTSON, N. A. (1974). Glycerol lysis time of incubated erythrocytes in the diagnosis of hereditary spherocytosis. *Journal of Laboratory and Clinical Medicine*, **84**, 746.

[22] GOTTFRIED, E. L. and ROBERTSON, N. A. (1974). Glycerol lysis time as a screening test for erythrocyte disorders. *Journal of Laboratory and Clinical Medicine*, **83**, 323.

[23] GRIMES, A. J., LEETS, I. and DACIE, J. V. (1968). The autohaemolysis test: appraisal of the method for the diagnosis of pyruvate kinase deficiency and the effect of pH and additives. *British Journal of Haematology*, **14**, 309.

[24] GUNN, R. B., SILVERS, D. N. and ROSSE, W. F. (1972). Potassium permeability in β-thalassaemia minor red blood cells. *Journal of Clinical Investigation*, **51**, 1043.

[25] HILL, A. V. (1910). The possible effect of the aggregation of the molecules of haemoglobin on its dissociation curves. *Journal of Physiology*, **40**, 4.

[26] International Committee for Standardization in Haematology. (1979). Recommended methods for the characterisation of red cell pyruvate kinase variants. *British Journal of Haematology*, **43**, 275.

[27] JACOB, H. S. and JANDL, J. H. (1964). Increased cell membrane permeability in the pathogenesis of hereditary spherocytosis. *Journal of Clinical Investigation*, **43**, 1704.

[28] JACOB, H. S. and JANDL, J. H. (1966). A simple visual screening test for glucose-6-phosphate dehydrogenase deficiency employing ascorbate and cyanide. *New England Journal of Medicine*, **274**, 1162.

[29] KRIMSKY, I. (1965). D-2, 3-Diphosphoglycerate. In *Methods of Enzymatic Analysis*. Ed. H. U. Bergmeyer, p. 238. Academic Press, New York and London.

[30] LUBIN, B. H. and OSKI, F. A. (1967). An evaluation of screening procedures for red cell glucose-6-phosphate dehydrogenase deficiency in the newborn infant. *Journal of Pediatrics*, **70**, 788.

[31] LUZZATTO, L., ESAN, G. J. F. and OGIEMUDIA, S. E. (1970). The osmotic fragility in newborns and infants. *Acta Haematologica* (Basel), **43**, 248.

[32] LUZZATTO, L. and MEHTA, A. (1989). Glucose-6-phosphate dehydrogenase deficiency. In *The Metabolic Basis of Inherited Disease*. Eds. C. R. Scriver, A. L. Beaudet, W. S. Sly and D. Valle, pp. 2237–2265. McGraw-Hill, New York.

[33] LYON, M. F. (1961). Gene action in the X-chromosomes of the mouse. (Mus musculus L.) *Nature* (London), **190**, 372.

[34] MIWA, S., FUJII, H., TAKEGAWA, S. et al (1980). Seven pyruvate kinase variants characterised by the ICSH recommended methods. *British Journal of Haematology*, **45**, 575.

[35] MIWA, S., NAKASHIMA, K., ARIYOSHI, K., SHINOHARA, K., ODA, E. and TANAKA, T. (1975). Four new pyruvate kinase (PK) variants and a classical PK deficiency. *British Journal of Haematology*, **29**, 157.

[36] MURPHY, J. R. (1967). The influence of pH and temperature on some physical properties of normal erythrocytes and erythrocytes from patients with hereditary spherocytosis. *Journal of Laboratory and Clinical Medicine*, **69**, 758.

[37] PARPART, A. K., LORENZ, P. B., PARPART, E. R., GREGG, J. R. and CHASE, A. M. (1947). The osmotic resistance (fragility) of human red cells. *Journal of Clinical Investigation*, **26**, 636.

[38] PETERS, J. P. and VAN SLYKE, D. D. (1931). Hemoglobin and oxygen. In *Quantitative Clinical Chemistry, Vol 1, Interpretations*, p. 525. Williams and Wilkins, Baltimore.

[39] ROSE, Z. B. and LIEBOWITZ, J. (1970). Direct determination of 2,3-diphosphoglycerate. *Annals of Biochemistry and Experimental Medicine*, **35**, 177.

[40] ROSSI-FANELLI, A. and ANTONINI, E. (1958). Studies on the oxygen and carbon monoxide equilibria of human myoglobin. *Archives of Biochemistry and Biophysics*, **77**, 478.

[41] SELWYN, J. G. and DACIE, J. V. (1954). Autohemolysis and other changes resulting from the incubation in vitro of red cells from patients with congenital hemolytic anemia. *Blood*, **9**, 414.

[42] SUESS, J., LIMENTANI, D., DAMESHEK, W. and DOLLOFF, M. J. (1948). A quantitative method for the determination and charting of the erythrocyte hypotonic fragility, *Blood*, **3**, 1290.

[43] TORRANCE, J. D. and LENFANT, C., (1969–70). Methods for determination of O_2, dissociation curves, including Bohr effect. *Respiration Physiology*, **8**, 127.

[44] VAN SLYKE, D. D. and NEILL, J. M. (1924). The determination of gases in blood and other solutions by vacuum extraction and manometric measurement. *Journal of Biological Chemistry*, **61**, 523.

[45] VULLIAMY, T. J., D'URSO, M., BATTISTUZZI, G. et al (1988). Diverse point mutations in the human glucose-6-phosphate dehydrogenase gene cause enzyme deficiency and mild or severe hemolytic anemia. *Proceedings of the National Academy of Sciences of the U.S.A.*, **85**, 5171.

[46] World Health Organization Scientific Group (1967). Standardization of procedures for the study of glucose-6-phosphate dehydrogenase. Technical Report series, No. 366. WHO, Geneva.

[47] World Health Organization Scientific Group on glucose-6-phosphate dehydrogenase (1990). In Press.

[48] YUNIS, J. J. (1969). *Biochemical Methods in Red Cell Genetics*, Academic Press, New York.

[49] ZANELLA, A., IZZO, C., REBULLA, P., ZANUSO, F., PERRONI, L. and SIRCHIA, G. (1980). Acidified glycerol lysis test: a screening test for spherocytosis. *British Journal of Haematology*, **45**, 481.

[50] ZINKHAM, W. H. (1959). An in-vitro abnormality of glutathione metabolism in erythrocytes from normal newborns: mechanism and clinical significance. *Pediatrics*, **23**, 18.

15. Investigation of the abnormal haemoglobins and thalassaemia

(Written in collaboration with J. M. White and G. W. Marsh)

THE HAEMOGLOBIN MOLECULE

Some knowledge of the chemical nature of the human haemoglobin molecule is necessary for an understanding of the abnormal haemoglobins. A short summary is given below.

Human haemoglobin is formed of two pairs of globin chains to each of which is attached one molecule of haem. Six variants are normally formed: three are transient embryonic haemoglobins referred to as Hb Gower 1, Hb Gower 2 and Hb Portland; Hb F is the predominant haemoglobin of fetal life, and Hb A (more than 95%) and Hb A_2 (2.5–3.5%) are the characteristic haemoglobins of adults. Hb F, although present in large amounts at birth (65–95%), is normally formed subsequently only in traces.

The individual chains formed in post-natal life are designated α, β, γ and δ. Hb A is formed of two α chains and two β chains ($\alpha_2\beta_2$); Hb F is formed of two α chains and two γ chains ($\alpha_2\gamma_2$), and Hb A_2 of two α chains and two δ chains ($\alpha_2\delta_2$). The α chain is thus common to all three types of haemoglobin molecule.

The α chain is directed by two α genes, $\alpha1$ and $\alpha2$, on chromosome 16, and the β and δ chains by single genes on chromosome 11. The γ chain is directed by two genes, $^G\gamma$ and $^A\gamma$, also on chromosome 11.

The α chains are formed of 141 amino acids and the β, γ and δ chains of 146; their exact sequence is known. They are arranged in a long right-handed spiral or α-helix folded to give rise to eight long helical segments joined by short non-helical segments or corners. The long segments have been named A to H and the non-helical sequences between the long segments NA, AB, CD, EF and so on to GH. (BC and DE do not exist as non-helical sequences.) Each amino-acid is numbered according to its position in its

227

chain or alternatively in its segment of chain, e.g. $\beta^6(A3)$.

The four chains are associated in the form of a tetramer: the $\alpha_1\beta_1$ contact is the strongest and involves many amino-acids with many interlocking side chains; the $\alpha_1\beta_2$ contact is less extensive, while the contacts between like chains are relatively weak. The binding of a molecule of haem into a 'haem pocket' in each chain is vital for the oxygen-carrying capacity of the molecule and stabilizes the whole molecule. If the haem attachment is weakened, the globin chains dissociate into dimers or monomers.

It is now realized that many naturally occurring genetically determined (inherited) variants of human haemoglobin structure exist and that although many are harmless some have serious clinical effects. Sickle cell disease, for instance, results from the synthesis of an abnormal haemoglobin molecule. Another group of genetically determined defects leads not to the formation of structurally abnormal haemoglobins but to the complete or almost complete failure to form normal haemoglobin (Hb A). This type of abnormality is the cause of thalassaemia.

Collectively, the clinical syndromes resulting from disorders of haemoglobin synthesis are referred to as 'haemoglobinopathies'. In reality, they are disorders of *globin* synthesis. Genetically-determined disorders of *haem* synthesis do exist: they are rare and lead to sideroblastic anaemias (see p. 115) and are not considered further in this Chapter.

The haemoglobinopathies can be grouped into three main categories:

1. Those due to structural variants of haemoglobin, e.g. Hb S.

2. Those due to failure to form Hb A normally, e.g. as in the thalassaemias.

3. Those due to failure to complete the normal neonatal switch from fetal haemoglobin (Hb F) to adult haemoglobin (Hb A). This leads to a group of disorders referred to as hereditary persistence of fetal haemoglobin (HPFH).

Structural variants of haemoglobin

The alterations in the structure of normal adult haemoglobin referred to above are brought about by mutations which result in the replacement usually of a single amino-acid (rarely two amino-acids) in either the α or β chains of the globin part of the haemoglobin molecule. Hb S is, for instance, caused by the substitution of valine for glutamic acid, the 6th residue in the β chain. Hb S can thus be written $\alpha_2\beta_2^{6\,Glu\rightarrow Val}$, and Hb Torino is caused by the substitution of valine for phenylalanine, the 43rd residue in the α chain, and can be written $\alpha_2^{43\,Phe\rightarrow Val}\beta_2$.

Less commonly, mutations result in one or a sequence of amino-acids being deleted, as for instance, in Hb Gun Hill in which five amino acids in the β chain (91–95) are deleted. A few haemoglobins result from extension of a globin chain. In Hb Constant Spring (named after a village in Jamaica) 31 residues are added to the α chain. Rarely, two chains are fused. Hb Lepore is an example of a fusion chain haemoglobin: Hb Lepore Washington (= Boston) is thus formed of δ chain residues 1–87 and β chain residues 116–146—the exact point of crossing over is uncertain, as residues 88–115 are the same in both chains.

All these categories contain variants which fail to cause any clinical or haematological abnormalities, but each category also contains variants which result in changes to the functional and physical properties of the haemoglobin molecule that bring about clinical and haematological abnormalities in either homozygotes (individuals who have inherited the same abnormality from both parents) or in heterozygotes (individuals who have inherited an abnormality from one parent only). In addition it is quite common for one structurally abnormal haemoglobin to be inherited from one parent and another different structurally abnormal haemoglobin or thalassaemia to be inherited from the other parent. Such individuals are referred to as compound heterozygotes.

An individual who is a homozygote or a compound heterozygote may have severe clinical manifestations (e.g. Hb SS, Hb SC). Some variants in contrast produce only mild clinical problems in the homozygous state (e.g. Hb DD, Hb EE). Other variants may lead to important problems in heterozygotes, e.g. stable high oxygen affinity haemoglobins that cause absolute polycythaemia (e.g. Hb Chesapeake, Hb J Capetown and Hb Heathrow)

Table 15.1 The β-thalassemias: the effect of simple and compound heterozygosity and of homozygosity for β-thalassaemia genes on clinical presentation and haemoglobin.

'Genotype'	Clinical presentation	Hb A (%)	Hb A_2 (%)	Hb F (%)	Hb Lepore (%)
β^+/β^A	Thal minima or normal	c 95	3.5–7.0	0–6	
β^0/β^A	Thal minor	c 95	3.5–7.0	0–6	
β^+/β^+	Thal intermedia	25–65	1–4	30–70	
β^0/β^0	Thal major	0	1–4	>95	
β^0/β^+	Thal major or intermedia	<20	1–4	>75	
$\delta\beta^0/\beta^A$	Normal	80–85	<2.5	10–18	
$\delta\beta^0/\beta^+$	Thal intermedia	0–50	<2.5	45–95	
$\delta\beta^0/\beta^0$	Thal intermedia	0	0	100	
Lepore/β^A	Normal	80–85	2.0–2.5	1–13	5–18
Lepore/Lepore	Thal intermedia	0	0	70–90	9–30
Lepore/β^0	Thal major or intermedia	0	c 2.5	c 90	5–15

The figures given for percentages of haemoglobin are approximate; their wide range reflects genotypic heterogeneity. The 'genotypes' given are also only approximate: β^0 denotes a thalassaemia gene resulting in complete failure to form β chains; β^+ a thalassaemia gene resulting in partial failure to form β chains. β^A represents the normal haplotype.

The Table illustrates the fact that thalassaemia may result from defects of the δ gene as well as the β gene (δβ-thalassaemia), and that the presence of an abnormal Lepore haemoglobin can lead to thalassaemia.

and unstable variants that result in chronic haemolytic anaemia (e.g. Hb Hammersmith and Hb Köln).

The thalassaemias

Two main types of thalassaemia exist, β-thalassaemia and α-thalassaemia, according to whether the genetic abnormality responsible for the reduced rate of synthesis of Hb A affects the synthesis of β or α chains of haemoglobin. Within each type there are many sub-types (Tables 15.1 and 15.2). The clinical syndromes (thalassaemia minima, minor, intermedia or major) reflect the degree to which the formation of Hb A is impaired. Heterozygotes for β-thalassaemia do not as a rule suffer from serious disabilities, but homozygotes often suffer from severe anaemia (Cooley's anaemia). Heterozygotes for α-thalassaemia are usually free from any symptoms, but homozygotes, if two defective α genes are inherited from each parent, usually die in utero (Hb Bart's hydrops fetalis). Three defective α genes, two inherited from one parent and one from the other parent, lead to Hb-H disease.

Hereditary persistence of fetal haemoglobin (HPFH)

A number of different types of HPFH exist, depending on the nature of the causal genetic defect. However, the presence of large amounts of Hb F persisting into adult life does not give rise to clinical problems, even in homozygotes in whom Hb F alone is present, no Hb A or Hb A_2 being detectable. Compound heterozygotes for HPFH and a structurally abnormal haemoglobin (e.g. Hb S or Hb C) or thalassaemia are known; they, too, do not as a rule have any symptoms attributable to their haemoglobinopathy.

INVESTIGATION OF PATIENTS SUSPECTED OF SUFFERING FROM A HAEMOGLOBINOPATHY

It is outside the scope of this chapter to offer detailed guidelines as to when an individual requires investigation for the possible presence of an abnormal haemoglobin or thalassaemia. An ade-

Table 15.2   Genotypes and nomenclature of the α-thalassaemias and clinical and haematological presentation of the main types

Genotype	Conventional nomenclature	WHO nomenclature[64]	Lehmann and Carroll's nomenclature[63]	Clinical haematological presentation	Haemoglobins present
αα/αα	Normal	Normal	Normal	Normal	Hb A, Hb A² (2–3.5%)
– α/αα	α-thal-2	α^+-thalassaemia	1α-thalassaemia	Silent trait. Blood picture: almost normal	Hb A, Hb A₂ Hb Bart's (0–3%, at birth) Hb H trace only
– α/– α (trans) ––/αα (cis)	α-thal-1	α^0-thalassaemia	2α-thalassaemia	Thalassaemia minor (trait). Blood picture: slightly to moderately abnormal	Hb A, Hb A₂ Hb Bart's (2–8%, at birth) Hb H (<2%)
– –/– α	Hb H disase	α^0/α^+-thalassaemia	3α-thalassaemia	Moderately severe haemolytic anaemia. Blood picture: markedly abnormal	Hb A, Hb A₂ (1–2%) Hb Bart's (<5%) Hb H (2–40%)
– –/– –	Hb Bart's fetal hydrops	α^0/α^0-thalassaemia	4α-thalassaemia	Death in utero or shortly after birth. Blood picture: markedly abnormal	Hb A absent or trace Hb Bart's (70–80%) Hb H (<5%) Hb Portland (10–15%)

The figures for haemoglobin percentages are approximate, their wide range reflects genotypic heterogeneity.

quate knowledge of the world-wide distribution of these conditions is certainly a necessary requirement and the investigator should also be familiar with the clinical manifestations that variants may produce in heterozygotes and homozygotes and in compound heterozygotes.

Investigation of persons considered to be possibly suffering from a haemoglobinopathy is usually carried out to establish, first, if a haemoglobinopathy is present and, if so, to ensure that patients who have a haemoglobinopathy of clinical significance are correctly managed and that, whether with or without clinical problems, they receive, if necessary, adequate genetic counselling. Genetic counselling implies discussions with both partners and, where appropriate, consideration of the possibility of the pre-natal diagnosis of an affected fetus.

In the majority of patients the presence of a haemoglobinopathy may be accurately diagnosed from knowledge of the patient's ethnic group, clinical history (including family history) and the results of physical examination combined with a few simple haematological tests. The peripheral blood picture should always be considered first, and the quantitative data must include a red cell count, calculation of red cell indices and measurement of haemoglobin and haematocrit. In some instances a reticulocyte count and a search for red cell inclusions give valuable information. Most important, however, is the detailed examination of a well-stained blood film. Assessment of iron status by estimation of serum iron or ferritin or bone-marrow aspiration is sometimes necessary. Other important basic tests are haemoglobin electrophoresis, assessment of haemoglobin solubility and measurement of Hb A₂ and Hb F percentage. If it is possible to carry out the above tests accurately, a reliable diagnosis can usually be made without the need for more sophisticated investigations.

The majority of errors occurring in the detection and identification of a haemoglobinopathy are due either to failure to obtain correct laboratory data or failure to interpret the data correctly. To avoid laboratory error, quality control guidelines must be observed, and participation in local or national quality assessment schemes should be mandatory. Controls must be set up with all electrophoretic procedures and each laboratory must establish its own normal range for quantitative tests. Interpretation of laboratory findings is a skill only fully achieved after much practice. A number of different procedures have usually been undertaken to establish a diagnosis and it requires judgement and experience to select the most appropriate tests and then to integrate the results obtained.

In this chapter a sequence of investigations is suggested based on procedures which should be available in any hospital laboratory. Isoelectric focusing[1,42] has not been included, but a brief description has been given of the technique of in-vitro globin chain synthesis as this procedure, although unlikely to be generally employed, is now available in an increasing number of laboratories. Fingerprinting and high-pressure liquid chromatography (HPLC) for the detection of aberrant peptides is outside the scope of this chapter and the reader is referred to the relevant literature.[26,46,48,49]

Laboratory investigation of a suspected haemoglobinopathy should follow a definite but flexible protocol. The data obtained from the clinical findings, blood picture and electrophoresis on cellulose acetate will almost invariably indicate in which direction to proceed and with further procedures such as citrate agar electrophoresis, solubility testing, and Hb A_2 and F estimation a definitive diagnosis will usually be possible.

A list of the various procedures described is given below. These have been divided into three groups.

(A) Initial tests

  (i)   Blood count and film.
  (ii) Cellulose acetate electrophoresis at alkaline pH.
  (iii) Hb S sickling and solubility tests.
  (iv) Estimation of Hb A_2.
  (v)   Estimation of Hb F.
  (vi) Intracellular distribution of Hb F.
  (vii) Demonstration of inclusion bodies.

(B) Further tests

  (i)   Citrate agar electrophoresis.
  (ii) Electrophoresis at neutral pH for Hb H and Hb Bart's.
  (iii) Globin chain electrophoresis.
  (iv) Starch block electrophoresis.
  (v)   Starch gel electrophoresis.

(C) Additional tests

  (i)   Detection of unstable haemoglobins.
  (ii) Detection of Hb M.

  (iii) Detection of altered oxygen affinity haemoglobins.

Globin chain synthesis was described in the previous (6th) edition of this book and will not be included here.

Gene mapping of globin peptides and amino-acid sequencing are not described. Readers are referred to Old and Higgs[40] and to Weatherall and Clegg.[55] A comprehensive list of the haemoglobin variants and relevant references has recently been published by Wrightstone.[60]

COLLECTION OF BLOOD AND PREPARATION OF HAEMOLYSATES

Blood can be collected into any anticoagulant and even red cells from a clotted sample can be used, although less satisfactorily, if anticoagulated blood is not available. ACD is the most suitable anticoagulant if the samples have to be transported.

For routine analysis wash the red cells three times in 9.0 g/l NaCl (saline) and then lyse them by adding to the packed cells 2 volumes of water and 1 volume of carbon tetrachloride (CCl_4). Alternatively, lyse by freezing and thawing and then add 2 volumes of CCl_4. After shaking in a mechanical agitator, centrifuge the mixture at 3000 rpm (1200 g) for 30 min and transfer the clear solution to a clean tube and adjust the haemoglobin concentration to c 100 g/l by adding water.

In a routine laboratory, if many samples are to be analysed, a practical rapid alternative for qualitative tests is to lyse 1 volume of unwashed packed cells with 4 volumes of 50 mmol/l EDTA. However, this type of haemolysate does not keep for more than 1–2 days at 4°C or at room temperature (c 20°C) as it tends to gel.

Storing specimens prepared by either procedure at −20°C is satisfactory for a few weeks, but lysates can be stored almost indefinitely in liquid nitrogen.

INITIAL TESTS

BLOOD COUNT AND FILM

A full blood count, including red cell count, haemoglobin level, mean cell volume and mean cell haemoglobin, provides valuable information with respect to the diagnosis of both α and β thalas-saemia (Chapter 5) whilst examination of blood films may show characteristic red cell changes, e.g. target cells with Hb C and sickle cells with Hb S (see Chapter 8).

CELLULOSE ACETATE ELECTROPHORESIS AT ALKALINE PH

For routine work, the best method for separating abnormal haemoglobins is by electrophoresis on cellulose acetate membrane. This method is simple, rapid and sensitive. It is generally satisfactory for distinguishing the common haemoglobin variants.

At alkaline pH (8.4–8.6) haemoglobin is a nega-tively charged protein and in an electric field will migrate toward the anode (+). Most structural variants of haemoglobin will separate due to surface charge differences, thus allowing identification of abnormal forms.

Equipment

1. *Electrophoresis tank and power supply.* Any horizontal electrophoresis tank is suitable which will allow a bridge gap of 7 cm. (Tanks with an adjustable bridge gap have the advantage of allow-ing different electrophoretic procedures to be car-ried out.) A direct current power supply capable of delivering 350 V at 10 mA is recommended for cellulose acetate. If the supply is also to be used for agar gel electrophoresis, 350 V at 80 mA is recommended as agar has a higher conductivity than cellulose acetate.

2. *Wicks of filter paper or chromatography paper.*
3. *Blotting paper.*
4. *Applicators.* These are available from com-mercial sources, but fine microcapillary tubes are also suitable.
5. *Cellulose acetate.* Cellulose acetate membranes are widely available from many sources including the manufacturers of electrophoresis tanks. Plastic backed membranes (7.6 × 6.0 cm) are recom-mended.[15,44]
6. *Staining equipment and oven.*
7. *Balance and pH meter.*

Reagents

1. *Electrophoretic buffer (Tris/EDTA/Borate (TEB), pH 8.5).* Tris-(hydroxymethyl)-amino-methane 10.2 g; ethylenediaminetetra-acetic acid (EDTA) 0.6 g; boric acid 3.2 g; water to 1 litre.

The buffer may be repeatedly used without significant deterioration. It may be stored at 4°C. The pH should be checked before each use. Commercially-produced buffers are also satisfac-tory.

2. *Protein stain.* Ponceau S (5 g/l) in trichlor-acetic acid (7.5 g/l).
3. *Destaining solution.* 5% (v/v) acetic acid, 50 ml/l.
4. *Absolute methanol.*
5. *Clearing solution.* Methanol 4 volumes, glacial acetic acid, 2 volumes. 50 ml of polyethylene glycol, mol wt 400,* may be added to 20% (v/v) acetic acid in methanol for better clearing.

Method

The procedure described below may require mod-ification to comply with the instructions given by the various manufacturers of specific products.

1. Fill the compartments of the electrophoresis tank with TEB buffer. Soak and position the wicks.
2. In a separate dish soak the cellulose acetate membranes in TEB buffer for at least 5 min. It is important to immerse the membranes slowly so as to avoid trapping air bubbles.
3. Blot the membranes between two pieces of absorbent paper, but do not allow them to dry out before applying the haemolysates.
4. Dilute the haemolysate (p. 231) 1 in 4 or 1 in 5 (c 20 g Hb/l). Place a small volume (10 μl) of each diluted sample in a sample well into which the applicator is dipped in order to transfer the sample to the cellulose acetate membrane.
5. Apply the haemolysate samples to the cellu-lose acetate approximately 2 cm from one end of the strip. Allow the applicator tips to remain in contact with the strip for approximately 3 s.
6. Place the strip upside down in the tank so that the wicks are in contact with the buffer and the cellulose acetate so that the application line is toward the cathode.
7. Apply the power and run at 250–350 V for c 20 min or until adequate separation is obtained.

---

*E.g. Carbowax 400, BDH.

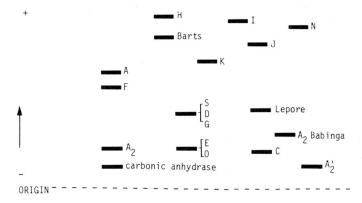

Fig. 15.1 **Relative mobilities of some abnormal haemoglobins on cellulose acetate.** Tris buffer, pH 8.5.

8. Switch off the power, remove the strips from the tank and stain for 3–5 min with Ponceau S.

9. Remove the strips, drain and elute the excess stain with three consecutive 2 min washes with 50 ml/l acetic acid.

10. Dehydrate in absolute methanol for 3–5 min.

11. Clear in 20% (v/v) acetic acid in methanol for 6–8 min.

12. Dry in a 65°C oven for 4–6 min.

13. Make certain the strips are adequately labelled and place in a protective container, e.g. a plastic envelope.

Control preparation

The pattern given by unknown samples must be compared with that given by control haemolysates of known abnormal haemoglobins applied to each membrane alongside the unknown samples. Thus, a control sample containing Hbs A, F, S and C should be included with each electrophoretic run. Blood from a person with sickle cell trait (Hbs A, S, A_2), a normal baby (Hbs A, F) and a person with Hb C trait (Hbs A, C) provides this combination.

1. Obtain these fresh blood samples (in any anticoagulant).

2. Wash the cells three times with saline. Lyse the cells with water and CCl_4 as described on p. 231. Mix vigorously and then centrifuge for 10 min at 3000 rpm (1200 g).

3. Add a few drops of 0.3 mol/l (20 g/l) KCN to the haemolysate to stabilize the haemoglobin as cyanmethaemoglobin (HiCN).

4. Adjust the concentrations of the haemolysates with water to 120–140 g/l.

5. Mix equal volumes of the three haemolysates.

6. Check the mixture by electrophoresis.

7. Dispense in 0.5 ml volumes. If stored at 4°C they should be stable for several weeks; in liquid nitrogen they should be stable almost indefinitely.

Interpretation and comments

Figure 15.1 shows the relative electrophoretic mobility of some haemoglobins at pH 8.5 using cellulose acetate as the support medium.

Satisfactory separation of Hbs F, A, S and C is obtained (Fig. 15.2), but it is not possible to

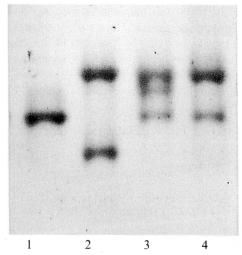

Fig. 15.2 **Separation of Hbs A, F, S and C on cellulose acetate.** (1) Hb 55, (2) Hb AC, (3) Hb AS + F, (4) Hb AS. Tris buffer, pH 8.5.

differentiate between Hbs S, D and G or between Hbs C, E and O for which citrate agar electrophoresis at acid pH (p. 243) is required.

It may be difficult to detect small amounts of Hb F in the presence of large amounts of Hb A or small amounts of Hb A in the presence of large amounts of Hb F. In the latter situation, if distinction is required between β^+ and β° homozygous thalassaemia, citrate agar electrophoresis (p. 243) should be performed.

The small volume of haemolysate applied by many commercially available applicators may lead to difficulty in detecting minor bands unless the concentration of the haemolysate is carefully controlled (e.g. with Hb Constant Spring, Hb A_2, Hb Bart's, Hb H). This is particularly relevant to the detection of raised Hb A_2 levels which should be clearly visible by comparison with normal samples on the same membrane. Such a qualitative estimate, however, must not be used for diagnostic purposes, for which the estimation of Hb A_2 has to be precise.

TESTS FOR Hb S

Tests to detect the presence of Hb S depend on the decreased solubility of the abnormal Hb at low oxygen tensions.

SICKLING IN WHOLE BLOOD

The sickling phenomenon may be simply demonstrated in a thin wet film of blood sealed between slide and cover-glass by means of a petroleum jelly/paraffin wax mixture. Sickling develops in the various types of sickle cell disease and also in Hb S trait. In homozygous Hb S disease (or Hb SC disease or Hb S/β-thalassaemia) marked sickling is usually visible after incubation for 1 h or less at 37°C and filamentous forms are conspicuous (Fig. 15.3). In Hb S trait the process is slower and the changes are less severe (Fig. 15.4), and incubation for as long as 12 h may be necessary for the changes to develop. They can, however, be hastened by the addition of reducing agents to the blood, e.g. sodium dithionite (see below).

METHOD USING REDUCING AGENT[29]

Reagents

(A) *Sodium dithionite ($Na_2S_2O_4$), 0.114 mol/l (19.85 g/l).* Prepare freshly just before use.
(B) *Disodium hydrogen phosphate (Na_2HPO_4), 0.114 mol/l (16.2 g/l).* For use, mix 2 volumes of A with 3 volumes of B to obtain a final pH of *c* 6.8.

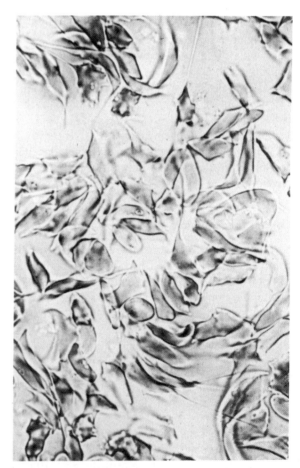

Fig. 15.3 Photomicrograph of sickled red cells. Hb SS. Sealed preparation of blood. Fully sickled filamentous forms predominate.

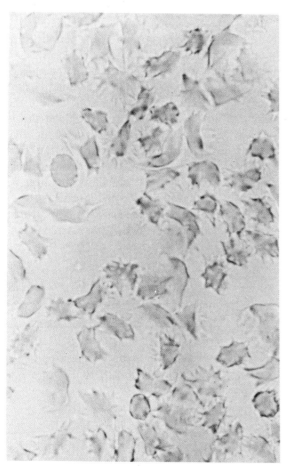

Fig. 15.4 Photomicrograph of sickled red cells. Hb AS. Similar preparation to that shown in Fig. 15.3. 'Holly leaf' sickling is present.

Method

Add 5 drops of the freshly prepared reagent to 1 drop of anticoagulated blood on a slide. Cover immediately with a cover-glass and seal with petroleum jelly/paraffin wax mixture. Sickling takes place almost immediately in Hb S disease and should be obvious in Hb S trait within 1 h.

Hb S SOLUBILITY TEST

Principle. A number of abnormal haemoglobins have an electrophoretic mobility similar to that of Hb S. The solubility test allows other haemoglobins to be differentiated from Hb S, as only variants with valine substituted for glutamic acid at the β6

position precipitate in the reduced state when placed in a high molarity phosphate buffer.[38]

Reagents

Phosphate buffer, pH 7.1. Potassium dihydrogen phosphate (KH_2PO_4) 33.78 g, dipotassium hydrogen phosphate (K_2HPO_4) 59.33 g, white saponin 2.5 g, water to 250 ml.

Working solution. Dissolve 0.1 g of sodium dithionite in 10 ml of buffer just prior to use.

Method[25]

1. Place 1 ml of working buffer in a test tube and allow to warm to room temperature.
2. Add 0.05 ml of whole blood, mix well and leave to stand for 5 min.
3. The resulting solution will be clear if the test is negative and cloudy if it is positive.
4. Any positive, or any suspected positive, sample must be centrifuged at 1200 *g* for 5 min. Positive tests will show a dark band at the top while the subnatant will be pink or colourless.
5. A positive (Hb AS) and negative control must be run with each batch of solubility tests.

Interpretation and comments

Positive results are given by the presence of Hb S and not by other haemoglobin variants with the same electrophoretic mobility such as Hb D and Hb G.

False negative results may be obtained if old or outdated reagents are used; they may also be given by the blood of children under the age of 6 months when only small amounts of Hb S are present. They may also occur in severe anaemia following recent blood transfusion and in heterozygotes when the proportion of Hb S is less than 20%. False positive results can be given by blood with a low haemoglobin and they have also been reported in severe leucocytosis, in hyperproteinaemia and in the presence of unstable haemoglobins especially after splenectomy.[25] Positive results may also be produced by other 'sickling' haemoglobins such as Hb C Harlem and Hb S Travis but the electrophoretic mobility of these rare variants on cellulose acetate at alkaline pH is different from that of Hb S.

A positive solubility test merely indicates the presence of Hb S and does not differentiate between sickle cell trait and the various forms of sickle cell disease. However, if the tube is centrifuged at c 4000 g for 5 min a colourless or only slightly pink supernatant usually indicates the presence of Hb S alone, and that the patient suffers from sickle cell disease. Whenever a solubility test is positive, haemoglobin electrophoresis must be performed before a definitive diagnosis is made.

An emergency sometimes makes it necessary to decide if an individual suffers from sickle cell disease before the results of haemoglobin electrophoresis are available. In these circumstances the solubility test can provide useful information, but a positive result must not be considered in isolation and must always lead to electrophoresis being performed at the earliest opportunity. If the test is positive and electrophoresis cannot be immediately undertaken, the following procedure should be adopted. A provisional diagnosis of sickle cell trait is made if the peripheral blood picture, including the blood film, is normal. If the blood film shows sickle or target cells, irrespective of the haemoglobin concentration, a provisional diagnosis of sickle cell disease is made. Always remember that the solubility test may be negative in infants with sickle cell disease.

A number of kits for the detection of Hb S, which are based on the insolubility of this haemoglobin, are available from commercial sources.

ESTIMATION OF Hb A$_2$

A raised Hb A$_2$ level is characteristic of heterozygous β-thalassaemia, and its accurate measurement is an essential requirement for the diagnosis of β-thalassaemia traits.

Two methods are available for the estimation of Hb A$_2$ and in experienced hands either gives reliable results.[43] The first technique uses elution after cellulose acetate electrophoresis while the second method employs microcolumn chromatography.

ESTIMATION OF Hb A$_2$ BY ELUTION FROM CELLULOSE ACETATE

Principle. Hb A$_2$ is separated from other haemoglobins by electrophoresis on cellulose acetate at pH 8.9, eluted into buffer and the percentage of Hb A$_2$ calculated by measuring and comparing the absorbence of the Hb A$_2$ eluate and an eluate prepared from the remaining haemoglobins.

Equipment

1. *Electrophoresis tanks and power supply.* Apparatus similar to that used for cellulose acetate electrophoresis (p. 232)

2. *Wicks of double layer filter paper.*

3. *10 μl microcapillary pipette.*

4. *Cellulose acetate membranes.* 10 × 5 cm is a suitable size.

Buffer

Electrophoresis buffer [Tris/EDTA/Borate (TEB), pH 8.9]. Tris-(hydroxymethyl)-aminomethane 14.4 g; ethylenediaminetetra-acetic acid (EDTA) 1.5 g; boric acid 0.9 g; water to 1 litre.

The buffer should be stored at 4°C and the pH checked before each use.

Method[36,58]

1. Fill the compartments of the electrophoresis tank with TEB buffer. Soak and position a double layer of filter paper wicks.

2. In a separate dish soak the cellulose acetate membranes in TEB buffer for at least 5 min. It is important to immerse the membranes slowly so as to avoid trapping air bubbles.

3. Blot the menbranes, but do not allow them to dry out before application of the haemolysates.

4. Stretch the strips across the bridges of the electrophoresis tank so that they are connected to

the buffer chambers by a double-layered wick of filter paper.

5. Apply 10 µl of haemolysate (100 g/l) to the cathode end of the strip by a micropipette. The application should stretch to within 0.5 cm of the edge of the strip.

6. Apply the power and run at 3 mA for 30–40 min per strip or until good separation is obtained.

7. Switch off the power. Remove the membranes and cut the Hb A and Hb A_2 zones into small pieces and elute into 15 ml and 1.5 ml, respectively, of buffer.

8. Allow to elute with occasional shaking or on a mechanical mixer for 20–30 min.

9. Remove the eluted strips and centrifuge the eluates at 1200 g for 5 min to sediment debris.

10. Determine the absorbence of each eluate at 413 nm using a spectrophotometer.
Use TEB buffer as a blank.

Calculation

$$\% \text{ Hb } A_2 = \frac{A^{413} \text{ Hb } A_2}{(10 \times A^{413} \text{ Hb A}) + A^{413} \text{ Hb } A_2} \times 100.$$

Interpretation and comments

Difficulties in cutting out the Hb A_2 band precisely may result in considerable variation in the normal range but in general values below 3% are normal and those above 3.5% are abnormal.

Prolonged storage of samples does not seem to affect the Hb A_2 level unduly but methaemoglobin formation may cause less clear definition between the bands.

Raised levels of Hb A_2 occur in β-thalassaemia trait (minor) and in the β unstable haemoglobinopathies.[57] Some overlap between normal subjects and those with β-thalassaemia trait has, however, been reported.[12] The levels are variable in β-thalassaemia major and thalassaemia intermedia. Decreased levels have been reported in Hb H disease[53] δβ-thalassaemia,[50] hereditary persistence of fetal haemoglobin (HPFH)[10] and Hb Lepore.[37] Decreased levels have also been reported in severe iron deficiency[31] but this has not been confirmed.

There is some evidence to suggest that persons with Hb S trait may have elevated Hb A_2 levels.

Increased levels are well documented in Hb S/β-thalassaemia but normal Hb A_2 levels are usually found in patients who have unusually high Hb F levels.[41] Some investigators have reported slightly raised Hb A_2 levels in patients who have both homozygous sickle cell disease and α-thalassaemia.[14,22,61] It is, however, important to take particular care when cutting the strips of samples with a band in the position of Hb S as this diminishes the separation between Hb A_2 and other haemoglobins.

Estimation of the percentage of Hb A_2 by elution from cellulose acetate cannot be used in the presence of Hb C, Hb E, Hb O Arab and Hb C Harlem, because those haemoglobins have a similar electrophoresis mobility to that of Hb A_2 at pH 8.9.

Densitometry of stained strips as a means of the quantitative estimation of different haemoglobins is unsatisfactory as many undefined factors influence the amount of dye attached to the different proteins.

ESTIMATION OF Hb A_2 BY MICRO-COLUMN CHROMATOGRAPHY

Principle. Micro-column chromatography depends on the interchange of charged groups on the ion exchange resin with charged groups on the haemoglobin molecule. When a mixture of haemoglobins is adsorbed onto the resin a particular haemoglobin component may be eluted from the column using a buffer (developer) with a specific pH and/or ionic strength while a second component (either a single haemoglobin or a mixture of haemoglobins) may be eluted by changing the pH or ionic strength of the buffer (developer). The separation of haemoglobin components in such a system will depend on such factors as the pH and ionic strength of the developers used for equilibration of the column and for elution, the type of resin, the volume of the sample applied, the size of the column, the gradient and the flow rates.

The methods described below use the anion exchange resin diethylaminoethyl (DEAE) cellulose (Whatman DE-52 microgranular and preswollen), with tris-HCl developers[13] or glycine-KCN developers.[24]

ESTIMATION OF Hb A$_2$ BY MICRO-COLUMN CHROMATOGRAPHY WITH TRIS-HCl DEVELOPERS[13]

Buffers

Stock buffer, 1.0 mol/l tris. Tris-(hydroxymethyl)-aminomethane 121.1 g; water to 1 litre).
Working buffers, 0.05 mol/l tris-HCl, pH 8.5, 8.3 and 7.0.

For each buffer add 200 mg of KCN to 100 ml of stock 1.0 mol/l tris buffer, and make up with water to 2 litres. Adjust the pH with concentrated HCl. If the buffers have been kept at 4°C they must be allowed to return to room temperature before use. Columns should be prepared in Pasteur pipettes using a pre-swollen microgranular anion exchange resin, e.g. Whatman DE 52 (diethylaminoethyl cellulose).

Method

To prepare the slurry, add 10 g of DE 52 to 200 ml of tris/HCl buffer, pH 8.5. Mix gently for a few min, then adjust the pH of the thoroughly suspended resin to 8.5 with concentrated HCl. Allow the resin to settle, remove the supernatant and resuspend the resin in a further 200 ml of pH 8.5 buffer. Check that the pH is steady at 8.5, which it normally is in *c* 10 min. Then allow the resin to settle and remove enough of the buffer so that the settled resin constitutes about half the total volume.

Set up disposable Pasteur pipettes with short stems vertically in stands. Place either a 3 mm glass bead for a very small piece of cotton wool in the tapered part of the pipette to act as a base for the column. If cotton wool is used, it should not be packed tightly and should be moistened with pH 8.5 buffer. Fill the pipette with thoroughly resuspended slurry allowing the column to pack under gravity to a height of about 6 cm.

Dilute 1 drop of haemolysate with 5 drops of pH 8.5 buffer. When all the excess buffer has drained from the column, gently apply the haemoglobin solution to the top of the column, and allow a few minutes for it to be absorbed onto the resin. Then apply buffer at pH 8.3 gently to the column with a piece of polythene tubing attached to the top of the pipette acting as a reservoir. About 9 ml of pH 8.3

buffer should be used to elute the Hb A$_2$ band, the greater part of which should elute between 4 and 6 ml. Collect the eluate in a 10 ml flask or cylinder and make up the volume to 10 ml with the pH 8.3 buffer.

Then elute the remaining Hb A, using 10 ml of pH 7.0 buffer; collect the eluate and make up the volume to 25 ml with pH 7.0 buffer. If, at any stage, the flow through the column stops, it should be discarded.

The amount of haemoglobin applied to the column must be carefully controlled. Overloading of the column with more than 7–8 mg of haemoglobin will cause contamination of the Hb A$_2$ fraction with Hb A. Less than 2 mg of haemoglobin will result in an eluate with an absorbance too low for accurate measurement.

The flow-rate of the column may be adjusted by altering the height of the reservoir above the column. A flow-rate of 10–20 ml per hour is satisfactory. Raising the reservoir increases the flow-rate and broadens the Hb A$_2$ band on the column but does not affect its elution or quantity.

MODIFIED PROCEDURE FOR SAMPLES CONTAINING SLOW-MOVING HAEMOGLOBIN VARIANTS

The above procedure may be modified to make it suitable for samples containing slow-moving haemoglobins such as Hb S. A longer exchange column is required.[12] The column is packed with the prepared slurry to a height of 16 cm. The Hb A$_2$ is eluted using a tris HCl developer pH 8.3, and the effluent collected in a 10 ml volumetric flask, as previously described. The slow-moving haemoglobin is then eluted using a tris HCl developer pH 8.2, and if the proportion of the variant is to be estimated the effluent is collected in a 10 ml volumetric flask. The remaining haemoglobin is then eluted with the tris HCl developer pH 7.0 and collected in a 25 ml volumetric flask. The percentages of Hb A and Hb S may be calculated as follows:

$$\% \; Hb \; S = \frac{2.5 \times A^{413} \, Hb \; S}{A^{413}HbA_2 + (2.5 \times A^{415}HbS) + (2.5 \times A^{413}HbR)} \times 100;$$

% Hb A_2 =

$$\frac{2.5 \times A^{413} \text{Hb } A_2}{A^{413}\text{HbA}_2 + (2.5 \times A^{413}\text{HbS}) + (2.5 \times A^{413}\text{HbR})} \times 100;$$

where A^{413} Hb R is the absorbence of the remaining haemoglobin.

Interpretation and comments

A normal and high Hb A_2 control should be tested with each batch of samples. Each laboratory must establish its own normal range and this should not differ significantly from that determined by cellulose acetate electrophoresis. Efremov[12] quotes a normal range of 1.5 to 3.5%, mean 2.5 $\pm$ 0.15%.

By this method, the percentage of Hb A_2 is usually raised in β-thalassaemia, range 4.0–7.0%; and in the β unstable haemoglobinopathies.[57] However, in some types of β-thalassaemia, i.e. δβ-thalassaemia, the Hb A_2 percentage is normal or low. It is also normal or low in α_1-thalassaemia trait and is usually low in Hb H disease. In some acquired disorders, too, the Hb A_2 percentage may be altered,[22] e.g. raised in pernicious anaemia; lowered in iron-deficiency anaemia, sideroblastic anaemia and aplastic anaemia. More than 8–10% 'Hb A_2' suggests the presence of another haemoglobin that is not Hb A_2.

Hb E does not separate from Hb A_2; however, when present it usually constitutes more than 25% of the total haemoglobin. Hb E can be separated from Hb C by column chromatography. Hb C will also elute with Hb A. In Hb AC heterozygotes Hb C usually exceeds 35% of the total, and can be identified by citrate agar gel electrophoresis.

ESTIMATION OF Hb A_2 BY MICRO-COLUMN CHROMATOGRAPHY WITH GLYCINE-POTASSIUM CYANIDE DEVELOPERS[24]

The method described is suitable for samples containing slow-moving variants such as Hb S. The elution of Hb A_2 is dependent on the pH of the ion exchanger and is relatively less sensitive to the pH of the developer.

Reagents

(i)   Developer A: Glycine 15.0 g; KCN 0.1 g; water to 1 litre.

(ii)   Developer B: 9 g/l NaCl.

(iii)   Diethylaminoethyl (DEAE) anion exchange medium, microgranular, preswollen.

Method

1. *Preparation of ion exchanger.* Add *c* 250 ml of Developer A to *c* 50 g of DEAE cellulose. Mix gently and allow the material to settle (the slurry). Remove the supernatant and repeat the process at least twice. Then adjust the pH of the resuspended DEAE cellulose to 7.6 with 0.1 mol/l HCl. As a check, the DEAE column should be tested with a Hb AS lysate. The Hb A_2 should elute in the first 3–4 ml and Hb S in the next 15–20 ml of the developer. The slurry may be stored for up to 3–4 weeks but the pH should be checked and if necessary readjusted before use, and the stored slurry should also be checked with a control of known Hb A_2 content.

2. *Preparation of column.* Disposable Pasteur pipettes are set up as described on p. 238 for the tris HCl method, the column being filled to a height of 6–7 cm with the slurry prepared with DE-52 and Developer A which may also be used to moisten the cotton wool plug. Prepared columns may be stored after topping up with Developer A and closing both ends. Before use remove excess buffer.

3. Dilute 1 drop of haemolysate (*c* 100 g/l) with 6 drops of water and apply gently to the top of the column. Allow the haemoglobin to absorb onto the ion exchanger and then fill the column with Developer A and connect to the reservoir. Hb A_2 is eluted with 3–4 ml of Developer A and collected in a 5 ml volumetric flask. After all the Hb A_2 has been eluted, remove the flask and make up the volume to 5 ml.

4. Replace Developer A with 15–20 ml of Developer B and collect the remaining haemoglobin (Hb A or Hbs A + S) in a 25 ml volumetric flask. After collecting the effluent, make up the volume in the flask to 25 ml.

5. Read the absorbence of the eluted haemoglobin in the flask at 413 nm in a spectrophotometer using water as a blank. Calculate the

---

*E.g. Whatman DE 52.

percentage of Hb A$_2$ as follows:

$$\% \text{ HB A}_2 = \frac{A^{413} \text{ Hb A}_2}{A^{413} \text{ Hb A}_2 + (5 \times A^{413} \text{ Hb A})} \times 100.$$

Interpretation and comments

In general, similar comments apply to both the tris HCl and glycine KCN methods. Hb A$_2$ percentages tend to be slightly lower with the former, but with either procedure there should be no overlap between normal and β-thalassaemia trait subjects.[12] An advantage of the glycine KCN method is a reduced sensitivity to minor changes in the pH of the developer; an added advantage is that it may be used for samples containing Hb S.

To estimate the percentage of Hb S and the remaining haemoglobin as well as that of Hb A$_2$, Hb A$_2$ is eluted in the first 3–4 ml with Developer A, Hb S is eluted in the next 15–20 ml with the same Developer A and the remaining haemoglobin is eluted with Developer B. The effluent containing Hb A$_2$ is diluted to 5 ml and effluents containing Hb S and the remaining haemoglobin diluted to 25 ml. To ensure elution of all the Hb A$_2$ in the first 3–4 ml and all the Hb S in the next 15–20 ml, the pH of the ion exchanger may need adjustment following a test chromatogram.[24]

ESTIMATION OF THE PERCENTAGE OF SLOW-MOVING HAEMOGLOBIN VARIANTS IN MIXTURES OF HAEMOGLOBIN

Blood transfusion has an important role in the management of sickle cell disease. In such patients achieving and when necessary maintaining a Hb A level of 80–90% has been a factor in reducing morbidity and mortality. The successful use of transfusion or exchange transfusion requires accurate estimation of the percentage of Hb S present.

The estimation of Hb S (or Hb C) may be carried out either by elution after cellulose acetate electrophoresis or by microchromatography. The principles involved in the estimation of Hb S (or Hb C) by cellulose acetate electrophoresis are similar to those employed for the estimation of Hb A$_2$. The equipment and reagents differ only in the need for longer cellulose acetate strips, a size of 20 × 5 cm being suitable.

Carry out electrophoresis at 250–300 V for *c* 2–3 h or until good separation is obtained. As with the estimation of Hb A$_2$, the separation should be carried out at least in duplicate and preferably in triplicate. The volume of buffer into which each haemoglobin band is eluted will depend on the amount of haemoglobin present.

We recommend that the bands from triplicate strips be eluted into 25 ml of buffer or water. However, the volume of eluting fluid should be smaller than this when only a very small quantity of a particular haemoglobin is visible on the strip. Any estimation of Hb C will include any Hb A$_2$ that is present.

Determine the absorbance of each eluate at 413 nm using a spectrophotometer, using TEB buffer as a blank. Calculate the percentage of Hb A, and of Hb S or Hb C from the following formulae, remembering to make the relevant correction if the haemoglobin bands have not been eluted into equal volumes:

$$\% \text{ Hb A} = \frac{A^{413} \text{ Hb A}}{A^{413} \text{ Hb A} + A^{413} \text{Hb S} + A^{413} \text{HbA}_2} \times 100.$$

$$\% \text{ Hb S} = \frac{A^{413} \text{ Hb S}}{A^{413} \text{ Hb A} + A^{413} \text{ Hb S} + A^{413} \text{HbA}_2} \times 100.$$

$$\% \text{ Hb C}\star = \frac{A^{413} \text{ Hb C}}{A^{413} \text{ Hb A} + A^{413} \text{ Hb S} + A^{413} \text{ Hb C}} \times 100.$$

ESTIMATION OF Hb F

Hb F may be estimated by several methods, all of which are based on its resistance to denaturation at alkaline pH.

For small amounts of haemoglobin (below 10–

15%) the method of Betke et al[2] is reliable, whilst for levels of over 50%, and in cord blood, the

---

$\star$ In a patient with Hb SC disease.

method of Jonxis and Visser[30] is preferable; it is, however, not reliable at levels below 10%.

Ion exchange chromatography has been recommended for the estimation of Hb F but it is unsuitable for routine use.[23,47] More recently, immunological methods have been devised to measure Hb F by immunodiffusion[9]—there are commercially available kits—and by enzyme-linked immunoassay (ELISA).[34] It is likely that radioimmuno-assay may prove to be the most accurate method for measuring Hb F levels over the complete range.[19] At present, however, the specific Hb F antibodies which are required for immunological methods are not easily obtainable.

MODIFIED BETKE METHOD FOR THE ESTIMATION OF PERCENTAGE Hb F[2]

Principle. To measure the percentage of Hb F in a mixture of haemoglobins, sodium hydroxide is added to a haemolysate and after a set time denaturation is stopped by adding saturated ammonium sulphate. The ammonium sulphate lowers the pH and precipitates the denatured haemoglobin. After filtration, the quantity of undenatured (unprecipitated) haemoglobin is measured. The proportion of alkali-resistant (i.e. fetal) haemoglobin is then calculated as a percentage of the total amount of haemoglobin present.

Method

Prepare a cyanmethaemoglobin (HiCN) solution by adding 0.6 ml of red cell lysate to 10 ml of a solution of 0.2 g potassium cyanide and 0.2 g potassium ferricyanide per litre.*

To 2.8 ml of the HiCN solution add 0.2 ml of 1.2 mol/l NaOH; mix thoroughly and leave for exactly 2 min at room temperature (c 20°C). Then add 2.0 ml of saturated ammonium sulphate; mix thoroughly. Allow to stand for 10 min. Filter through a Whatman No. 42 filter paper.

Read the absorbence of both test and standard at 413 nm.** Use the rest of the HiCN solution as a standard.

Calculate the percentage of Hb F as follows:

$$\% \text{ Hb F} = \frac{A^{413} \text{ test} \times 100}{A^{413} \text{ standard} \times 20}.$$

METHOD OF JONXIS AND VISSER[30]

Principle. Increased resistance of Hb F to denaturation by alkali is detected by placing the sample in a spectrophotometer cuvette and recording the absorbence at 576 nm each minute for up to 15 min. At this wavelength the absorption of oxyhaemoglobin differs from that of the alkali haemochromogen which is formed on denaturation.

When the logarithm of the percentage of haemoglobin remaining undenatured is plotted against time a straight line is obtained. By extrapolation to zero time the percentage of Hb F in the original sample can be calculated.

Method

Add 0.1 ml of blood or haemolysate (approximately 100 g/l) to 10 ml of water; then add 2 drops of 10% NH_4OH solution. Measure the absorbence at 576 nm (A_B). Then add 0.1 ml of the same blood or lysate to 10 ml of 0.06 mol/l NaOH; add 2 drops of 10% NH_4OH solution at room temperature. Mix thoroughly and measure the absorbence every min for 15 min (A_T). Then place the solution at 37°C for 15 min, cool to room temperature and measure the absorbence (A_E). The ratio $A_B:A_E$ should be constant.

Calculate the percentage of undenatured haemoglobin at each minute:

$$\frac{A_T^{576} - A_E^{576}}{A_B^{576} - A_E^{576}} \times 100.$$

Then plot the percentage on the logarithmic scale of semi-logarithmic paper against time. This should produce a straight line from which the original amount of Hb F, i.e. that at zero time, can be found by extrapolation.

Significance

In infants aged 1 yr the level of Hb F should not be more than 1%. The normal range for adults is 0.2–1.0%. Each laboratory should, however, estab-

---

*The reagents used should not contain any detergent as this can reduce the resistance of Hb F to alkali denaturation, leading to falsely low results.

**Absorbence can also be measured satisfactorily at 540 nm.

lish its own normal range. Controls of known normal and known raised Hb F percentages must be run with each batch. The raised Hb F control should not contain more than 10% Hb F. It can be prepared easily by mixing cord blood and normal blood.

Zago et al[62] reported variability in the capacity of different batches of filter paper to absorb haemoglobin from the filtrate which in some instances may be responsible for a distinct drop in the normal range. Increased levels are found in many disorders, notably in β-thalassaemia trait and sickle-cell disease. But any haematological condition, congenital or acquired, may be associated with a slight increase.

The method of Jonxis and Visser requires an accurate spectrophotometer as the maximum absorption peak at 576 nm is very narrow and the difference in extinction between oxyhaemoglobin and alkali haemochromogen is relatively small.

INTRACELLULAR DISTRIBUTION OF Hb F

Differences in the intracellular distribution of Hb F are often used to differentiate between heterozygotes for δβ-thalassaemia and hereditary persistence of fetal haemoglobin (HPFH). In the former not all the red cells can be shown to contain Hb F (heterocellular distribution), while in the latter every cell contains Hb F (pancellular distribution), although there is some variability from cell to cell. The value of such a differentiation is questionable and it has been suggested that a heterocellular distribution may be more apparent than real and merely reflects the threshold for detection of Hb F by the particular technique used. Higher levels of Hb F give a more even (pancellular) distribution than lower levels. For these reasons results should be treated with caution and never used to make a diagnosis in isolation.

Two techniques have been widely used for measuring intracellular Hb F distribution. That most frequently used is the acid elution test of Kleihauer[32] which was originally developed for the detection of fetal red cells in maternal blood following transplacental haemorrhage. Less frequently employed is the more sensitive immunofluorescent technique using specific anti-Hb F antibodies.[59] With the latter technique the proportion of cells reacting positively has been reported to correlate well with the percentage of Hb F measured by alkali denaturation at levels between 0.5 and 5.0%. Immunofluorescent labelling is capable of detecting cells with as little as 1 pg of Hb F per cell (c 0.5% Hb F). The method can thus detect positively reacting cells in clinical syndromes with modest increases in Hb F and this gives the immunofluorescent technique an advantage over acid elution. A possible drawback of its increased sensitivity is that because positivity is achieved at relatively low Hb F levels per cell a heterocellular distribution may appear to be pancellular if the proportion of Hb F is greater than 10%.[16]

The acid elution method is described on p. 121.

RED CELL INCLUSIONS

The most important red cell inclusions found in the haemoglobinopathies are Hb H inclusions in α-thalassaemia,[54] α-chain inclusions in β-thalassaemia major[17,54] and Heinz bodies in unstable haemoglobin diseases.[21,56]

Precipitated α chains are found in the cytoplasm of nucleated red cell precursors of patients with β-thalassaemia major; they stain readily supravitally with methyl violet (as do Heinz bodies) and appear usually as irregularly shaped bodies close to the nucleus of normoblasts. After splenectomy they may also be found, too, in peripheral blood normoblasts and reticulocytes. Heinz bodies (insoluble denatured globin chains) form as a result of chemical poisoning and drug intoxication, and develop spontaneously in G6PD deficiency and in the unstable haemoglobin diseases. They are usually only readily discernible in the peripheral blood if the spleen has been removed. When due to the presence of an unstable haemoglobin they may be demonstrated in the peripheral blood of patients with intact spleens if their blood is kept at 37°C for 24–48 h. The use of methyl violet and of brilliant cresyl blue in the demonstration of α-chain inclusions and Heinz bodies is described in Chapter 9.

DEMONSTRATION OF Hb H INCLUSIONS

Hb H inclusions develop in the Hb Bart's hydrops fetalis syndrome and in Hb H disease. In Hb H disease many red cells develop inclusions but in α-thalassaemia-2 trait (α^+-thalassaemia) only 1 in 1000 to 1 in 10 000 red cells develop inclusions. Although usually more numerous in α-thalassaemia-1 trait (α^0-thalassaemia), the number of cells developing inclusions does not help in differentiating between the various gene deletion patterns seen in α-thalassaemia, and the absence of demonstrable inclusions does not preclude a diagnosis of α-thalassaemia trait. The relative value of testing for Hb H inclusions in different racial groups has been reviewed by Walford et al.[52]

Method

Mix 2 volumes of fresh blood added to any blood anticoagulant with 1 volume of 1% New methylene blue in saline. Then incubate at 37°C for 1 h. Make a film of the suspension and when dry examine microscopically unfixed, using a 2 mm objective as for a reticulocyte count. The inclusions appear as multiple greenish-blue bodies like the pitted pattern on a golf ball. They are readily distinguished from the precipitated dots and filaments in reticulocytes (see Fig. 9.7).

FURTHER TESTS FOR THE IDENTIFICATION OF ABNORMAL HAEMOGLOBINS

When an abnormal haemoglobin has been demonstrated by haemoglobin electrophoresis at an alkaline pH on cellulose acetate membrane, other electrophoretic techniques may be useful in making a presumptive identification. It is useful to measure the percentage of a variant Hb, and this can usually be done using the buffer and procedure recommended on p. 236 for Hb A_2 estimation by electrophoresis. The elution volume should be adjusted according to the proportion of the variant being investigated.

Of the fast-moving variants, Hb Bart's and Hb H can be distinguished by their movement on cellulose acetate membrane with a phosphate buffer at pH 6.5. Variants moving in a similar manner to Hb S, but with a negative solubility test, can be separated from Hb S on citrate agar electrophoresis at pH 6.0. This technique is useful when investigating compound heterozygotes, e.g. Hb SD or Hb SG; it can also be used to distinguish between Hb E, Hb C and Hb O, which move similarly at an alkaline pH on cellulose acetate, and also to separate Hb A from Hb F. This is particularly useful as an aid to the diagnosis of abnormal haemoglobins in cord blood, and to detect small amounts of Hb A in thalassaemia.

Globin-chain separation at both acid and alkaline pH is a useful technique for identifying the abnormal chain (p. 247). Starch gel electrophoresis is a very sensitive method which, too, gives good results (p. 245).

CITRATE AGAR ELECTROPHORESIS, pH 6.0[35]

Buffer

Stock citrate buffer. Sodium citrate 147 g; water 600 ml. Adjust the pH to 6.0 with 50% citric acid and then make the volume to 1 litre with water.

Working buffer. Dilute the stock buffer 1 in 10 for preparation of the gel and for use in the chambers.

Method

Make a 1% agar solution by adding 1 g of agar powder to 100 ml of working buffer and melt in a boiling water-bath. Keep unused stock and working buffer at 4°C.

Smear a few drops of hot agar over glass slides, 7.5 cm × 10 cm, and dry on a hot plate for 5 min. Place the pre-coated slides on a level surface and pipette approximately 9 ml of hot agar on to each one and spread it to cover the slide evenly. Allow to set before moving the slide. A firm plastic film may be used as an alternative to the glass slides; it has proved very satisfactory in use and is easy to store.

Dilute the haemolysates to be tested to 10–30 g haemoglobin per litre, matching their haemoglobin content closely to that of control samples. For detection of minor haemoglobin components, as in cord blood, a 100 g/l haemolysate is preferable. Samples may be applied using a commercial applicator. Load the plate wells with a drop of diluted lysate, prime the applicator and gently place the applicator on to the agar, without cutting the gel surface. Leave the applicator in contact with the gel for c 15 s.

Prepare the tank with cold buffer and filter paper or sponge wicks, and place the slides, agar side down, on to the filter paper or wicks. Apply a constant current of 50 mA. Separation should be complete within approximately 1 h.

Stain the agar gel with Ponceau S or bromophenol blue for 2–5 min. Rinse the plates in running water. Then dry the agar in an 80°C oven for $1\frac{1}{2}$–2 h or allow to dry at room temperature.

Stains

Bromophenol blue. Dissolve 100 mg of bromophenol blue in 1 litre of water containing 10 ml of glacial acetic acid.

Ponceau S. 20 g/l in 30 g/l trichloracetic acid.

The value of citrate agar in the differentiation of Hb S and Hb C from variants with similar electrophoretic mobilities on cellulose acetate has already been discussed (p. 234). Citrate agar electrophoresis also allows the demonstration of even small amounts of Hb F.

Successful citrate agar electrophoresis presents greater technical problems than electrophoresis with cellulose acetate and controls are essential. The haemolysates must not have a haemoglobin concentration greater than 30 g/l and for cord samples a concentration of not more than 15 g/l is recommended. The electrophoresis tank must be kept cool throughout the procedure. Commercial kits for citrate agar electrophoresis are available and contain detailed descriptions of the method.

The relative mobilities of some haemoglobins on citrate agar gel are shown in Fig. 15.5.

CELLULOSE ACETATE ELECTROPHORESIS, pH 6.5

Hb H and Hb Barts can be distinguished from other fast-moving variants by their movement towards the anode when using cellulose acetate membrane with phosphate buffer, pH 6.5.

Buffer

0.1 mol/l phosphate, pH 6.5. KH_2PO_4 3.11 g; $Na_2HPO_4.2H_2O$ 1.87 g; water to 1 litre.

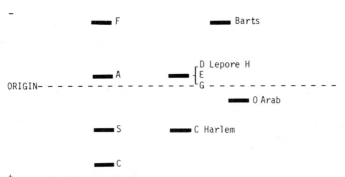

Fig. 15.5 Relative mobilities of some abnormal haemoglobins on agar gel. Citrate buffer, pH 6.0.

Method

Soak cellulose acetate strips in buffer, blot and place across the bridges. Apply the haemolysate at the centre of the strip and carry out electrophoresis at 250–350 V for 10–15 min. Stain with Ponceau S (p. 232).

The amount of Hb H or Hb Bart's can be estimated by eluting the haemoglobin bands in measured volumes of water (see method for Hb A_2, p. 236).

Controls

These should, if possible, include a cord-blood sample containing Hb Bart's, a sample containing Hb H and a normal sample. If possible, too, a fast-moving haemoglobin, other than Hb H or Bart's, should be included.

Comments

Most fast-moving haemoglobins may be differentiated from Hb H and Hb Bart's by this method. Hb H migrates further toward the anode than Hb Bart's. As Hb H is unstable and denatures readily, it is important to use haemolysates that have been prepared from fresh blood.

STARCH-GEL ELECTROPHORESIS

This is a very sensitive but complex method for the detection of abnormal haemoglobins. Starch-gel trays are now commercially available for both horizontal and vertical systems, and they can be made very cheaply from Perspex (Fig. 15.6). The vertical system is to be preferred as the bands, especially minor ones, are better resolved.

Tris/EDTA/borate (TEB) buffer similar to that used for cellulose acetate electrophoresis is suitable

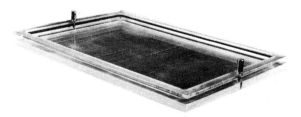

Fig. 15.6 Perspex tray for starch gel electrophoresis.

for the separation of Hbs H or Bart's and for the detection of Hb M a phosphate buffer at neutral pH gives satisfactory results. The system can also be adapted for globin chain separation using acid and alkaline barbitone buffers.[18]

Buffers

Continuous tris buffer system, pH 8.6, 0.08 mol/l. Tris-(hydroxymethyl)-aminomethane 110 g; EDTA 5.85 g; boric acid 30.9 g; water to 1 litre.

Dilute the buffer 1 in 20 for making gels, 1 in 5 for the anodal chamber and 1 in 7 for the cathodal chamber.

This is the most useful continuous buffer for routine work.

Discontinuous tris and sodium borate buffer system, pH 8.5, 45 mmol/l. Gels. Tris-(hydroxymethyl)-aminomethane 49.5 g; citric acid 5.0 g; water to 5 l. *Chambers.* Boric acid 92.5 g; 10 mol/l NaOH 25.0 g; water to 5 l.

This buffer system has the advantage that minor components are resolved more easily. However, major components tend to diffuse and the gels are less easy to handle.

Phosphate, pH 7.1, 5.4 mmol/l.[18] Titrate 40 mmol/l disodium hydrogen phosphate to pH 7.1 with syrupy phosphoric acid. Dilute 40 ml of the buffer with 300 ml of water.

The undiluted buffer is used for the electrode chambers and the diluted buffer is used for the gel. Separation takes about 4 h. This buffer is the most satisfactory one available for demonstrating Hb Bart's and Hb H, especially when they are present in low concentrations.

Method

Make up hydrolysed starch in buffer at a concentration of about 90–120 g/l. The volume should be more than sufficient to fill the tray. Thoroughly shake the mixture in a 1 litre Erlenmeyer flask and heat over a flame, continuously shaking, until the gel becomes translucent. Remove the dissolved air by applying a vacuum to the side arm of the flask, and in this way a mixture containing only small bubbles will be obtained. Excessive degassing should be avoided as this can result in dry gels. Pour the molten gel into the tray, allowing some to overflow the sides. After cooling, cut slots of 1 cm length through the gel with a razor. Soak filter papers of similar size in haemolysates (20–40 g/l), insert into the slots and leave in position. Place the gel mould in the two buffer chambers with strips of Whatman No. 3 paper, four layers thick, soaked in the buffer, at either end. Cover the system with a thin sheet of polythene and a glass plate, secured with elastic bands. Carry out electrophoresis for 2 h at 30 mA, or overnight at 8 mA. Remove the top section and slice the gel in half longitudinally with a cheese wire. Then stain one half with a protein stain, such as amido black, or with a haemoglobin stain such as orthotolidine (see below).

Stains

Amido black stain. Diluent: glacial acetic acid 200 ml; methanol 900 ml; water 900 ml. Add 0.8 g of amido black to 1 litre of the diluent.

Pour the stain over the gel and leave for 5 min. Then wash the gel with several changes of the diluent. The stained gel will keep indefinitely if sealed under Cellophane.

Orthotolidine. Orthotolidine 0.5 g; sodium nitroprusside 1 g; glacial acetic acid 50 ml.

Add a sufficient volume of the solution to cover the gel completely. Then add 30% hydrogen peroxide (100 vol) (5 ml/l stain) and leave the mixture until the desired intensity of staining is obtained, usually in 5 min. Then wash the gel several times with water. The stain is more readily retained if the gel is kept at 4°C.

Interpretation and comments

The migration of common haemoglobin variants on starch gel is similar to that obtained on cellulose acetate electrophoresis. With properly washed red cell lysates the only non-haemoglobin proteins capable of producing an abnormal band are the two iso-enzymes of carbonic anhydrase which migrate more slowly than Hb A_2. Haemolysates which contain traces of plasma may produce additional bands which will stain even with orthotolidine.

As with cellulose acetate electrophoresis, Hbs A_2, C, E and O migrate identically and the same is true of the faster-moving Hbs S, D Lepore and G. In samples from normal adults Hb F is not usually

detectable and when Hb F predominates small amounts of Hb A ($< 10\%$) may be difficult to detect. Raised levels of Hb A_2 should be clearly visible by comparison with normal samples. Controls must include at least two different known abnormal haemoglobins.

STARCH BLOCK ELECTROPHORESIS

This medium provides a sensitive method for separating haemoglobins but the process is time-consuming and unsuitable for routine use. It can be used for the estimation of Hb A_2 or for the separation and estimation of other haemoglobin variants.

Buffers

Barbitone, pH 8.9. Sodium diethylbarbiturate 10.3 g; diethylbarbituric acid 0.92 g; water to 1 litre.

This is the most suitable buffer for routine use, e.g. for the separation of Hb S from Hb C and for the isolation of Hb A_2.

Phosphate, pH 7.0. Titrate 40 mmol/l disodium hydrogen phosphate to pH 7.0 with syrupy phosphoric acid.

This buffer is recommended for the separation and estimation of Hb Bart's and Hb H. Migration is rapid and separation is adequate in 8–12 h at 30–40 mA and 250 V.

Method

Wash potato starch four times in the appropriate buffer and pour the mixture into trays, 25 × 30 × 0.5 cm, containing three thicknesses of Whatman No. 3 paper which have been soaked in the buffer and placed in the trays with half left outside to make contact with the buffer. Soak up excess buffer with large sheets of filter paper until the starch is just moist when pressed. Cut slits measuring 1 cm into the block, one-third of the way from the cathode, and pipette in the haemolysate (Hb *c* 100 g/l). Each should hold about 1 ml. Cover the whole with a sheet of polythene and a thick glass plate and secure with thick clamps on either side. Carry out electrophoresis at 4°C and, using barbitone buffer, continue this for 18 h at 30 mA and 250 V. Inspect the bands by trans-illumination and cut out fractions if desired. Elute the haemoglobin by allowing the fractions to stand in barbitone buffer at 4°C. Filter the eluate through a sintered glass funnel.

GLOBIN CHAIN ELECTROPHORESIS[39,45]

Introduction and principle. Initially, globin chain electrophoresis was largely employed in the investigation of an abnormal haemoglobin as a means of determining whether the substitution had occurred in either the α or β (or non-α) chains. More recently it has been used at both alkaline and acid pH as part of the systematic identification of a suspected abnormal haemoglobin.[28]

The preliminary screening for variants by electrophoresis on cellulose acetate at alkaline pH, followed by citrate agar electrophoresis at an acid pH, makes possible the presumptive identification of many haemoglobins, e.g. Hb S and Hb C. Globin chain electrophoresis at alkaline and acid pH is then a useful additional test; its particular value is, however, that it provides a means of identifying abonormal haemoglobins with differing mobilities in acid and alkaline buffers that cannot be identified by routine electrophoretic methods. Hb D (Punjab) is one such haemoglobin. It migrates like Hb S on cellulose acetate at alkaline pH and like Hb A on citrate agar. On globin electrophoresis at alkaline pH it is difficult to distinguish from Hb S but at acid pH it migrates closer to the anode. This variation in mobility of the globin chains with pH similarly has value in the diagnosis of Hb O Arab and Hb G Philadelphia.

Earlier methods for globin electrophoresis were time-consuming because of the time required to prepare the globin. This is, however, not essential as whole-blood haemolysates may be used and the haem groups and globin chains dissociated with DL-dithiothreitol (DL-DTT) and urea. The method described below employs electrophoresis on cellulose acetate gel using a TEB/urea buffer at pH 8.5 and pH 6.0–6.2.

ALKALINE GLOBIN CHAIN ELECTROPHORESIS

Reagents

1. Tris-EDTA-borate (TEB) buffer, pH 8.9, Ponceau S stain and 5 g/dl acetic acid, as described on pp. 232 and 236.
2. Urea.
3. DL-dithiothreitol (DL-DTT).

Method

1. Prepare fresh working buffer by dissolving 108 g of urea in 210 ml of TEB buffer. This should be sufficient for filling the tank and for soaking the cellulose acetate strip.
2. Mix 0.5 ml of haemolysate, 0.5 ml of working buffer and 0.5 ml of DL-DTT in a small test tube. Allow to stand at room temperature (c 20°C) for 30 min.
3. Add 2 ml of DL-DTT to the remainder of the working buffer and mix thoroughly. Soak the cellulose acetate strips in the buffer for 20 min, immersing the membranes slowly so as to avoid air bubbles.
4. Fill the compartments of the electrophoresis tank with buffer, blot the membranes and apply the previously prepared samples to the centre of the strip. Touching the applicator tips on a piece of card will remove an excess of the sample and ensure the light application necessary for good resolution.
5. Mark the cathode end of the strip and place in the tank ensuring that the ends are immersed in buffer. Apply 150 V for 90 min. Switch off the power, remove from the tank and stain with Ponceau S for at least 30 min. Rinse with 50 g/l acetic acid until clear and allow to dry in the air.

ACID GLOBIN CHAIN ELECTROPHORESIS

Procedure

Working buffer is prepared as described above, but the pH is adjusted to 6.0–6.2 with 300 g/l citric acid. The procedure then follows that detailed for alkaline globin chain electrophoresis except that the acid buffer replaces the alkaline buffer.

Preparation of globin

Although satisfactory results may be obtained by the method already described, the prior preparation of globin still has its advocates. The method described below is recommended.

Add 500 µl of whole haemolysate (40 g/l) to 10 ml of acid/acetone mixture (acetone 98 volumes, concentrated HCl 2 volumes) kept at – 20°C. The globin will immediately form a white precipitate leaving the haem in solution. Centrifuge at about 100 g for 5 min at – 20°C. Remove the supernatant and wash twice with acetone at – 20°C. Then wash once with ether at – 20°C, remove the ether and allow the precipitate to dry at room temperature (c 20°C). The whole procedure must be performed in a well-ventilated environment. Dissolve 10 mg of globin in 0.5 ml of a solution prepared by dissolving 12.0 g of urea in water, adding 0.5 ml of DL-DTT and diluting with water to 15 ml.

SEPARATION IN CELLOGEL*

Globin chain separation can be carried out at acid and alkaline pH, and the differences in mobility under these conditions can give a good indication of the identity of a variant haemoglobin.

Alkaline Buffer

Barbitone buffer, pH 8.6. Sodium diethyl barbiturate 51.5 g; barbitone (diethyl barbituric acid) 9.2 g; thiomersal (preservative) 0.5 g; water to 5 litres.

For use, add 240 g of urea to 400 ml of buffer and dilute with an equal volume of water.

Acid buffer

Tris-EDTA borate-citrate, pH 6.0. Tris 10.2g; EDTA 0.6 g; borate 3.2 g; water to 1 litre.

For use, add 240 g of urea to 400 ml of buffer and adjust to pH 6.0 with saturated citric acid.

Dissolve 10 mg of globin, prepared as above, in 0.5 ml of a 2-mercaptoethanol in urea solution, prepared by dissolving 12.0 g of urea in water, adding 0.5 ml of 2-mercaptoethanol, then diluting to 15 ml with water.

Alternatively, the following quick method may be used for the preparation of the globin sample. The method appears to present no disadvantages.

---

*Whatman

Mix 20 µl of haemolysate, 20 µl of the urea buffer and 20 µl of 2-mercaptoethanol in a small glass tube. Allow to stand for 2 h at 4°C. (This mixture is stable up to 4 h.)

At the same time, soak the Cellogel strip in urea buffer and place with the penetrable surface, as indicated by the manufacturer, uppermost on to the bridges. Secure the soaked filter paper strips. Apply the sample across the strip in a thin line with a pen nib about 2 cm from the anode. Control samples should be set up with each test sample. Apply a constant voltage (200 V) across the strip. Separation of globin chains will be complete within 1½–2 h.

It should be noted that when the quick sample preparation method is used, the coloured haem component of the mixture will migrate rapidly along the strip into the anode buffer, within about 15 min. The globin component is colourless.

Stain the strip with Ponceau S and remove the excess stain by immersion in 7% (v/v) acetic acid for 10 min, with two changes of the acetic acid. Then immerse the Cellogel strip in absolute methanol for 1 min, and subsequently in a clearing solution (87 ml of methanol, 12 ml of glacial acetic acid, 1 ml of glycerol) for 2 min. Place the strip on a glass plate and warm at 50–60°C on a hot plate until the strip is dry and translucent. It can then be peeled off the glass and stored at room temperature.

SEPARATION OF GLOBIN CHAINS ON STARCH GEL[8]

Barbitone buffer.

Dissolve 18.4 g of diethyl barbituric acid in 500 ml of boiling water; add 60 ml of 1 mol/l NaOH and make up the volume to 1 litre with water. Adjust the pH to 8.0 with 1 mol/l NaOH.

Method

Prepare gels by adding about 100 g of starch to 300 ml of barbitone buffer containing 180 g of urea. Warm the mixture at 70°C for 5–10 min, constantly shaking, and then pour into the gel mould, as described on p. 245.

Dissolve 1–3 mg of globin in 0.1 ml of urea-barbitone buffer containing 2-mercaptoethanol

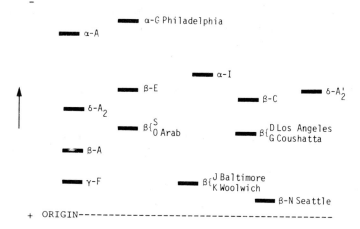

Fig. 15.7 Relative mobilities of some abnormal globin chains. TEB-urea-citrate buffer, pH 6.0.

(50 µl/5 ml of buffer). Then centrifuge the solution and apply the supernatant to the gel. Fill the buffer chambers with urea-barbitone buffer (containing 2-mercaptoethanol). Carry out electrophoresis at 4°C for 22 h at 33–45 mA and 250 V. Finally, stain the gels with amido black, in the usual way (see p. 246).

Interpretation and comments

The direction of migration of the globin chains in globin separation is from the anode to the cathode, whilst in electrophoresis at an alkaline pH on cellulose acetate whole haemoglobins migrate from the cathode to the anode. If the mobility of a whole haemoglobin is known on electrophoresis at pH 8.6, then abnormal α and β chains can be differen-

tiated. If an abnormal haemoglobin moves *faster* than Hb A on electrophoresis at an alkaline pH, the abnormal chain will migrate on globin separation more slowly than its normal counterpart. The α chains move faster than the β chains and migrate nearer to the cathode. Thus, a haemoglobin which migrates rapidly on electrophoresis at an alkaline pH due to an abnormal α chain will produce a *slow-moving* band of α chains on globin separation, which will migrate between the normal α and β chains. Under the same circumstances, a *fast-moving* haemoglobin due to an abnormal β chain will produce a *slow-moving* band of β chains migrating behind the normal β chain.

The relative mobilities of various α chain and β chain mutant globins are shown in Figs. 15.7 and 15.8.

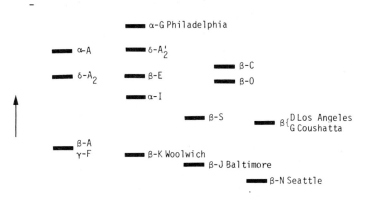

Fig. 15.8 Relative mobilities of some abnormal globin chains. Urea-barbitone buffer, pH 8.6.

DIAGNOSIS OF AN UNSTABLE HAEMOGLOBIN HAEMOLYTIC ANAEMIA (UHbHA): LABORATORY DEMONSTRATION OF HAEMOGLOBIN INSTABILITY

Although uncommon, the UHbHAs constitute a large group of hereditary haemolytic anaemias. 'Apparent (congenital) idiopathic Heinz-body anaemia' had been recognized in the early 1950s,[7] but it was not until the early 1960s that it was realized that the pathological basis of the haemolysis was the spontaneous breakdown (instability) of the haemoglobin molecule.[20,21] Since then a very large number of unstable haemoglobin variants have been recognized. Some of these variants (e.g. Hb Hammersmith) are very unstable; others far less so, and the associated haemolytic anaemias likewise vary in intensity from severe to mild and easily compensated for (see below).

The clinical and laboratory features of the UHbHAs were reviewed by White and Dacie[57] and more recently and extensively by Dacie.[11] Carrell[3] reviewed the ways in which haemoglobin instability may be demonstrated in the laboratory. He pointed out that these mutations may cause such diverse clinical findings as polycythaemia, haemolytic anaemia, cyanosis, microcytic anaemia and pseudo-thalassaemia and stressed that the cause of such clinical conditions may remain undiagnosed unless a patient's haemoglobin is tested for its stability as well as by electrophoresis. Approximately one-third of cases have been found to be due to de-novo mutations.[51]

Many of the unstable variants have an altered oxygen affinity, either increased or decreased. The combination of instability and increased oxygen affinity may result in a situation in which a near normal haemoglobin level may actually mask the existence of increased haemolysis (e.g. with Hb Köln). In contrast, the combination of instability and decreased oxygen affinity may produce a situation in which a low haemoglobin is able to provide an adequate oxygen delivery to the tissues (e.g. with Hb Hammersmith), the patient being quite severely anaemic but almost free from symptoms of anaemia.

The severity of a patient's increased haemolysis appears to be directly proportional to the instability of the variant haemoglobin, and with extremely unstable mutants intramedullary haemolysis may occur with the bone marrow exhibiting marked dyserythropoietic features. The majority of variants, however, cause only moderate or slightly increased haemolysis. Often, however, there are intermittent exacerbations: sometimes these have been associated with the use of oxidant drugs such as a sulphonamide; more frequently, however, they are caused by infections, especially viral, resulting in pyrexia and subsequent increased precipitation of haemoglobin, probably as the result of a rise in body temperature. Such a situation is often first encountered in infancy, and as the majority of the causal amino-acid substitutions are in the β chain of haemoglobin the disease often first becomes apparent at around 4–6 months. If due to an α chain substitution, increased haemolysis may be noticeable at birth. Rare variants are known, too, in which the γ chain has been affected.

The UHbHAs may be confused diagnostically with thalassaemia: β-chain variant UHbHAs may have raised Hb A_2 levels and Heinz-body inclusions may be confused with those of Hb H disease.

The discovery that some genetically-determined haemoglobin variants are unstable corresponded in time to a period when much basic research was being undertaken into the molecular structure of the haemoglobin molecule; it focused attention particularly on the forces which normally hold the haemoglobin monomers together, and bind a molecule of haem to each globin monomer, and the ways in which amino-acid substitutions or deletions may weaken these forces and lead to the break-up of the molecule's tetramer.

Normal globin is soluble because in aqueous solution it takes up a configuration that allows its hydrophilic side chains to interact with water while its hydrophobic side chains are closely packed internally with exclusion of water. This stable configuration is maintained by weak van der Waals bonds between the hydrophobic residues both in the interior of the globin monomer and also in the subunit interface that binds the αβ diamer. The stability of normal haemoglobin is further strengthened by the side chains of the hydrophobic amino-acids which line the haem pocket on the surface of the globin and form van der Waals bonds with the haem. Unstable haemoglobins result from abnormalities at these sites, and if the instability is sufficient to cause a break-up of the haemoglobin molecule in-vivo haemolytic anaemia may result. Over one-third of identified unstable haemoglobins result from mutations in the vicinity of the haem pocket. Any factor that tends to weaken the van der Waals bonds, especially those of the haem pocket, will result in oxidation of haemoglobin with methaemoglobin formation. This is followed by the production of haemichromes, a break-up of the haemoglobin molecule and Heinz-body formation and premature removal of the red cell from the circulation, particularly during splenic transit.

DIAGNOSIS OF AN UNSTABLE HAEMOGLOBIN HAEMOLYTIC ANAEMIA

A firm diagnosis of an UHbHA depends upon demonstrating in the laboratory that the patient's haemoglobin is abnormally unstable. There are several ways of testing for stability (see below). First, however, the clinical picture provided by the patient may provide clues, e.g. the presence of cyanosis due to methaemoglobinaemia, as well as anaemia and jaundice, and the passage of dark brown to almost black urine (dipyrroluria). The dark discolouration is due to the presence of dipyrrylmethenes (mesobilifuscins), derived from haem molecules partly broken down after separation from globin. Careful inspection of blood films may also suggest the diagnosis of an UHbHA (Figs. 8.35–8.36), especially if splenectomy has been carried out (Fig. 8.58), while the presence of many Heinz bodies in the blood of a haemolytic anaemia patient after splenectomy (Fig. 9.3) makes the presence of an unstable haemoglobin almost certain.

Autohaemolysis

In a patient whose spleen has not been removed, an autohaemolysis test may provide an important pointer to the presence of an UHbHA. If an unstable haemoglobin is present, the serum may appear brown or opaque after incubation for 48 h. This is due to the presence of methaemoglobin (Hi) and Heinz bodies, and numerous Heinz bodies will be seen if the incubated red cells are stained with methyl violet. Normal cells do not form Heinz bodies under these conditions.

Starch-gel electrophoresis at pH 8.6

Electrophoresis often fails to demonstrate the presence of an unstable haemoglobin. However, with some unstable haemoglobins haem-depleted components may be seen which migrate in the position of Hb S or just in front of Hb A_2; and, in addition, free α chains that have migrated towards the cathode may be visible.

DEMONSTRATION OF HAEMOGLOBIN INSTABILITY

Several methods are available for the demonstration of a haemoglobin's instability, e.g. sensitivity to heat[20,21] and precipitation by isopropanol[4] or zinc acetate.[6] The heat and isopropanol tests are described below.

HEAT INSTABILITY TEST

Principle. When haemoglobin in solution is heated the hydrophobic van der Waals bonds are weakened and the stability of the molecule is decreased. Under suitable controlled conditions unstable haemoglobins precipitate while normal haemoglobin remains in solution.[5,20,21]

Reagent

Tris HCl buffer, pH 7.4, 50 mmol/l. Tris-(hydroxymethyl-aminomethane) 6.05 g; water to 1 litre; concentrated HCl to adjust the pH to 7.4.

Method

1. Add 0.2 ml of haemolysate, freshly prepared by the water/carbon tetrachloride method, to a test-tube containing 1.8 ml of 0.05 mol/l tris HCl buffer, pH 7.4.

2. Place the tube in a 50°C water-bath together with a normal control haemolysate of the same age as the test sample and a haemolysate of a haemoglobin known to be unstable, if one is available. Keep the tubes at 50°C for 60–120 min and examine them periodically for turbidity and fine flocculation.

If a precipitate is present, to estimate the percentage of haemoglobin that has been precipitated, centrifuge the suspension and then add 1 volume of the supernatant to 20 volumes of cyanide-ferricyanide reagent (p. 241). Treat the original (unheated) haemolysate in the same way and read their absorbence at 280 nm.

Calculation:

% unstable Hb

$$= \frac{A^{280} \text{ of unheated sample} - A^{280} \text{ of heated sample}}{A^{280} \text{ of unheated sample}}$$
$$\times 100.$$

Interpretation and comments

The normal control haemolysate may give minimal cloudiness at 60 min but a major unstable haemoglobin will have undergone marked precipitation at 60 min and gross flocculent precipitation at 120 min.

ISOPROPANOL PRECIPITATION TEST[4]

Principle When haemoglobin is dissolved in a solvent such as isopropanol which is more nonpolar than water, the van der Waals bonds are weakened and the stability of the molecule is decreased. This results in precipitation of unstable haemoglobins while normal haemoglobin remains in solution.

Reagents

(i) Tris HCl buffer, pH 7.4, 100 mmol/l. Tris-(hydroxymethyl-aminomethane) 12.11 g; water to 1 litre; add concentrated HCl to adjust the pH to 7.4.

(ii) 100% isopropanol. 17 volumes of isopropanol are made up to 100 volumes with the tris HCl buffer. The resultant 17% isopropanol solution may be stored for several months at 4°C in a stoppered glass bottle.

Method

1. Blood samples for preparation of haemolysates may be stored at 4°C for up to 1 week. On the day of the test prepare the haemolysates by the water/carbon tetrachloride method described on p. 231 and adjust the haemoglobin concentration to c 100 g/l. KCN should not be added.

2. A normal blood sample of approximately the same age as the test specimen should be used as a negative control. If available, a haemoglobin known to be unstable should be used as a positive control. Alternatively, a haemolysate of cord blood containing a high percentage of Hb F can be used.

3. Add 0.2 ml of the test haemolysate and of normal and positive controls, respectively, to 2 ml volumes of buffered isopropanol in stoppered tubes. Mix by inverting each tube and place in a 37°C water-bath. Examine the tubes at 5, 20 and 30 min.

Interpretation and comments

The normal control haemolysate will remain clear at 20 min. At 30 min slight cloudiness should be apparent but significant precipitation will not occur until 40 min. A clinically significant unstable haemoglobin will undergo precipitation at 5 min and gross flocculent precipitation will have developed by 20 min. A slightly unstable haemoglobin such as Hb E will undergo diffuse precipitation at 20 min. Cloudiness may develop at 30 min if Hb F is present at levels greater than 5%.

'False positive' results may be given by samples containing large amounts of Hb F or by samples containing increased methaemoglobin as a result of prolonged storage or by haemolysates that have not been freshly prepared. If the normal sample undergoes premature precipitation the temperature of the water-bath is likely to have been higher than 37°C. 'False negative' results should be avoided by continuing the incubation until the normal control undergoes precipitation.

DETECTION OF HAEMOGLOBIN M

Methaemoglobin has iron present in the ferric form. Genetically determined variants of haemoglobin, which undergo oxidation to methaemoglobin more readily than does normal Hb A, are referred to as Hb Ms. They are the cause of one variety of a rather rare condition—congenital methaemoglobinaemia. Clinically, their presence is associated with cyanosis and in some cases with mild haemolytic anaemia. Methaemoglobin levels vary but may be as high as 40% of the total haemoglobin. The variants have been found in all ethnic groups, with the Japanese being perhaps most frequently affected.

Methaemoglobin variants can be detected electrophoretically but almost all can be distinguished from methaemoglobin A (Hi A) by their absorption spectra.

SPECTROPHOTOMETRIC DETECTION OF HAEMOGLOBIN M

Each methaemoglobin has its own distinct absorption spectrum. Methaemoglobin A (Hi A) has two absorption peaks at 502 nm and 632 nm while the peaks for the variant Hb M methaemoglobins are shifted to slightly shorter wavelengths (Fig. 15.9).

Preparation of methaemoglobin A

Lyse washed red cells with water to give a concentration of about 1 g haemoglobin per litre. Then convert the haemoglobin to Hi by the addition of 5 μl of 0.1 mol/l potassium ferricyanide per ml of lysate. Leave for 10 min at room temperature (c 20°C). Then record the spectrum of Hi A on an automatic scanning spectrophotometer.

Next, scan the spectrum of a water lysate of the suspected Hb M. If a Hb M is present, the spectrum will reflect the admixture of Hb A with the Hb M. If the spectrophotometer is set to a fixed wavelength of 630 nm, then conversion of Hi to HiCN can be followed by the addition of 50 μl of 1 mol/l KCN per ml of lysate.

ELECTROPHORETIC SEPARATION OF Hb Ms

If a Hb M is suspected, prepare a lysate at a concentration of 20 g/l haemoglobin without KCN,

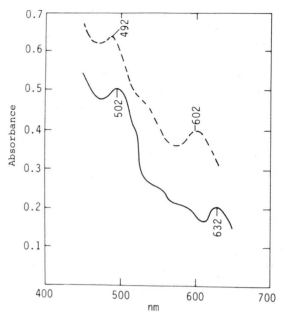

Fig. 15.9 Absorption maxima of methaemoglobins in the range 450–650 nm.
—Normal methaemoglobin; ---- Hb M Saskatoon (Reproduced with permission from Lehmann, H. and Huntsman, R. G. (1974). *Man's Haemoglobins*, 2nd edn, p. 214. North-Holland Publishing Company, Amsterdam).

thus avoiding any conversion to HiCN. Compare the sample against Hb A and Hi A. Some Hb Ms can be separated on alkaline electrophoresis, on which Hi A runs slightly cathodally to Hb A. Clearer results can be obtained by starch gel electrophoresis in phosphate buffer at pH 7.1. Prepare Hi A by adding 1 volume of 50 g/l potassium ferricyanide to 9 volumes of haemolysate at a concentration of 20 g/l, and allow to stand at room temperature (c 20°C) for 10 min.

Buffers

Stock buffer, pH 7.1. Disodium hydrogen phosphate (Na_2HPO_4) 13.3 g; potassium dihydrogen phosphate (KH_2PO_4) 2.15 g; water to 2 litres.

Working buffer. Stock buffer 60 ml; water to 300 ml.

Method

Starch should be mixed with the working buffer and the gel prepared as described on p. 245. Fill the electrode compartments of the system with undiluted stock buffer and then carry out electrophoresis.

In addition to the test and control methaemoglobin samples, additional controls comprising a normal oxyhaemoglobin sample and the test sample (without the addition of potassium ferricyanide) should be set up. Methaemoglobins migrate more slowly than does oxyhaemoglobin and Hb M variants more slowly than Hi A.

ALTERED AFFINITY HAEMOGLOBINS

Electrophoresis techniques may or may not be helpful, depending on whether the amino-acid substitution has involved a charge change.

The most important investigation is the measurement of the oxygen dissociation curve (p. 219). The most significant finding is a decreased Hill's constant ('n' value), since this can only come about by a change in the structure of haemoglobin. The p_{50} may be either increased or decreased. It has to be borne in mind that the p_{50} alone may be modified by other factors, e.g. by the high concentration of 2,3 DPG in pyruvate kinase deficiency.

SUGGESTED USE OF ELECTROPHORETIC TECHNIQUES IN THE ANALYSIS OF HAEMOGLOBINS

1. Routine analysis

Cellulose acetate: tris buffer, pH 8.5.

2. Demonstration and estimation of Hb A$_2$

a. Cellulose acetate: tris buffer, pH 8.9.
b. Microcolumn chromatography.

3. Demonstration and estimation of Hb Bart's and Hb H

Cellulose acetate or starch block, phosphate buffer, pH 6.5.

4. Separation of Hb S from Hb C

Starch block: barbitone buffer, pH 8.9.

5. Separation of Hb S from Hb D and Hb G

Agar: citrate buffer, pH 6.0.

6. Separation of Hb C from Hb E and Hb O

a. Agar: citrate buffer, pH 6.0.
b. Isopropanol stability test.

7. Separation of Hb I from Hb H

Cellulose acetate: phosphate buffer, pH 7.0.

8. Detection of Hb M

Starch gel: phosphate buffer, pH 7.1.

9. Identification of variant chains

Globin-chain separation at pH 8.6 and pH 6.0.

The relative mobilities of some abnormal haemoglobins by various methods are shown in Fig. 15.10.

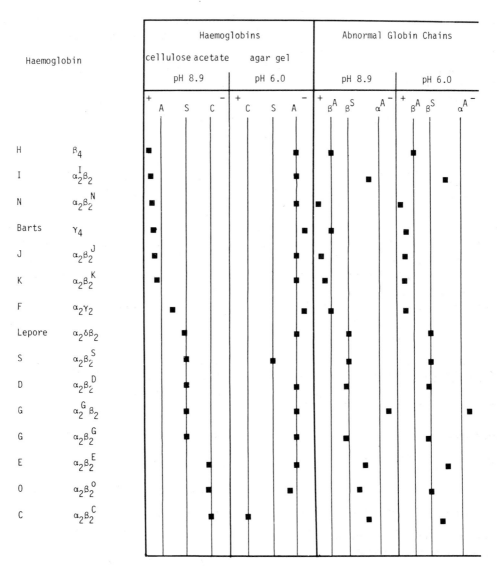

Fig. 15.10 Comparison of relative mobilities of some abnormal haemoglobins by different methods. The positions of Hb A, Hb S and Hb C and their corresponding chains are indicated by the vertical lines (adapted from ICSH[27]).

REFERENCES

[1] BASSET, P., BEUZARD, Y., GAREL, M. C. and ROSA, J. (1978). Isoelectric focusing of human hemoglobins: its application to screening, to characterization of 70 variants and to study of modified fractions of normal hemoglobins. *Blood*, **51**, 971.

[2] BETKE, K., MARTI, H. R. and SCHLICT, L. (1959). Estimation of small percentages of foetal haemoglobin. *Nature* (London), **184**, 1877.

[3] CARRELL, R. W. (1986). The hemoglobinopathies: methods of determining hemoglobin instability (unstable hemoglobins). *Methods in Hematology*, **15**, 109.

[4] CARRELL, R. W. and KAY, R. (1972). A simple method for the detection of unstable haemoglobins. *British Journal of Haematology*, **23**, 615.

[5] CARRELL, R. W. and LEHMANN, H. (1969). The unstable hemoglobin hemolytic anemias. *Seminars in Hematology*, **6**, 116.

[6] CARRELL, R. W. and LEHMANN, H. (1981). Zinc acetate as a precipitant of unstable haemoglobins. *Journal of Clinical Pathology*, **34**, 796.

[7] CATHIE, I. A. B. (1952). Apparent idiopathic Heinz body anaemia. *Great Ormond Street Journal*, No. 3, 43.

[8] CHERNOFF, A. I. and PETTIT, N. M. (1964). The amino acid composition of hemoglobin III. A qualitative method for identifying abnormalities of the polypeptide chains of hemoglobin. *Blood*, **24**, 750.

[9] CHUDWIN, D. S. and RUCKNAGEL, D. L. (1974).

Immunological quantification of hemoglobins F and A[2].
Clinica Chimica Acta, **50**, 413.

[10] CONLEY, C. L., WEATHERALL, D. J., RICHARDSON, S. N., SHEPARD, M. K. and CHARACHE, S. (1963). Hereditary persistence of fetal hemoglobin: a study of 79 affected persons in 15 Negro families in Baltimore. *Blood*, **21**, 241.

[11] DACIE, J. V. (1988). *The Haemolytic Anaemias, 3rd edn., Vol. 2: The Hereditary Haemolytic Anaemias*, Part 2, p. 322. Churchill Livingstone, Edinburgh.

[12] EFREMOV, G. D. (1986). The hemoglobinopathies: quantitation of hemoglobins by microchromatography. *Methods in Hematology*, **15**, 72.

[13] EFREMOV, G. D., HUISMAN, T. H. J., BOWMAN, K., WRIGHTSTONE, R. and SCHROEDER, W. A. (1974). Microchromatography of hemoglobins: II A rapid method for the determination of Hb A[2]. *Journal of Laboratory and Clinical Medicine*, **83**, 657.

[14] EMBURY, S. H., DOZY, A. M., MILLER, J. et al (1982). Concurrent sickle-cell anemia and thalassemia: effect on severity of anemia. *New England Journal of Medicine*, **306**, 270.

[15] FAIRBANKS, V. F. (1980). *Hemoglobinopathies and Thalassemias. Laboratory methods and case studies.* B.C. Decker, New York.

[16] FELICE, A. E. (1986). The hemoglobinopathies: quantitation of fetal hemoglobin. *Methods in Hematology*, **15**, 91.

[17] FESSAS, P. (1963). Inclusions of hemoglobin in erythroblasts and erythrocytes of thalassemia. *Blood*, **21**, 21.

[18] GAMMACK, D. B., HUEHNS, E. R., LEHMANN, H. and SHOOTER, E. M. (1961). The abnormal polypeptide chains in a number of haemoglobin variants. *Acta Genetica et Statistica Medica*, **11**, 1.

[19] GARVER, F. A., JONES, C. S., BAKER, M. M. et al (1976). Specific radioimmunochemical identification and quantitation of hemoglobins A[2] and F. *American Journal of Hematology*, **1**, 459.

[20] GRIMES, A. J. and MEISLER, A. (1962). Possible cause of Heinz bodies in congenital Heinz body anaemia. *Nature* (London), **194**, 190.

[21] GRIMES, A. J., MEISLER, A. and DACIE, J. V. (1964). Congenital Heinz-body anaemia: further evidence on the cause of Heinz-body production in red cells. *British Journal of Haematology*, **10**, 281.

[22] HIGGS, D. R., ALDRIDGE, B. E., LAMB, J. et al (1982). The interaction of alpha-thalassemia and homozygous sickle-cell disease. *New England Journal of Medicine*, **306**, 1441.

[23] HUISMAN, T. H. J. and JONXIS, J. H. P. (1977). The hemoglobinopathies: techniques of identification. *Clinical and Biochemical Analysis*, **6**, Dekker, New York.

[24] HUISMAN, T. H. J., SCHROEDER, W. A., BRODIE, A. R., MAYSON, S. M. and JAKURAY, J. (1975). Microchromatography of hemoglobins III. A simplified procedure for the determination of hemoglobin A[2]. *Journal of Laboratory and Clinical Medicine*, **86**, 700.

[25] HUNTSMAN, R. G., BARCLAY, G. P. T., CANNING, D. M. and YAWSON, G. I. (1970). A rapid whole blood solubility test to differentiate the sickle cell trait from sickle-cell anaemia. *Journal of Clinical Pathology*, **23**, 781.

[26] INGRAM, V. M. (1959). Abnormal human hemoglobins III. The chemical difference between normal and sickle cell hemoglobins. *Biochimica et Biophysica Acta*, **36**, 402.

[27] International Committee for Standardization in Hematology (1978). Simple electrophoretic system for presumptive identification of abnormal hemoglobins. *Blood*, **52**, 1058.

[28] Internatioanl Committee for Standardization in Hematology (1978). Recommendations of a system for identifying abnormal hemoglobins. *Blood*, **52**, 1065.

[29] ITANO, H. A. and PAULING, L. (1949). A rapid diagnostic test for sickle cell anemia. *Blood*, **4**, 66.

[30] JONXIS, J. H. P. and VISSER, H. K. A. (1956). Determination of low percentages of fetal hemoglobin in blood of normal children. *American Journal of Diseases of Children*, **92**, 588.

[31] JOSEPHSON, A. M., MASRI, M. S., SINGER, L., DWORKIN, D. and SINGER, K. (1958). Starch block electrophoretic studies on human hemoglobin solutions II. Results in cord blood, thalassemia and other hematologic disorders: comparison with Tiselius electrophoresis. *Blood*, **13**, 543.

[32] KLEIHAUER, E. (1974). Determination of fetal hemoglobin: elution technique. In *The Detection of Hemoglobinopathies*. Eds. Schmidt, R. M., Huisman, T. H. J. and Lehmann, H., p. 20. CRC Press, Cleveland, Ohio.

[33] KUNKEL, H. G., CEPPELLINI, R., MÜLLER-EBERHARD, U. and WOLF, J. (1957). Observations on the minor basic hemoglobin component in the blood of normal individuals and patients with thalassemia. *Journal of Clinical Investigation*, **36**, 1615.

[34] MAKLER, M. T. and PESCE, A. J. (1980). ELISA assay for measurement of human hemoglobin A and hemoglobin F. *American Journal of Clinical Pathology*, **74**, 673.

[35] MARDER, V. J. and CONLEY, C. L. (1959). Electrophoresis of hemoglobin on agar gels. Frequency of hemoglobin D in a Negro population. *Bulletin of the Johns Hopkins Hospital*, **105**, 77.

[36] MARENGO-ROWE, A. J. (1965). Rapid electrophoresis and quantitation of haemoglobins on cellulose acetate. *Journal of Clinical Pathology*, **18**, 790.

[37] MARINUCCI, M., MAVILIO, F., MASSA, A. et al (1979). Haemoglobin Lepore trait: haematological and structural studies in the Italian population. *British Journal of Haematology*, **42**, 557.

[38] NALBUNDIAN, R. M., NICHOLS, B. M., CAMP, F. R., LUSHER, J. M., CONTE, N. F. and HENRY, R. T. (1971). Dithionite tube test—a rapid inexpensive technique for the detection of hemoglobin S and non S sickling hemoglobin. *Clinical Chemistry*, **17**, 1028.

[39] NEDA, S. and SCHNEIDER, R. G. (1969). Rapid identification of polypeptide chains of hemoglobin by cellulose acetate electrophoresis of hemolysates. *Blood*, **34**, 230.

[40] OLD, J. M. and HIGGS, D. R. (1983). The thalassemias: gene analysis. *Methods in Hematology*, **6**, 74.

[41] PEMBREY, M. E., PERRINE, R. P., WOOD, W. G. and WEATHERALL, D. J. (1980). Sickle cell β° thalassemia in Eastern Saudi Arabia. *American Journal of Human Genetics*, **32**, 41.

[42] RIGHETTI, P. G., GIANAZZA, E., BIANCHI-BOSISIO, A. and COSSU, G. (1986). The hemoglobinopathies: conventional isoelectric focussing and immobilized pH gradients for hemoglobin separation and identification. *Methods in Hematology*, **15**, 47.

[43] SCHMIDT, R. M., RUCKNAGEL, D. L. and NECHELES, T. F. (1975). Comparison of methodologies for thalassemia screening by Hb A[2] qua ntitation. *Journal of Laboratory and Clinical Medicine*, **86**, 873.

[44] SCHNEIDER, R. G. (1974). Identification of hemoglobin by electrophoresis. In: *The Detection of Hemoglobinopathies*. Eds. Schmidt, R.M., Huisman, T. H. J. and LEHMANN, H., p. 11. CRC Press, Cleveland, Ohio.

[45] SCHNEIDER, R. G. (1974). Differentiation of electrophoretically similar hemoglobins—such as S, D, G and P or A_2, C, E and O—by electrophoresis of the globin chains. *Clinical Chemistry*, **20**, 1111.

[46] SCHROEDER, W. A. (1986). The hemoglobinopathies: HPLC of globin chains and of peptides in the identification of hemoglobin variants. *Methods in Hematology*, **15**, 143.

[47] SCHROEDER, W. A. and HUISMAN, T. H. J. (1980). The chromatography of hemoglobin. *Clinical and Biochemical Analysis*, **9**, M. Dekker, New York.

[48] SCHROEDER, W. A., SKELTON, J. B. and SKELTON, J. R. (1980). Separation of hemoglobin peptides by high performance liquid chromatography (HPLC). *Hemoglobin*, **4**, 551.

[49] SCHROEDER, W. A., SKELTON, J. B., SKELTON, J. R. and POWANS, D. (1979). Separation of peptides by high pressure liquid chromatography for the identification of a hemoglobin variant. *Journal of Chromatography*, **174**, 385.

[50] SILVESTRONI, E., BIANCO, I., GRAZIANI, B. and CARBONI, C. (1978). Heterozygous β-thalassaemia with normal haemoglobin pattern. *Acta Haematologica* (Basel), **59**, 332.

[51] STAMATOYANNOPOULOS, G. and NUTE, P. E. (1984). Cases of unstable hemoglobin and methemoglobin produced by de novo mutation. *Hemoglobin*, **8**, 85.

[52] WALFORD, D. M. and DEACON, R. (1976). Alpha-thalassaemia trait in various racial groups in the United Kingdom. Characterization of a variant of alpha-thalassaemia in Indians. *British Journal of Haematology*, **34**, 193.

[53] WASI, P., Na-NAKORN, S., POOTRAKUL, S. et al (1969). Alpha- and beta-thalassemia in Thailand. *Annals of New York Academy of Sciences*, **165**, 60.

[54] WEATHERALL, D. J. (1983). The thalassemias: hematologic methods. *Methods in Hematology*, **6**, 27.

[55] WEATHERALL, D. J. and CLEGG, J. B. (1981). *The Thalassemia Syndromes*, 3rd edn. Blackwell Scientific Publications, Oxford.

[56] WHITE, J. M. (1974). The unstable haemoglobin disorders. *Clinics in Haematology*, **3**, 333.

[57] WHITE, J. M. and DACIE, J. V. (1971). The unstable haemoglobins—molecular and clinical features. *Progress in Hematology*, **7**, 69.

[58] WOOD, W. G. (1983). The thalassemias: hemoglobin analysis. *Methods in Hematology*, **6**, 31.

[59] WOOD, W. G., STAMATOYANNOPOULOS, G., LIM, G. and NUTE, P. E. (1975). F cells in the adult: normal values and levels in individuals with hereditary and acquired elevations of Hb F. *Blood*, **46**, 671.

[60] WRIGHTSTONE, R. N. (1986). The Hemoglobinopathies: Abnormal properties of hemoglobin variants: a summary. *Methods in Hematology*, **15**, 160.

[61] WRIGHTSTONE, R. N. and HUISMAN, T. H. J. (1974). On the levels of Hb F and A_2 in sickle cell anemia and some related disorders. *American Journal of Clinical Pathology*, **61**, 375.

[62] ZAGO, M. A., WOOD, W. G., CLEGG, J. B., WEATHERALL, D. J., O'SULLIVAN, M. and GUNSON, H. (1979). Genetic control of F-cells in human adults. *Blood*, **53**, 977.

[63] LEHMANN, H. and CARRELL, R. W. (1984). Nomenclature of the α-thalassaemias. *Lancet*, **i**, 552.

[64] WHO Working Group (1982). Hereditary anaemias: genetic basis, clinical features, diagnosis, and treatment. *Bulletin of the World Health Organization*, **60**, 643.

16. Laboratory methods used in the investigation of paroxysmal nocturnal haemoglobinuria (PNH)

Paroxysmal nocturnal haemoglobinuria is an acquired disorder in which the patient's red cells are abnormally sensitive to lysis by normal constituents of plasma. In its classical form it is characterized by haemoglobinuria during sleep (nocturnal haemoglobinuria), jaundice and haemosiderinuria. Not uncommonly, however, PNH presents as an obscure anaemia without obvious evidence of intravascular haemolysis or develops in a patient suffering apparently from aplastic anaemia or more rarely from myelosclerosis or leukaemia.[11,17,45]

PNH red cells are unusually susceptible to lysis by complement.[16,40] This can be demonstrated in vitro by a variety of tests, e.g. the acidified-serum (Ham),[16,21] sucrose,[19,21] thrombin,[9] cold-antibody lysis,[12] inulin[5] and cobra-venom[22] tests. In the acidified-serum, inulin and cobra-venom tests complement is activated via the alternative (Pillemer) pathway, while in the cold-antibody test, and probably in the thrombin test, complement is activated by the classical sequence initiated through antigen-antibody interaction. In the sucrose lysis test a low ionic strength is thought to lead to the binding of IgG molecules non-specifically to the cell membrane and to the subsequent activation of complement via the classical sequence. In addition, the alternative pathway appears to be activated.[26] In each test PNH cells undergo lysis because of their greatly increased sensitivity to lysis by complement.

Minor degrees of increased lysis may be observed in the cold-antibody lysis and sucrose tests with the red cells from a variety of dyserythropoietic anaemias, e.g. aplastic anaemia, megaloblastic anaemia and myelosclerosis.[6,24] Weak positive results in these tests have thus to be interpreted with care. PNH red cells, however, almost always undergo major amounts of lysis in these tests which thus have considerable value as screening procedures. A positive acidified-serum test is probably specific for the PNH red cell abnormality and the cobra-venom test can also be carried out in such a way as to make positive test specific for PNH.[22] A characteristic feature of positive test for PNH is that not all the patient's cells undergo lysis, even if the conditions of the test are made optimal for lysis (Fig. 16.1). This implies that only a proportion of any patient's PNH red cell population is hypersensitive to lysis by complement. This population varies from patient to patient, and there is a direct relationship between the proportion of red cells that can be lysed (in any of the diagnostic tests) and the severity of in-vivo haemolysis.

The phenomenon of some red cells being sensitive to complement lysis and some insensitive was studied quantitatively by Rosse and Dacie who obtained two-component complement sensitivity curves in a series of PNH patients.[40] Later, Rosse and his co-workers reported that in some cases

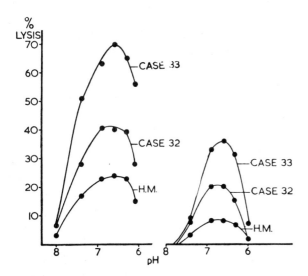

Fig. 16.1 Effect of pH on lysis in vitro of PNH red cells by human sera. The red cells of three patients (Cases 32, 33 and H.M. of different sensitivity) were used, and two fresh normal sera, one serum being more potent than the other.

three populations of red cells could be demonstrated.[36,37,39]

1. Very sensitive (Type-III) cells, 10–15 times as sensitive as normal cells.
2. Cells of medium sensitivity (Type-II), 3–5 times as sensitive as normal cells.
3. Cells of normal sensitivity (Type-I).

In vivo, the proportion of Type-III cells parallels the severity of the patient's illness, and it is these Type-III cells which are lysed in the acidified-serum test. In the sucrose and cold-antibody lysis tests, however, both Type-III and Type-II cells undergo lysis. Both types of cells bind on more complement component C3 than normal, but with Type-III cells there is, in addition, increased sensitivity to the terminal complement components C5b–C9.[32] It is this double mechanism of increased sensitivity which makes Type-III cells so hypersensitive to complement lysis. Further information as to the relative sensitivity of the two types (II and III) of PNH red cells to lysis by complement has more recently become available.[32,35] Rosse and Parker's[41] review of the nature of the PNH abnormality or abnormalities is an admirable summary of a complex situation.

PNH is an acquired clonal disorder of stem cells,[31] and it is possible to demonstrate that granulocytes and platelets, as well as red cells, are hypersensitive to complement lysis in appropriate immune systems.

Another feature of PNH is diminished activity of the red cell enzyme acetylcholinesterase (AChE).[2,7,13,27,48] It seems, however, that the two phenomena—increased sensitivity to lysis by complement and diminished activity of AChE—are not directly connected. It is interesting to note that the red cells in PNH patients that resist lysis by complement have a normal AChE content.[14]

A further important abnormality, more recently discovered[29,30,33,42] is deficiency of the decay accelerating factor (DAF), a protein thought normally to protect red cells (and leucocytes and platelets, too) from damage by complement. In addition, the glycophorin-α in the PNH red cell membrane has been reported to be abnormal.[34] The PNH red cell thus suffers from at least three abnormalities—increased sensitivity to lysis by complement, deficiency in acetylcholinesterase and abnormal glycophorin-α.[38] PNH neutrophils are deficient in alkaline phosphatase.[3,23] Whether all these abnormalities can be explained by a single primary lesion (a somatic mutation[10]) remains to be determined.

Remarkably, it has been found that a variety of chemicals, in particular sulphydryl compounds, can act on normal red cells in vitro so as to increase their complement sensitivity. In this way PNH-like red cells can be created in the laboratory and can be used as useful reagents (p. 264).

ACIDIFIED-SERUM TEST (HAM TEST)

Principle. The patient's red cells are exposed at 37°C to the action of normal or the patient's own serum suitably acidified to the optimum pH for lysis (pH 6.5–7.0) (Fig. 16.1).

The patient's red cells can be obtained from defibrinated, heparinized, oxalated, citrated or EDTA blood, and the test can be satisfactorily carried out even on cells which have been stored at 4°C for up to 2–3 weeks in ACD or Alsever's solution, if kept sterile. The patient's serum is best obtained by defibrination, for if in PNH it is obtained from blood allowed to clot in the ordinary way at 37°C or at room termperature it will almost certainly be found to be markedly lysed. Normal serum should similarly be obtained by defibrination, but serum derived from blood allowed to clot spontaneously at room termperature or at 37°C can be used. Normal serum known to be strongly lytic to PNH red cells is to be preferred to patient's serum, the lytic potentiality of which is unknown. However, if the test is positive using normal serum it is important, particularly if the patient appears not to be suffering from overt intravascular haemolysis, to obtain a positive result using the patient's serum, in order to exclude HEMPAS (see p. 262). The variability between the sera of individuals in their capacity to lyse PNH red cells is shown in Figure 16.1. The activity of a single individual's serum also varies from time to time[32] and it is always important to include in any test, as a positive control, a sample of known PNH cells or artifically created 'PNH-like' cells (see p. 264).

The sera should be fresh, i.e. used within a few hours of collection. Their lytic potency is retained for several months at $-70°C$, but at 4°C, and even at $-20°C$, this deteriorates within a few days.

Method

Deliver 0.5 ml samples of fresh normal serum, group AB or ABO-compatible with the patient's blood, into six (three pairs) of 75×12 mm glass tubes. Place two tubes at 56°C for 10–30 min in order to inactivate complement. Keep the other two pairs of tubes at room temperature and add to the serum in two of the tubes one-tenth volumes (0.05 ml) of 0.2 mol/l HCl. Add similar volumes of acid subsequently to the inactivated serum samples. Then place all the tubes in a 37°C water-bath.

While the serum samples are being dealt with, wash samples of the patient's red cells and of control normal red cells (compatible with the normal serum) twice in 9.0 g/l NaCl and prepare 50% suspensions in the saline. Then add one-tenth volumes of each of these cells suspensions (0.05 ml) to single tubes containing unacidified fresh serum, acidified fresh serum and acidified inactivated serum, respectively (Table 16.1). Mix the contents carefully and leave the tubes at 37°C. Centrifuge them after about 1 h.

Add 0.05 ml of each cell suspension to 0.55 ml of water so as to prepare a standard for subsequent quantitative measurement of lysis and retain 0.5 ml of serum for use as a blank. For the measurement of lysis, deliver 0.3 ml volumes of the supernatants of the test and control series of cell-serum suspensions, and of the blank serum and of the lysed cell suspension equivalent to 100% lysis, respectively, into 5 ml of 0.4 ml/l ammonia or Drabkin's reagent. Measure the lysis in a photoelectric colorimeter using a yellow-green (e.g. Ilford 625) filter or in a spectrophotometer at a wave-length of 540 nm.

If the test cells are from a patient with PNH, they will undergo definite, although, as already mentioned, incomplete lysis in the acidified serum. Very much less lysis, or even no lysis at all, will be visible in the unacidified serum. No lysis will be brought about by the acidified inactivated serum. The normal control sample of cells should not undergo lysis in any of the three tubes.

In PNH 10–50% lysis is usually obtained, when lysis is measured as liberated haemoglobin. Exceptionally, there may be as much as 80% lysis or as little as 5%.

The red cells of a patient who has been transfused will undergo less lysis than before the trans-

Table 16.1 The acidified-serum test

Reagents	Test (ml) 1	2	3	Controls (ml) 4	5	6
Fresh normal serum	0.5	0.5	0	0.5	0.5	0
Heat-inactivated normal serum	0	0	0.5	0	0	0.5
0.2 mol/l HCl	0	0.05	0.05	0	0.05	0.05
50% patient's red cells	0.05	0.05	0.05	0	0	0
50% normal red cells	0	0	0	0.05	0.05	0.05
Lysis (in a positive test)	Trace (2%)	+ + + (30%)	–	–	–	–

fusion, because the normal transfused cells, despite circulation in the patient, behave normally. In PNH, it is characteristic that a young cell (reticulocyte-rich) population, such as the upper red cell layer obtained by centrifugation, undergoes more lysis than the red cells derived from mixed whole blood.

Significance of the acidified-serum test

A positive acidified-serum test, carried out with proper controls, denotes the PNH abnormality (or abnormalities), and unless the test is positive PNH cannot be diagnosed. The only other disorder which at first sight may appear to give a clear-cut positive test is a rare congenital dyserythropoietic anaemia, CDA Type II or HEMPAS.[8,49] In contrast to PNH, however, HEMPAS red cells undergo lysis in only a proportion (about 30%) of normal sera; moreover, they do not undergo lysis in the patient's own acidified serum and the sucrose lysis test is negative. In HEMPAS, lysis appears to be due to the presence on the red cells of an unusual antigen which reacts with a complement-fixing IgM antibody ('anti-HEMPAS') present in many but not in all normal sera.[49]

Heating at 56°C inactivates the lytic system and, if there is lysis in inactivated serum, the test cannot be considered positive. Markedly spherocytic red cells or effete normal red cells may lyse in acidified serum, probably due to the lowered pH, and such cells may lyse, too, in acidified inactivated serum.

It must be stressed that PNH red cells are not unduly sensitive to lysis by a lowered pH per se. The addition of the acid adjusts the pH of the serum-cell mixture to the optimum for the activity of the lytic system. As is shown in Fig. 16.1, it is possible to construct pH-lysis curves, if different concentrations of acid are used. The optimum pH for lysis is between pH 6.5 and 7.0 (measurements made after the addition of the red cells to the serum).

THROMBIN TEST[9]

Crosby observed that PNH red cells undergo more lysis in acidified serum if thrombin is added. He suggested that this reaction might be a useful test for PNH. Much of the effect seems to be due to

anit-human-red-cell antibodies present in varying amounts in commercial preparations of thrombin[4] or to the presence of complement components. In practice, the thrombin test is seldom if ever positive when the simple acidified-serum test is completely negative.

COBRA-VENOM TEST[22]

In this test complement is activated via the alternative pathway by the addition to serum of partially purified cobra venom. In Kabakçi, Rosse and Logue's hands the percentage of lysis of a series of PNH red cell samples was almost identical with the PNH 'sensitive-cell' percentage as determined by the complement lysis test.[22] The parallelism between the results of the cobra-venom test and the acidified-serum test was less close. Lysis was observed only in patients thought on other grounds to have PNH and the results in patients with myeloproliferative disorders or aplastic anaemia were strictly negative.

On the basis of the above-quoted results, the cobra-venom test seems to be useful and reliable in the diagnosis of PNH. As, however, cobra venom contains factors, probably phospholipases, which lyse normal red cells in the absence of serum, the test has the disadvantage that the factor in the venom activating C3 proactivator in serum has to be separated from the crude venom by column chromatography before it can be used. Details were given by Kabakçi et al.[22]

SCREENING TESTS FOR PNH

Several simple tests are available which, although less specific than the acidified-serum and cobra-venom tests, are useful screening tests for PNH.

'HEAT RESISTANCE TEST'[20]

Allow blood to clot at 37°C and inspect for spontaneous lysis. A positive test is not specific for PNH although, characteristically, PNH blood lyses rapidly and markedly, i.e. haemoglobin can be seen diffusing from the clot into the serum as soon as the clot has retracted. Exceptionally, in patients with auto-immune haemolytic anaemia in whom there is very marked spherocytosis, the clot may undergo almost as rapid lysis.

INULIN TEST[5]

Place 1 drop (50 µl) of inulin (100 g/l in saline) in one of two 75 × 12 mm glass tubes. Deliver 3 ml of freshly collected blood into each of the tubes, which are then stoppered, gently mixed and allowed to stand at 37°C for at least 30–45 min until the blood has clotted and the clot has retracted. Then centrifuge the tubes and inspect the supernatant serum for lysis. Lysis in the inulin-containing tube with less lysis (or no lysis) in the tube not containing inulin constitutes a positive test. A control test using normal blood should always be set up at the same time. There should be no lysis or no difference in lysis between the two tubes of the control.

'COLD-ANTIBODY LYSIS' TEST

The greatly increased sensitivity of PNH red cells to complement can be dramatically demonstrated if the cells are suspended in dilutions of a high-titre cold agglutinin (anti-I) in the presence of fresh human serum complement.[12] Using suitable dilutions of the reagents, PNH red cells undergo marked lysis whereas normal red cells undergo little or no lysis. This reaction, the basis of the cold-antibody lysis test, is however, not quite specific for PNH as the red cells from some patients with various types of dyserythropoietic anaemia may undergo minor, or rarely moderate, amounts of lysis.[24]

An anti-I serum is required (titre at 4°C, >8000), which when used unacidified fails to lyse at room temperature most normal human red cells, i.e. a typical anti-I serum from a patient suffering from the cold haemagglutinin disease. Such sera keep their properties for years if frozen at −20°C. The serum should be distributed in 0.5–1.0 ml volumes in a number of tubes to avoid repeated thawing and freezing.

Method

Make a 1 in 50 or 1 in 100 dilution of the anti-I serum in undiluted fresh normal group AB or ABO-compatible serum. Deliver two 0.5 ml volumes of the serum into 75 × 12 mm tubes and add 0.5 ml volumes of a 5% suspension of washed normal and test (? PNH) red cells, respectively, to the serum samples. Add a further 0.5 ml volume of the washed test cells to a tube containing 0.5 ml of saline to serve as a standard for the quantitative measurement of lysis. Retain 0.5 ml of the serum mixture as a blank. After 1 h at room temperature centrifuge the two tubes containing the serum-cell suspensions, and add 0.3 ml volumes of their supernatants to 5 ml of 0.4 ml/l ammonia or Drabkin's reagent. Measure lysis in a photoelectric colorimeter using a yellow-green (e.g. Ilford 625) filter or in a spectrophotometer at a wavelength of 540 nm. Add 0.3 ml of the diluted red cell suspension to a further 5 ml of the diluent to give a standard for 100% lysis.

If a potent complement-fixing (i.e. lytic) antiserum is available, a very sensitive anti-I lysis test can be carried out using diluted human AB serum as complement. This is the basis of the complement lysis sensitivity test and the less elaborate 'four-tube complement lysis sensitivity' test.[40] These tests are probably more specific for PNH than is the original and very simple cold-antibody lysis test.

SUCROSE LYSIS TEST[18,19,21]

An iso-osmotic solution of sucrose (92.4 g/l) is required. This can be stored at 4°C for up to 2–3 weeks.

For the test, set up two tubes, one containing 0.05 ml of fresh normal group AB or ABO-compatible serum diluted in 0.85 ml of sucrose solution and the other containing 0.05 ml of serum diluted in 0.85 ml of saline. Add to each tube 0.1 ml of a 50% suspension of washed red cells. After incubation at 37°C for 30 min, centrifuge the tubes and examine for lysis. If lysis is visible in the sucrose-containing tube, measure this in a photoelectric colorimeter or a spectrophotometer (see above), using the tube containing serum diluted in saline as a blank and a tube containing 0.1 ml of the red cell suspension in 0.9 ml of 0.4 ml/l ammonia in place of the sucrose-serum mixture as a standard for 100% lysis.

Interpretation

The sucrose lysis test is based on the fact that red cells absorb complement components from serum at low ionic concentrations.[26,28] PNH cells, because of their great sensitivity will undergo lysis but normal red cells do not. The red cells from some cases of leukaemia[6] or myelosclerosis[47] may undergo a small amount of lysis, almost always <10%; in such cases the acidified-serum test is usually negative and PNH should not be diagnosed. In PNH, lysis varies from 10% to 80%, but exceptionally may be as little as 5%. Sucrose lysis and acidified-serum lysis[25] of PNH red cells are fairly closely correlated. The sucrose lysis test is typically negative in HEMPAS (see p. 262).

PNH-LIKE RED CELLS

By treating normal red cells with certain chemicals it is possible to increase their complement sensitivity so that they take on many of the characteristics of PNH cells.[43] The chemicals include sulphydryl compounds such as L-cysteine, reduced gluthathione (GSH), 2-aminoethyl*iso*thiouronium bromide (AET) and 2-mercaptobenzoic acid (MBA). AET and MBA cells can be used conveniently as a positive control for in-vitro lysis tests for PNH.[46]

Preparation of AET cells[44]

Prepare an 8 g/l solution of AET and adjust its pH to 8.0 with 5 mol/l NaOH. Collect normal blood into ACD and wash it twice in 9 g/l NaCl (saline).

Add 1 volume of the packed cells to 4 volumes of the AET solution in a 75 × 12 mm glass tube which is then stoppered. Mix the contents gently and place the tube at 37°C for 10–20 min. (According to Jenkins, the optimal time of incubation varies from red cell sample to red cell sample.[21]) Then wash the cells repeatedly with large volumes of saline until the supernatant is colourless. The red cells are now ready to use.

RED CELL ACETYLCHOLINESTERASE (AChE) IN PNH

As already referred to (p. 260), red cell AChE activity is dimished in PNH.[2,13,27] It seems likely that the activity of the enzyme is zero in sensitive (Type-III) PNH red cells, but because only a proportion, often a minority, of the red cells are abnormal in PNH, a lowered red cell AChE activity may not be demonstrable in whole blood.[27] AChE assay has, therefore, only limited diagnostic value. The AChE activity of AET cells is reduced but, in contrast to PNH, the reduced activity is not correlated with lysis in acidified serum or sucrose.[43]

Assay of acetylcholinesterase (AChE) activity

In the 4th edition of this book (p. 506), Michel's electrometric method was described. An alternative method that depends on the release by AChE of sulphydryl (SH) groups from a substrate of acetylthiocholine was described in the 6th edition (p. 205).

REFERENCES

[1] ASTER, R. H. and ENRIGHT, S. E. (1969). A platelet and granulocyte membrane defect in paroxysmal nocturnal hemoglobinuria: usefulness for the detection of platelet antibodies. *Journal of Clinical Investigation*, **48**, 1199.

[2] AUDITORE, J. V. and HARTMANN, R. C. (1959). Paroxysmal nocturnal hemoglobinuria: II. Erythrocyte acetylcholinesterase defect. *American Journal of Medicine*, **27**, 401.

[3] BECK, W. S. and VALENTINE, W. N. (1965). Biochemical studies on leucocytes. II. Phosphatase activity in chronic lymphatic leucemia, acute leucemia and miscellaneous hematologic conditions. *Journal of Laboratory and Clinical Medicine*, **38**, 245.

[4] BLUM, S. F. and GARDNER, F. H. (1967). Paroxysmal nocturnal hemoglobinuria. Mechanism of the enhancement of hemolysis by bovine thrombin. *Blood*, **30**, 352.

[5] BRUBAKER, L. H., SCHABERG, D. R., JEFFERSON, D. H. and MENGEL, C. E. (1973). A potential rapid screening test for paroxysmal nocturnal hemoglobinuria. *New England Journal of Medicine*, **288**, 1059.

[6] CATOVSKY, D., LEWIS, S. M. and SHERMAN, D. (1971). Erythrocyte sensitivity to in-vitro lysis in leukaemia. *British Journal of Haematology*, **21**, 541.

[7] CHOW, F.-L., TELEN, M. J. and ROSSE, W. F. (1985). The acetylcholinesterase defect in paroxysmal nocturnal hemoglobinuria: evidence that the enzyme is absent from the cell membrane. *Blood*, **66**, 940.

[8] CROOKSTON, J. H., CROOKSTON, M. C., BURNIE, K. L., FRANCOMBE, W. H., DACIE, J. V., DAVIS J. A. and LEWIS, S. M. (1969). Hereditary erythroblastic multinuclearity associated with a positive acidified-serum test: a type of congenital dyserythropoietic anaemia. *British Journal*

of Haematology, **17**, 11.

[9] Crosby, W. H. (1950). Paroxysmal nocturnal hemoglobinuria. A specific test for the disease based on the ability of thrombin to activate the hemolytic factor. Blood, **5**, 843.

[10] Dacie, J. V. (1963). Paroxysmal nocturnal haemoglobinuria. Proceedings of the Royal Society of Medicine, **56**, 587.

[11] Dacie, J. V. and Lewis, S. M. (1972). Paroxysmal nocturnal haemoglobinuria: clinical manifestations, haematology and nature of the disease. Series Haematologica, **5**, 3.

[12] Dacie, J. V., Lewis, S. M. and Tills, D. (1960). Comparative sensitivity of the erythrocytes in paroxysmal nocturnal haemoglobinuria to haemolysis by acidified normal serum and by a high-titre cold antibody. British Journal of Haematology, **6**, 362.

[13] De Sandre, G. and Ghiotto, G. (1985). Über die Bedeutung der Acetycholinesterase der Erythrocyten. Helvetica Medica Acta, **25**, 235.

[14] Dockter, M. E. and Morrison, M. (1986). Paroxysmal nocturnal hemoglobinuria erythrocytes are of two distinct types: positive or negative for acetylcholinesterase. Blood, **67**, 540.

[15] Francis, D. A. (1983). Production of PNH-like red cells using 2-mercaptobenzoic acid. Medical Laboratory Sciences, **40**, 33.

[16] Ham, T. H. and Dingle, J. H. (1939). Studies on destruction of red blood cells. II. Chronic hemolytic anemia with paroxysmal nocturnal hemoglobinuria: certain immunological aspects of the hemolytic mechanism with special reference to serum complement. Journal of Clinical Investigation, **18**, 657.

[17] Hansen, N. E. and Killman, S.-A. (1968). Paroxysmal nocturnal haemoglobinuria. A clinical study. Acta Medica Scandinavica, **184**, 525.

[18] Hartmann, R. C. and Jenkins, D. E. Jnr (1966). The 'sugar water' test for paroxysmal nocturnal hemoglobinuria. New England Journal of Medicine, **275**, 155.

[19] Hartmann, R. C., Jenkins, D. E. Jnr and Arnold, A. B. (1970). Diagnostic specificity of sucrose hemolysis test for paroxysmal nocturnal hemoglobinuria. Blood, **35**, 462.

[20] Hegglin, R. and Maier, C. (1944). The 'heat resistance' of erythrocytes. A specific test for the recognition of Marchiafava's anemia. American Journal of Medical Sciences, **207**, 624.

[21] Jenkins, D. E. Jnr. (1979). Paroxysmal nocturnal hemoglobinuria hemolytic systems. In A Seminar on Laboratory Management of Hemolysis, p. 45–49. American Association of Blood Banks, Washington.

[22] Kabakçi, T., Rosse, W. F. and Logue, G. L. (1972). The lysis of paroxysmal nocturnal haemoglobinuria red cells by serum and cobra factor. British Journal of Haematology, **23**, 693.

[23] Lewis, S. M. and Dacie, J. V. (1965). Neutrophil (leucocyte) alkaline phosphatase in paroxysmal nocturnal haemoglobinuria. British Journal of Haematology, **11**, 549.

[24] Lewis, S. M., Dacie, J. V. and Tills, D. (1961). Comparison of the sensitivity to agglutination and haemolysis by a high-titre cold antibody of the erythrocytes of normal subjects and of patients with a variety of blood diseases including paroxysmal nocturnal haemoglobinuria. British Journal of Haematology, **7**, 64.

[25] Lewis, S. M. And Sirchia, G. (1972). PNH: disease or defect? British Journal of Haematology, **23**, (suppl.), 71.

[26] Logue, G. L., Rosse, W. F. and Adams, J. P. (1973). Mechanisms of immune lysis of red blood cells in vitro. I.

Paroxysmal nocturnal hemoglobinuria cells. Journal of Clinical Investigation, **52**, 1129.

[27] Metz, J., Bradlow, B. A., Lewis, S. M. and Dacie, J. V. (1960). The acetylcholinesterase activity of the erythrocytes in paroxysmal nocturnal haemoglobinuria in relation to the severity of the disease. British Journal of Haematology, **6**, 372.

[28] Mollison, P. L. and Polley, M. J. (1964). Uptake of γ-globulin and complement by red cells exposed to serum at low ionic strength. Nature (London), **203**, 535.

[29] Nicholson-Weller, A., March, J. P., Rosenfield, S. I. and Austen, K. F. (1983). Affected erythrocytes of patients with paroxysmal nocturnal hemoglobinuria are deficient in the complement regulatory protein, decay accelerating factor. Proceedings of the National Academy of Sciences of the United States of America, **80**, 5066.

[30] Nicholson-Weller, A., Spicier, D. B. and Austen, K. F. (1985). Deficiency of the complement regulating protein 'decay accelerating factor' on membranes of granulocytes, monocytes, and platelets in paroxysmal nocturnal hemoglobinuria. New England Journal of Medicine, **312**, 1091.

[31] Oni, S. B., Osunkoya, B. O. and Luzzatto, L. (1970). Paroxysmal nocturnal hemoglobinuria: evidence for monoclonal origin of abnormal red cells. Blood, **36**, 145.

[32] Packman, C. H., Rosenfeld, S. I., Jenkins, D. E. Jnr, Thiem, P. A. and Leddy, J. P. (1979). Complement lysis of human erythrocytes. Differing susceptibility of two types of paroxysmal nocturnal hemoglobinuria cells to C5b-9. Journal of Clinical Investigation, **64**, 428.

[33] Pangburn, M. K., Schreiber, R. D. and Müller-Eberhard, H. F. (1983). Deficiency of an erythrocyte membrane protein with complement regulatory activity in paroxysmal nocturnal hemoglobinuria. Proceedings of the National Academy of Sciences of the United States of America, **80**, 5430.

[34] Parker, C. J., Soldato, C. M., Telen, M. J. and Rosse, W. F. (1984). Abnormality of glycophorin-α on paroxysmal nocturnal hemoglobinuria erythrocytes. Journal of Clinical Investigation, **73**, 1130.

[35] Parker, C. J., Wiedmer, T., Sims, P. J. and Rosse, W. F. (1985). Characterization of the complement sensitivity of paroxysmal nocturnal hemoglobinuria erythrocytes. Journal of Clinical Investigation, **75**, 2074.

[36] Rosse, W. F. (1972). The complement sensitivity of PNH cells. Series Haematologica, **5**, 101.

[37] Rosse, W. F. (1973). Variations in the red cells in paroxysmal nocturnal haemoglobinuria. British Journal of Haematology, **24**, 327.

[38] Rosse, W. F. (1986). The control of complement activation by the blood cells in paroxysmal nocturnal hemoglobinuria. Blood, **67**, 268. (Brief review).

[39] Rosse, W. F., Adams, J. P. and Thorpe, A. M. (1974). The population of cells in paroxysmal nocturnal haemoglobinuria of intermediate sensitivity to complement lysis: significance and mechanism of increased immune lysis. British Journal of Haematology, **28**, 281.

[40] Rosse, W. F. and Dacie, J. V. (1966). Immune lysis of normal human and paroxysmal nocturnal hemoglobinuria (PNH) red blood cells. I. The sensitivity of PNH red cells to lysis by complement and specific antibody. Journal of Clinical Investigation, **45**, 736.

[41] Rosse, W. F. and Parker, C. J. (1985). Paroxysmal nocturnal haemoglobinuria. Clinics in Haematology, **14**, 105.

[42] SCHREIBER, A. D. (1983). Paroxysmal nocturnal hemoglobinuria revisited. *New England Journal of Medicine*, **309**, 723. (Editorial).

[43] SIRCHIA, G. and FERRONE, S. (1972). The laboratory substitutes of the red cell of paroxysmal nocturnal haemoglobinuria (PNH): PNH-like red cells. *Series Haematologica*, **5**, 137.

[44] SIRCHIA, G., FERRONE, S. and MERCURIALI, F. (1965). The action of two sulfhydryl compounds on normal human red cells. Relationship to red cells of paroxysmal nocturnal hemoglobinuria. *Blood*, **25**, 502.

[45] SIRCHIA, G. and LEWIS, S. M. (1975). Paroxysmal nocturnal haemoglobinuria. *Clinics in Haematology*, **4**, 199.

[46] SIRCHIA, G., MARUBINI, E., MERCURIALI, F. and FERRONE, S. (1973). Study of two *in vitro* diagnostic tests for paroxysmal nocturnal haemoglobinuria. *British Journal of Haematology*, **24**, 751.

[47] STRATTON, F. and EVANS, D. I. K. (1967). Lysis of P.N.H. cells in solutions of low ionic strength. *British Journal of Haematology*, **13**, 862.

[48] SUGARMAN, J., DEVINE, D. V. and ROSSE, W. F. (1986). Structural and functional differences between decay-accelerating factor and red cell acetylcholinesterase. *Blood*, **68**, 680.

[49] VERWILGHEN, R. L., LEWIS, S. M., DACIE, J. V., CROOKSTON, J. H. and CROOKSTON, M. C. (1973). HEMPAS: congenital dyserythropoietic anaemia (Type II). *Quarterly Journal of Medicine*, **42**, 257.

[50] WEBER, H. (1966). Rasche und einfache Ultramikromethode zur Bestimmung der Serumcholinesterase. *Deutsche Medizinische Wochenschrift*, **91**, 1927.

17. Investigation of haemostasis

(By M. Brozović)

The haemostatic mechanisms have two primary functions: to ensure that circulating blood remains fluid while in the vascular bed, and to arrest bleeding at the site of an injured blood vessel. Normal haemostasis depends on a delicate balance and complex interreactions between at least five components: blood vessels, platelets, plasma coagulation proteins, inhibitors and the fibrinolytic system, as shown in Fig. 17.1.

In this chapter a brief review of normal haemostasis is presented, followed by a discussion on the general principles of tests used to investigate haemostasis.

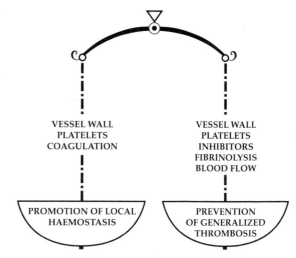

Fig. 17.1 Haemostatic balance.

VASCULAR HAEMOSTASIS

General structure of the blood vessel

The blood vessel wall has three layers: intima, media and adventitia. The intima consists of endothelium and subendothelial connective tissue and is separated from the media by the elastic lamina interna. *Endothelial cells* form a continuous monolayer lining all blood vessels. The structure and the function of the endothelial cells varies according to their location in the vascular tree, but they all share three important characteristics: they are 'non-thrombogenic', that is do not react with plasma or the cellular elements of the blood; they play an active role in supplying nutrients to the subendothelial structures, and act as a barrier to macromolecules and particulate matter circulating in the blood stream.

Endothelial cell function[2,9,10]

The luminal surface of the endothelial cell is covered by the glycocalyx, a proteoglycan coat. It contains heparin sulphate and other glycosaminoglycans which are capable of activating antithrombin III, an important inhibitor of coagulation enzymes. Beneath the glycocalyx, there is a trilaminar membrane containing ADPase, an enzyme which degrades ADP which is a potent platelet agonist (see p. 269). There are also various membrane-lined structures, such as vesicles and 'pits', which participate in transport across the membrane.

The endothelial cell also participates in vasoregulation: on one hand it metabolizes and inactivates vasoactive peptides; on the other hand, the endothelial cell can produce prostacyclin and thus inhibit platelet aggregation (see later). It can also generate angiotensin II, a local vasoconstrictor.

Thrombin generated at the site of injury (p. 271) is rapidly bound to a specific cofactor of the endothelial cell, thrombomodulin. When bound to this protein, thrombin can activate the protein C system to degrade and inhibit factors Va and VIIIa. Thrombin also stimulates the endothelial cell to produce plasminogen activator.

Finally, the endothelial cell produces von Willebrand factor (vWF), essential for platelet adhesion to the subendothelium. vWF is secreted partly into the circulation and partly towards the subendothelial matrix.

The subendothelium[13]

The subendothelium consists of connective tissues composed of collagen, elastic tissues, proteoglycans and non-collagenous glycoporteins, including fibronectin and vWF. After endothelial damage has taken place, components of the subendothelium are exposed and platelets adhere to various elements including collagen of the basement membrane and microfibrils. The adhesion of platelets is regulated by the specific properties of the platelet membranes and the biochemical characteristics of the subendothelial structures. Other factors, such as the plasma concentration of vWF and the characteristics of the blood flow also affect adhesion.

Vasoconstriction[13]

Vessels with muscular coats contract following injury, thus assisting haemostatic plug formation by reducing the blood flow. Vasoconstriction occurs, however, even in the microcirculation in vessels without smooth muscle cells. Endothelial cells themselves can produce vasconstrictors such as angiotensin II; in addition, activated platelets produce prostaglandins (TXA_2) with vasoconstricting properties.

PLATELETS

Platelet structure

Platelets circulate as non-nucleate discs and consist of a trilaminar lipoprotein *membrane* with submembrane contractile filaments, three types of *granules* and an irregular internal network of canaliculi, through which the granule contents can be released on to the platelet surface. The granule types are: dense granules which release adenosine diphosphate (ADP), adenosine triphosphate (ATP), serotonin and calcium ions; alpha granules, whose release constituents include platelet-derived growth factor, platelet factor 4 with heparin neutralizing ability, beta thromboglobulin, vWF, factor V, fibrinogen and fibronectin; and lysosomal granules.

The platelet membrane. This is the site of interaction with the plasma environment and with damaged vessel wall. It consists of phospholipids, cholesterol, glycolipids and at least nine glycoproteins, Gp I–IX. The membrane phospholipids are asymmetrically distributed, with sphingomyelin and phosphatidylcholine predominating in the outer leaflet, and phosphatidylethanolamine, inositol and serine in the inner leaflet.

The contractile system of the platelet. This consists of the dense microtubular system and the circumferential microfilaments which maintain the disc shape. Actin is the main constituent of the contractile system, but myosin and a regulatory protein, calmodulin, are also present.

Platelet function in the haemostatic process

When the vessel wall is damaged, the subendothelial structures, including basement membrane, collagen and microfibrils, are exposed. Circulating platelets react with exposed collagen fibres, and their adherence to the damaged surface is mediated by high molecular weight multimers of vWF, and possibly fibronectin. Once activated, platelets immediately change shape from a disc to a tiny sphere with numerous projecting pseudopods. After adhesion of a single layer of platelets to the exposed subendothelium, platelets stick to one another to form aggregates. Fibrinogen and fibronectin are essential at this stage to increase the cell to cell contact and facilitate aggregation. Certain substances (agonists) react with specific platelet membrane receptors and initiate platelet aggregation and further activation. The agonists include: exposed collagen fibres, ADP, adrenaline, serotonin, certain arachidonic acid metabolites including thromboxane $A_2(TXA_2)$. In areas of non-linear blood flow such as may occur at the site of an injury, locally damaged red cells release ADP which further activates platelets.

Platelet aggregation

Platelet aggregation may occur by at least two independent but closely linked pathways.[16] The first pathway involves arachidonic acid metabolism. Activation of phospholipase enzymes releases free arachidonic acid from the membrane phospholipids. About 50% of free arachidonic acid is converted by a lypo-oxygenase enzyme to a series of products including leucotrienes which are important chemoattractants of white cells. The remaining 50% of arachidonic acid is converted by the enzyme cyclooxygenase into labile cyclic endoperoxides, most of which are in turn converted by thromboxane synthetase into TXA_2. TXA_2 has profound biological effects, causing platelet granule release and local vasoconstriction, as well as further local platelet aggregation. It exerts these effects by raising intracellular cytoplasmic free calcium concentration and binding to specific granule receptors. TXA_2 is very labile with a half-life of less than 1 minute, before being degraded into the inactive thromboxane B_2 (TXB_2) and malonyldialdehyde.

The second pathway of activation and aggregation can proceed completely independently from the first one: various platelet agonists, including thrombin and collagen, produce a brisk increase in the free cytoplasmic calcium to cause the release reaction. Calcium is released from the dense tubular system to form complexes with calmodulin; this complex and the free calcium act as co-enzymes for the release reaction, for the activation of different regulatory proteins, as well as of actin and myosin and the contractile system, and also to liberate arachidonic acid from membrane phospholipids and generate TXA_2.

The aggregating platelets align together into loose reversible aggregates, but after the release reaction of the platelet granules, a larger, firmer aggregate forms. Changes in the platelet membrane configuration now occur: 'flip-flop' rearrangement of the surface brings the negatively charged phosphatidylserine and inositol onto the outer leaflet, thus generating platelet factor 3 (procoagulant) activity.

Platelets are not activated if in contact with healthy endothelial cells. The 'non-thrombogenicity' of the endothelium is due to a combination of control mechanisms exerted by the endothelial cell: synthesis of prostacyclin,[8] capacity to bind thrombin and activate the protein C system,[5] ability to inactivate vasoactive substances, etc (see p. 268). Prostacyclin released locally binds to specific platelet membrane receptors and then activates the membrane-bound adenylate cyclase (c-AMP). c-AMP inhibits platelet aggregation by inhibiting arachidonic acid metabolism and the release of cytoplasmic free calcium ions.

Platelets promote coagulation in a number of ways: by enhancing contact activation through a specific factor XI receptor, by generating tissue factor through membrane 'flip-flop', and by providing the phospholipid surfaces necessary for the activation of factor X and prothrombin.

BLOOD COAGULATION

At the site of vascular damage the coagulation cascade is rapidly activated to produce thrombin and finally to generate solid fibrin from soluble fibrinogen, reinforcing the primary platelet plug. The coagulation cascade is shown in Fig. 17.2. Two separate pathways of coagulation, intrinsic and extrinsic, are defined by the two commonly used coagulation tests, the activated partial thromboplastin time and the prothrombin time. It has become increasingly obvious over the years that the two pathways are closely linked and interdependent. The components of the cascade are coagulation enzymes, membrane phospholipid surfaces, protein cofactors and calcium ions. The coagulation proteins can conveniently be divided into three groups on the basis of their biochemical properties and function: (vitamin-K-dependent proteins, contact proteins and thrombin-sensitive proteins (Table 17.1). Tables 17.2–4 list the biochemical properties of the three families of coagulation proteins.

Vitamin-K-dependent coagulation proteins

Vitamin-K-dependent proteins are all synthesized by the liver and include prothrombin, factor VII, factor IX, factor X, and proteins C and S (Table 17.2). The characteristic chemical feature of these proteins is a unique amino-acid residue called

Table 17.1 Biochemical properties of the three 'families' of coagulation proteins

Property	Vit-K-dependent factors	Contact factors	Thrombin sensitive factors
Mol wt	57–69 000	variable	300 000 +
Stability	heat stable		labile
Consumed in coagulation	No (except Factor II)	No	Yes
Adsorbed by BaSO$_4$, Al(OH)$_3$	Yes	No	No
Reagent for correction	serum (except factor II)	plasma or serum	serum
Present in platelets	No	No	Yes
Acute phase reactants	No	No	Yes

γ-carboxyglutamic acid. γ-carboxyglutamic acid results in the presence of vitamin K.[5,14]

The γ-carboxyglutamic acid residues enable the K-dependent proteins to bind calcium ions and form calcium bridges with acidic phospholipids. Prothrombin and factors VII, IX and X are procoagulant, whereas proteins C and S are anticoagulant.

The zymogen or proenzyme forms of the K-dependent factors are either single chain proteins (prothrombin, factor VII and IX, protein S) or double chain proteins (factor X and protein C). Each zymogen contains several γ-carboxyglutamic acid residues at the amino terminal end. The active site is located nearer the carboxy terminal end. As a result of proteolytic cleavage a small activation peptide is released and the active serine protease generated.

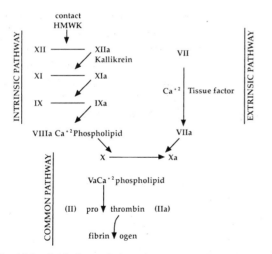

Fig. 17.2. Intrinsic, extrinsic and common pathways of coagulation.

Table 17.2 Properties of vitamin-K-dependent factors

Factor	Mol wt	Half-life	Concentration in plasma (mg/dl)
Prothrombin (II)	72 000	60 h	10–15
Factor VII	48 000	4–6 h	0.1
Factor IX	57 000	12 h	0.01
Factor X	58 000	24 h	0.75
Protein C	62 000	6 h	0.5
Protein S	69 000		0.01

Table 17.3   Properties of contact factors

Factor	Mol wt	Half-life	Concentration in plasma (mg/dl)
Factor XI	160 000	40 h	1.2
Factor XII	80 000	48–52 h	0.4
Prekallikrein	85 000	48–52 h	0.3
HMWK*	110 000	6.5 days	2.5

*High mol wt kininogen.

Contact factors

Contact factors are: factor XII or Hageman factor, prekallikrein or Fletcher factor, factor XI and High Molecular Weight Kininogen (HMWK) or Fitzgerald factor. Their physical properties are shown in Table 17.3; they are produced by the liver. Factor XII is a single chain glycoprotein which is bound to, and can be non-enzymatically activated by, collagen fibres and other negatively charged surfaces. HMWK is required for optimum binding of factor XII to the negatively charged surfaces. The enzyme generated in this way is called α XIIa and it can in turn activate factor XI. Factor XIa will then cleave a peptide from factor XII and give rise to a slightly different active form called β XIIa. β XIIa activates prekallikrein, plasminogen activators and HMWK.[12]

Thrombin-sensitive coagulation proteins

The thrombin-sensitive proteins are: fibrinogen, factor XIII, factor V and factor VIII protein complex (see Table 17.4).

Fibrinogen is a large six-chain molecule. Thrombin removes only less than 5% of its molecular mass by releasing first two A, then two B peptides.[5,7] The fibrin monomers formed in this way are able to polymerize non-enzymatically and become a gel. This early fibrin is relatively easily solubilized and

digested by the fibrinolytic system. A tough, insoluble fibrin is formed after interaction with factor XIII. *Factor XIII* is the only transamidase amongst the coagulation enzymes: it is converted to its active form in the presence of calcium and thrombin.

The native *factor V* in plasma is a pro-cofactor. Thrombin cleaves the molecule to give rise to active cofactor, Va, essential for rapid conversion of prothrombin into thrombin.

Factor VIII protein complex consists of two proteins:[17] factor VIII:C or factor VIII procoagulant protein, and vWF, von Willebrand factor. Factor VIII:C in plasma is a pro-cofactor. Like factor V it is cleaved by thrombin to give rise to active cofactor, VIIIa, necessary for optimal activation of factor X by factor IX. Further cleavage by thrombin leads to inactivation. Factor VIII:C and vWF circulate in plasma as a complex and probably stabilize and protect each other.

von Willebrand factor makes up over 99% of the VIII:C/vWF complex. The basic vWF subunit has a mol wt of about 200 000, and each molecule consists of multimers varying in mol wt from 800 000 to over 14 000 000. vWF facilitates the platelet adhesion to the subendothelium particularly in small blood vessels where there is a rapid blood flow creating high shear rates, and serves as a carrier and stabilizer for factor VIII:C.

Other components of the coagulation cascade

Tissue factor or thromboplastin is an important cofactor of the extrinsic pathway. It is a lipoprotein, present in many tissues and is required for activation of factor VII. The negatively-charged phospholipids from the inner leaflet of platelet and other cellular membranes are essential for the activation of other vitamin-K-dependent factors.

Table 17.4   Properties of thrombin-sensitive factors

Factor	Mol wt	Half-life	Concentration in plasma (mg/dl)	Site of synthesis
Fibrinogen	340 000	90 h	150–400	liver
Factor XIII	320 000	3–5 days	2.5	liver
Factor V	330 000	12–36 h	0.5–1.0	liver
Factor VIII:C	c200 000	12 h	<0.01	liver
von Willebrand factor	800 000–14 000 000	24 h	0.5–1.0	endothelium, platelets

Table 17.5 Some properties of serpines

Serpine	Mol wt	Rate of inhibition	Concentration in plasma (mg/dl)	Main substrate
Antithrombin III*	54 000	slow	23–40	Xa, thrombin plasmin
Heparin cofactor II*	65 000	slow	7–14	thrombin
α_2-macroglobulin	725 000	rapid	190–330	thrombin, plasmin
C_1-inhibitor	104 000	slow	14–30	contact factors
α_2-antitrypsin	54 000	rapid	250–340	non-haemostatic proteases
α_2-antiplasmin	70 000	rapid	10–14	plasmin

* Action potentiated by heparin.

LOCALIZATION OF THE HAEMOSTATIC PLUG

The uncontrolled growth of thrombi is limited by three mechanisms. First, *blood flow* removes activated coagulation enzymes and platelet activating substances from the site of injury. They are rapidly inactivated after their passage through the liver; the clearance mechanism involves complexing with inhibitors and interaction with macrophages. Secondly, *serine proteases* generated during coagulation not only activate coagulation factors but also degrade them. The degradation can be due to a direct proteolytic effect, e.g. degradation of Xa by thrombin, or result from activation of an inhibitory system as is the case with the protein C system. Thrombin forms a complex with an endothelial cell protein, thrombomodulin, to activate protein C.[6] Activated protein C, in the presence of phospholipid and protein S, rapidly degrades factor Va and VIII:Ca. The third mechanism of control involves naturally occurring serine protease inhibitors (*serpines*) in plasma.[11] The major ones are: alpha-2-macroglobulin, alpha-1-antitrypsin, antithrombin III, heparin cofactor II, C_1-esterase inhibitor and alpha-2-antiplasmin. Their physical characteristics are shown in Table 17.5. Antithrombin III is crucial in neutralizing the coagulation enzymes. It inactivates all serine proteases of the cascade by forming high mol wt complexes. Heparin and contact with damaged endothelial cells markedly accelerate these reactions.

THE FIBRINOLYTIC SYSTEM

The deposition of fibrin and its removal from circulation are regulated by the fibrinolytic system. It is also a multicomponent system (Fig. 17.3) composed of a circulating pro-enzyme, plasminogen, plasminogen activators and inhibitors.[15] Plasminogen is a single-chain glycoprotein with an amino terminal glutamic acid residue which is easily cleaved by limited proteolysis to a modified form with a terminal lysine, valine or methionine. Plasminogen with amino terminal lysine is called lys-plasminogen and has an increased affinity for fibrin and for plasminogen activators. The plasminogen molecule contains a region rich in lysine which is essential for binding to fibrin and to alpha-2-macroglobulin, and the region where the active site is situated. The activators cleave a peptide from plasminogen and generate the two-chain plasmin. Activation into plasmin may occur via one of the three pathways (see Fig. 17.3): (1) the intrinsic pathway involving activation of circulating proactivators via factor XIIa; (2) the extrinsic pathway in which the activators are released into the blood stream from damaged tissues, cells or vessel walls (all activators are also serine proteases); (3) a third pathway, not shown in Fig 17.3, is called the exogenous pathway, through which plasminogen is

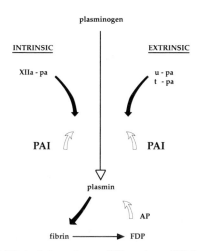

Fig. 17.3 Fibrinolytic pathways. XII-pa: factor-XII-dependent plasminogen activator, present in circulating blood. u-pa: urokinase-like plasminogen activator. t-pa: tissue plasminogen activator. Both these activators are released from activated or damaged cells. PAI: plasminogen activator inhibitors. AP: α_2-antiplasmin, a potent inhibitor of plasmin.

activated in the presence of a thrombolytic drug, e.g. streptokinase (for details see Chapter 21).

Plasmin hydrolyses numerous bonds in fibrin to dissolve it into fibrin degradation products (FDP). Plasmin also degrades factors V and VIII:C. Explosive fibrinolysis is prevented by a potent inhibitor, alpha-2-antiplasmin, and to a lesser extent by alpha-2-macroglobulin. Free plasmin in plasma is immediately inactivated by alpha-2-antiplasmin, whereas plasmin adhering to fibrin within the local haemostatic plug is protected from alpha-2-antiplasmin and can digest fibrin into FDP. Inhibitors of plasminogen activators also play an important role in regulating fibrinolysis and limiting it to the site of injury.

INVESTIGATION OF THE HAEMOSTATIC MECHANISM

INVESTIGATION OF THE DISORDERS OF VASCULAR HAEMOSTASIS

Disorders of vascular haemostasis may be due to increased vascular permeability, reduction of vessel 'strength' and failure to contract on injury. An accurate history and a careful clinical examination are almost always the keystones of diagnosis. Tests of defective vascular function are difficult to perform and interpret. The only test of value is the bleeding time and its modifications (see p. 285). Tests of capillary resistance are of limited value. In some cases skin biopsy with specific staining or even biochemical analysis of the micro-sample may be helpful.

LABORATORY INVESTIGATION OF PLATELETS AND PLATELET FUNCTION

The peripheral blood platelet count and the skin bleeding time are the first-line tests of platelet function. If the results of these two tests are within the normal limits, it is unlikely that a clinically important platelet defect is responsible for the bleeding tendency. Additional information may be

obtained by inspecting a fresh blood film which may show abnormalities of platelet size or morphology which may be of diagnostic importance.

If the screening procedures suggest a disorder of platelet function, further tests should be organized. Drugs and certain foods (Table 17.6) may affect platelet function tests, and the patient must be asked to refrain from taking such substances for at least seven days before the test.

Platelet function tests can be divided into five main groups (Table 17.7): adhesion tests, aggegation tests, assessment of the granular content and the release reaction, investigation of the prostaglandin pathways and tests of platelet coagulant activity.

Tests of *platelet retention or adhesion* by a glass bead column are rarely used today because of the lack of specificity. More sophisticated tests based on the Baumgartner technique of passing whole blood over everted rabbit aorta denuded of endothelial cells are very useful research tools, but unsuitable for the routine laboratory.

In contrast, studies of *platelet aggregation* are mandatory in investigating platelet function, particularly in patients with a normal platelet count

Table 17.6 Substances which commonly affect platelet function.

Agents which affect prostanoid synthesis
  Aspirin
  Non-steroidal anti-inflammatory drugs
  Corticosteroids

Membrane stabilizing agents
  α antagonists
  β blockers
  Antihistamines
  Tricyclic antidepressants
  Local anaesthetics

Antibiotics
  Penicillin
  Cephalosporins

Agents which increase c-AMP activity
  Dipyridamole
  Aminophylline
  Prostanoids

Others
  Heparin
  Dextran
  Ethanol
  Clofibrate
  Phenothiazine
  Garlic

---

and a prolonged bleeding time. A turbidometric technique using patient's own platelet-rich plasma is commonly used; numerous platelet activating agents or agonists can be applied. Details of the technique and the agonists, as well as the diagnostic patterns encountered, are discussed in detail in Chapter 19.

The *granular content* of the platelets can be assessed by electron microscopy or by measuring the substances released (Table 17.7). Adenine nucleotide and serotonin release from the dense granules are probably best measured by a specialist laboratory. The release of β-thromboglobulin and platelet factor 4 can be measured using commercial radio-immunoassay kits, but there are problems with reproducibility and interpretation of the results. The release from the α granules is mostly investigated as a marker of in-vivo platelet activation and thrombotic tendency. Platelet vWF is measured to diagnose variants of von Willebrand disease. Platelet-derived growth factor can also be measured by some specialized laboratories.

If the initial aggregation studies suggest a defect in the prostaglandin pathways, TXB_2 can be estimated quantitatively by radio-immune assay. Highly specific assays of various steps in arachidonic acid metabolism are also available but are outside the scope of a routine laboratory.

Platelet coagulant activity—the completion of the membrane 'flip-flop'—can be indirectly measured using the prothrombin consumption index (see p. 299).

Table 17.7 Platelet function tests

Adhesion tests	
Retention in a glass-bead column	
Baumgartner's technique	
Aggregation tests	
Turbidometric technique using	
ADP	Adrenaline
Collagen	Thrombin
Ristocetin	Arachidonic acid
	Endoperoxide analogues U44069, U46619
	Calcium ionophore A21387
Investigation of granular content and release	
Dense bodies:	electron microscopy
	ADP and ATP content (bioluminescence)
	serotonine release
Granules:	β-thromboglobulin
	platelet factor 4
	vWF
Prostaglandin pathways	
TXB_2 radio-immune assay	
MDA assay using thiobarbituric acid	
Studies with radioactive arachidonic acid	
Platelet coagulant activity	
Prothrombin consumption index	

Modified from Yardumian et al.[16]; reproduced by permission.

Calcium is an extremely important regulator of platelet functions (p. 269). It has recently become possible to measure the concentrations of intra-cellular calcium, but it remains primarily a research technique.

INVESTIGATION OF BLOOD COAGULATION

Coagulation tests are necessary in patients with an acute or chronic haemorrhagic tendency as well as in those with a family history of coagulation factor defect or deficiency. The first step, however, in the diagnostic process is to obtain a detailed history, including the family history. The type, location, frequency, duration and severity of bleeding, whether spontaneous or traumatic, must be estab-lished. Physical examination is also essential and may help either by revealing manifestations of other, systemic, diseases or by the discovery of characteristic features such as the joint deformities of haemophilia.

Every laboratory should be capable of performing screening or first-line coagulation tests. These are: activated partial thromboplastin time, one-stage prothrombin time, and the measurement of fibrin-ogen by one of the techniques listed in Chapter 18. A platelet count should always be carried out and the skin bleeding time performed whenever von Willebrand's disease is suspected. The data obtained from these tests usually allow a tentative diagnosis to be made.

By defintion screening tests are non-specific and lack sensitivity. It does not always follow that a patient in whom the results of screening tests are normal has an entirely normal haemostatic mech-anism. Nevertheless, if the screening tests are entirely normal and the history unremarkable, it is unlikely that such an individual has a clinically severe haemorrhagic tendency. If, however, the history and clinical findings are consistent with a haemorrhagic tendency, further investigations, par-ticularly to exclude a variant von Willebrand's disease, must be carried out even if the screening tests are entirely normal. In the presence of an abnormality in the screening tests, detailed investi-gation of the likely defect must follow.

Detailed investigation of coagulation proteins can be divided into four categories (Table 17.8).

Coagulation assays. These are bioassays and comparative in nature: the test preparation with an unknown level of the activity to be measured is compared with a control (standard) preparation with a known level of activity. The assay can be performed using either a one-stage or a two-stage system. In the one-stage system optimal amounts of all the clotting factors are present except the one to be determined, which should be as near to nil as possible. The best one-stage system is provided by a substrate plasma either obtained from a severely congenitally deficient patient or artificially depleted by immuno-adsorption. In the two-stage assay, the coagulation enzyme is generated in a two-step system and there is no requirement for a 'factor'-deficient substrate plasma. The principles of bioas-say, its standardization and limitations are consid-ered in detail in Chapter 19.

Coagulation techniques are also used in mixing tests to identify a missing factor in an emergency, or to identify and estimate quantitatively an inhibitor or anticoagulant.

Immunological methods.[3] These have become important tools in investigating coagulation dis-orders. They are usually carried out in parallel with coagulation or functional assays in order to detect the presence of abnormal proteins. Immunological techniques used in coagulation include immuno-diffusion, immuno-electrophoresis, radio-immuno-metric assays, latex agglutination tests and tests using enzyme-linked antibodies. Many of these techniques are simple slide tests which require no complex instrumentation or expertise.

Assays using chromogenic peptide substrates (amidolytic assays). The serine proteases of the coagulation cascade have narrow substrate specific-ities. Various amino-acid sequences have a high affinity for these proteases and it is possible to synthesize short peptides containing the specific sequence for each enzyme.[1,4] The synthetic tri-or tetra-peptides have a dye, p-nitroaniline (pNA), attached to the terminal amino-acid. When the synthetic peptide reacts with the specific enzyme, the dye is released and the rate of its release or the total amount released can be measured photomet-rically.

Chromogenic substrate assays can be classified into direct and indirect assays. Direct assays can be further sub-classified into primary assays in which a

Table 17.8 Techniques used for the measurement of coagulation factors

Factor	Coagulation assay	Immunoassay	Chromogenic assay*	Other assay
Fibrinogen	Clot opacity Clot weight	ID IE		Chemical tests
Prothrombin	Two-stage	ID	Specific substrate	Taipan venom
Factor V	One-stage		Non-specific	
Factor VII	One-stage	ID ELISA	Specific substrate	
Factor VIII:C	One-stage Two-stage	IRMA	Non-specific	
von Willebrand factor		IE, CIE, ELISA, IRMA		Ristocetin cofactor
Factor IX	One-stage	IRMA, ELISA	Non-specific	
Factor X	One-stage	ID, IE, ELISA	Specific substrate	Russell viper venom (RVV)
Factor XI	One-stage	ID		
Factor XII	One-stage	IE	Non-specific	
Prekallikrein	One-stage		Specific substrate	
HMWK	One-stage	ID		
Factor XIII	Clot solubility	IE		Incorporation of synthetic amines

IE = immuno-electrophoresis; CIE = crossed immuno-electrophoresis;
ID = immunodiffusion; IRMA = immunoradiometric assay;
ELISA = enzyme-linked saturation analysis; HMWK = high mol wt. kininogen.
* All chromogenic assays for coagulation factors are direct (for explanation, see p. 275).

substrate specific for the enzyme to be measured is used and secondary assays in which the enzyme or pro-enzyme measured is used to activate a second protease for which a specific substrate is available. Specific substrates are available for kallikrein, Xa, thrombin, activated protein C, plasmin and urokinase. Indirect assays are used to measure naturally occurring inhibitors and some platelet factors.

It should be remembered that the measurement of amidolytic activity is not the same as the measurement of biological activity in a coagulation assay. This is particularly important when dealing with the molecular variants of various coagulation factors. Nevertheless, the continuing development of more specific substrates with good solubility and high affinity for individual enzymes, together with rapid advances in automation, make chromogenic substrate assays increasingly popular. The assays can be carried out in a tube when a spectrophotometer is used to measure the intensity of the colour development, or in a microtitre plate when the colour is noted by eye.

Other assays. These include measurement of coagulation factors using snake venoms, assay of ristocetin cofactor and the clot solubility test for factor XIII.

INVESTIGATION OF THE FIBRINOLYTIC SYSTEM

The fibrinolytic system is assessed most commonly in patients with recurrent thrombotic phenomena; rarely, its assessment is necessary as a part of investigations into an unusual haemorrhagic tendency in some cases of acute haemostatic failure. The assays used can be classified into functional

Table 17.9 Components of the fibrinolytic system and tests used in their assay

Component	Functional assay	Immunoassay	Chromogenic assay
Plasminogen activators	Whole-blood clot lysis Dilute clot lysis Euglobulin lysis Fibrin plate lysis	ELISA	Non-specific substrate
Plasminogen	Caseinolytic assay	ELISA, IE	Specific substrate
Plasminogen activator inhibitor		IRMA, ELISA	Non-specific substrate
α₂-antiplasmin		IE, IRMA	Specific substrate
FDP	Thrombin time	Latex agglutination, IE	
D-dimer		Latex agglutination, IRMA, ELISA	

IE = immuno-electrophoresis; ID = immunodiffusion;
IRMA = immunoradiometric assay;
ELISA = enzyme-linked saturation assay.

assays, immunological methods, chromogenic peptide assays and other tests including the venous occlusion and DDAVP tests.[15] The various components of the fibrinolytic system and some of the tests used in their assay are set out in Table 17.9.

The tests used as a screen in an emergency, e.g. disseminated intravascular coagulation (DIC) or acute hyperfibrinolysis due to a malignant tumour, are few and of relatively limited value: they include estimation of fibrinogen and FDP concentration, and one of the paracoagulation tests such as the ethanol gelation test (see p. 291). Exceptionally, the euglobulin or dilute whole blood lysis time may be required.

INVESTIGATION OF SERPINES AND OTHER INHIBITORY PROTEINS

The plasma concentration of serpines and proteins C and S is usually measured in individuals with a thrombotic tendency. The assays can, yet again, be divided into functional, amidolytic (using chromogenic peptides) and immunological. The assays using commercially available kits with chromogenic peptide substrates are by far the most widely used as the initial screening procedure. Immunological tests and functional assays are generally used only by specialist laboratories when investigating affected kindreds or as research tools. For details see Chapter 20.

REFERENCES

[1] BLOMBACK, M. and EGBERG, M. (1987). Chromogenic peptide substrates in the laboratory diagnosis of clotting disorders. In *Haemostasis and Thrombosis*. Eds. Bloom, A. L. and Thomas, D. P., p. 967. Churchill Livingstone, Edinburgh.
[2] CHESTERMAN, C. N. and BERNDT, M. C. (1986). Platelet and vessel wall interaction and the genesis of atherosclerosis.

Clinics in Haematology, **15**, 323.
[3] GIDDINGS, J. C. (1987). Immunoanalysis of haemostatic components. In *Haemostasis and Thrombosis*. Eds. Bloom, A. L. and Thomas, D. P., p. 982. Churchill Livingstone, Edinburgh.
[4] HUTTON, R. A. (1987). Chromogenic substrates in haemostasis. *Blood Reviews*, **1**, 201.

[5] LAMMLE, B. and GRIFFIN, J. H. (1985). Formation of fibrin clot: the balance of procoagulant and inhibitory factors. *Clinics in Haematology*, **14**, 281.

[6] MANNUCCI, P. M. and OWEN, W. G. (1987). Basic and clinical aspects of proteins C and S. In *Haemostasis and Thrombosis*. Eds. Bloom, A. L. and Thomas, D. P., p. 452. Churchill Livingstone, Edinburgh.

[7] MARDER, V. J., FRANCIS, C. W. and DOOLITTLE, R. F. (1982). Fibrinogen. Structure and physiology. In *Haemostasis and Thrombosis*. Eds. Coleman, R. W., Hirsh, J., Marder, V. J. and Salzman, E. W., p. 145. J. B. Lippincott Co, Philadelphia.

[8] MONCADA, S. and HIGGS, E. A. (1986). Arachidonate metabolism in blood cells and the vessel wall. *Clinics in Haematology*, **15**, 273.

[9] NAWROTH, P. P., HANDLEY, D. A. and STERN, D. M. (1986). The multiple levels of endothelial cell-coagulation factor interactions. *Clinics in Haematology*, **15**, 293.

[10] NAWROTH, P. P., KISIEL, W. and STERN, D. M. (1985). The role of endothelium in the homeostatic balance of haemostasis. *Clinics in Haematology*, **14**, 531.

[11] SALEM, H. T. (1986). The natural anticoagulants. *Clinics in Haematology*, **15**, 371.

[12] SCHMAIER, A. H. and COLEMAN, R. W. (1985). The contact phase of coagulation: a review and specific techniques to study its components. In *Blood Coagulation and Haemostasis. A Practical Guide*. Ed. Thomson, J. M., p. 22. Churchill Livingstone, Edinburgh.

[13] SIXMA, J. J. (1987). Role of platelets, plasma proteins and vessel wall in haemostasis. In *Haemostasis and Thrombosis*. Eds. Bloom, A. L. and Thomas, D. P., p. 283. Churchill Livingstone Edinburgh.

[14] TRIPLETT, D. A. (1985). *Hemostasis. A Case Oriented Approach*. Igaku-Schoin, New York & Tokyo.

[15] WALKER, I. D. and DAVIDSON, I. F. (1985). Fibrinolysis. In *Blood Coagulation and Haemostasis. A Practical Guide*. Ed. Thomson, J. M., p. 208. Churchill Livingstone, Edinburgh.

[16] YARDUMIAN, D. A., MACKIE, I. J. and MACHIN, S. J. (1986). Laboratory investigation of platelet function: a review of methodology. *Journal of Clinical Pathology*, **39**, 701.

[17] ZIMMERMAN, T. S. and MEYER, D. (1987). Structure and function of factor VIII and von Willebrand factor. In *Haemostasis and Thrombosis*. Eds. Bloom, A. L. and Thomas, D. P., p. 131. Churchill Livingstone, Edinburgh.

18. Investigation of acute haemostatic failure

(By M. Brozović)

Acute haemostatic failure is a common emergency in surgical, medical and obstetric practice. There is usually no time for complicated tests: all investigations must be simple, quick and reliable. Their significance should be familiar to both the laboratory and the clinical emergency staff. The tests used can be divided into *first-line tests* available at all times and designed to confirm the more common causes of acute haemostatic failure as shown in Table 18.1, and *second-line tests* performed when more time is on hand or in cases where the cause of acute bleeding remains unclear after the first-line screen.

FIRST-LINE TESTS

General notes on first-line tests

First-line coagulation techniques appear deceptively easy, because they require simple apparatus: a water-bath, test tubes, pipettes and stop-watches or a coagulometer. Nevertheless, accurate results are not possible unless particular attention is given to blood collection and processing, selection, preparation and storage of reagents and the use of appropriate controls and standards. To ensure the reliability of local methodology, most laboratories participate in local, national or commercial quality assessment schemes (see p. 35).

Collection of venous blood

Venous blood samples should be obtained whenever possible even from the neonate. Capillary blood tests require careful modification of the techniques, experienced operators and locally established normal ranges; they are not an easy alternative to tests on venous blood.[16]

Blood is withdrawn without undue venous stasis and without frothing, into a plastic syringe fitted with a butterfly or short needle of 19 to 21 SWG for adults and 23 to 25 SWG for young children. The venepuncture must be 'clean'; blood from indwell-

Table 18.1 First-line tests used in investigating acute haemostatic failure.

PT	PTTK	TT	Platelet count	Condition
1. N	N	N	N	Disorder of platelet function Factor XIII deficiency Disorder of vascular haemostasis Normal haemostasis
2. Long	N	N	N	Factor VII deficiency Early oral anticoagulation
3. N	Long	N	N	Factors VIII:C, IX, XI, XII, prekallikrein, HMWK deficiency von Willebrand's disease Circulating anticoagulant
4. Long	Long	N	N	Vitamin K deficiency Oral anticoagulants Factors V, VII, X and II deficiency
5. Long	Long	Long	N	Heparin Liver disease Fibrinogen deficiency Hyperfibrinolysis
6. N	N	N	Low	Thrombocytopenia
7. Long	Long	N	Low	Massive transfusion Liver disease
8. Long	Long	Long	Low	DIC Acute liver disease

N = normal

ing catheters should never be used for tests of haemostasis. For investigation of acute haemostatic failure, 10 ml of citrated blood (9 volumes of blood to 1 volume of 3.13% aqueous trisodium citrate dihydrate or 3.8% aqueous trisodium citrate pentahydrate) are required as well as an appropriate amount of blood taken into a screw-cap container containing dried EDTA so that a full blood count and platelet count can be carried out and a blood film made. The blood is thoroughly mixed with the anticoagulant by inverting the container several times. The samples should be brought to the laboratory as soon as possible. If urgent fibrinolysis tests are contemplated, the blood samples should be kept on crushed ice until delivered to the laboratory.

Preparation of platelet-poor plasma

Platelet-poor plasma (PPP) is prepared by centrifugation at 2000 *g* for 15 min at 4°C (approximately 4000 rpm in a standard bench centrifuge). It should be kept at room temperature if it is to be used for prothrombin time tests, factor VII assays or platelet function testing, and at 4°C for other assays; the testing should preferably be completed within 2 h of collection. The samples may be frozen at −40°C for several weeks without a significant loss of activity for most of the haemostatic components to be assayed.

Control blood samples

Control blood samples, obtained from a healthy subject, are treated as described above. Care should be taken when handling all plasma samples, whether test or control, because of the risk of transmission of hepatitis and HIV. Alternatively, commercial freeze-dried control plasma samples tested for HIV and hepatitis B virus can be used (see also p. 24)

Equipment

Water-baths set at 37°C should have a tolerance of no more than ±0.5°C as temperature markedly affects the speed of clotting reactions. A water-bath with plastic or glass sides is preferable and some type of cross-illumination helps to determine the exact time of appearance of fibrin. At least four stop-watches are needed unless the laboratory is equipped with an automatic coagulometer. Disposable plastic Pasteur pipettes marked at 0.1 and 0.2 ml, or automatic pipettes, are also required.

If coagulometers are used, it is important to ensure that their temperature control and the mechanism for detecting the end-point are functioning properly. Although such instruments reduce observer error when a large number of samples are tested, it is important to apply stringent control to the instrument at all times to ensure accuracy and precision.[4]

Reagents

Some reagents are common to most if not all first-line tests. They are described here, whereas the reagents specific for one test or assay only are described with the details of the relevant test.

CaCl₂. The working solution is best prepared from a commercial molar solution. Small volumes of 0.025 mol/l concentration should be frequently prepared and stored for short periods of time to avoid proliferation of microorganisms. Pre-warmed $CaCl_2$ should always be discarded at the end of the working day.

Kaolin (light). 5 g/l in barbitone buffered saline.

Barbitone buffered saline, pH7.4. See p. 537.

Glyoxaline buffer. Dissolve 2.72 g of glyoxaline (imidazole) and 4.68 g of NaCl in 650 ml of water. Add 148.8 ml of 0.1 mol/l HCl and adjust the pH to 7.4. Adjust the volume to 1 litre with water.

Handling of samples and reagents

All plasma samples should be kept in plastic or siliconized glass tubes and placed on melting ice or at 4°C until used, except when cold activation of factor VII and platelets is to be avoided. The plasma is then kept at room temperature. All pipetting should be performed using disposable plastic pipettes or automatic pipette tips. The actual clotting tests are performed at 37°C in new round-bottom glass tubes of standard size (10 or 12 mm external diameter). Ideally all glassware should be disposable. If the tubes have to be re-used, scrupulous cleaning using chromic acid and a detergent such as 2% Decon 90 is essential.

Eliminating a time trend

The potential instability of biological reagents used in tests of haemostasis makes it desirable to arrange results so as to reduce bias related to time. Thus, if there is a significant length of time between the results with the patient's plasma and the results with the control sample, the difference may be due to the deterioration of one or more of the reagents or of the plasma itself rather than to a true defect or deficiency. In the simplest case, if there are two samples A and B, the readings should be carried out in the order A_1, B_1, B_2, A_2. Additional specimens are allowed for by inserting further letters into the design.[4]

The end-point

The visual properties of a clot depend to some extent on the rate of its formation: the shorter the clotting time the more opaque and easier it is to detect the clot. A slowly forming clot may appear as mere fibrin wisps. In manual work, the observer must try to adopt a uniform convention in selecting the moment in clot formation which will be accepted as the end-point. It is also important to ensure that the tube can be watched with its lower part under the water or while quickly dipped in and out so as to avoid cooling and a slowing down of the clot formation. Bubbles also make the determination of the end-point difficult. In instrumental work the coagulometer must be shown to detect long clotting times reliably and reproducibly.

Some common 'technical' errors

An artefactual prolongation of clotting time occurs in the following situations:

1. Faulty collection of the sample, resulting in it undergoing partial clotting.

2. Excess citrate or insufficient blood so that the volume of citrate in relation to the blood is incorrect.

3. An unsuitable anticoagulant, such as EDTA, used to collect the sample.

4. An unduly high PCV, so that there is less plasma than normal per unit volume of blood and consequently an excess of anticoagulant.

5. A hole in the $CaCl_2$ or other reagent tube may also cause unexpected prolongation in the clotting times.

6. Collection of blood through a line that has at some stage been in contact with heparin. This leads to a marked prolongation of the partial thromboplastin time with kaolin.

7. Incorrect water-bath temperature.

ONE STAGE PROTHROMBIN TIME

Principle. The test measures the clotting time of plasma in the presence of an optimal concentration of tissue extract (thromboplastin) and indicates the overall efficiency of the extrinsic clotting system.[13] Although originally thought to measure prothrombin, the test is now known to depend also on reactions with factors V, VII and X, and on the fibrinogen concentration of the plasma.

Reagents

Patient's and control plasma samples. Platelet-poor plasma from the patient and control (see below) is obtained as described on p. 279. Note that plasma stored at 4°C may have a shortened pro-thrombin times as a result of factor VII activation in the cold.[10]

Thromboplastin. Thromboplastins are tissue ex-tracts obtained from different species and different organs. Because of the potential hazard of slow viral and other infections from handling human brain, its use as a source of thromboplastin is no longer recommended. The majority of thromboplastins now in use are extracts of rabbit brain or lung. Each preparation has a different sensitivity of clotting factor deficiencies and defects, in particular to the defect induced by oral anticoagulants (see Chapter 21, p. 337). In addition, even the same type of thromboplastin may show variation between batches. Whenever possible, a preparation cali-brated against the International Reference Throm-boplastin should be used; a calibrated commercially available thromboplastin will have its International Sensitivity Index (ISI) determined and clearly la-belled. For further details, see p. 339. It is also important to remember that some thromboplastins are not sensitive to an isolated factor VII deficiency. If the manufacturer does not state in the accompanying literature that the reagent is sensitive to factor VII, it is advisable to check whether it is capable of detecting this deficiency by performing a prothrombin time on a known factor-VII-deficient plasma.

CaCl$_2$.0.025 mol/l.

Method

Deliver 0.1 ml of plasma into a glass tube placed in a water-bath and add 0.1 ml of thromboplastin. Wait 1 to 3 min to allow the mixture to warm. Then add 0.1 ml of warmed CaCl$_2$ and mix the contents of the tube. Start the stop-watch and record the end-point. Carry out the test in duplicate on the patient's and control plasma. When a number of samples are to be tested as a batch, the samples and controls must be suitably staggered to eliminate the time bias.

Expression of results

The results are expressed as the mean of the duplicate readings in seconds or as the ratio of the mean patient's time to the mean normal control time. The control value is obtained from 20 normal men and women (non-pregnant and not on oral contraceptives). If the thromboplastin is calibrated in ISI (see p. 337, the results can be expressed as the International Normalized Ratio (INR). This is the ratio which would have been obtained had the International Reference Preparation been used in the test system. For further details and a discussion of the importance of the one-stage prothrombin time test in oral anticoagulant control, see also Chapter 21.

Normal values

Normal values depend on the thromboplastin used, the exact technique and whether visual or instru-mental end-point reading is used. With most rabbit thromboplastins the normal range of the prothrom-bin time is between 11 and 16 s with an INR of 1.0 to 1.3.

Interpretation

The common causes of prolonged one-stage pro-thrombin times when investigating acute haemo-static failure are:

1. The administration of oral anticoagulant drugs.
2. Liver disease, particularly obstructive.
3. Vitamin K deficiency.
4. Disseminated intravascular coagulation.
5. Rarely, a previously undiagnosed factor VII, X, V or prothrombin deficiency or defect (see pp. 302 and 313).

PARTIAL THROMBOPLASTIN TIME WITH KAOLIN (PTTK)[8,12]

This test is also known as the Activated Partial Thromboplastin Time (APTT) and the Kaolin Cephalin Clotting Time (KCCT).

Principle. The test measures the clotting time of plasma after the activation of contact factors but without added tissue thromboplastin, and so indicates the overall efficiency of the intrinsic pathway. To standardize the activation of contact factors, the plasma is first pre-incubated with kaolin. A standardized phospholipid is provided to allow the test to be performed on platelet-poor plasma. The test depends not only on the contact factors and on factors VIII and IX, but also on the reactions with factors X, V, prothrombin and fibrinogen. It is also sensitive to the presence of circulating anticoagulants (inhibitors) and heparin.

Reagents

Platelet-poor plasma from the patient and a control, stored as described previously.

Kaolin. 5 g/l (laboratory grade) in barbitone buffered saline, pH 7.4 (p. 537). Add a few glass beads to aid resuspension. The suspension is stable at room temperature indefinitely. Other surface active insoluble substances such as celite or ellagic acid can also be used.

Phospholipid. Many reagents are available; these contain different phospholipids. Each laboratory should use the reagent it is familiar with. When choosing a phospholipid reagent for the PTTK, it is important to establish that the reagent is sensitive to deficiencies of factors VIII:C, IX and XI at concentrations of 20 to 25 iu/dl[11] and preferably as high as 50 iu/dl. Reagents which fail to detect this reduction in Factor VIII:C are too insensitive for routine use.

CaCl₂. 0.025 mol/l.

Method

Mix equal volumes of the phospholipid reagent and the kaolin suspension and leave in a glass tube in the water-bath at 37°C. Place 0.1 ml of plasma into a new glass tube. Add 0.2 ml of the kaolin-phospholipid solution, mix the contents and start the stop-watch simultaneously. Leave at 37°C for 10 min with occasional shaking. At exactly 10 min add 0.1 ml of pre-warmed CaCl₂ and start a second stop-watch. Record the time taken for the mixture to clot. Repeat the test at least once on both the patient's and the control plasma. It is possible to do

four tests at 2 min intervals if sufficient stop-watches are available.

Expression of results

Express the results as the mean of the paired clotting times.

Normal range

30–40 s. The actual times depend on the reagents used. Whenever possible pooled normal plasma (see p. 301) should be used as a control in preference to a single random plasma sample. The difference between the patient's and the control means should not exceed 6 s. If the difference is greater than 10 s, the patient's plasma is clearly abnormal.

Interpretation

The common causes of a prolonged PTTK in acute haemostatic failure are:

1. Disseminated intravascular coagulation.
2. Liver disease.
3. Massive transfusion with stored blood.
4. Administration of heparin or contamination with heparin.
5. A circulating anticoagulant.

The PTTK is also moderately prolonged in patients on oral anticoagulant drugs and in the presence of vitamin K deficiency. Occasionally, a patient with previously undiagnosed haemophilia or another congenital coagulation disorder presents with a prolonged PTTK (see Chapter 19).

If the patient's PTTK is abnormally long, the equal mixture test must be set up (see below).

Deficiency or circulating anticoagulant?

In cases with a long PTTK, a 50:50 mixture of normal and test plasma should be tested. If the PTTK of the mixture is reduced by more than 50% of the difference between the two individual clotting times, i.e. the normal plasma corrects the prolonged time, the patient probably has a deficiency of one or more clotting factors. If, however, the normal plasma fails to correct, an inhibitor or anticoagulant may be present. For details of testing for inhibitors, see p. 311.

Modifications of the PTTK

Commercial reagents with a recommended incubation time shorter than 10 min are widely available but, while they are more sensitive to the abnormalities of contact factors, they are generally less sensitive to factor VIII:C deficiency than the tests with longer pre-incubation times. For correction tests, see p. 287.

THROMBIN TIME

Principle. Thrombin is added to plasma and the clotting time measured. The thrombin time is affected by the concentration and reaction of fibrinogen, and by the presence of inhibitory substances, including fibrinogen/fibrin degradation products (FDP) and heparin. The clotting time and the appearance of the clot are equally informative.

Reagents

Platelet-poor plasma. From the patient and a control.

Thrombin solution. A commercial bovine thrombin is used. It is stored frozen as a 50 NIH unit solution, and freshly diluted in barbitone buffered saline in a plastic tube so as to give a clotting time of normal plasma of 13–15 s (usually *c* 7–8 NIH thrombin units per ml). Shorter times with normal plasma may fail to detect mild abnormalities.

Method

Place 0.1 ml of barbitone buffered saline, pH 7.4 (p. 537) and 0.1 ml of control plasma in a glass tube at 37°C. Add 0.1 ml of thrombin and start the stop-watch. Measure the clotting time and observe the nature of the clot, e.g. whether transparent or opaque, firm or wispy, etc. Repeat the procedure with two tubes containing patient's plasma in duplicate, and then with a second sample of control plasma. A variation of 1 to 2 s between duplicate samples is not uncommon.

Expression of results

The results are expressed as the mean of the duplicate clotting times in seconds for the control and the test plasma.

Normal range

A patient's thrombin time should be within 2 s of the control. Times of 20 s and over are definitely abnormal.

Interpretation of results

The common causes of prolonged thrombin time are:

1. Hypofibrinogenaemia as found in disseminated intravascular coagulation and, more rarely, in a congenital defect or deficiency.

2. Raised concentrations of FDP, as encountered in disseminated intravascular coagulation or liver disease.

3. Presence of heparin which interferes with the thrombin–fibrinogen reaction. If the presence of heparin is suspected, a Reptilase time test should be carried out (see p. 289).

A transparent bulky clot is found if fibrin polymerization is abnormal, as is the case in liver disease and some congenital dysfibrinogenaemias.

A gross elevation of the plasma fibrinogen concentration may also prolong the thrombin time. Correction can be obtained by diluting the patient's plasma with saline (see p. 289).

As an alternative to the thrombin time, the fibrinogen titre can be estimated.

FIBRINOGEN TITRE (SEMI-QUANTITATIVE ASSAY)[14]

Principle. Serial dilutions of both normal and test plasma sample are clotted with thrombin. The highest dilution in which fibrin clots can be observed are compared.

Reagents

Platelet-poor plasma. From the patient and a control.

Thrombin solution. Freshly reconstituted to 50 NIH units per ml in tris or barbitone buffer, pH 7.4.

Method

Prepare two sets of seven glass tubes. Into each tube place 0.5 ml of barbitone buffered saline, pH 7.4 (p. 537). Add 0.5 ml of control plasma to the first tube of the first set. Mix the contents and transfer 0.5 ml to the second tube, and so on, so as to give final concentrations of plasma from 1 in 2 to 1 in 128. Repeat the procedure with the patient's plasma. Add 0.1 ml of thrombin solution to each tube, mix well and leave undisturbed at 37°C for 15 min. Inspect for the presence of fibrin.

Expression of results

The dilution of plasma in the last tube containing an obvious fibrin clot is noted and the results are expressed as a titre (reciprocal of dilution). Both the control and the patient's titre are reported.

Normal range

Normally fibrin clots are seen in all plasma dilutions up to 1 in 128. A titre of 32 is definitely abnormal, and it is advisable to estimate the fibrinogen concentration by a more accurate method if a titre is 64 or less.

Interpretation

An absence of a fibrin clot in the first few tubes (1 in 2, 1 in 4, etc), but its presence in the subsequent tubes is a typical finding in patients receiving heparin or in samples contaminated with heparin. The fibrinogen titre is insensitive to most dysfibrinogenaemias and to moderate increases in FDP concentration. If a high concentration of FDP is anticipated, its inhibitory effect may be neutralized by adding 0.5 ml of 0.4 mg/ml protamine sulphate to the first tube in place of saline. The titre in the presence and in the absence of protamine sulphate can then be compared. A much higher titre is noted with protamine if FDP are present in the patient's plasma.

Comment

It is important to keep automatic pipettes used for thrombin separate from all the other equipment used in coagulation work in order to avoid contamination. Plastic pipettes and automatic pipette tips must also be discarded immediately after use to prevent contamination.

SECOND-LINE INVESTIGATIONS

Relevant second-line investigations are discussed with each of the possible patterns of abnormalities detected by the first-line tests.

1. PT: normal
   PTTK: normal
   Thrombin time: normal
   Platelet count: normal

If all the first-line investigations are normal in a patient who continues to bleed from the site of injury or after surgery, there are four possible diagnoses:

1. A disorder of platelet function, either congenital or acquired.

2. Factor XIII deficiency.
3. A disorder of vascular haemostasis.
4. Bleeding from a severed or damaged blood vessel or vessels with normal haemostasis.

The second line investigations required in this situation are the bleeding time and the clot solubility test.

THE BLEEDING TIME

Principle. A standard incision is made on the volar surface of the forearm and the time the incision bleeds is measured. Cessation of bleeding indicates the formation of haemostatic plugs which are in turn dependent on an adequate number of platelets and on the ability of the platelets to adhere to the subendothelium and to form aggregates.

STANDARDIZED TEMPLATE METHOD[9]

Materials

Sphygmomanometer.
Cleansing swabs.
Template bleeding time device, such as 'Simplate' (General Diagnostics).
Filter paper 1 mm thick.
Stop-watch.

Method

Place a sphygomomanometer cuff around the patient's arm above the elbow, inflate to 40 mm Hg and keep it at this pressure throughout the test. Clean the volar surface of the forearm with 70% ethanol and choose an area of skin which is devoid of visible superficial veins. Press a sterile metal template with a linear slit 7–8 mm long firmly against the skin and use a scalpel blade with a guard so arranged that the tip of the blade protrudes 1 mm through the template slit. In this way make an incision 6 mm long and 1 mm deep. Modifications of the template and blade are commercially available.

Blot off gently but completely with filter paper at 15 s intervals the blood exuding from the cut. When bleeding has ceased, carefully oppose the edges of the incision and apply an adhesive strip to lessen the risk of keloid formation and an unsightly scar.

Normal range

2.5–9.5 min.

IVY'S METHOD[5]

The test is similar to the template method, but instead of a standardized incision two separate punctures, 5–10 cm apart, are made in quick succession using a disposable lancet. Any micro-

lance with a cutting depth of 2.5 mm and width of just over 1 mm is suitable; it can be inserted to its maximum depth without fear of penetrating too deeply. A source of inaccuracy with Ivy's method is the tendency for the puncture wound to close before bleeding has ceased.

Normal range

2–7 min. Ideally, each laboratory should determine its own normal range.

Interpretation of results

A prolonged bleeding time may be due to:

1. Thrombocytopenia. It is advisable to check the platelet count before carrying out the bleeding time test. Patients with a platelet count below 50 × 10^9/l may have a very long bleeding time and the bleeding may be difficult to arrest.

2. Disorders of platelet function. They may be congenital, such as thrombasthenia, storage pool defect, etc (see p. 295), or acquired, due to drugs, the presence of a paraprotein, or platelet abnormalities per se as in myelodysplastic syndromes.

3. von Willebrand's disease, due to defective platelet adherence to the subendothelium in the absence of a normal amount or of normally functioning von Willebrand factor (vWF) (see Chapter 19, p. 305).

4. Vascular abnormalities, as found in Ehler-Danlos's syndrome, or in pseudoxanthoma elasticum.

5. Occasionally in severe deficiency of factors V and XI.

CLOT SOLUBILITY TEST

Principle. Clots formed in the presence of factor XIII and Ca^{2+} are stable (due to cross-linking) for at least 1 h in 1% monochloracetic acid solution and in 5 mol/l urea, whereas clots formed in the absence of factor XIII dissolve rapidly.

Reagents

Platelet-poor plasma. From the patient and a control.

CaCl₂. 0.025 mol/l.
Monochloracetic acid. 10 g/l.
Urea. 5 mol/l in 9 g/l NaCl.

Method

Place 0.5 ml of the two plasma samples in glass tubes, add an equal volume of $CaCl_2$ solution to each and incubate for 30 min. Tap the tube gently to loosen the clot from the sides of the tube and add 3 ml of monochloracetic acid solution or 5 mol/l urea so that the clot is suspended. Leave at room temperature (*c* 20°C). Inspect the clot at 4 h if monochloracetic acid is used, and at 24 h if urea is used.

Interpretation

The control clot, if normal, shows no sign of dissolving. If the patient's factor XIII concentration is grossly defective (<2% average normal), the clot will completely dissolve. The presence of deficiency or defect must be confirmed by a combination of immunological and functional techniques, such as the incorporation of synthetic radioactive or fluorescein-labelled ester.[15,17]

2. PT: long
   PTTK: normal
   Thrombin time: normal
   Platelet count: normal

This combination of results is only found in:
1. The rare congenital factor VII deficiency.
2. At the start of oral anticoagulant therapy.

Factor VII assay is described in Chapter 19 (p. 302). It is usually possible to establish from the history whether or not the patient has been given oral anticoagulant drugs within the preceding 12 to 36 h.

3. PT: normal
   PTTK: long
   Thrombin time: normal
   Platelet count: normal

An isolated prolonged PTTK is found in:

1. Congenital deficiencies or defects of the intrinsic pathway, i.e. haemophilia A, haemophilia B, and factor XI and factor XII deficiency, as well as in prekallikrein and high molecular weight kininogen deficiencies.

2. von Willebrand's disease, when it is usually associated with a prolonged bleeding time.

3. In the presence of circulating anticoagulants (inhibitors).

4. As the result of the presence of heparin in the sample, either because the patient is on treatment, or because of sample contamination.

The next diagnostic step is to establish whether the patient has a deficiency or an inhibitor by performing the 50:50 mixture test described on p. 311. Mixing tests should be done immediately, followed by the specific assay, as described in Chapter 19, p. 312.

MIXING EXPERIMENTS IN THE PTTK SYSTEM

Principle. Plasma samples found to have a prolonged PTTK are further investigated to define the abnormality by performing mixing or correction tests. Correction of the abnormality by the additive indicates that the reagent must contain the substance deficient in the test sample. An abnormal PTTK is repeated on 50:50 mixtures of a known congenitally deficient plasma and the test plasma, or on 50:50 mixtures of aged/adsorbed plasma and test plasma until correction is obtained and the missing factor identified.

Reagents

Platelet-poor plasma. From the patient and a control.

Plasma deficient in factors VIII, IX and XI. Note that individuals deficient in factor XII, prekallikrein or high molecular weight kininogen rarely if ever bleed despite a prolonged PTTK.

Aged plasma. Platelet-poor plasma from a healthy donor is collected into a one-ninth volume of potassium oxalate (14 g potassium oxalate per litre), and separated under sterile conditions and incubated at 37°C for 2–3 days. The prothrombin time at the end of this time should not exceed 90 s. Volumes of plasma are then delivered into plastic tubes and stored at −40°C. Aged plasma is deficient in factors V and VIII:C.

Adsorbed plasma. Aluminium hydroxide gel (alumina) is prepared by mixing 1 g of moist gel* with 4 ml of water to a smooth suspension. A one-tenth volume of aluminium hydroxide suspension is added to platelet-poor plasma prepared from a healthy subject, mixed and incubated for 2 min at 37°C. The mixture is then centrifuged to sediment the gel. The supernatant plasma is placed in plastic containers and stored at −40°C. It is stable for several weeks. Adsorbed plasma is deficient in factors II (prothrombin), VII, IX and X.

Other reagents, as described under Partial Thromboplastin Time with Kaolin (p. 282).

Method

Perform a PTTK on control, patient's and a known deficient plasma, followed by a PTTK on 50:50 (0.05 ml of each) mixtures of the control and known deficient plasma and of patient's and known deficient plasma. Perform all the tests in duplicate using a balanced order to avoid time bias; or perform a PTTK on mixtures of control, test, aged and adsorbed plasma.

Interpretation

The failure to correct by a plasma with a known congenital defect indicates that the factor missing in the patient is the same as that missing in the known deficient plasma. Correction indicates that the factor missing in the known plasma and that missing in the patient's plasma are not identical. In many instances only a partial correction is possible because the congenitally deficient plasma samples have been stored for long periods of time or are freeze-dried commercially obtained preparations. It is therefore essential always to include a control normal plasma and mixtures with a control normal plasma in every experiment.

The interpretation of mixing tests with aged and adsorbed plasma is shown in Table 18.2.

---

* eg. BDH Ltd.

Table 18.2 Interpretation of mixing experiments with PTTK

PTTK of test plasma corrected with		Interpretation
Aged plasma	Al(OH)$_3$ plasma	
No	Yes	Factor VIII:C deficiency
Yes	No	Factor IX deficiency
Yes	Yes	Factor XI or XII deficiency

4. PT: long
PTTK: long
Thrombin time: normal
Platelet count: normal

The main causes of a prolonged prothrombin and partial thromboplastin time in a patient who is bleeding either from a single site or has a generalized bleeding tendency are:

1. Lack of vitamin K. In this case the prothrombin time is usually relatively more prolonged than is the PTTK.
2. The administration of oral anticoagulant drugs. The prothrombin time is usually more prolonged than is the PTTK.
3. Liver disease.
4. Rare congenital defects of factors V, X, prothrombin, and combined V and VIII:C deficiency.

Mixing experiments using the prothrombin time may be useful if there is no history of anticoagulant therapy and no obvious reason for vitamin K deficiency, e.g. a breast-fed neonate or baby, malabsorption, parenteral feeding, long-term antibiotic treatment etc.

MIXING EXPERIMENTS IN THE PROTHROMBIN TIME SYSTEM

Principle. The test plasma is mixed with aged and adsorbed plasma to establish which factor is lacking.

Reagents

Platelet-poor plasma. From the patient and a control.
Adsorbed plasma. See above.
Aged plasma. See p. 287.
Other reagents. As for prothrombin time.

Table 18.3 Interpretation of mixing experiments using the prothrombin time

PT of test plasma corrected with		Interpretation
Aged plasma	Al (OH)$_3$ plasma	
No	Yes	Factor V deficiency
Yes	No	Factor X or VII deficiency
No	Partial	Prothrombin deficiency

Method

Measure the prothrombin time of 50:50 mixtures of test plasma and control plasma with aged and adsorbed plasma in a balanced order.

Interpretation

The results can be interpreted using Table 18.3.

5. PT: long
   PTTK: long
   Thrombin time: long
   Platelet count: normal

Abnormalities in all three screening tests are found:

1. In the presence of heparin.
2. In hypo- and dys-fibrinogenaemias.
3. In some cases of liver disease.
4. In systemic hyperfibrinolysis.

To distinguish between these conditions, carry out thrombin time correction tests, the Reptilase or ancrod time, and measure the FDP concentration in plasma.

CORRECTION TESTS USING THE THROMBIN TIME

Principle. The tests utilize certain physico-chemical properties of reagents to bind to inhibitors or abnormal molecules and normalize the prolonged thrombin time. Protamine sulphate has a net electro-positive charge and interacts with heparin, as well as binding to FDP, neutralizing the inhibitory effects of both. Toluidine blue is also a charged reagent which will neutralize heparin but has no effect on FDP. Interestingly, toluidine blue normalizes the thrombin time in some dysfibrinogenaemias, probably by interacting with the excess of sialic acid attached to these molecules.

Table 18.4 Interpretation of correction tests using the thrombin time (TT)

TT of test plasma corrected with				Interpretation
Saline	Normal plasma	Protamine sulphate	Toluidine blue	
No	Yes	No	No	Deficiency
Yes	No	No	No	High fibrinogen
No	Var	No	Yes	Dysfibrino-genaemia of liver disease
No	Var	Yes	Yes	High concentration of FDP

Var = variable

Reagents

Patient and control plasma.
Protamine sulphate. 1% and 10% in 9 g/l NaCl.
Toluidine blue. 0.05 g in 100 ml of 9 g/l NaCl.
Bovine thrombin. As described under Thrombin Time (p. 284).

Method

Perform the test as described for Thrombin Time, replacing 0.1 ml of saline in the test with protamine sulphate or toluidine blue solution. Also perform a thrombin time on a 50:50 mixture of control and test plasma.

Interpretation

See Table 18.4.

Comment

The end-point may be difficult to see in samples with a low fibrinogen content in the presence of toluidine blue owing to the dark colour of the reagent. Grossly elevated fibrinogen concentrations or the presence of a paraprotein can cause a prolonged time not corrected by either protamine or toluidine blue; diluting the test plasma in saline will shorten the thrombin time.

REPTILASE OR ANCROD TIME[2]

Reptilase[R], a purified enzyme from the snake *Bothrops atrox,* and ancrod (Arvin), a similar enzyme from the snake *Agkistrodon rhodostoma,* may be used to replace thrombin in the thrombin time test.

The venoms are reconstituted as directed by the manufacturers, and the test is performed exactly as described for the thrombin time. The snake venoms are not inhibited by heparin and will give normal times for the clotting of normal plasma in the presence of heparin. The clotting times will, however, remain prolonged in the presence of raised FDP or abnormal or reduced fibrinogen.

DETECTION OF FIBRINOGEN/FIBRIN DEGRADATION PRODUCTS (FDP) USING A LATEX AGGLUTINATION METHOD[3]

Principle. A suspension of latex particles is sensitized with specific antibodies to the purified FDP fragments D and E. The suspension is mixed on a glass slide with a dilution of the serum to be tested. Aggregation indicates the presence of FDP in the sample. By testing different dilutions of the unknown sample, a semi-quantitative assay can be performed.

Reagents

Venous blood. Collected into a special tube (provided with the kit) containing the antifibrin-olytic agent and thrombin.
*Thrombo-Wellcotest kit.**
Positive and negative controls. Provided by the manufacturer.
Glycine buffer. Part of the kit.

Method

Allow the tube with blood to stand at 37°C until clot retraction commences. Then centrifuge the tube and withdraw the serum for testing.

Make 1 in 5 and 1 in 20 dilutions of serum in glycine buffer. Mix one drop of each serum dilution with one drop of latex suspension on a glass slide. Rock the slide gently for 2 min while looking for macroscopic agglutination. If a positive reaction is observed in the higher dilution, make doubling dilutions from the 1 in 20 dilution until macroscopic agglutination can no longer be seen.

---

* Wellcome Reagents, Beckenham, Kent.

Table 18.5 Interpretation of results obtained with Reptilase or ancrod time and FDP measurement.

| Result of test | | Interpretation |
Reptilase time	FDP level	
normal	normal	Heparin
long	normal	Fibrinogen abnormality
long	high	Hyperfibrinolysis

Interpretation

Agglutination with a 1 in 5 dilution of serum indicates a concentration of FDP in excess of 10 µg/ml; agglutination in a 1 in 20 dilution indicates FDP in excess of 40 µg/ml.

Normal range

Healthy subjects have an FDP concentration less than 10 µg/ml. Concentrations between 10 and 40 µg/ml are found in a variety of conditions including acute venous thrombo-embolism, acute myocardial infarction, severe pneumonia and after major surgery. For detection and measurement of the D-dimer see Chapter 20 (p. 328).

For the interpretation of the second-line investigations in patients giving prolonged thrombin times, see Table 18.5.

6. PT: normal
   PTTK: normal
   Thrombin time: normal
   Platelet count: low

If the only abnormality is a low platelet count, its possible causes must be investigated. The usual approach is to perform an aspirate of bone marrow to exclude acute leukaemia and/or aplastic anaemia. If the number of megakaryocytes in the bone marrow is normal (see also p. 163), further investigations into the nature of the presumed peripheral destruction of platelets are undertaken as described on p. 393.

7. PT: long
   PTTK: long
   Thrombin time: normal
   Platelet count: low

This pattern of abnormalities in the screening tests is found:

1. After massive transfusion with stored blood which contains adequate amounts of fibrinogen, but does not contain factors VIII:C or V, or platelets.

2. In some cases of chronic liver disease, especially cirrhosis.

8. PT: long
   PTTK: long
   Thrombin time: long
   Platelet count: low

All the first-line tests are abnormal in:

1. Acute disseminated intravascular coagulation.

2. Some cases of acute liver necrosis with disseminated intravascular coagulation.

It is only exceptionally necessary to confirm the diagnosis of DIC with additional tests; e.g. by estimating FDP concentration and by carrying out a screening test for the presence of fibrin monomers.

SCREENING TESTS FOR FIBRIN MONOMERS[1,6]

Principle. When thrombin acts on fibrinogen, some of the monomers do not polymerize but give rise to soluble complexes with plasma fibrinogen and FDP. These complexes can be dissociated in vitro by ethanol or protamine sulphate.

Reagents

Platelet-poor plasma. From the patient and a control.
Positive control. This is prepared by adding 0.1 ml of thrombin (0.2 NIH units/ml) to 0.9 ml of control plasma and incubating at 37°C for 30 min. Fibrin threads formed during the incubation are removed by centrifugation.
Protamine sulphate. 1% (10 g/l).
Ethanol. 50% (v/v) in water.

Method

Protamine sulphate test. Add 0.05 ml of protamine sulphate to 0.5 ml of patient's plasma and 0.5 ml of positive control plasma. Incubate undisturbed at 37°C for 30 min. A positive result is indicated by the formation of a fine fibrin network or fibrin strands. The presence of amorphous material only is a negative result.

Ethanol gelation test. Add 0.15 ml of ethanol to 0.5 ml of patient's plasma and to 0.5 ml of the positive control plasma at room temperature (c 20°C). After gentle agitation, inspect the tubes at 1 min intervals. A positive result is the formation of a definite gel within 3 min.

Interpretation

Positive gelation tests are found in:

1. The early stages of acute disseminated intravascular coagulation.
2. After major surgery.
3. Severe inflammatory illness, in particular lobar pneumonia.
4. Liver disease.

TESTS USED FOR MONITORING THE THERAPY OF ACUTE HAEMOSTATIC FAILURE

The tests commonly used to monitor the effects of replacement or drug therapy are shown in Table 18.6.

Table 18.6 Tests used for monitoring the therapy of acute haemostatic failure

Cause of haemostatic failure	Test of choice	Therapy	Earliest time of improvement
DIC	TT or PT	FFP or blood	30–60 min
Massive transfusion	PTTK, PT	FFP	immediate
Vit K deficiency	PT	FFP	immediate
	PT	Vit K	6–8 h
Heparin	PTTK	protamine	immediate

TT = thrombin time. PT = prothrombin time.
PTTK = partial thromboplastin time with kaolin.
FFP = fresh frozen plasma.

REFERENCES

[1] BREEN, F. A. Jnr and TULLIS, J. L. (1968). Ethanol gelation: a rapid screening test for intravascular coagulation. *Annals of Internal Medicine*, **69**, 1197.

[2] FUNK, C., GMUR, J., HEROLD, R. and STRAUB, P. W. (1971). Reptilase-R—a new reagent in blood coagulation. *British Journal of Haematology*, **21**, 43.

[3] GARVEY, M. B. and BLACK, J. M. (1972). The detection of fibrinogen/fibrin degradation products by means of a new antibody coated latex particle. *Journal of Clinical Pathology*, **25**, 680.

[4] INGRAM, G. I. C., BROZOVIC, M. and SLATER, N. (1982). *Bleeding Disorders*, p. 243. Blackwell Scientific Publications, Oxford.

[5] IVY, A. C., NELSON, D. and BUCHER, G. (1940). The standardization of certain factors in the cutaneous 'venostasis' bleeding time technique. *Journal of Laboratory and Clinical Medicine*, **26**, 1812.

[6] LIPINSKI, B. and WOROWSKI, K. (1969). Detection of soluble fibrin monomer complexes in blood by means of protamine sulphate test. *Thrombosis et Diathesis Haemorrhagica*, **20**, 44.

[7] LORAND, L., SIEFRING, G. E. Jnr, TONG, Y. S., BRUNER LORAND, J. and GRAY, A. J. Jnr (1979). Dansylcadaverine specific staining for transamidase enzymes. *Analytical Biochemistry*, **93**, 453.

[8] MACPHERSON, J. C. and HARDISTY, R.M. (1961). A modified thromboplastin screening test. *Thrombosis et Diathesis Haemorrhagica*, **6**, 492.

[9] MIELKE, C. H., KENESHIRO, M. M., MAHER, I. A., WIENER, J. M. and RAPAPORT, S. I. (1969). The standardized normal Ivy bleeding time and its prolongation by aspirin. *Blood*, **34**, 204.

[10] MILLER, G. J., SEGATCHIAN, M. J., WALTER, S. J. et al (1986). An association between the factor VII coagulant activity and thrombin activity induced by surface/cold exposure of normal human plasma. *British Journal of Haematology*, **62**, 379.

[11] O'BRIEN, P. F. NORTH W. R. S. and INGRAM, G. I. C. (1981). The diagnosis of mild haemophilia by the partial thromboplastin time. WFH/ICTH study of the Manchester method. *Thrombosis and Haemostasis*, **45**, 162.

[12] PROCTOR, R. R. and RAPAPORT, S. I. (1961). The partial thromboplastin time with kaolin. A simple screening test for first stage plasma clotting factor deficiencies. *American Journal of Clinical Pathology*, **36**, 212.

[13] QUICK, A. J. (1942). *The Hemorrhagic Diseases and the Physiology of Hemostasis*. Thomas, Illinois.

[14] SHARP, A. A., HOWIE B., BIGGS, R. and METHUEN, D. T. (1958). Defibrination syndrome in pregnancy: value of various diagnostic tests. *Lancet*, **ii**, 1309.

[15] STENBERG, P. and STENFLO, J. (1979). A rapid and specific fluorescent activity staining procedure for transamidating enzymes. *Analytical Biochemistry*, **93**, 445.

[16] STUART, J. PICKEN, A. M., BREEZE, G. R. and WOOD, B. S. B. (1973). Capillary blood coagulation profile in the newborn. *Lancet*, **ii**, 1467.

[17] TYLER, H. M. (1966). A comparative study of the solvents commonly used to detect fibrin stabilization. *Thrombosis et Diathesis Haemorhagica*, **16**, 61.

19. Investigation of a bleeding tendency

(By M. Brozović and I. Mackie)

A chronic or insidious bleeding tendency, whether inherited or acquired is a relatively uncommon condition. It rarely causes acute haemorrhage unless the patient is subjected to surgical or accidental trauma. Comprehensive clinical evaluation, including the patient's history, the family history and the family tree, as well as the details of the site, frequency and the character of haemorrhagic manifestations (purpura, bruising, large haematomata, haemarthroses, etc), is required to establish a definitive diagnosis. It is also desirable to undertake a series of screening tests before proceeding to more specific tests. The results of the screening investigations, taken in conjunction with clinical information, usually point to the additional appropriate method of analysis.

The common patterns of results obtained on screening investigations are shown in Table 19.1.

INVESTIGATION OF A SUSPECTED DISORDER OF PLATELET FUNCTION, INHERITED OR ACQUIRED

(For investigation assays of von Willebrand's disease, see p. 305; for diagnosis of thrombocytopenia, see p. 58).

Abnormalities of platelet function all lead to signs and symptoms characteristic of defects of primary haemostasis: bleeding into the mucous membranes and small skin ecchymoses. The patient may also suffer from abnormal intra-operative bleeding and oozing from small cuts or wounds. The usual sequence of investigation is shown in Table 19.2. in the form of a flow chart.

PLATELET AGGREGATION[4,5,7,18,19]

Principle. The absorbence of platelet-rich plasma falls as platelets aggregate. The amount and the rate of fall are dependent on platelet reactivity to the added agonist if other variables, such as

Table 19.1 Common patterns of the results of screening tests in patients with chronic bleeding tendency

PT	PTTK	TT	Bleeding time	Conditions
N	N	N	L	Platelet dysfunction, disorders of vascular haemostasis
N	L	N	L*	von Willebrand's disease (vWD)
L	N	N	N	Factor VII deficiency
N	L	N	N	Factor VIII:C deficiency, vWD, factor IX deficiency, factor XI, XII, PK or HMWK deficiency, circulating anticoagulants
L	L	N	N	Factor V, factor X or prothrombin deficiency, liver disease
L	L	L	N	Deficiency or defect of fibrinogen

* Occasionally found in severe factors XI and V deficiency. L: prolonged. N: normal. PK: prekallikrein. HMWK: high molecular weight kininogen.

temperature, platelet count and mixing speed are controlled. The absorbence changes are monitored on a chart recorder, using a technique originally developed by Born.[4,5]

Reagents

Test and control platelet-rich plasma. The patient and control should be off all drugs, beverages and foods which may affect aggregation for at least 10 days (see Chapter 17, p. 274) and preferably should have fasted as the presence of chylomicra may also disturb the aggregation patterns. Twenty ml of venous blood are collected with minimal venous occlusion and added to a one-tenth volume of 3.13% or 3.8% trisodium citrate (see p. 280) contained in a plastic or siliconized container. The blood should not be chilled because cold activates platelets. Platelet-rich plasma (PRP) is obtained by centrifuging at room temperature (c 20°C) for 10–15 min at 150–200 g. The PRP is carefully removed, avoiding contamination with red cells or buffy coat, and placed in a stoppered plastic tube. PRP should be stored at room temperature until tested and is stable for about 3 h. It is important test all samples after a similar interval of time (say

1 h) and to store them at the same temperature in order to minimize variation.

Test and control platelet-poor plasma (PPP). The remaining blood is centrifuged at 2000 g for 20 min to obtain platelet-poor plasma (PPP).

Standardization of PRP. A platelet count is performed on the PRP. The number of platelets will influence aggregation responses if the count falls outside 200–400 × 10^9/l. For very high PRP counts, the count should be adjusted by diluting the PRP in the patient's PPP. Platelet counts below 200×10^9/l give rise to diminished aggregation responses. Further centrifugation of PRP is not recommended because it induces platelet activation. The control PRP should be diluted to the same count and tested as a comparison.

PRP should always be stored in tightly stoppered tubes which are filled nearly to the top, to avoid changes in pH which also affect platelet aggregation and tests of nucleotide release.

Aggregating agents. The five aggregating agents listed below should be sufficient for the diagnosis of most functional disorders. For research purposes and when investigating unusual kindreds, other agonists listed in Table 17.7. may also be used.

ADP. The anhydrous sodium salt of adenosine 5-diphosphate is used. A stock solution is prepared by dissolving 4.93 mg of the trisodium salt or 4.71 mg of the disodium salt in 10 ml of 9 g/l NaCl, pH 6.8. This makes a 1 mmol/l solution. It is stored in 0.5 ml volumes at – 40°C until use and remains stable for up to 3 months at this temperature. Once thawed, the solution must be used within 3 h and then discarded. For aggregation testing, prepare 100, 50, 25 and 10 μmol/l solutions as shown in Table 19.2.

Collagen (Hormon-Chemie, Munich). This is a 1 mg/ml stock solution. For use it is diluted in the buffer supplied with the collagen or in 5% dextrose to obtain concentrations of 10 and 40 μg/l. The final concentrations achieved in PRP will be 1 and 4 μg/ml.

Ristocetin sulphate (H. Lundbeck, Copenhagen). Each vial contains 100 mg of ristocetin and should be stored at 4°C until dissolved; 8 ml of 9 g/l NaCl are added to each vial so as to obtain a 12.5 mg/ml solution. This is then stored at – 40°C in 0.5 ml

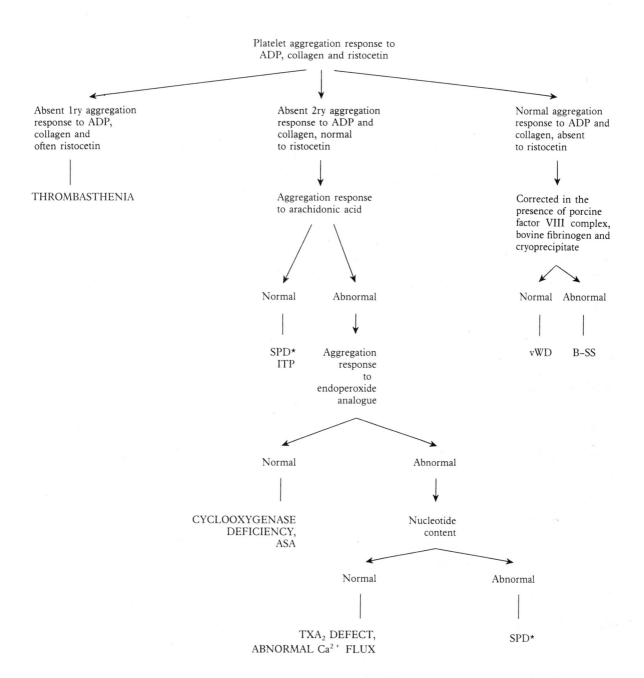

Fig. 19.1 Flow chart for investigation of suspected platelet dysfunction. SPD: storage pool defect. ITP: coating of platelets by auto-antibodies in idiopathic thrombocytopenic purpura. vWD: von Willebrand's disease. B-SS: Bernard Soulier syndrome. ASA: effect of aspirin ingestion. *some cases.

Table 19.2 Platelet aggregation test: dilutions used with various aggregating reagents

Agonist	Stock solution	Working concentration	Final concentration
ADP	1 mmol/l in saline pH 6.8	100, 50, 25, 10 and 5 μmol/l in saline	10, 5, 2.5 and 1 μmol/l
Collagen	1 mg/ml	10, 40 μg/ml in buffer*	1, 4 μg/ml
Ristocetin sulphate	12·5 mg/ml (add 8 ml saline) 10 mg/ml (add 10 ml saline) 5 mg/ml (add 20 ml saline)		1.2 mg/ml 1.0 mg/ml 0.5 mg/ml
Arachidonic acid	20 mmol/l (add 1·5 ml water to 10 mg vial)	5 and 10 mmol/l in saline	50 and 100 μmol/l
Adrenaline	1 mmol/l in water with 0.1% sodium bisulphite	20, 200 μmol/l in saline with 0.1% sodium bisulphite	2, 20 μmol/l

* provided by the manufacturers.
Saline = 9 g/l NaCl.

volumes until used. Ristocetin may be refrozen after use. It should never be used in concentrations of greater than 1.4 mg/ml as protein precipitation may occur in plasma and give rise to false results.

Arachidonic acid. Na-salt, 99% pure. The contents of a 10 mg vial are dissolved in 1.5 ml of sterile water by gentle mixing to give a 20 mmol/l stock solution. This may be frozen in 0.5 ml volumes at −20°C for later use. A working solution is prepared by making doubling dilutions of the stock in saline to give 5 and 10 mmol/l solutions.

Adrenaline. l-epinephrine bitartrate. 3.33 mg are dissolved in 10 ml of water to prepare a 1 mmol/l stock solution. It is stored in 0.5 ml volumes at −40°C. 20 and 200 μmol/l solutions are prepared for use in barbitone buffered saline, pH 7.4.
All aggregation reagents should be kept on ice until used.

Method

Centrifugation may cause cellular release of ADP and platelet refractoriness to aggregation, and the actual aggregation test should not be started within 30 min of preparing the PRP. However, the tests should be completed within 3 h and whenever possible within 2 h of preparing the PRP. Platelets left standing at room temperature (c 20°C) become increasingly reactive to adrenaline and in some cases to collagen; the rate of change increases after 3 h.

Switch the aggregometer on about 30 min before the tests are to be performed to allow the heating block to warm up to 37°C. Set the stirring speed to 900 rpm. Pipette the appropriate volume of PRP, usually 270 μl (this varies depending on the make of the aggregometer used), into a plastic tube or cuvette. Place the tube in the heating block. After 1 min insert the stirrer into the plasma. Set the transmission to 0 on the chart recorder. Replace with a cuvette containing 300 μl of PPP and set the transmission to 100%. Repeat this procedure until no further adjustments are needed and the pen traverses most of the width of the chart paper in response to the difference in absorbence between the PRP and PPP.

Allow the PRP to warm up to 37°C for 2 min and then add 30 μl of the agonist. Record the change in absorbence until the response reaches a plateau or for 3 min (whichever is sooner). Repeat this procedure for each agonist. The starting concentration for each agonist is underlined in Table 19.2. If no release is obtained, increase the concentration until a satisfactory response is obtained.

Interpretation

Normal platelet aggregation curves are shown in Fig. 19.2.

ADP. Low concentrations of ADP (<0·5 to 2·5 μmol/l) cause primary or reversible aggregation. First, ADP binds to a membrane receptor and releases Ca^{2+} ions. A reversible complex with extracellular fibrinogen forms and the platelets undergo a shape change reflected by a slight increase in absorbance. After this, the bound fibrinogen adds to the cell-to-cell contact and reversible aggregation occurs. At very low concentrations of ADP, platelets may disaggregate after the first phase. In the presence of higher concentrations of ADP an irreversible secondary wave aggregation is

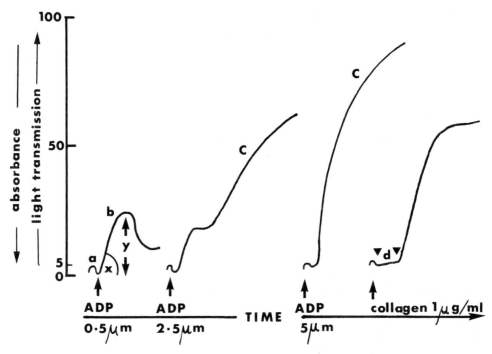

Fig. 19.2   Traces obtained during the aggregation of platelet-rich plasma. a: shape change, b: primary wave aggregation. c: secondary wave aggregation. x°: angle of the initial aggregation slope. y: height of the aggregation trace. d: lag phase. μm = μmol/l Reproduced with the permission of authors and publisher from Yardumian et al.[18]

associated with the release of dense and α granules due to activation of the arachidonic acid pathway. If only high doses of ADP are used, defects in the primary wave (measuring the second pathway described on p. 269) will be missed.

Collagen. The aggregation response to collagen is preceded by a short 'lag' phase lasting between 10 and 60 s. The duration of the lag phase is inversely proportional to the concentration of collagen used and to the responsiveness of the platelets tested. This phase is succeeded by a single wave of aggregation due to the activation of the arachidonic acid pathway and the release of the granules. Higher doses of collagen (>2 μg/ml) cause a sudden increase in intra-platelet calcium concentration and this may bring about the release reaction without activating the prostaglandin pathway. Collagen responses should therefore always be measured using 1 and 4 μg/ml concentrations.

Ristocetin. Ristocetin reacts with vWF and the membrane receptor to induce platelets to clump together ('agglutination'). It does not activate any of the three aggregation pathways and does not initially cause granule release. The response is assessed on the basis of the angle of the initial slope. The platelet response to 1.2 mg/ml is initially studied. Concentrations above 1.4 mg/ml may cause nonspecific platelet 'agglutination' due to an interaction between ristocetin and fibrinogen and protein precipitation. For a detailed discussion on ristocetin 'agglutination' in von Willebrand's disease, see p. 308.

Arachidonic acid. Arachidonic acid induces thromboxane A_2 generation and granule release even if there is a defect of agonist binding to the surface membrane or of the phospholipase-induced release of endogenous arachidonate. If steps further along the pathway are impaired, such as absence or inhibition of cyclooxygenase, arachidonic acid will not produce normal aggregation.

Adrenaline. No shape change precedes aggregation, but the response thereafter resembles the ADP response. Such a response is usually obtained with concentrations of 2–10 μmol/ml. Some clinically normal people have severely reduced responses to adrenaline.[17]

Table 19.3 Differential diagnosis of disorders of platelet function

Condition	Platelet		ADP	Aggregation with			
	Count	Size		Col	Ri	AA	FVIII
Thrombasthenia	N	N	0	0	Ab	0	Ab
Bernard-Soulier syndrome	L	Large	N	N	0	N	0
Storage pool defect	N	N	1	Ab	1/0	1/0	1/0
Cyclooxygenase deficiency	N	N	1/N	Ab	N	Ab	–
Thromboxane synthetase deficiency	N	N	1/N	Ab	N	Ab	–
Aspirin ingestion	N	N	1	Ab	N/Ab	Ab	N/Ab
Ehler-Danlos syndrome	N	N	N	Ab	N	N	–
von Willebrand disease	N	N	N	N	0	N	N

N: normal. 0: absent. 1: primary wave only. Ab: abnormal. Col: collagen. Ri: ristocetin. AA: arachidonic acid. FVIII: porcine factor VIII complex/bovine fibrinogen.
Note that many other defects, such as found in oculo-cutaneous albinism, Chediak-Higashi syndrome, grey platelet syndrome, etc, have also been described.

The pattern of responses in various disorders of platelet function is shown in Table 19.3. For a discussion of hyperaggregability, see Chapter 20, p. 328)

Calculation of results[18,19]

Results can be expressed in one of three ways:

1. As a percentage fall in absorbence measured at 3 min after the addition of an agonist (see Fig. 19.2, y). This does not provide any information on the shape of the curve.

2. By the initial slope of the aggregation tracing (see Fig. 19.2, x°). This indicates the rate of aggregation but does not show whether or not secondary aggregation has occurred.

3. By the minimum amount of agonist required to induce a secondary response.

Normal range

The platelets of normal subjects usually produce a single reversible primary wave with 1 μmol/l ADP or less, biphasic aggregation with ADP at 2.5 μmol/l, and a single irreversible wave at 5 or 10 μmol/l. A single phase response is observed after a lag phase lasting not more than 1 min with 1 and 4 μg/ml of collagen. A single phase or biphasic response is seen with 1.2 mg/ml of ristocetin and after 50 and 100 μmol/l of arachidonic acid. Biphasic aggregation is observed with 2–10 μmol/l of adrenaline.

Some common technical problems associated with platelet aggregation are shown in Table 19.4.

Table 19.4 Technical factors which may influence platelet aggregation tests

Centrifugation. At room temperature, *not* at 4°C. Should be sufficient to remove red cells and white cells but not the largest platelets.

Time. For 30 min after the preparation of PRP, platelets are refractory to the effect of agonists. Progressive increase in reactiveness occurs thereafter, more marked from 2 h onward.

Platelet count. Slow and weak aggregation observed with platelet counts below 150 or over 400 × 10⁹/l.

pH. <7.7 inhibits aggregation; pH >8.0 enhances aggregation.

Mixing speed. <800 rpm or >1200 rpm slows aggregation.

Haematocrit. >0.55 is associated with less aggregation, especially in the 2ry phase due to the increased concentration of citrate in PRP. It may also be difficult to obtain enough PPP. Centrifuging twice may help.

Temperature. <35°C causes decreased aggregation except to low dose ADP which may be enhanced.

Dirty cuvette. May cause spontaneous platelet aggregation or interfere with the optics of the system.

Air bubbles in the cuvette. Cause large irregular oscillations even before the addition of agonists.

No stir bar. No response to any agonist obtained.

FURTHER INVESTIGATION OF PLATELET FUNCTION

If an abnormal aggregation pattern is observed it is advisable to check the assessment on at least one further occasion. If the aggregation tests are persistently abnormal, and the patient is not taking any drugs or substances known to interfere with platelet function, the following tests should be done (see also Fig 19.1 and Table 19.3):

1. If thrombasthenia or the Bernard-Soulier syndrome is suspected, an analysis of membrane glycoproteins is necessary.

2. If a release abnormality is suspected, additional agonists including synthetic endoperoxide analogues and calcium ionophores should be used in testing for aggregation. In addition, the total adenine nucleotide content of the platelets and the amount released after maximal stimulation should be measured using a firefly bioluminescence technique.[8,19]

3. Whenever possible electron microscopic studies of platelet ultrastructure should be carried out.

4. Factor VIII:C, vWF:Ag and ristocetin cofactor assay should be carried out on all patients investigated for an abnormality of platelet function who show abnormal ristocetin 'agglutination', or in whom all platelet function tests are normal.

5. Plasma assays of β-thromboglobulin and platelet factor 4 are described in Chapter 20 (p. 328) as tests of hypercoagulability. They are also used to detect α-granule deficiency states, such as the grey platelet syndrome.

THE PROTHROMBIN CONSUMPTION INDEX (PCI)

Principle. During normal coagulation, prothrombin consumption and thrombin production continue after the blood or plasma has clotted. If the serum is tested 1 h after coagulation, it will be found that practically all the prothrombin has been 'consumed'. If there is a deficiency of any of the factors required for the coagulation of blood or plasma in glass, the prothrombin will be incompletely consumed and more than normal will be present in the serum 1 h after coagulation. This is so even if the blood or plasma clots in the normal time.

The PCI is a non-specific test of overall coagulation. If the coagulation factors are quantitatively and qualitatively normal, the PCI can be taken as a measure of the contribution of platelets to coagulation, or the 'coagulant' activity of platelets.

Reagents

Platelet-poor plasma. From the patient and a control.

Serum. 1 ml of patient's and control blood are delivered into standard glass clotting tubes, kept at 37°C and the serum separated 1 h after the blood has clotted. If the PCI cannot be done immediately, the serum may be citrated with a one-ninth volume of 3.13 g/l trisodium citrate dihydrate.

Rabbit thromboplastin.

Calcium chloride. 0.025 mol/l.

Bovine fibrinogen. 1.5–2.0 g/l.

Method

Place the $CaCl_2$ and the fibrinogen solution in a 37°C water-bath. Pipette into a glass clotting tube 0.1 ml of thromboplastin and 0.1 ml of plasma. Warm at 37°C. Add 0.1 ml of $CaCl_2$. Start a stop-watch and mix. After exactly 60 s sub-sample 0.1 ml of the mixture into 0.4 ml of pre-warmed bovine fibrinogen, start a second stop-watch and record the clotting time. At a time after recalcification of the plasma corresponding to the prothrombin time, the plasma will clot. This clot has to be removed on a swab stick (by slowly turning it inside the tube) before sub-sampling.

Repeat the procedure using the serum. In this instance there will be no clot to remove before sub-sampling, except in some cases of severe haemophilia.

Results

The relationship between the plasma and serum clotting times is expressed as an index:

$$PCI(\%) = \frac{\text{plasma clotting time}}{\text{serum clotting time}} \times 100.$$

Normal range

0–10%.

Interpretation

Note that normal values are low. In the absence of a coagulation factor defect or deficiency, a high PCI implies a defect in platelet procoagulant activity.

INVESTIGATION OF A BLEEDING DISORDER DUE TO A COAGULATION FACTOR DEFICIENCY OR DEFECT

When the screening tests indicate that an individual has a coagulation defect, the plasma concentration of the coagulation factors should be assayed. Such assays not only establish the diagnosis of the deficiency or defect, they also assess its severity, and can be used to monitor replacement therapy and to detect the carrier state in families in which one or more members are affected by a congenital bleeding disorder.

Assays of coagulation factors (whether functional or immunological) are discussed in subsequent pages according to the abnormality found in the screening tests. Assays used to diagnose the cause of an isolated long one-stage prothrombin time are presented first; those used to elucidate a long PTTK are discussed next, and so on. The general principles of coagulation assays and the standards used are reviewed first. Techniques for detecting inhibitors are presented next. Finally, the methods used for detecting carriers are reviewed and there is a general discussion on assays used to monitor replacement therapy.

An individual may have a deficiency of a coagulation factor because of impaired synthesis or because a variant of the molecule is synthesized which is deficient in clotting activity. In both instances the results of assays based on coagulation tests will be subnormal, but when a variant molecule is being produced, the result of an immunological assay may be normal or near normal. In many congenital bleeding disorders, immunological assays form an important part of the diagnostic procedure and of management.

GENERAL PRINCIPLES OF PARALLEL LINE BIOASSAYS OF COAGULATION FACTORS.[1,12]

If two materials containing the same coagulation factor are assayed in a specific assay system in a range of dilutions, and the clotting times are plotted against the plasma concentration on linear graph paper, curved dose response lines are obtained. If the plot is redrawn on double-log paper, a sigmoid curve with a straight middle section is obtained (Fig. 19.3).

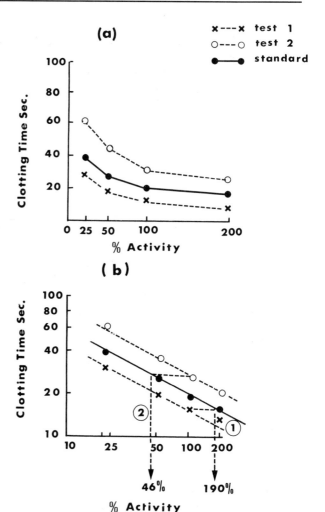

Fig. 19.3   Parallel line bioassay of factor VII. a) Clotting times with 1 in 5, 1 in 10, 1 in 20 and 1 in 40 dilutions of test and standard plasma plotted on linear graph paper. b) The same data plotted on double log paper. Three parallel straight lines are obtained. The horizontal shift of the test line represents the difference in potency. In this case test 1 has a potency of 190% and test 2 a potency of 46%.

If the dilutions of the test and standard materials are chosen carefully, it should be possible to draw two straight parallel lines. The horizontal distance between the two lines represents the difference in potency ('strength' or concentration) of the factor assayed. If the test line is to the right of the standard it contains less of the factor than the standard; if to the left, it contains more.

When setting up and performing a parallel line assay, a number of measures must be taken to ensure that the assay is valid and reliable.

1. *Dilution range.* This should be chosen so that the coagulation times lie on the linear portion of the sigmoid curve. For example, when assaying factor VIII:C by one-stage assay, dilutions giving times between 60 and 100 s are chosen if the blank clotting time is over 120 s. (The blank consists of a mixture of buffer and substrate or deficient plasma which provides all factors except the one to be measured.)

2. *Number of dilutions.* At least three dilutions of the standard and at least two dilutions of the test are assayed to give the best graphical or mathematical solution.

3. *Responses.* Dilutions of the test sample should be chosen so that the clotting times fall within the range obtained for the standard. The standard curve should not be extrapolated beyond this range.

4. *Duplicates and replicates.* Duplicates are obtained from the same dilution of the sample and sometimes by sub-sampling from the same incubation mixture. Replicates are true repeats involving a fresh dilution and fresh reagents. Normally, coagulation times are measured on duplicates. Replicates are sometimes used for particularly difficult assays.

5. *Temporal drift.* This has already been discussed in Chapter 18, p. 281. Duplicates in a coagulation assay should always be tested in a balanced order, e.g. ABCCBA.

Standard plasma

The use of a suitable standard is crucial for an accurate assay. The concentration of some coagulation factors may vary as much as fourfold in different normal plasma samples and it is therefore inadvisable to use plasma from any one person as representing 100% clotting activity. A normal plasma pool is the only satisfactory standard for coagulation factor assays. The larger the number of donors in the pool, the more likely the pool clotting activity will be *c* 100% or 100 units/dl.

Collection of blood samples and preparation of the pool. Add 9 volumes of venous blood to 1 volume of citrate (see p. 279). Prepare platelet-poor plasma by centrifuging at 2000 *g* for 15 min. Remove the supernatant carefully without disturbing the buffy coat or red cells. Pool the plasma samples in a plastic container and store in 1.0 ml volumes frozen, preferably at $-40°C$ or below.

Most pools are made from between 6 and 40 donors. Larger pools are preferable and it is best to include individuals of both sexes, aged between 20 and 60. Women taking oestrogen-containing oral contraceptives should not contribute to the standard pool.

Calibration of standard pools. Whenever possible, the normal pool should be calibrated against a freeze-dried reference material already calibrated against the international standard. The reference material may be a national standard or a commercial standard. The international standards and reference preparations for factor VIII:C, vWF:Ag and factor IX are available from the National Institute of Biological Standards and Control, Potters Bar, England, which holds them on behalf of the WHO.

In the absence of reference materials the laboratory should follow the procedure set out below to calibrate its own normal pool and assign it a value of 100 u/dl.

Suggested calibration procedure. The most important principle of calibration is repetition needed to minimize possible errors at each stage of calibration. It is necessary to carry out at least four independent assays, and preferably six. An independent assay is an assay for which a new ampoule of standard is opened, or if a freeze-dried standard is not available, for which a new set of dilutions are prepared from frozen or fresh previous reference plasma. Each plasma must be tested in duplicate; two replicate assays should be carried out each day, and the procedure repeated on at least 4 days (four independent assays). Whenever possible more than one operator should be involved.

Comparison should always be made with the previous normal pool. The potency of the new normal pool is calculated for each replicate assay on each day and an overall mean value calculated. The calibration also enables an assessment of the precision of the method used.

Calculation of results

The results can be worked out graphically or mathematically. For a graphical solution, mean values for duplicate clotting times are plotted against the dilutions on double-log paper. The dilutions are converted to decimals; the lowest dilution of the standard is assigned a value of 100% or 1.0 (see Fig. 19.3). Best-fit lines (Fig 19.3) are drawn through each set of points. Non-parallel or grossly curved lines indicate an invalid assay and should be discarded (see p. 304). To obtain the actual potency of the test sample in terms of the standard, a horizontal line is drawn through both dose response lines to cut the test sample line where it crosses 1.0 or 100%. A vertical line is then dropped on to the concentration axis and the relative potency of the test sample read directly off the concentration scale.

Mathematical solutions are better than graphical ones, as they provide exact criteria for parallelism and curvature. Computer or calculator programmes can be used to calculate the results.

Variability of coagulation assays

Within one laboratory, variability is most commonly due to a dilution error, differences in the composition of reagents, failure to take the time-trend into account, and because of differences in experience and technique between operators. A coefficient of variation of 15–20% is not uncommon for factor VIII:C assay. Furthermore, the variability increases if like is not compared to like: e.g. if concentrate preparations are assayed against plasma.

Variability between laboratories is much higher. Apart from the factors described for the within-laboratory variability, there is the major effect of differences in methods and in the composition of reagents. Comparability between laboratories improves if standardized reagents are used.

The unavoidable variability associated with coagulation assays makes the use of reliable reference materials imperative.

INVESTIGATION OF A SUSPECTED FACTOR VII DEFICIENCY OR DEFECT

The investigation of an isolated prolonged one-stage prothrombin time in an individual with a life-long history of bleeding includes a one-stage factor VII assay. If a reduced concentration of factor VII is found, further tests should include immuno-assays of factor VII and whenever possible a family study.

ONE-STAGE ASSAY OF FACTOR VII[7]

Principle. The assay of factor VII is based on the prothrombin time. The assay compares the ability of dilutions of the patient's plasma and of a standard plasma to correct the prothrombin time of a substrate plasma.

Reagents

Platelet-poor plasma from the patient.
Standard plasma. (For details see p. 301).
Factor VII deficient plasma. Commercial or from a patient with known severe deficiency. Plasma from dogs with severe congenital deficiency can also be used.

Barbitone buffered saline. (See p. 537.)
Thromboplastin. Rabbit brain thromboplastin known to be sensitive to factor VII deficiency (see p. 282). The thromboplastin should be diluted 1 in 20 in buffered saline.
CaCl$_2$. 0.025 mol/l.

Method

Prepare 1 in 5, 1 in 10, 1 in 20 and 1 in 40 dilutions of the standard and test plasma in buffered saline. Transfer 0.1 ml of each dilution to a glass tube and add to it 0.1 ml of deficient (substrate) plasma, and 0.1 ml of dilute thromboplastin. Mix and allow to warm to 37°C. Add 0.1 ml of CaCl$_2$ and start the stop-watch. Record the clotting time. A blank must be included with every assay and all tests carried out in duplicate, and in balanced order.

Calculation of results

Plot the clotting times of the test and standard against the concentration of factor VII on 3 cycle × 2 cycle log paper. Read the concentration as shown in Fig. 19.3. (Some automated coagulometers produce computed values using mathematical formulae).

Normal range

50–200 u/dl (for discussion of units see p. 301).

Interpretation

Patients with a congenital deficiency have factor VII levels of 30 u/dl and less. The concentration measured varies according to the thromboplastin used in the assay. A small proportion of patients have normal factor VII antigen despite abnormal functional activity.

INVESTIGATION OF A PATIENT WITH A SUSPECTED INTRINSIC PATHWAY DEFICIENCY OR DEFECT

An isolated prolongation of the PTTK in a patient with a lifelong bleeding disorder may be due to a deficiency or defect of one the following factors: factor VIII:C or vWF, factor IX or factor XI. Individuals with factor XII, prekallikrein and HMWK deficiencies do not usually bleed and the prolonged PTTK is most often an accidental finding. The first step would be to carry out mixing experiments in order to discover which factor is lacking (see p. 287) and whether an inhibitor is present (see Fig. 19.4). The missing factor should then be estimated quantitatively using a coagulation assay. Further tests may become necessary to elucidate the nature of the disorder.

ONE-STAGE ASSAY OF FACTOR VIII:C[7,11,12]

Principle. The one-stage assay for factor VIII:C is based on the PTTK. It consists of comparing the ability of dilutions of the patient's plasma and of a standard plasma to correct the PTTK of a plasma known to be severely deficient in factor VIII:C, but containing all other factors required for normal coagulation. An identical principle applies to the assays of factors IX, XI and XII. Assays of von Willebrand factor are described separately.

Reagents

Platelet-poor plasma. From the patient.
Standard plasma. (p. 301).
Factor VIII deficient plasma (substrate plasma). If using a commercial plasma, the reagent should be reconstituted according to the manufacturer's instructions. If a haemophiliac donor is used, his factor VIII:C concentration should be less than 1% and his plasma should be free of inhibitors. The plasma should be stored in suitable volumes, e.g. 2 ml, at −40°C until used. All samples obtained from patients must be considered potentially HIV positive. In addition, the plasma must be hepatitis B-virus negative. Alternatively, plasma depleted of factor VIII:C by immuno-adsorption can be used.

Kaolin. 5 mg/ml in barbitone buffered saline.
Barbitone buffered saline. (See p. 537).
Phospholipid solution (platelet substitute). (As described on p. 544).
CaCl$_2$. 0.025 mol/l.
Ice-bath.

Method

Place the kaolin, phospholipid and CaCl$_2$ at 37°C, and the patient's, standard and substrate plasma in the ice-bath until used.

Make 1 in 10 dilutions of the test and standard plasma in buffered saline in plastic tubes in the ice-bath. If the test plasma is suspected of having a very low factor VIII:C content make a 1 in 5 dilution instead. Using 0.2 ml volumes, make doubling dilutions in buffered saline to obtain 1 in 20 and 1 in 40 dilutions. Place 0.1 ml of the three dilutions (1 in 10, 1 in 20 and 1 in 40) in glass tubes.

Add to each dilution 0.1 ml of freshly reconstituted or thawed substrate plasma and warm up at

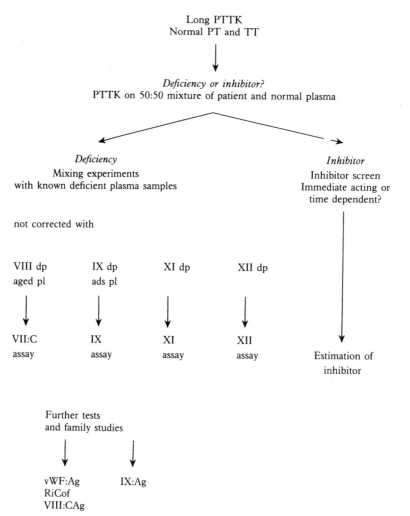

Fig. 19.4 Flow chart for investigating a prolonged PTTK. dp: deficient plasma. aged pl: aged plasma. ads pl: adsorbed plasma. vWF:Ag: von Willebrand factor antigen. IX:Ag: factor IX antigen. VIII:CAg: factor VIII:C antigen.

37°C. Add 0.2 ml of the phospholipid/kaolin mixture, mix the contents of the tube and start a master stop-watch. At 10 min exactly add the CaCl₂ and start a second stop-watch. Record the clotting time.

The dilutions should be tested at 3 min intervals on the master watch. The assay must end with a blank consisting of 0.1 ml of buffered saline and 0.1 ml of substrate plasma. A balanced order of testing should be followed.

Calculation of results

Plot the clotting times of the test and standard against the concentration of factor VIII:C on 4

cycle × 3 cycle log paper. Read the concentration as shown in Fig. 19.3. It is important to obtain straight and parallel lines if the result is to be accurate. The reasons for non-parallelism and curvature are:

1. Technical error. Repeat the assay with new dilutions.

2. Activation of the plasma by poor collection. A new sample should be collected.

3. A low concentration of factor VIII:C in the test plasma gives rise to non-parallel lines. Stronger concentrations of plasma should be prepared and tested.

4. The presence of an inhibitor. The tests described on p. 311 should be carried out.

Some automated coagulometers produce computed values using mathematical formulae. If the standard plasma is calibrated in terms of international units, the result can be expressed in iu. For example, if the standard plasma has a factor VIII:C concentration of 65 iu/dl and the test is shown to have 20% of the activity of the standard, the test plasma will have a factor VIII concentration of 13 iu/dl (20% of 65 iu).

Normal range

50–200 iu/dl.

Interpretation

Some clinically normal people have factor VIII:C concentrations of 35–50 iu/dl. Values below 30 iu/dl are unequivocally abnormal; values below 50 iu/dl are significant in carriers (see p. 317).

A reduced factor VIII:C concentration is found in:

1. Haemophilia A.
2. Some carriers of haemophilia A.
3. von Willebrand disease, types I and III, and some cases of type II.
4. Rare congenital combined deficiency of factors VIII:C and V.
5. Disseminated intravascular coagulation.
6. Circulating anticoagulant.

Further tests in haemophilia A

Factor VIII:CAg (IRMA) and vWF:Ag (immunoassay, described below) should be measured and the patient's family investigated.

Other one-stage assays based on the PTTK

Factors IX, XI and XII can be measured in an identical manner using an appropriate substrate plasma. The normal values for these factors are given in Table 19.5. If low values are detected in a patient with a history of bleeding, immunoassays should be undertaken to establish whether there is any cross-reacting material, and family studies should be carried out.

Isolated factor IX or XII deficiency may be acquired as a result of a selective urinary loss in the nephrotic syndrome. An acquired low factor IX concentration has also been described in Sheehan's syndrome.

Table 19.5 Normal range and some causes of increased plasma concentration for factors of the intrinsic pathway

Factor	Normal range	Increased
Factor VIII:C	50–200 iu/dl	In acute phase reaction, stress, exercise, pregnancy, chronic liver disease, vasculitic diseases.
Factor IX	40–160 iu/dl	In pregnancy, in women taking oestrogen-containing contraceptives.
Factor XI	40–160 iu/dl	
Factor XII	30–150 iu/dl	

INVESTIGATION OF A SUSPECTED VON WILLEBRAND'S DISEASE[2,7,12,19]

A diagnosis of von Willebrand's disease should be contemplated in individuals with a history of bleeding who show a prolonged bleeding time and PTTK in screening tests. All factor VIII activities, that is VIII:C concentration, vWF:Ag concentration and ristocetin cofactor activity (RiCoF), should be measured. If an abnormality is detected, further investigations, such as crossed immuno-electrophoresis (CIE) of vWF:Ag and the multimer analysis of the plasma should be performed. In normal plasma, each multimer of vWF (a large molecule consisting of four to over 20 subunits of vWF) is seen to be composed of a 'triplet', a dark central band sandwiched between two lighter bands; high molecular weight multimers predominate. In von Willebrand's disease, there may be either no vWF:Ag detectable, or the high molecular weight forms necessary for normal platelet adhesion may be lacking, or the triplet pattern may be abnormal. On the basis of these results von Willebrand's disease can be classified as shown in Table 19.6.

IMMUNOELECTROPHORETIC ASSAY OF vWF:Ag[7]

Principle. A precipitating rabbit anti-serum to human vWF:Ag is incorporated into an agarose

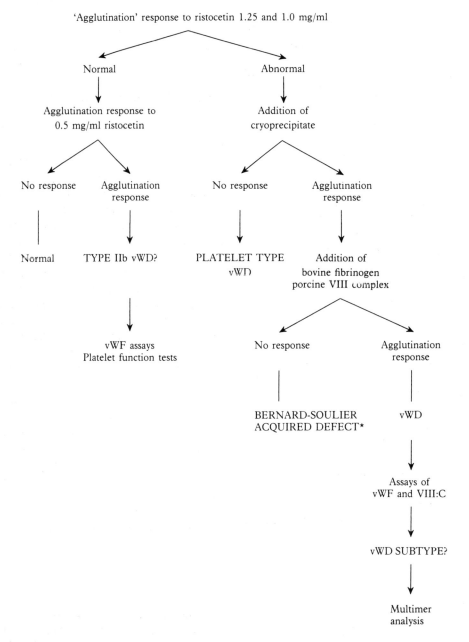

Fig. 19.5   Flow chart for investigating von Willebrand's disease.
*Acquired defect of platelet 'agglutination' response to ristocetin, most commonly found in myelodysplastic syndromes.

plate the wells of which are filled with dilutions of test and standard plasma. An electric current is applied; precipitation peaks are obtained, the height of which is proportional to the concentration of vWF:Ag in the samples.

Reagents

Barbitone buffer. 0.05 mol/l, pH 8.4. Dissolve 85g of sodium diethyl barbiturate in 116 ml of HCl and add water to 10 litres.

Agarose. 1% in barbitone buffer. Low electro-endoosmosis (LE) type should be used.

NaCl. 9 g/l and 30 g/l.

Coomassie Blue stain. Add 5 g of Coomassie Brilliant Blue R (Kenacid Blue) to a mixture containing 450 ml of 96% methanol (industrial methylated spirit) and 100 ml of acetic acid. Mix and leave at room temperature (c 20°C) overnight. Filter the solution and add 450 ml of water.

Destainer. Mix 250 ml of 96% methanol, 100 ml of acetic acid and 450 ml of water.

Platelet-poor plasma. Samples from the patient may be frozen at −40°C.

Standards. Normal pool, commercial freeze-dried plasma, or a national/international reference material.

Antisera. These are commercially available. The amount of antiserum per agarose plate varies from antiserum to antiserum and from batch to batch. To obtain the optimum dilution of antiserum, make a series of plates with varying dilutions of antiserum in agarose: 1 in 10, 1 in 20, 1 in 50, 1 in 80, 1 in 100, 1 in 200, 1 in 300, etc. These are tested using normal, known vWF-deficient and known haemophilic plasma. The correct dilution of the antiserum gives a clear, well-defined peak. The dilution of the antiserum is also dependent on the size of the plate, the diameter of the well and the depth of the agar. Once the optimum dilution is established, it should not alter for the same batch of antiserum.

Apparatus

56°C water-bath.
Glass plates. 90 × 110 × 1.5 mm.
Well cutter to give 3 mm wells.
Micropipetting system. 10 µl adjustable.
Electrophoresis apparatus.

Filter paper. Whatman No 1.
Wicks. Surgical Lambskin lint.
Applicator sticks.

Method

Dissolve 1 g of agarose in 100 ml of buffer by boiling in a glass tube or in a conical flask. Transfer to a 56°C water-bath. Clean glass plates with methylated spirit to remove dust and grease. Place on a level tray. Pipette a selected amount of anti-serum into a plastic container and add 13 ml of agarose. Carefully pour the agarose onto the plate and quickly spread it using an applicator stick to ensure an even film. Allow to cool and, when set, store in a moist chamber at 4°C until ready for use.

Fill the electrophoresis tank with barbitone buffer and insert the wicks.

Make dilutions of the plasma standard in 9 g/l NaCl: 1 in 2 = 50 u/dl, 1 in 4 = 25 u/dl, 1 in 8 = 12.5 u/dl. Make two dilutions of each patient's plasma. The dilutions chosen depend on the expected vWF:Ag concentration. Peak height should be within the range of the standard peaks.

Cut 17 equidistant wells in the agarose plate. Apply 5 µl to each well. Place the plates, two per tank, agar side down, on the wicks, with the wells on the cathode side so that the peaks migrate towards the anode. Pass the current at approximately 16 mA per tank for 18 h at room temperature (c 20°C).

After electrophoresis, remove the plates from the tank and immerse in 30 g/l NaCl for up to 24 h to elute out any excess protein. Then immerse in 9 g/dl NaCl and finally water, and then dry the agar by covering the plate with filter paper and place in a hot-air oven. As the agar dries the paper will lift off the plate.

Stain with Coomassie Blue for 5–10 min. Wash out excess stain with the destainer. Allow the plates to dry in air.

Results

Measure the height in mm of the peak from the top of the well to the tip of the peak. Plot the height in mm against the concentration of vWF:Ag in the standard on log/log paper (Fig. 19.6). For each

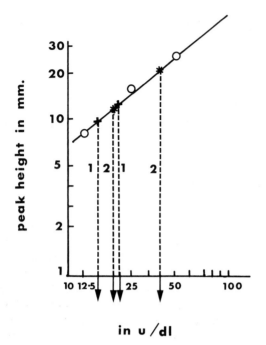

in u /dl

Fig. 19.6 Calculation of vWF: Ag concentration from the peak height. The peak heights for the standard plasma, continuous line (o), are: 23 mm for a 1 in 2 dilution, 14 mm for a 1 in 4 dilution, and 8 mm for a 1 in 8 dilution. Plasma 1 (+) was tested in two dilutions: 1 in 2 which gave a peak height of 10 mm = 15 u, and undiluted which gave a peak of 13 mm = 23 u. To calculate the vWF:Ag concentration the values must be multiplied by the dilution factor (15 × 2 = 30; 23 × 1 = 23) and their mean taken as the value: 23 + 30 ÷ 2 = 26.5. The concentration of vWF:Ag in this plasma is 26.5 u/dl. Plasma 2 (*): 1 in 2 dilution gave a peak of 20 mm = 42 u (× 2 dilution factor) = 84 u/dl); 1 in 4 dilution gave a peak of 12 mm = 22 (× 4) = 88 u/dl. The mean is 86 u/dl.

dilution of patient's plasma read the concentration of vWF:Ag from the graph. Multiply by the dilution factor.

Normal range

50–200 u/dl.

Interpretation

The results must be interpreted in conjunction with the results of factor VIII:C assay and the ristocetin cofactor assay (Table 19.6). VWF:Ag can also be measured by ELISA in a microplate or tube.[19]

RISTOCETIN COFACTOR ASSAY[7, 15]

Principle. Washed platelets do not 'agglutinate' in the presence of ristocetin unless normal plasma is added as a source of vWF. 'Agglutination' follows a dose response curve dependent upon the amount of plasma added. Fresh washed platelets or formalin-fixed platelets can be used in the assay. Fixed platelets take longer to prepare, but are not susceptible to aggregation (as distinct from 'agglutination') with ristocetin, and they can be stored so that they are available for emergency use. Fresh washed platelets are quicker to prepare, and retain a functional platelet membrane, but they cannot be retained for later use. Commercial lyophilized washed platelet preparations are also available. The type of platelet preparation which best suits an individual laboratory depends on the work-load and urgency of the test. Where there are large batches of non-urgent assays, there may be no advantage in using fixed platelets. Commercial preparations may not be economical.

ASSAY USING FRESH PLATELETS

Preparation of platelets

Reagents

K_2EDTA. 0.134 mol/l.
Citrate-saline. One volume of 31.1 g/l trisodium citrate + 9 volumes of 9 g/l NaCl.
EDTA-citrate-saline. One volume of 0.134 mol/l K_2EDTA + 9 volumes of citrate-saline.

Method

Collect 40–60 ml of normal blood into a one-tenth volume of EDTA-saline in flat-bottom plastic universal containers. Do not use conical bottom containers. Centrifuge at 150–200 *g* at room temperature (*c* 20°C) for 15 min.

Pipette, using a plastic pipette, the platelet-rich plasma into a plastic container. Mark the level of plasma on the tube. Centrifuge at 1500–2000 *g* to obtain a platelet button.

Discard the platelet-poor plasma. Resuspend the platelet button in a pipetteful of EDTA-citrate-saline by gently squeezing the liquid up and down

Table 19.6 Classification of von Willebrand's disease

Type	Inheritance	VIII:C	vWF:Ag	RiCoF	CIE	Multimer analysis
I	Autos. dominant	L	L	L	N	Normal pattern
IIa*	Autos. dominant	L or N	L or N	L	Abn	Large and intermediate multimers absent from plasma and platelets, abnormal triplets.
IIb	Autos. dominant	L or N	L or N	L or N	Abn	Large multimers absent from plasma only, normal triplets.
IIc	Autos. recessive	N	N	L	Abn	Large multimers absent from plasma and platelets, abnormal triplets.
III	Autos. recessive	L	L	0	ND	None detected

L: low. N: normal. 0: absent. ND: none detected. autos: autosomal. CIE: crossed immuno-electrophoresis.
* Types IId, e, and f are also described with different abnormalities of the multimeric structure.
Some forms of vW disease Type II may show normal or even enhanced ristocetin 'agglutination' in platelet-rich plasma (see Fig. 19.5).

the pipette until a smooth suspension is formed. Add EDTA-citrate-saline to the 20 ml mark.

Centrifuge at 1500–2000 *g* for 15 min. Discard the supernatant. Resuspend in EDTA-citrate-saline and leave at room temperature for 20 min to elute the ristocetin cofactor off the platelets.

Centrifuge again, discard the supernatant, resuspend in EDTA-citrate-saline two more times to a total of four washes.

Centrifuge at 1500–2000 *g* for 15 min. Discard the supernatant and resuspend in citrate-saline using a volume slightly under the original plasma volume (marked on the container). Centrifuge at 800 *g* for 5 min to remove platelet clumps, white cells and red cells.

Remove the platelet-rich supernatant carefully. Perform a platelet count and dilute the platelet-rich suspension with citrate-saline until the platelet count is about $200 \times 10^9/l$.

Leave the platelets at room temperature for 30–45 min to allow the platelets to recover from the trauma of washing and centrifugation

Reagents for assay

Citrate-saline.
Ristocetin. 100 mg/ml. Stored frozen in 1 ml volumes.
Plasma standard.
Platelet-poor plasma. From the patient or patients.

Assay method

Confirm that the washed platelets do not 'agglutinate' with ristocetin in the absence of added plasma.

Deliver 0.5 ml of citrate-saline into an aggregometer cuvette and 0.4 ml of the platelet suspension + 0.1 ml of citrate-saline into another cuvette. Place in the warming block and allow to warm. Add 5 μl of ristocetin and record at 1 cm/min for 2 min. The absorbence due to citrate-saline alone is taken to represent 100% agglutination, and that due to platelets alone represents zero (0%) agglutination (blank). The absorbence due to the platelet suspension must not exceed 5 divisions on the chart paper. If it is greater, the platelets must be washed again and the procedure repeated. The reading of this blank must be repeated every hour.

All plasma samples and ristocetin should be kept in an ice-bath.

Standard curve. A standard curve is obtained by making doubling dilutions, 1 in 2 to 1 in 32 in citrate-saline, of the standard plasma (donor pool, commercial reference plasma or other reference materials). The absorbence due to a mixture of 0.4 ml of citrate-saline and 0.1 ml of plasma dilution is taken to represent 100% agglutination and that due to the mixture of 0.4 ml of platelet suspension and 0.1 ml of plasma dilution zero (0%) agglutination.

Add 5 μl of ristocetin to the cuvette containing the mixture giving zero agglutination and record the agglutination for 2 min. Test each dilution of the standard plasma in a similar way.

The patient's plasma is tested at two dilutions, depending on the expected concentration of vWF in the plasma. Both dilutions should give agglutination within the range of that of the standard curve.

Reset 100% and zero aggregation for each patient.

A reading of the platelet blank should be repeated at hourly intervals. If the reading differs from the original, the difference must be subtracted from the results of subsequent tests.

Results

Measure 'agglutination' at 1 or 2 min depending on the strength of 'agglutination'. All responses must be compared on the same time scale and not read at maximum 'agglutination'.

Plot the standard curve on semi-log paper with 'agglutination' on the linear scale and the concentration of vWF in u/dl on the log scale (see Fig. 19.7). For assay purposes, assign the 1 in 2 dilution of standard plasma a value of 50 u/dl. (Each batch

of standard is precalibrated as described on p. 301 and may not necessarily be 100 μ/dl.)

Read the patient's vWF concentration directly off the standard curve, correct for the dilution factor and average the two results from the different dilutions.

Normal

50–200 u/dl.

Interpretation

The vWF concentration measured by ristocetin cofactor assay can only be interpreted in conjunction with other factor VIII:C and vWF:Ag assays, as shown in Figure 19.7.

ASSAY USING FORMALIN-FIXED PLATELETS

Preparation of platelets

Reagents

Sodium citrate solution. 32 g/l trisodium sodium citrate ($Na_3C_6H_5O_7$. $2H_2O$).
K_2EDTA. 0.134 mol/l.
2% formalin (40% formaldehyde). In 9 g/l NaCl.
0.05% sodium azide. In 9 g/l NaCl.

Method

Citrated blood in a blood donation bag, obtained from a normal individual or from a therapeutic venesection carried out on a patient with a normal platelet count can be used. ACD or CPD solution from the donor bag is ejected through the taking needle and replaced by the equivalent volume of sodium citrate. Collect *c* 500 ml of blood.

Centrifuge the blood at 300 *g* for 15 min at room temperature. Separate the platelet-rich plasma (PRP) and add 9 volumes of PRP to 1 volume of EDTA solution. Incubate for 1 h at 37°C to reverse the effect of ADP released during the preparation. Add an equal volume of 2% formalin and leave at 4°C for 1 h. Centrifuge at 200 *g* for 10 min at 4°C. Decant the supernatant and recentrifuge it at 250 *g* for 20 min at 4°C. Discard the supernatant and

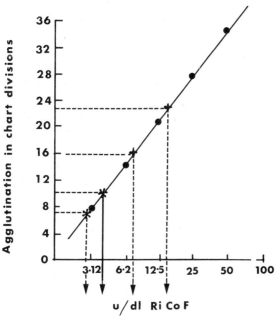

Fig. 19.7 Ristocetin cofactor assay. The standard curve is plotted on semi-log paper. Each test plasma is assayed in two dilutions. Plasma 1 (+) produces the following readings: 1 in 4 dilution: 16 divisions of the chart paper = 7 u (× 4 (dilution factor) = 28 u/dl); 1 in 2 dilution: 22 divisions = 13 u/dl (× 2 (dilution factor) = 26 u/dl). The mean of the two readings is 27 u/dl. Plasma 2 (*) gave the following results. 1 in 2 dilution: 7 divisions = 2.5 u (× 2 dilution factor) = 5 u/dl). 1 in 4 dilution: 5 divisions (not shown on the fig.) This result was similar to the blank and the plasma was next tested undiluted, giving a reading of 10 divisions = 4 u/dl. The mean is 4.5 u/dl (very low).

resuspend the platelet sediment in chilled (4°C) 9 g/l NaCl. Wash the platelets twice more. After the final wash resuspend the platelets in the sodium azide solution. Adjust the platelet count to 300–500 $\times 10^9$/l. The suspension is stable for 1 month at 4°C.

Reagents for assay

Buffer for plasma dilutions. Barbitone buffer, pH 7.4, containing 40 mg/ml of bovine serum albumin.

Ristocetin, plasma standard and patient's platelet-poor plasma. As described in the previous assay.

Assay method

Follow the method described for washed fresh platelets. Prepare all plasma dilutions in the albumin-containing buffer.

Results, interpretation and normal range

As described for the washed platelet assay.

INVESTIGATION OF A PATIENT WITH A CIRCULATING ANTICOAGULANT (INHIBITOR)[3,7,13]

Circulating anticoagulants or acquired inhibitors of coagulation factors are immunoglobulins arising either in congenitally deficient individuals as a result of the administration of the missing factor or in previously haemostatically normal subjects as a part of an auto-immune process.

Of the anticoagulants which cause a bleeding tendency, antibodies to factor VIII:C are most common. They develop in approximately 12% of haemophiliacs. Inhibitors directed against vWF and factors IX, V, XI, XII, etc. are very rare. The commonest anticoagulant in haemostatically normal people is the lupus anticoagulant, but despite the prolongation of clotting tests in vitro, this anticoagulant predisposes to thrombosis and its diagnosis and investigation is therefore considered in Chapter 20 (p. 319). Only the factor VIII:C inhibitor assays are described in detail in this section. Inhibitors against factors VIII:C fall into two general categories: those with simple kinetics, and those with complex kinetics. Patients with haemophilia usually develop antibodies with simple kinetics; this inhibitor reacts with factor VIII:C in a linear fashion and the antigen/antibody complex has no factor VIII:C activity. Complex inhibitors usually arise in non-haemophilic individuals. Inactivation of factor VIII:C is at first rapid, but it then slows as the antigen/antibody complex either dissociates or displays some factor VIII:C activity. In some patients diluted plasma can neutralize more factor VIII:C than an undiluted sample.

INHIBITOR (ANTICOAGULANT) SCREEN BASED ON THE PTTK[7,13]

Principle. Circulating anticoagulants or inhibitors affecting the PTTK may act immediately or be time-dependent. Normal plasma mixed with a plasma containing an immediately acting inhibitor will have little or no effect on the prolonged clotting time. In contrast, if normal plasma is added to a plasma containing a time-dependent inhibitor, the clotting time of the latter will be substantially shortened. However, after 1–2 h, correction will be abolished, and the clotting time will become long again. In order to detect both types of inhibition, normal plasma and test plasma samples are mixed and tested immediately and then after incubation at 37°C for 60 min.

Reagents

Normal plasma. A pool of 20 donors as described on p. 301.
Platelet-poor plasma. From the patient.
Reagents for the PTTK.

Method

Prepare three plastic tubes as follows: place 0.5 ml of normal plasma in a first tube, 0.5 ml of the patient's plasma in a second tube, and a mixture of 0.25 ml of normal and 0.25 ml of patient's plasma in a third tube. Incubate the tubes for 60 min at 37°C and then place all three tubes in an ice-bath or on crushed ice.

Make a 50:50 mixture of the contents of tubes 1 and 2: this tube serves to check for the presence of an immediate inhibitor. Perform PTTKs in duplicate on all four tubes.

Results and interpretation

See Table 19.7.

QUANTITATIVE MEASUREMENT OF FACTOR VIII:C INHIBITORS[7,13]

Principle. Factor VIII inhibitors are time-dependent. Thus if factor VIII:C is added to plasma containing an inhibitor and the mixture is incubated, factor VIII:C will be progressively neutralized. If the amount of factor VIII:C added and the duration of incubation are standardized, the strength of the inhibitor may be measured in units according to how much of the added factor VIII:C is destroyed.

In the Bethesda method described below, the unit is defined as the amount of inhibitor which will neutralize 50% of 1 unit of factor VIII:C in 2 h at 37°C.

Dilutions of test plasma are incubated with an equal volume of the normal plasma pool at 37°C. The normal plasma pool is taken to represent 1 unit of factor VIII:C. Dilutions of a control normal plasma containing no inhibitor are treated in the same way. An equal volume of normal plasma mixed with buffer is taken to represent the 100% value.

At the end of the incubation period the residual factor VIII:C is assayed and the inhibitor strength calculated from a graph of residual factor VIII:C activity versus inhibitor units.

Reagents

Glyoxaline buffer (See p. 281.)
Kaolin. 5 mg/ml.
Factor VIII:C deficient plasma.
Standard plasma. Normal plasma pool.
Platelet substitute. Phospholipid (see p. 544); also available commercially.

Method

Pipette into each of a series of plastic tubes 0.2 ml of normal pool plasma. Add 0.2 ml of glyoxaline buffer to the first tube (this tube serves as the 100% value); add 0.2 ml of test plasma dilutions in glyoxaline buffer to each of the other tubes. If the patient's inhibitor has been assayed previously, this can be used as a guide to the dilutions that should be used. If the patient has not been tested before, a range of dilutions should be set up ranging from undiluted plasma to a 1 in 50 dilution.

Cap, mix and incubate all the tubes for 2 h at 37°C. Then immerse all the tubes in an ice-bath. Perform factor VIII:C assays on all the incubation mixtures.

Calculation of results

Record the residual factor VIII:C percentage for each mixture assuming the assay value of the control to be 100%. The dilution of test plasma that gives the residual factor VIII:C percentage nearest to 50% (between 30 and 60%) is chosen for calculating the strength of inhibitor. How the

Table 19.7   Interpretation of the inhibitor screen based on the PTTK

Tube	Content	PTTK		
1	Normal plasma	normal	normal	normal
2	Patient's plasma	long	long	long
3	50:50 mixture, patient:normal, incubated 1 h	normal	long	long
4	50:50 mixture, patient:normal, no incubation	normal	long	normal
Interpretation:		deficiency	immediately acting inhibitor	time-dependent inhibitor

Table 19.8 Example of the calculation of Bethesda units in three plasma samples

Patient	Plasma dilution	% residual VIII:C	Calculation u × dilution	Inhibitor in Bethesda u
A	undiluted	61	0.70 × 1	= 0.07
B	1 in 5	33	1.60 × 5	= 8.0
	1 in 10	55	0.85 × 10	= 8.5
	1 in 15	68	0.55 × 15	= 8.3
C	1 in 5	40	1.30 × 5	= 6.5
	1 in 10	55	0.85 × 10	= 8.5
	1 in 15	61	0.70 × 15	= 10.5
	1 in 20	65	0.60 × 20	= 12

Patient A has a mild inhibitor, patient B an inhibitor with simple kinetics and patient C an inhibitor with complex kinetics. All values are chosen for the percent residual factor VIII:C activity close to 50%. The units are calculated from Fig 19.8. (modified from Kasper & Ewing[13]).

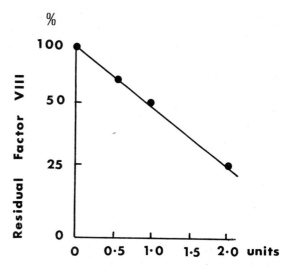

Fig. 19.8 Measurement of factor VIII:C inhibitors.
Relationship between the residual factor VIII:C activity in a standard plasma and the inhibitor activity of a test plasma can be read off this plot. At 50% inhibition the test plasma contains 1 Bethesda inhibitor unit per ml. See also Table 19.8.

results are calculated is shown in Table 19.8 and Fig. 19.8 for three different patients: one had a mild inhibitor only detected in undiluted plasma, one a stronger inhibitor with simple kinetics and one an inhibitor with complex kinetics.

Interpretation

If the residual factor VIII:C activity is between 80 and 100%, the plasma sample does not contain an inhibitor. If the residual activity is less than 60% the plasma unequivocally contains an inhibitor. Values between 60 and 80% are borderline and repeated testing on additional samples is needed before the diagnosis can be established.

Tests for other inhibitors

Factor IX inhibitors can be measured in a system identical to that described above. Because factor IX inhibitors act immediately, there is no need for prolonged incubation: the mixtures can be assayed after 5 min at 37°C.

INVESTIGATION OF A PATIENT WHOSE PTTK AND PT ARE PROLONGED

A prolonged PTTK and PT in a patient with a bleeding disorder may be due to a defect or deficiency of one of the factors of the common pathway: factor X, factor V or prothrombin. In addition, the patient could be suffering from the much rarer combined deficiency of factors V and VIII:C. Liver disease and vitamin K deficiency should always be excluded, even in the presence of a family history of bleeding. Mixing tests illustrated on p. 304 may help to pinpoint the defect; the missing factor or factors should be estimated quantitatively. Further tests (including chromogenic and immunoassays as well as immuno-electrophoresis) may be necessary to elucidate the nature of the defect.

TAIPAN VENOM ASSAY FOR PROTHROMBIN[7]

Principle. The venom of the snake *Oxyuranus scutellatus*, or Taipan venom, converts prothrombin into thrombin in the presence of calcium and phospholipid. This action is not dependent on factors V or X. If a source of fibrinogen is included into the system, the resultant clotting times are proportional to the concentration of prothrombin in the plasma tested.

The best source of fibrinogen is adsorbed oxalated bovine plasma: it provides antithrombin in excess and eliminates the effect of antithrombins in the test plasma.

Reagents

Taipan venom. Commercially available.
Adsorbed oxalated bovine plasma.
Platelet substitute (see p. 544); also available commercially.
Barbitone buffered saline.
Platelet-poor plasma. From the patient.
Standard plasma.
$CaCl_2$. 0.025 mol/l.

Method

Prepare 1 in 5, 1 in 10, 1 in 20, 1 in 40 and 1 in 80 dilutions of the test and standard plasma in buffered saline in plastic tubes. Place 0.1 ml of each dilution in a glass tube, add 0.1 ml of platelet substitute and 0.1 ml of bovine plasma. Warm at 37°C; then add 0.2 ml of a mixture of equal volumes of $CaCl_2$ and Taipan venom, start a stop-watch and record the clotting time. Repeat for each dilution of the standard and test plasma.

Calculation

Plot the clotting times against the reciprocal of the dilutions on *linear* graph paper. Straight but not necessarily parallel lines should be obtained. To calculate the result, express the result with each dilution of the test sample in relation to the standard and calculate the mean of all the readings.

Normal range

50–200 u/dl.

Interpretation

Congenital prothrombin deficiency is very uncommon. Its basis is the presence of an abnormal prothrombin molecule. The condition has been described as dysprothrombinaemia. Before making this diagnosis it has, however, to be differentiated from various acquired disorders and the presence of the lupus anticoagulant (see p. 319).

A two-stage assay for prothrombin was described in the 6th edition of this book.

FACTOR X ASSAY[9]

Principle. Factor X is assayed by a one-stage procedure using Russell Viper venom (RVV). RVV is insensitive to factor VII deficiency and if the venom is used instead of thromboplastin, prolongation of the prothrombin time reflects a deficiency of factors X, V and prothrombin. By incorporating an excess of factor V and prothrombin in the system, the concentration of factor X can be sensitively measured.

Reagents

Platelet-poor plasma. From the patient.
Standard plasma.
$CaCl_2$. 0.025 mol/l.
Barbitone buffered saline.
Factor X deficient plasma. Commercially available.
Platelet substitute. (see p. 544); also commercially available.
Russell viper venom (Burroughs Wellcome). Add 2 ml of buffered saline to the vial: this results in a 1 in 10 000 dilution of the venom. To provide the working reagent the venom is combined with platelet substitute. Dilute the platelet substitute 1 in 5 with buffered saline. Add 0.1 ml of the solution of the venom to 2.9 ml of platelet substitute so as to achieve a final dilution of 1 in 300 000. This mixture must be prepared fresh before every assay.

Method

Prepare in plastic tubes 1 in 5, 1 in 10, 1 in 20 and 1 in 40 dilutions of both the test and the standard plasma in buffered saline. Transfer 0.1 ml of each dilution into a glass tube and add 0.1 ml of factor X deficient plasma. Warm to 37°C. Then add 0.1 ml of the RVV/platelet substitute mixture, start the stop-watch and mix. At exactly 30 sec add 0.1 ml of $CaCl_2$. Record the clotting time. Repeat for each dilution of the test and standard plasma. Always include a blank containing buffered saline instead of a plasma dilution. Test in balanced order to avoid time-trend.

Results

Plot the clotting times against factor X concentration using 2 cycle × 3 cycle log paper. The lines should be straight and parallel. Read the factor X concentration of the test from the intercept with the standard curve, as shown previously.

Normal range

50–200 u/dl.

Interpretation

Factor X deficiency is a rare disorder and affected families have abnormal, variant proteins. Immunoassays and tests of factor X activation are necessary to confirm the diagnosis. Isolated acquired factor X deficiency has also been described in association with amyloidosis and investigations to exclude amyloidosis and paraproteinaemia may be required.

FACTOR V ASSAY[7]

Principle. Factor V assay is a one-stage procedure based on the prothrombin time. It is carried out in the same way as the assay of factor VII. Factor V deficient plasma is, however, used as substrate.

Reagents

Factor V deficient plasma. This is prepared by ageing normal plasma. Blood from a healthy individual is collected into a one-ninth volume of 14 g/l potassium oxalate. Plasma is separated by centrifuging at 2000*g* for 15 min. The plasma is kept at 37°C under sterile conditions for 3 days, then stored in 2 ml volumes at −30°C until used.

Other reagents are described on p. 302.

Normal range

50–200 u/dl.

Interpretation

It is important to ensure that the test sample is fresh and that a low result is not due to ageing of the patient's plasma. Factor V deficiency is very rare, combined deficiency of factors V and VIII:C even rarer. Factor VIII:C assays should be carried out in all individuals found to have a deficiency of factor V. Acquired factor V deficiency is also uncommon; it has been found as part of the consumption coagulopathy resulting from DIC and very rarely in untreated chronic granulocytic leukaemia.

INVESTIGATION OF A PATIENT SUSPECTED OF AFIBRINOGENAEMIA, HYPOFIBRINOGENAEMIA OR DYSFIBRINOGENAEMIA

The patient usually has a prolonged PTTK, PT and thrombin time. The prolongation of the PT is usually less marked than that of the PTTK and thrombin time. There may be either a history of bleeding or of recurrent thrombotic events. Fibrinogen should be measured quantitatively using a clot weight method or a thrombin-based estimation.

FIBRINOGEN ESTIMATION (DRY CLOT WEIGHT)[7]

Principle. Fibrinogen in plasma is converted into fibrin by clotting with thrombin and calcium. The resulting clot is weighed.

Reagents

Citrated platelet-poor plasma.

CaCl₂. 0.025 mol/l.
Bovine thrombin. 50 NIH u/ml.

Method

Pipette 1 ml of plasma into a 12×75 mm glass tube and warm to $37°C$. Place a wooden applicator or swab stick in the tube, add 0.1 ml of $CaCl_2$ and 0.9 ml of thrombin and mix. Incubate for 15 min at $37°C$.

Gently wind the fibrin clot onto the stick, squeezing out the serum. Wash the clot in a tube containing at first 9 g/l NaCl, then water. Blot the clot carefully with filter paper, remove the fibrin from the stick and put into acetone for 5–10 min. Dry the clot in a hot air oven or over a hot lamp for 30 min. Allow it to cool and weigh.

Results

The fibrinogen level is expressed as g/l, i.e. the weight of fibrin obtained from 1 ml of plasma $\times 1000$.

Normal range

1.5–4.0 g/l.

FIBRINOGEN ASSAY[6]

Principle. The clotting time of plasma after the addition of thrombin in excess is proportional to the concentration of fibrinogen.

Reagents

Platelet-poor plasma. From the patient and from a normal pool.

Bovine thrombin. Dissolve the thrombin to obtain a final concentration of *c* 250 NIH units per ml. The solution may be stored at $-20°C$.

Barbitone buffered saline.

Fibrinogen. Freeze-dried human fibrinogen powder should be dissolved in buffered 9 g/l NaCl to give a master solution containing 40 mg/dl.

Method

Dilute the fibrinogen solution further with buffered saline so as to obtain concentrations of 10, 20 and 30 mg/dl. Place 0.1 ml of each dilution in a glass tube in a water-bath at $37°C$. Add to each tube in turn 0.2 ml of thrombin solution, rapidly mix and record the clotting times. Repeat the procedure once. Plot the mean clotting time for each dilution against the fibrinogen concentration on double-log graph paper. A straight line should be obtained.

Dilute the patient's plasma and the normal plasma 1 in 10 with buffered saline. To 0.2 ml of this dilution add 0.2 ml of thrombin and record the clotting times. Repeat the test and average the times. Read off the concentration of fibrinogen from the standard line.

Calculation

Multiply the concentration read off the graph by 10, the dilution factor. If the test plasma gives clotting times which do not fall within the range of 10 and 40 mg fibrinogen per dl, repeat the test using an appropriate dilution.

Normal range

1.5–4.0 g/l.

Further investigations

Whenever a congenital fibrinogen abnormality is suspected, DIC and hyperfibrinolysis must be excluded: FDP should not be in excess and there should be no evidence of the consumption of other coagulation factors and platelets (see Chapter 18, p. 290).

Immunological or chemical determination of fibrinogen is the next step in investigation. In dysfibrinogenaemias there is often a normal or even raised plasma fibrinogen concentration using these methods although the functional assays indicate a deficiency. Other tests which may be helpful are the Reptilase time, fibrinopeptide release, factor XIII cross-linking, tests of polymerization, binding to thrombin and lysis by plasmin. In some cases genomic DNA analysis can be performed.[14]

INVESTIGATION OF CARRIERS OF A CONGENITAL COAGULATION DEFICIENCY OR DEFECT [2,10,16]

Carrier detection is important in genetic counselling, and antenatal diagnosis may enable heterozygotes to consider abortion of a severely affected fetus. The information of value in carrier detection is derived from family studies, phenotype investigations and the determination of genotype.

Family studies. Haemophilia A and B (factor VIII:C and factor IX deficiency) are inherited by X-linked genes. This means that all the sons of a haemophiliac will be normal and all his daughters carriers. The children of a carrier have a 0.5 chance of being affected if they are sons, and a 0.5 chance of being carriers if they are daughters. The other coagulation factor defects are inherited as autosomal traits. Heterozygotes possess approximately half the normal concentration of the coagulation factor and are generally not affected clinically; only homozygotes have a significant bleeding tendency.

A detailed family study is important in all coagulation factor defects in order to establish the true nature of the defect and its severity. Patients often describe any familial bleeding tendency as haemophilia, and it is therefore essential to prove the exact defect in every new patient and family. In some inbred kindreds more than one coagulation defect may be simultaneously inherited.

When a detailed family study has been carried out it may be possible to establish the statistical chance of inheriting a coagulation defect. For a review, see Graham et al.[10]

Phenotype investigation. Theoretically, the average concentration of the affected coagulation factor in the heterozygote or carrier is half of that found in normal individuals. It is, however, not always easy to establish that the plasma concentration of a coagulation factor is truly lower than normal: this is particularly difficult in the carriers of haemophilia because factor VIII:C is an acute phase reactant and its concentration may be increased as a result of an intercurrent illness or stress. Factor VIII:C concentration also varies with age and blood group and even healthy young adults may show a fourfold difference in its concentration. Determination of vWF:Ag may be helpful: the ratio of factor VIII:C to vWH:Ag is reduced in most carriers of haemophilia and the ratio may be used as a diagnostic tool. Nevertheless, approximatey 16% of haemophilia carriers cannot be diagnosed with certainty using coagulation and immunological assays.[2]

Variability in the plasma concentration is less marked for other coagulation factors, and it is usually (but not always) possible to establish the presence of the heterozygous state, especially if a combination of functional and immunological assays is used in the family study.

Genotype assignment. Genotype can be assigned by linkage studies or by direct gene probing. This has been successfully achieved for many families with haemophilia A and B. The diagnosis of the heterozygous state is definitive in such cases.

TESTS REQUIRED FOR MONITORING REPLACEMENT THERAPY IN COAGULATION FACTOR DEFECTS AND DEFICIENCIES

Replacement therapy requires the following:

1. Calculation of the dose of the material to be administered and its frequency.
2. Assessment of the response to the dose.
3. Monitoring of any untoward effects.

The *dose* to be administered is calculated from the patient's body weight and the rise in the plasma concentration of the defective coagulation factor that is desired. Thus, the patient's plasma concentration of the factor and the potency or strength of the therapeutic material must be known. For the vast majority of patients whose defect is known and its plasma concentration has been measured, and for whom a commercial freeze-dried factor concentrate is used, this means a calculation based on the following formulae:

For factor VIII:C the dose in iu per kg body weight = rise required in iu per dl divided by 2. For factor IX, the formula is dose in iu per kg body weight = rise required in iu per dl.

The rise required depends on the type of bleeding, the half-life and stability of the clotting factor used, and on the concentration of the defective factor in the patient's plasma prior to treatment. For details, see Rizza and Jones.[16]

Assessment of the response to the therapy requires regular measurements of the plasma concentration of the coagulation factor infused by means of a functional assay. The response can be assessed from the formula:

Rise in iu per dl divided by dose in iu per kg body weight = K, which is approximately 2 for haemophilia A, and approximately 1 for haemophilia B (if concentrates are used).

The response is usually measured immediately after the administration of the therapeutic material. If the response is inadequate, this may have been due to an error in calculating the dose, or because the potency of the therapeutic material is less than expected, or because the patient is developing an inhibitor.

The main *untoward effects* are transmission of infection and the development of inhibitors. If the presence of an inhibitor is suspected, it must be confirmed using the tests described on p. 311, and later assessed quantitatively. For monitoring replacement and other types of therapy in patients with inhibitors, see Bloom.[3]

REFERENCES

[1] BARROWCLIFFE, T. W. and CURTISS, A. D. (1987). Principles of bioassay. In *Haemostasis and Thrombosis*. Eds. Bloom, A. L. and Thomas, D. P., 2nd edn, p. 996. Churchill Livingstone, Edinburgh.

[2] BLOOM, A. L. (1987). Inherited disorders of blood coagulation. In *Haemostasis and Thrombosis*. Eds. Bloom, A. L. and Thomas, D. P., 2nd edn, p 393. Churchill Livingstone, Edinburgh.

[3] BLOOM, A. L. (1987). The treatment of factor VIII inhibitors. In *Thrombosis and Hemostasis*. Eds. Verstraete, M., Vermylen, J., Lijnen, H. R. and Arnout, J., p. 108. International Society on Thrombosis and Haemostasis and Leuven University Press, Leuven.

[4] BORN, G. V. R. (1962). Aggregation of blood platelets by adenosine diphosphate and its reversal. *Nature*, **194**, 927.

[5] BORN, G. V. R. (1962). Quantitative investigations into the aggregation of blood platelets. *Journal of Physiology*, **162**, 67.

[6] CLAUSS, A. (1957). Rapid physiological coagulation method in determination of fibrinogen. *Acta Haematologica (Basel)*, **17**, 237.

[7] *Coagulation Manual*. (1989). Katharine Dormandy Haemophilia Centre, Royal Free Hospital, London.

[8] DAVID, J. L. and HERION, F. (1972). Assay of platelet ADP and ATP by the luciferase method. *Advances in Experimental Medicine and Biology*, **34**, 341.

[9] DENSON, K. W. E. (1961). The specific assay of Prower-Stuart Factor and Factor VII. *Acta Haematologica* (Basel), **25**, 105.

[10] GRAHAM, J. B., ELSTON, R. C., BARROW, E. S., REISNER, H. M. and NAMBOODIRI, K. K. (1982). The hemophilias:statistical methods for carrier detection in hemophilias. *Methods in Hematology*, **5**, 156.

[11] HARDISTY, R. M. and MACPHERSON, J. C. (1962). A one stage factor VIII (antihaemophilic globulin) assay and its use on venous and capillary plasma. *Thrombosis et Diathesis Haemorrhagica*, **7**, 215.

[12] INGRAM, G. I. C., BROZOVIC, M. and SLATER, N. (1982). *Bleeding Disorders*. Blackwell Scientific Publication, Oxford.

[13] KASPAR, C. K. and EWING, N. P. (1982). The Hemophilias: Measurement of inhibitor to factor VIII C (and IX C). *Methods in Hematology*, **5**, 39.

[14] LANE, D. A. and SOUTHAN, C. (1987). Inherited abnormalitites of fibrinogen synthesis and structure. In *Haemostasis and Thrombosis*. Eds. Bloom, A. L. and Thomas, D. P., 2nd edn, p. 442. Churchill Livingstone, Edinburgh.

[15] MACFARLANE, D. E., STIBBE, D. E., KIRBY, J., ZUCKER, M. B., GRANT, R. A. and MCPHERSON, J. (1975). A method for assaying Willebrand Factor (ristocetin cofactor). *Thrombosis et Diathesis Haemorrhagica*, **34**, 306.

[16] RIZZA, C. R. and JONES, P. (1987). Management of patients with inherited blood coagulation defects. In *Haemostasis and Thrombosis*. Eds. Bloom, A. L. and Thomas, D. P., 2nd edn, p. 465. Churchill Livingstone, Edinburgh.

[17] SCRUTTON, M. C., CLARE, K. A., HUTTON, R. A. and BRUCKDORFEN, K. R. (1981). Depressed responsiveness to adrenaline in platelets from apparently normal human donors. A familial trait. *British Journal of Haematology*, **49**, 303.

[18] YARDUMIAN, D. A., MACKIE, I. J. and MACHIN, S. J. (1986). Laboratory investigation of platelet functions: a review of methodology. *Journal of Clinical Pathology*, **39**, 701.

[19] British Society for Haematology (1988). Guidelines on platelet function testing. *Journal of Clinical Pathology*, **41**, 1322.

20. Investigation of a thrombotic tendency

(By M. Brozović, and I. Mackie)

Investigations to exclude an acquired or inherited thrombotic tendency are carried out in neonates, children and young adults who develop venous thrombosis, or have a strong family history of such events, and in individuals of all ages with recurrent episodes of thrombo-embolism. These investigations are commonly instituted in venous thrombosis, but some unexplained arterial events, especially in young people, are also studied. In this chapter the investigations to diagnose or exclude an acquired thrombotic tendency are presented first, followed by a simplified battery of tests needed to establish the diagnosis of the more common inherited 'thrombophilias'.

INVESTIGATION OF A SUSPECTED ACQUIRED THROMBOTIC TENDENCY

An acquired thrombotic tendency is common and occurs in many conditions. An outline of appropriate investigations is described below and also shown as a flow chart in Table 20.1. A list of causes and probable mechanisms is outlined in Table 20.2.

INVESTIGATION FOR THE PRESENCE OF LUPUS ANTICOAGULANT

The lupus anticoagulant is an acquired auto-antibody found in a variety of autoimmune disorders and sometimes even in otherwise healthy individuals.[16] Lupus anticoagulants are immunoglobulins which bind to phospholipids active in coagulation and thus prolong the clotting times of phospholipid-dependent tests such as the PT or PTTK. The name 'anticoagulant' is a misnomer since patients do not have a bleeding tendency. Instead, there is a clear-cut association with recurrent venous thrombo-embolism, cerebrovascular accidents and other arterial events, and in women, with recurrent abortions in the second trimester.

Tests for the presence of the lupus anticoagulant should be carried out in all young individuals with

Table 20.1   Flow chart for investigating a suspected thrombotic tendency

First-line tests (PTTK, PT, TT and platelet count)	
1. Clotting times shorter than normal, platelet count raised	?*Acquired thrombotic tendency* To confirm or elucidate, measure: fibrinogen, VIII:C and vWF, fibrinolytic potential; inhibitors;* platelet hyperreactivity
2. Clotting times normal, either platelet count normal	*Acquired thrombotic tendency* Investigate as under 1.
or	*Congenital thrombophilia* Measure: plasma inhibitors and inactivators, plasminogen
3. PTTK prolonged, PT normal or long, with an inhibitor pattern of behaviour	Investigate for: *Lupus anticoagulant*
4. TT prolonged	Investigate for: *Dysfibrinogenaemia*
5. All clotting tests slightly prolonged, platelets low, normal or high	?*Chronic DIC* Measure: FDP and D-dimer; platelet hyperreactivity; inhibitors

*In some clinical situations such as nephrotic syndrome, in women taking oestrogen-containing contraceptive pill, etc.

unexplained thrombosis, especially if there is no family history, and also in women with recurrent second trimester fetal loss. The detection of lupus anticoagulant should not preclude further investigation for other prethrombotic defects, such as co-existent ATIII, protein C and protein S deficiency. When lupus anticoagulant is present, the first-line tests usually show a normal TT and a prolonged PTTK which cannot be corrected by the addition of normal plasma. The PT may be normal or prolonged. The results obtained in the PTTK will depend on the reagent and method used as well as on the potency and avidity of the antibody. Even the most sensitive PTTK method may fail to detect the lupus anticoagulant in a small number of patients. It is advisable to confirm or exclude its presence with one or more of the tests described below.

Tests for the lupus anticoagulant involving tissue thromboplastin are not recommended because many samples give false negative results. Some one-stage coagulation assays which utilize phospholipid reagents are also sensitive to the lupus anticoagulant.

It is essential that all the samples of plasma tested for the lupus anticoagulant should be as free of platelets as possible, especially if they are to be stored frozen before testing. This is achieved by further centrifugation of plasma at 2000 *g* or by passing the test plasma through a 0.2 μm microfilter under pressure using a syringe.

Patients with the lupus anticoagulant may show other abnormalities, including thrombocytopenia, a positive direct antiglobulin test and a positive antinuclear factor test. In some rare cases, specific antibodies against coagulation factors are also found. Such patients may have a bleeding tendency. The tests used are: the kaolin clotting time, the heat stability test, the dilute Russell's viper venom time and the platelet neutralization test. At least two of these tests must be performed when investigating a patient with a suspected lupus anticoagulant.

KAOLIN CLOTTING TIME[4,6]

Principle. When the PTTK is performed in the absence of platelet substitute reagent, it is particularly sensitive to the lupus anticoagulant. If the test is performed on a range of mixtures of normal and patient's plasma, different patterns of response are obtained indicating the presence of lupus anticoagulant, deficiency of one or more of the coagulation factors or the 'lupus cofactor' effect. (The lupus cofactor is a plasma protein necessary for the full inhibitory effect of the lupus anticoagulant.)

Reagents

Kaolin. 20 mg/ml in tris buffer, pH 7.4. (See p. 281).

Normal platelet-poor plasma. Depleted of platelets by second centrifugation or microfiltration.

Patient's plasma. Also platelet-depleted.

CaCl₂. 0.025 mol/l.

Method

Mix normal and patient's plasma in plastic tubes in the following ratios of normal to patient's plasma:

Table 20.2 Acquired thrombotic tendency. Aetiology, mechanisms of hypercoagulability and effects on haemostasis.

Aetiology	Mechanisms of hypercoagulability	Effect on first-line tests	Other haemostatic abnormalities
Acute phase reaction	Increase in VIII:C, vWF, fibrinogen and PAI	PTTK and PT often short	Increased plasma concentration of acute reactants
Malignancy	Acute phase reaction and/or DIC due to release of tumour products	PTTK, PT and TT may be long	Increased FDP, signs of activation of coagulation and of consumption
Myeloproliferative diseases	Increased blood viscosity and high platelet count with activation of haemostasis	PTTK and PT may be short	Increased β-TG and PF4; increased acute reactants
Oestrogen-containing pill	Increased levels of vitamin-K-dependent factors, reduced ATIII; dose related	PT may be short	Increased plasma conc. of VII, IX, and X; reduced ATIII concentration
Lupus anticoagulant	Anti-phospholipid antibodies interfering with coagulation	PTTK long, PT variable	Tests for lupus anticoagulant positive; ATIII and PC conc. may be low
Nephrotic syndrome	Loss of ATIII in urine	Normal	Reduced plamsa ATIII
Vasculitic diseases and angiopathies	Stimulation of endothelium with acute phase reaction, fibrinolytic shut-down and platelet activation	Variable	Very high plasma vWF, VIII:C and fibrinogen; increased PAI, FDP, βTG and PF4
ARDS*	Low grade DIC	Variable	Reduced ATIII, PC, increased FDP, variable levels of acute reactants

*ARDS: Adult Respiratory Distress syndrome.
vWF: von Willebrand factor. β-TG: B-thromboglobulin. PF4: platelet factor 4.
ATIII: antithrombin III. PC: protein C. PAI: plasminogen activator inhibitor.

10:0, 9:1, 8:2, 5:5, 2:8, 1:9 and 0:10. Pipette 0.2 ml of each mixture into a glass tube at 37°C. Add 0.1 ml of kaolin and incubate for 3 min, then add 0.2 ml of $CaCl_2$ and record the clotting time.

Results

Plot the clotting times against the proportion of normal : patient's plasma on linear graph paper as shown in Figure 20.1.

Interpretation

If pattern 1 is obtained, the patient has a classical lupus anticoagulant. Pattern 2 indicates a coagulation factor deficiency as well as a lupus anticoagulant. Pattern 3 is found in plasma containing the anticoagulant but also deficient in a cofactor necessary for the full inhibitory effect. Pattern 4 is seen in the absence of the lupus anticoagulant.

HEAT STABILITY TEST[1]

Principle. Immunoglobulins are not adsorbed to aluminium hydroxide and are stable at 56°C,

whereas most clotting factors are removed from plasma or inactivated by this treatment. When the adsorbed and heated plasma is mixed with fresh normal plasma and a PTTK performed, any immunoglobulin inhibitor will still be present and will prolong the clotting time. This test is particularly useful in patients receiving oral anticoagulants, since the test and control plasma are equally depleted of clotting factors by adsorption and heating.

Reagents

Platelet-poor plasma. From the patient and a control.
Fresh control plasma.
Aluminium hydroxide moist gel. 4 g of moist gel per 100 ml of water.
Kaolin. 0.05% in 0.2 mol/l tris buffer, pH 7.4 (see p. 281).
Phospholipid. Platelet substitute. (p. 544); also available commercially.
$CaCl_2$. 0.025 mol/l.

Equipment

56°C water-bath.

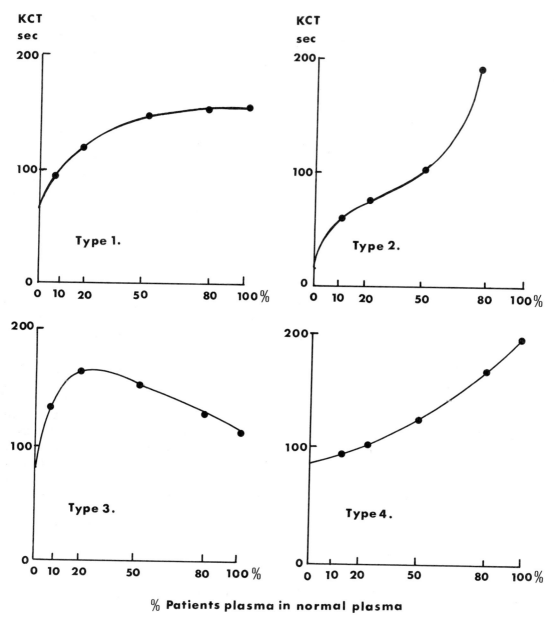

Fig. 20.1   Curves obtained using the kaolin clotting time to test for the presence of the lupus anticoagulant. For explanation see text.

Method

Place 0.5 ml of control plasma and 0.5 ml of patient's plasma in separate plastic round-bottom tubes. Add 0.05 ml of aluminium hydroxide suspension and incubate the tubes at 37°C for 3 min before centrifuging at 2000 g for 15 min. Carefully pipette the supernatants into fresh plastic tubes, which are capped and placed at 56°C for 30 min. Then centrifuge the tubes for 10 min at 2000 g and pipette the supernatant into clean plastic tubes.

Mix 0.1 ml of treated patient's or control plasma with 0.1 ml of fresh normal plasma in a glass clotting tube at 37°C, and carry out a PTTK.

Interpretation

If an immunoglobulin inhibitor is present, the clotting time of the mixture of treated patient's plasma and fresh control plasma will be at least 2 s longer than that of the treated and fresh control plasma. This test is not specific for lupus anticoagulant and is affected by anti-factor VIII:C and other inhibitors. It also has a poor sensitivity and gives some false negative results. It is not affected by oral anticoagulants and is useful when investigating patients receiving these drugs.

DILUTE RUSSELL'S VIPER VENOM TIME[17,18]

Principle. Russell's viper venom (RVV) activates factor X in the presence of phospholipid and calcium ions. The lupus anticoagulant prolongs the clotting time by binding to the phospholipid and preventing the action of RVV. In the test described below, dilution of the venom and phospholipid makes it particularly sensitive for detecting the lupus anticoagulant.[18] Since RVV activates factor X directly, defects of the contact system, and factor VIII:C and IX deficiencies will not influence the test.

Reagents

Platelet-poor plasma. From the patient and a control.

Pooled normal plasma.

Glyoxaline buffer. 0.05 mol/l, pH 7.4 (p. 281).

Russell's viper venom. Stock solution: 1 mg/ml in saline. For working solution dilute approximately 1 in 200 in imidazole buffer. The working solution is stable at 4°C for several hours.

Phospholipid. Platelet substitute (p. 544); also available commercially.

$CaCl_2$. 0.025 mol/l.

Reagent preparation

The RVV concentration is adjusted to give a clotting time of 30–35 s when 0.1 ml of RVV is added to the mixture of 0.1 ml of normal plasma and 0.1 ml of undiluted phospholipid. The test is then repeated using doubling dilutions of phospho-lipid reagent. The last dilution of phospholipid before the clotting time is prolonged by 2 s or more is selected for the test (thus giving a clotting time of 35–40 s).

Method

Place 0.1 ml of pooled normal plasma and 0.1 ml of dilute phospholipid reagent in a glass tube at 37°C. Add 0.1 ml of dilute RVV and, after warming for 30 s, add 0.1 ml of $CaCl_2$. Record the clotting time. Repeat the sequence using the test plasma. Calculate the ratio of the clotting times of the patient and control (normal pool) plasma.

Interpretation

The normal ratio should be determined in each laboratory: it is usually between 0.9 and 1.05. Ratios greater than 1.05 suggest the presence of the lupus anticoagulant, or an abnormality of factors II, V or X. The presence of the lupus anticoagulant should be confirmed by testing a mixture of equal volumes of patient's and control plasma, and/or using the platelet neutralization test described below. The addition of normal plasma will correct an abnormal dilute RVV test result due to factor deficiency or defect, but will not do so in the presence of the lupus anticoagulant. The platelet neutralization procedure will shorten the clotting time in the dilute RVV test of plasma containing the lupus anticoagulant (see next test).

False positive results may be obtained in patients on intravenous heparin, and the interpretation is difficult in patients receiving oral anticoagulants.

PLATELET NEUTRALIZATION TEST[18]

Principle. When platelets are used instead of phospholipid reagents in clotting tests, the tests become insensitive to the lupus anticoagulant. This may be partly due to the high concentration in the platelets, of phospholipids active in coagulation but it may also be due to the presence of other functional sites and receptors at the platelet membrane which favour the coagulation process rather than the binding of the anti-phospholipid immunoglobulins. To utilize this property of platelets, they must be washed to remove contaminating plasma proteins, and activated or 'fractured' to expose their coagulation factor binding sites.

Reagents

Commercial platelet extract reagent or *washed normal platelets.*

ACD anticoagulant solution, pH 5.4. (see p. 535) For use, one part of this anticoagulant is added to 6 parts of blood.

Na$_2$EDTA. 0.1 mol/l in saline.

Calcium-free Tyrode's buffer. To prepare dissolve 8 g NaCl, 0.2 g KCl, 0.625g Na$_2$HPO$_4$, 0.415 g MgCl$_2$ and 1.0 g NaHCO$_2$ in 1 litre of water. Adjust pH if necessary to 6.5 with 1 mol/l HCl.

Method

Collect normal blood into ACD and centrifuge at 270 *g* for 10 min. Pipette the supernatant platelet-rich plasma (PRP) into a plastic container, and centrifuge for a second time to obtain more PRP, which is added to the first lot. Dilute the PRP with an equal volume of the calcium free buffer, and add sufficient EDTA to give a final concentration of 0.01 mol/l. Centrifuge the mixture in a conical or round-bottom tube at 2000 *g* for 10 min, and discard the supernatant. Gently resuspend the platelet pellet in buffer and 0.01 mol/l EDTA, and centrifuge again. Again discard the supernatant, and resuspend the pellet in buffer alone. Then centrifuge the platelets a third time, and finally resuspend the pellet in buffer without EDTA to give a platelet count of at least 400 $\times$ 10^9/l. The washed platelets may be stored below $-20°$C in volumes of 1–2 ml. Before use, they must be activated by repeatedly thawing and refreezing 3–4 times.

Use the washed platelets or the commercial reagent in the dilute RVV test or in the PTTK in place of the usual phospholipid reagent. First, determine a suitable dilution by testing a range of doubling dilutions in the test system with control plasma. A suitable dilution will give a similar clotting time to that obtained using control plasma and the phospholipid reagent.

Interpretation

Since washed platelets are not inhibited by the lupus anticoagulant, their addition to the dilute RVV or PTTK system will shorten the clotting time when the lupus anticoagulant is present. It will not shorten the time when the prolongation is due to a factor deficiency or an inhibitor directed against a specific coagulation factor.

ANTI-CARDIOLIPIN ASSAY[7]

Individuals with the lupus anticoagulant almost always have other abnormalities due to the anti-phospholipid antibodies. The most frequent finding is the presence of anti-cardiolipin antibodies. These antibodies are detected using an immunoassay on microtitre plates or in coated polystyrene tubes. Commercial kits for the assay are available.

Care must be taken in the selection of control sera and in setting the cut-off point for normal values. It is also important to remember that anti-cardiolipin antibodies may be found in conditions other than the thrombotic tendency associated with lupus anticoagulant. They occur after vaccination, after viral infections, including glandular fever, and after myocardial infarction.

INVESTIGATION OF THE FIBRINOLYTIC SYSTEM

Investigation of the fibrinolytic system consists of the measurement of fibrinogen and plasminogen concentration and their functional integrity, and of the assessment of the 'fibrinolytic potential'.

INVESTIGATION OF A SUSPECTED DYSFIBRINOGENAEMIA

Congenital dysfibrinogenaemia associated with thrombosis should be suspected in individuals with a prolonged thrombin time and a slightly or moderately reduced fibrinogen concentration in plasma (see Table 20.1). For details of investigation see Chapter 19, p. 315.

INVESTIGATION OF A SUSPECTED PLASMINOGEN DEFECT OR DEFICIENCY

Inherited plasminogen deficiency or defect may account for about 2–3% of unexplained thromboses in young people.[11] The laboratory screening should be carried using a functional assay based on full transformation of plasminogen into plasmin by activators. Such assays can be caseinolytic, fibrin substrate or chromogenic.

CHROMOGENIC ASSAY FOR PLASMINOGEN[4]

Principle. In this two-step amidolytic assay plasminogen is first complexed with excess streptokinase. In the second step, the plasmin-like activity of the streptokinase-plasminogen complex is measured by its effect on a plasmin-specific peptide. The amount of the dye released is proportional to the amount of plasminogen available in the sample for complexing with streptokinase.

Reagents and method

Details can be found in the manufacturer's instructions. They vary from manufacturer to manufacturer and even from batch to batch of the same kit.

Normal range

80–120 u/dl.

Interpretation

Plasminogen concentration is reduced in the newborn, in patients with cirrhosis, with DIC and during and after thrombolytic therapy. Plasminogen is an acute phase reactant and in increased concentration is found in infection, trauma, myocardial infarction and malignant disease. The diagnosis of inherited plasminogen deficiency must be confirmed by functional tests using other activators, immunological assays and family studies.

INVESTIGATION OF 'FIBRINOLYTIC POTENTIAL'

The 'fibrinolytic potential' is measured as the combined effect of plasminogen activators and inhibitors. The concentration of activators may be increased by venous occlusion or by the adminstration of DDAVP. The tests used are, firstly, the assays of plasminogen activators, using a fibrin substrate (euglobulin lysis time, fibrin plate lysis and many others) or a chromogenic substrate or ELISA techniques; and secondly, assays of inhibitors. The commonly used tests for inhibitors are the chromogenic assays of plasminogen activator inhibitor (PAI) and of α_2 antiplasmin (AP).[14,20]

EUGLOBULIN LYSIS TIME[4,19]

Principle. When plasma is diluted and acidified, the precipitate which forms contains plasminogen activator (mostly t-PA), plasminogen and fibrinogen. Most of the inhibitors are left in the solution. The precipitate is redissolved, the fibrinogen clotted with thrombin and the time for clot lysis measured.

Reagents

Acetic acid. 0.01%.
Bovine thrombin. 10 NIH u/ml.
Fresh platelet-poor plasma from the patient and control. As t-PA is very labile, blood must be collected into cooled sample tubes, placed on ice and processed immediately.
Glyoxaline buffer, pH 7.4. (p.281).

Method

Place venous blood in a plastic tube containing citrate; after mixing, keep the tube in an ice-bath. Centrifuge the sample as soon as possible (never later than 30 min after collection) at 4°C at 1200–1500 *g*. Pipette 1.0 ml of plasma into 9 ml of acetic acid. Mix well and keep on ice for 15 min. Centrifuge at 4°C for 15 min, at a speed of 1500 *g*, to deposit the white euglobulin precipitate. Discard the supernatant, invert the tubes, then wipe the walls with cotton wool on an applicator stick until completely dry inside. Add 0.5 ml of glyoxaline buffer and dissolve the precipitate. Place duplicate

0.3 ml volumes of patient's and control dissolved euglobulin fraction in glass tubes and clot with 0.1 ml of thrombin. Leave undisturbed at 37°C and inspect for clot lysis at 15-min intervals.

Normal range

90–240 min.

Interpretation

The major cause of a long lysis time is the failure to maintain a low temperature throughout all the stages of the test. Exercise and prolonged venous stasis shorten the lysis times. There is also a significant diurnal variation: lysis time is longer in the morning than at noon or in the afternoon. Prolonged fibrinolysis (as found during fibrinolytic therapy) may result in plasminogen depletion and give rise to a falsely long time. In DIC, a low fibrinogen concentration in the patient's plasma gives a wispy clot which dissolves rapidly and results in a falsely short lysis time.

Long lysis times are found in the last trimester of pregnancy, in the post-operative period, after myocardial infarction, in obese individuals and in many cases of recurrent venous thrombosis. Very short lysis times are seen in some haematological or disseminated malignancies, and in cirrhosis.

LYSIS OF FIBRIN PLATES[4,13]

Principle. Most commercially available fibrinogen preparations are contaminated with plasminogen. If a standard fibrinogen solution is poured into a Petri dish and clotted with $CaCl_2$ and thrombin, a solid fibrin plate is obtained. If the euglobulin fraction under test is placed on the plate, the plasminogen in the plate will be converted into plasmin and a zone of lysis will appear around the sample. The area of lysis will be proportionate to the concentration of plasminogen activator in the euglobulin fraction.

Reagents

Bovine fibrinogen.
Bovine thrombin. 50 NIH u/ml.
Calcium. 0.025 mol/l.

Barbitone buffered saline.
Platelet-poor plasma. From the patient and a control collected as described for euglobulin lysis time.

Equipment

Plastic Petri dishes.

Method

To prepare the fibrin plate, dilute the fibrinogen in buffered saline to obtain a final concentration of 1.5 g/l. Pipette 10 ml of diluted fibrinogen into a Petri dish. Place it on a level tray. Add 0.5 ml of $CaCl_2$ and 0.2 ml of thrombin solution. Mix the contents by swirling quickly. The plate clots within 10 to 20 s; it must clot evenly to be suitable for the test. Leave the plate undisturbed for 20 min. The prepared plates can then be kept for 3–4 days at 4°C.

Carefully apply 30 µl of the euglobulin fraction, prepared as described in the previous test, to the surface of the plate. There is no need to cut a well. Place in an incubator at 37°C for 24 h.

Perform all tests (patient and control) in duplicate.

Results

Calculate the zone of lysis by measuring two diameters in mm at right angles to each other. Multiply the two values to obtain the approximate area of lysis in mm^2.

Normal range

Variable, but usually between 40 and 60 mm^2.

Interpretation

The area of lysis may be difficult to define because of incomplete lysis. Only areas of complete, clear lysis should be measured.

VENOUS OCCLUSION TEST[4,5]

Principle. Localized venous occlusion of an arm for a standardized period of time is used as a stimulus for release of t-PA from the vessel wall. Pre- and post-occlusion lysis times, using the above-described euglobulin lysis or the fibrin plate lysis tests, are measured. In normal subjects fibrinolysis is greatly enhanced by occlusion.

Method

Withdraw blood from the arm to be tested without stasis, place it in a citrate-containing tube and keep in an ice-bath. Inflate the sphygmomanometer cuff to a pressure midway between the systolic and diastolic (measured on the other arm). Leave the inflated cuff on for 10 min. Take a sample of venous blood from below the cuff immediately before deflation and place on ice. Measure the lysis in both samples as described previously. This test is uncomfortable and some patients may not be able to tolerate as much as 10 min occlusion.

Results

The post-occlusion lysis times should be shorter than the pre-occlusion times. Shortening by at least 30 min is found in most normal subjects.

Interpretation

Failure to enhance lysis is found in some cases of recurrent venous thrombosis, in obese people and after surgery, trauma or severe illness. It may also be due to a failure to release the activator because insufficient pressure was applied or the occlusion time was too short. Normal people vary in the degree of response: 'good' responders increase the concentration of t-PA by 3–4 fold, whereas 'poor' responders may consistently show only a very slight enhancement of fibrinolysis even with longer occlusion times.

TISSUE PLASMINOGEN ACTIVATOR (t-PA) AMIDOLYTIC ASSAY[8,10]

Principle. Different amidolytic assays for t-PA have been described. One relies on the activation of purified plasminogen to plasmin in the presence of fibrinogen fragments which stimulate the t-PA activity in the test plasma. The plasmin is measured using a specific chromogenic substrate. In the second method, t-PA is captured on specific antibodies bound to a solid phase matrix such as a microtitre plate; plasminogen is added together with a stimulator of t-PA activity, and the plasmin produced measured with chromogenic substrates. Alternatively, chromogenic substrates specific for t-PA may be used, but there are specificity problems especially in the plasma assays.

Tissue plasminogen activator can also be measured by ELISA using monoclonal antibodies on microtitre plates.

PLASMINOGEN ACTIVATOR INHIBITOR (PAI-1) ASSAY

Principle. A fixed amount of t-PA is added in excess to undiluted plasma. Part of it rapidly complexes with the t-PA inhibitor (PAI). Plasminogen in plasma is then activated into plasmin by the residual, uncomplexed t-PA. The amount of plasmin formed is directly proportional to the residual t-PA activity and inversely proportional to the PAI activity of the sample. The amount of plasmin generated is measured using a plasmin-specific substrate.

Reagents are available in a kit form and the manufacturer's instructions must be closely followed. The normal range is as yet poorly defined, and each laboratory should establish its own range until suitable normal values become available.

α_2-ANTIPLASMIN AMIDOLYTIC ASSAY

Principle. Plasma dilutions are incubated with excess plasmin, a proportion of which will be inhibited by antiplasmins. The residual, uninhibited plasmin is measured using a specific chromogenic substrate. α_2-antiplasmin is the major circulating inhibitor of plasmin and forms complexes much faster than other inhibitors: if the reaction times are short, the assay effectively measures α_2-antiplasmin only.

Different commercial kits are available containing all the necessary reagents. The manufacturer's instructions should be carefully followed.

The usual normal range is between 80 and 120%. Congenital α_2-antiplasmin deficiency is associated with a severe bleeding tendency. A reduced plasma concentration is found in liver disease, DIC and during thrombolytic therapy. α_2-antiplasmin increases with age and is higher in Caucasians than in Africans.

D-DIMER LATEX ASSAY (DIMERTEST)

Principle. During normal fibrin formation, fibrinogen chains are cross-linked by factor XIII, and if plasmin digestion of the clot occurs, the fragment D portions of two adjacent fibrin monomers remain cross-linked together as a D-dimer. This fragment is not generated during the degradation of fibrinogen or non-cross-linked fibrin, and is therefore specific to the lysis of fibrin clots, and may be detected by immunological techniques.

Patient's plasma or serum is mixed with latex particles coated with antibodies against the D-dimer fragment of fibrin. If D-dimer is present, it will bind to the latex, and agglutination may be visualized on a glass slide.

Reagents

Fresh citrated, heparinized or EDTA plasma; or serum. Collected with or without anti-fibrinolytic agent as described for fibrinogen/fibrin degradation products (Chapter 18, p. 290).

Commercial D-dimer kit. Comprises latex beads, phosphate buffer and positive and negative controls.

Method

Place 25 µl of latex beads on a glass slide and mix with 10 µl of undiluted test plasma or serum. Rock the slide gently for 3 min and observe any agglutination over a dark background. If the test is positive, make doubling dilutions of its plasma or serum in phosphate buffer, pH 7.4 and repeat the test until a negative result is obtained.

Calculation

Calculate the result in ng/ml according to the dilutions in which agglutination was observed, and the manufacturer's specifications.

Normal range

Less than 200 ng/ml.

Interpretation

Elevated concentrations are found in venous thrombosis and pulmonary embolism, in DIC and conditions associated with microvascular fibrin deposition. The test is not influenced by fibrinogen or non-cross-linked fibrin.

INVESTIGATION OF PLATELET 'HYPERREACTIVITY'

Platelets may be more reactive than normally as a consequence of in-vivo activation by thrombin or non-endothelial surfaces, such as prosthetic valves or Dacron grafts. This can sometimes be detected by a lowered threshold (increased sensitivity) for aggregating agents. Because there is considerable variation in response to aggregating agents in normal people, the attempts to show platelet hyperaggregability are rarely successful and the results are frequently inconsistent. Spontaneous aggregation of platelets in the blood can also be demonstrated.[21]

Platelets which have formed a part of a platelet thrombus and have been released into the circulation may show a measurable decrease in aggregability due to a loss of some of the granular content.

The released contents can be measured in plasma: the α-granule proteins, β-thromboglobulin and platelet factor 4 are the two proteins most commonly measured.[22] Shortened platelet survival using [111]Indium-labelled platelets can also be used as a marker of platelet activation by a thrombotic process (see p. 394).

β-THROMBOGLOBULIN (β-TG) AND PLATELET FACTOR 4 (PF4) ASSAYS

Principle. ELISA and RIA methods are available for the measurement of these proteins using specific anti-sera. In the former, a double antibody sandwich technique is used, in which the surface of a tube or microplate is coated with antibody against β-TG or PF4, and plasma is added. Protein is then bound to the antibody, and may be detected by the binding of a second antibody carrying an enzyme tag. In the RIA methods, there is competition between β-TG or PF4 from the test sample and radio-labelled (usually ^{125}I) tracer protein for binding to a specific antibody. A high plasma concentration of the protein released from the platelets displaces the tracer from the immune complex.

Sample collection

Blood has to be collected and handled carefully to avoid artefactual release of β-TG and PF4 from the platelets. Samples are collected from free-flowing blood, drawn without venous stasis, and the first 2–3 ml discarded. Blood is immediately added to a tube chilled in a beaker filled with melting ice, which contains a special mixture of inhibitors of platelet activation, as well as calcium chelators. Plasma must be separated strictly at 4°C.

Reagents and method

Sample collection tubes and reagents are provided with the commercial kits used for the two tests. It is important to follow the manufacturer's instructions carefully.

The calculation of results depends on whether an ELISA or a RIA method is used.

Interpretation

The normal concentration of β-TG is less than 50 ng/ml and that of PF4 less than 10 ng/ml. Falsely high results may be encountered in RIA methods if diagnostic isotope techniques (such as leg scanning for thrombosis using ^{125}I fibrinogen) have been used in the patient. The tests cannot be performed for a week or so after the scanning or until ^{125}I is cleared from the patient's plasma.

PF4 is rapidly cleared from plasma by the vascular endothelium; it may be displaced from the endothelial binding by heparin. Thus a high PF4 concentration may be found in patients receiving heparin. β-TG is cleared from plasma by the kidney, and its concentration is commonly high in renal failure. In patients without these clinical problems, both proteins should be measured in order to distinguish in-vivo release from an in-vivo artefact. With in-vivo activation of platelets, the plasma concentration of both proteins rises, but the concentration of β-TG remains much higher owing to the rapid endothelial clearance of PF4. The ratio of β-TG to PF4 is usually greater than 5:1. If venepuncture has been difficult or sample handling inadequate, in-vitro platelet release occurs and the concentration of both proteins is high (ratio less than 2:1).

INVESTIGATION OF SUSPECTED INHERITED THROMBOTIC SYNDROMES

The prevalence of inherited thrombotic syndromes in the general population may be as high as 1 in 2500 or 1 in 5000, deficiency of protein C (PC) and ATIII being the commonest.[12] It is becoming increasingly important to screen for such disorders. Screening must start by excluding the common causes of an acquired thrombotic tendency as described below. A careful family history must be taken next; however, a negative history does not exclude an inherited thrombotic tendency because the defects have a low penetrance or a fresh mutation may have been responsible. As with a bleeding tendency, laboratory investigation is a step-wise procedure, starting with the simpler, first-line tests (as shown in Table 20.1). The key tests at each step are described below.

MEASUREMENT OF ANTITHROMBIN III

Antithrombin III is the major physiological inhibitor of thrombin, and factors Xa, IXa and XIa and XIIa.[16] It is also known as heparin cofactor I since its inhibitory action is potentiated and accelerated in the presence of heparin. Antithrombin III deficiency is not uncommon and may be acquired (see Table 20.2) or congenital.

Table 20.3 Dilutions of serum for the antithrombin III assay

Buffer (ml)	Serum (ml)	ATIII (%)
0.8	0	0
0.75	0.05	25
0.70	0.10	50
0.65	0.15	75
0.60	0.20	100
0.55	0.25	125

A variety of methods are available for measuring either functional or antigenic activity of antithrombin III. The functional methods are based on the reaction with thrombin or factor Xa; they can be coagulation or chromogenic assays. A chromogenic and a thrombin-based coagulation assay are described below.

ANTITHROMBIN III ASSAY USING THROMBIN[4,9]

Principle. Antithrombin III is a progressive inhibitor. If serum is incubated with excess thrombin, any residual thrombin remaining at the end of incubation will reflect the concentration of antithrombin III in the serum.

Reagents

Thrombin. c 50 u/ml.
Reptilase-R.
Citrate-glyoxaline buffer. Add 1 volume of tri-sodium citrate to 5 volumes of glyoxaline buffer. The pH should be 7.4.
Bovine fibrinogen solution. Made according to the manufacturer's instructions.
Normal platelet-poor plasma. From the normal pool.
Patient's plasma.

Method

Clot 1 ml of patient's and of the normal plasma at 37°C for 10 min with 0.1 ml of Reptilase to remove fibrinogen. Gently remove the clots by winding onto a wooden applicator stick. Then dilute the serum as shown in Table 20.3.

Incubate 0.8 ml of each dilution for 4 min at 37°C with 0.1 ml of thrombin solution. The throm-

bin should be adjusted initially to give a clotting time of about 15–17 s with the blank. At 4 min pipette two 0.1 ml sub-samples into pre-warmed volumes of fibrinogen solution and note the clotting time.

Results

Plot the clotting times against the concentration of antithrombin III on semi-log graph paper. Draw best straight lines and calculate the ATIII concentration in the patient's sample by reading off at various points along the line and averaging the results.

Normal range

Between 75 and 125 u/dl.

Interpretation

In an inherited deficiency, the ATIII concentration is usually approximately 40–50 u/dl. Similar values are seen in acquired deficiencies; very low values are sometimes encountered in fulminant DIC. Normal newborns have a lower ATIII concentration (60–80 u/dl) than adults. In congenitally deficient neonates, very low values (30 u/dl and lower) may be found. Very high values are encountered after myocardial infarction and in some forms of vascular disease. If high values are measured, it is important to exclude the presence of heparin in plasma as heparin interferes with the assay and causes falsely high values.

ANTITHROMBIN III MEASUREMENT USING A CHROMOGENIC ASSAY[4,15]

Principle. In the presence of heparin, antithrombin III reacts rapidly to inactivate thrombin by forming a 1:1 complex. Chromogenic antithrombin III assay is a two-step procedure. In the first step the plasma sample is incubated with a fixed quantity of thrombin and heparin. The amount of thrombin inactivated is then proportional to the ATIII concentration in the plasma. In the second step the residual thrombin is measured spectrophotometrically by its action on a synthetic chromogenic substrate which results in the release of para-nitro-aniline dye (PNA).

Method

Carry out the procedure on dilutions of a standard plasma so as to construct a standard graph. Then test dilutions of the test plasma in an identical manner and read the results directly from the standard graph.

The reagents provided and details of the method vary from manufacturer to manufacturer and should be closely followed. There may also be variation between different batches of the same reagent.

Normal range

Generally between 75–125 u/dl. Some manufacturers, however, recommend a slightly narrower range, i.e. 80–120 u/dl. Repeated freezing and thawing of samples, as well as storage at or above $-20°C$ result in a reduction in ATIII concentration. It is also important to remember that oral anticoagulant therapy raises the ATIII concentration by c 10 u/dl in cases of congenital deficiency.

Further investigations

If an inherited ATIII deficiency is suspected more than one functional ATIII assay should be performed and the antigenic activity also determined. Family studies should always be performed.

INVESTIGATION OF PROTEIN C DEFICIENCY

Protein C (PC) is a vitamin-K-dependent protein; after thrombin activation which is accelerated in the presence of thrombomodulin and the vascular endothelium, PC complexes with phospholipids and protein S (PS) to degrade factors Va and VIII:C. Inherited protein C deficiency accounts for some 5–7% of all recurrent thrombo-embolic episodes in young adults.[2,12] Most such individuals are heterozygotes. The homozygous state has been occasionally reported in the neonate with massive visceral thrombosis and purpura fulminans.[3] Ac-

quired PC deficiency is found in all conditions associated with vitamin K deficiency or defect, including oral anticoagulant therapy. A low plasma concentration is also found in DIC, liver disease and in the early post-operative period.

PC can be measured using a chromogenic assay, a coagulation assay or an antigenic method.

MEASUREMENT OF FUNCTIONAL PROTEIN C (PC) BY THE PROTAC METHOD[4]

Principle. In the presence of a specific snake venom activator, PC is converted into its active form. Activated PC is measured by its action on one of the specific synthetic substrates (such as S-2366, CBS 65.25). The reaction is stopped by the addition of 50% acetic acid and the p-nitroalanine produced measured at 405 nm in a spectrophotometer.

Reagents

Platelet-poor plasma. Standard and test: samples are centrifuged at $1500–2000\,g$ for 15 min. After centrifugation, plasma can be stored indefinitely at $-40°C$ or below.

Protac C. This is an activator derived from the venom of *Agkistrodon contortix contortix*. This is obtained commercially; each vial contains lyophilized powder which is reconstituted and stored according to the manufacturer's instructions.

Specific chromogenic substrate. Reconstituted and stored according to the manufacturer's instructions.

Barbitone buffered saline.

Acetic acid. 50%.

Method

Construct the standard curve according to the instructions. Some manufacturers recommend the use of commercial calibrators or control plasma in preference to the normal pool.

The assay is carried out by a two-step method. In the first step plasma and activator are incubated for an exact period of time. In the second step the specific chromogenic substrate is added and the reaction is stopped with acetic acid again at a precise point in time. Read the amount of the dye produced at 405 nm against a blank obtained in the following way. Acetic acid, activator and chromogenic substrate are first mixed; then standard or patient's plasma is added to the mixture and the absorbence measured at 405 nm. The manufacturer's instructions must be closely followed. Plot the protein C % activity against the corresponding absorbence reading on linear graph paper.

Normal range

70–140%. Each laboratory should preferably establish its own normal range.

Further investigation

If the inherited PC deficiency is suspected, an immunological assay should also be carried out. It is also important to exclude vitamin K deficiency by assaying other vitamin-K-dependent factors which should be normal. Family studies should be carried out whenever possible.

INVESTIGATION OF PROTEIN S DEFICIENCY

Protein S is also a vitamin-K-dependent protein which acts as a cofactor of the activated PC. In plasma, 60% of PS is bound to C4b-binding protein and does not possess any anticoagulant activity; the remaining 40% is free and available to interact with PC. The functional assays of PS are based on the capacity of PS to prolong the one-stage factor Xa time or PTTK in the presence of activated purified PC. The reagents for the functional assay are not yet commercially available. Measurement of the total PS antigen by an immunoassay is possible using enzyme-linked immunoassays, or by the Laurell rocket technique, which is described below.

IMMUNO-ELECTROPHORETIC ASSAY OF PROTEIN S (PS)

Principle. The assay is based on the method of Laurell. The C4b complexed PS may be removed from plasma by precipitation with polyethylene glycol (PEG) allowing the measurement of free PS.

Reagents

Tris/tricine/EDTA buffer, pH 8.55. Dissolve 17.2 g tricine, 38.2 g tris, and 15.5 g disodium EDTA in 4 litres of water.

Agarose. 1% in buffer described above. Low electro-endo-osmosis (LE) type should be used.

Rabbit anti-human protein S. Commercially available.

25% PEG 6000.

Coomassie Blue stain. Dissolve 5 g of PAGE Blue 83 'Electran'* in a mixture of 450 ml methanol, 450 ml water and 100 ml glacial acetic acid.

Destaining solution. As described under Coomassie Blue stain, but without PAGE Blue.

Standard. Pooled normal plasma.

Test plasma. Platelet-poor plasma from the patient.

Equipment

The equipment is described in Chapter 19, p. 307. Additional apparatus required is described below.

Gelbond film. (ICN Biomedicals Ltd, High Wycombe, Bucks.)

56°C water-bath.

Electrophoresis tank with a cooling facility (cooling platten).

Well cutter 2.5 mm.

Method

For 'free' PS measurement, place 340 µl of the standard in a microcentrifuge tube and warm to 37°C. Add slowly 60 µl of 25% PEG while constantly gently agitating the tube. Place the tube on ice for 30 min. Then centrifuge the tube for 5 min and pipette the supernatant into a fresh tube. Treat the test samples in a similar fashion. Use the standard supernatant undiluted (100%), and after dilution in buffer to give 75, 50 and 25% solutions. Use the test samples as 100% and 50% solution. For 'total' PS measurement, prepare dilutions of the standard and test plasma as above, omitting the PEG precipitation step.

---

* BDH Ltd.

Place 1.5 g of agarose in a 250 ml conical flask and add 150 ml of the buffer. Place the flask on a hot plate, stirring magnetically while it heats. As soon as the agarose is dissolved leaving a clear solution, remove the flask and place it in the 56°C water-bath.

Pipette 13 ml of agarose into a pre-warmed glass test tube at 56°C. Add the antiserum (26 µl for 'free' PS or 75 µl for 'total PS), cover the tube and mix the contents by inverting the tube 5 or 6 times.

Cut a piece of gelbond film, 7.5 × 10 cm, and place on the levelling table, hydrophilic side up. Pour the agarose-antibody mixture onto the film and leave to set at room temperature. Store at 4°C for 30 min.

Place the gel with its gelbond backing flat on the bench, and cut a row of wells 150 mm from one end of the plate, using a 2.5 mm well cutter. Ensure that residual pieces of agarose are removed from the wells. Place the plate on the cooling platten of the electrophoresis tank so that the wells are at the cathodal end.

Attach wicks soaked in buffer to each side of the gel so that 1 cm strips of gel are covered. Place 1 litre of buffer in each side of the tank.

Place 6.5 µl of the standard and test dilutions in each well. Apply a voltage of 3 v/cm gel width at constant current overnight, cooling the platten at 10°C.

Turn the power off next morning. Remove the gel from the tank and wash it 3 times by immersion in saline. Remove the gel from the last saline wash, cover with filter paper and make holes through the paper over the wells using a hypodermic needle. Place several layers of paper towelling on top, then a flat board and a 1 kg weight. The paper towelling is changed 2 or 3 times until the gel is pressed flat and dried. Place the almost dry gel in a 37°C incubator until completely dry and the filter paper peels off.

Stain in Coomassie stain for 10 min. Destain until the precipitin lines are clearly visible.

Measure the height of each rocket from the well to the tip of the rocket. Plot the rocket height against PS concentration on double-log paper. Read off the test values from the standard curve. Convert the percentage of the standard value to u/ml by multiplying the percentage by the standard potency and dividing by 100.

Normal range

70–140%. Ideally, the normal range should be determined by each laboratory.

Interpretation

Protein S is reduced in the congenital deficiency, in patients on oral anticoagulants, in liver disease and vitamin K deficiency, as well as in some cases of DIC.[2,12]

Technical comments

1. Agarose should not be heated for too long, or at too high a temperature, because it may char and become brown.

2. Higher or lower test dilutions must be made if the plasma concentration is very high or very low.

3. The correct volume of antiserum to use must be determined for each batch of antiserum; it is usually c 100 µl per 100 ml of agarose.

INVESTIGATION OF HEPARIN COFACTOR II DEFICIENCY

A deficiency of heparin cofactor II is found in some individuals with recurrent thrombo-embolism. Its concentration is measured in the presence of a strong family history if the assays of other physiological inhibitors give normal results.

HEPARIN COFACTOR II ASSAY

Principle. Heparin cofactor II (HCII) present in test and standard plasma is activated by dermatan sulphate and incubated with human thrombin. The residual, uninhibited thrombin is then measured by cleavage of a chromogenic substrate.

Reagents

Reagents are commercially available in a kit form.

Buffer, pH 8.2. 0.05 mol/l tris, 0.15 mol/l NaCl, 6.8 mmol/l Na_2EDTA, 2 mg/l Polybrene, 10 g/l bovine serum albumin, pH adjusted with HCl.

Dermatan sulphate (free of heparin).

Human thrombin.

Chromogenic substrate for thrombin.

50% acetic acid.

Pooled normal plasma as standard.

Test plasma.

Method

It is important to follow the manufacturer's instructions which come with the kit. Prepare a range of dilutions of pooled normal plasma in order to construct a calibration curve. Prepare also a single dilution of each test plasma. Incubate the dilutions with dermatan sulphate at 37°C in a plastic tube or a microtitre plate. Then add thrombin, followed after a further incubation by the chromogenic substrate. After a suitable reaction time, add acetic acid to stop the reaction, and measure the absorbence at 405 nm in a spectrophotometer or a microtitre plate reader as appropriate.

Calculation

Read the absorbence of the test plasma from the calibration curve and express as percentage normal.

Normal range

Generally 55–145%.

Interpretation

The plasma concentration may be increased in healthy women on oral contraceptive pills. HCII is reduced in congenital deficiency, liver disease and DIC.

REFERENCES

[1] AUSTEN, D. E. G. and RHYMES, I. L. (1976). *A Laboratory Manual of Blood Coagulation.* Blackwell Scientific Publications, Oxford.

[2] BROEKMANS, A. W., VAN DER LINDEN, I. K., JANSEN-KOETER, Y. and BERTINA, R. M. (1986). Prevalence of protein C (PC) and protein S (PS) deficiency in patients with thromboembolic disease. *Thrombosis Research,* **Supplement VI,** 135.

[3] BRANSON, H. E., KATZ, J., MARBLE, R. and GRIFFIN, J. H. (1983). Inherited protein C deficiency and coumarin responsive chronic relapsing purpura fulminans in a newborn infant. *Lancet,* **ii,** 1165.

[4] *Coagulation Manual.* Katherine Dormandy Haemophilia Centre, Royal Free Hospital, London. By permission.

[5] DAVIDSON, J. F. and WALKER, I. D. (1987). Assessment of the fibrinolytic system. In *Haemostasis and Thrombosis.* Eds. Bloom, A. L. and Thomas, D. P., 2nd ed., p. 953. Churchill Livingstone, Edinburgh.

[6] EXNER, T., RICKARD, K. A. and KRONENBERG, H. (1978). A sensitive test demonstrating lupus anticoagulant and its behavioural patterns. *British Journal of Haematology,* **40,** 143.

[7] HARRIS, E. N., GHARAVI, A. E., PATEL, S. P. and HUGHES, G. R. V. (1987). Evaluation of the anticardiolipin antibody test: report of an international workshop held 4th April 1986. *Clinical and Experimental Immunology,* **68,** 215.

[8] HOLVOET, P., CLEEMPUT, H. and COLLEN, D. (1985). Assay of human tissue type plasminogen activator (t-PA) with an enzyme-linked immunosorbent assay (ELISA) based on three murine monoclonal antibodies. *Thrombosis and Haemostasis,* **54,** 684.

[9] HOWIE, P. W., PRENTICE, C. R. M. and McNICOL, G. P. (1973). A method of antithrombin III estimation using plasma defibrinated with ancrod. *British Journal of Haematology,* **25,** 101.

[10] MAHMOOD, M. and GAFFNEY, P. J. (1985). Bioimmunoassay (BIA) of tissue plasminogen activator (t-PA) and its specific inhibitor (t-PA/INH). *Thrombosis and Haemostasis,* **53,** 356.

[11] MANNUCCI, P. M., KLUFT, C., TRAAS, D. W., SEVESO, P. and D'ANGELO, A. (1986). Congenital plasminogen deficiency associated with venous thromboembolism: therapeutic trial with stanozolol. *British Journal of Haematology,* **63,** 753.

[12] MANNUCCI, P.,M. and TRIPODI A. (1987) Laboratory screening of inherited thrombotic syndromes. *Thrombosis and Haemostasis,* **57;** 247.

[13] MARSH, N. A. and AROCHA-PINANGO, C. L. (1972). Evaluation of the fibrin plate method for estimating plasminogen activators. *Thrombosis et Diathesis Haemorrhagica,* **28,** 75.

[14] NILSSON, I. M., LJUNGNER, H. and TENGBORN, L. (1985). Two different mechanisms in patients with venous thrombosis and defective fibrinolysis: low concentration of plasminogen activator or increased concentration of plasminogen activator inhibitor. *British Medical Journal,* **290, 1453.**

[15] ODEGARD, O. R., LIE, M. and ABILDGAARD, U. (1976). Heparin cofactor activity measured with an amidolytic method. *Thrombosis Research,* **6,** 287.

[16] SALEM, H. H. (1986). The natural anticoagulants. *Clinics in Haematology,* **15;** 371.

[17] THIAGARAJAN, P., PENGO, V. and SHAPIRO, S. S. (1986). The use of the dilute Russell Viper Venom time for the diagnosis of lupus anticoagulants. *Blood,* **68;** 869.

[18] THIAGARAJAN P. and SHAPIRO, S. S. (1983). Disorders of thrombin formation: lupus anticoagulants. *Methods in Hematology,* **7,** 121.

[19] VON KAULLA, K. N. (1963). *Chemistry of Thrombolysis: Human Fibrinolytic Enzymes.* Thomas, Illinois.

[20] WIMAN, B., LJUNGEBERG, B., CHMIELEWSKA, J., URDEN J., BLOMBACK, M. and JOHNSSON, H. (1985). The role of fibrinolytic system in deep vein thrombosis. *Journal of Laboratory and Clinical Medicine,* **105,** 265.

[21] WU, K. K. and HOAK, J. C. (1976). Spontaneous platelet aggregation in arterial insufficiency: mechanisms and implications. *Thrombosis and Haemostasis,* **46,** 702.

[22] YARDUMIAN, D. A., MACKIE, I. J. and MACHIN, S. J. (1986). Laboratory investigation of platelet function: a review of methodology. *Journal of Clinical Pathology,* **39,** 701.

21. Laboratory control of anticoagulant, thrombolytic and anti-platelet therapy

(By M. Brozović)

Anticoagulant therapy prevents thrombosis or the further propagation of an existing thrombus. Anticoagulant drugs have little if any effect upon an already formed thrombus. There are three main classes of anticoagulant drugs:

1. The oral anticoagulants, coumarins and indanediones, which act by interfering with the γ-carboxylation step in the synthesis of the vitamin-K-dependent factors (see p. 270).

2. Heparin and heparinoids (low molecular weight and synthetic compounds) which have a complex action on haemostasis, the main effect being the potentiation and acceleration of the effect of antithrombin III on thrombin and factor Xa.

3. Defibrinating agents such as ancrod (Arvin) and Reptilase which induce hypocoagulability by the removal of fibrinogen from the blood. The laboratory control of defibrinating agents is described in the previous edition of this book.

The anticoagulant drugs may be used to treat an acute episode of thrombosis or to prevent its onset in cases where there is a high risk of thrombosis, e.g. post-operatively or in pregnancy. Heparin may also be used to treat patients with DIC and some types of renal failure, as well as during haemodialysis and cardiopulmonary bypass.

ORAL ANTICOAGULANT TREATMENT

It is not possible to produce a therapeutic derangement of haemostasis without increasing the risk of haemorrhage. The purpose of laboratory control is to maintain a level of hypocoagulability—the therapeutic range—which is effective in preventing thrombosis but does not cause spontaneous bleeding. Oral anticoagulant treatment must be regularly and frequently controlled by laboratory tests to ensure that the results of the test remain within the therapeutic range. The therapeutic range differs from method to method, and from reagent to reagent used, and is affected by the laboratory technique. It also depends on the reason for anticoagulation: an individual with a prosthetic aortic valve may require more intensive anticoagulation than another who has experienced a simple calf vein thrombosis.

Selection of patients

Haemostasis is not as a rule investigated before starting oral anticoagulant treatment but it is advisable to perform the first-line coagulation screen (PT, PTTK, thrombin time and platelet count) in the elderly or frail or in those with a previous history of increased blood loss. A slight prolongation of the results of the first-line tests indicates that a lower dose should be given from the beginning of treatment. A marked prolongation must be investigated and is usually a contra-indication to the use of oral anticoagulants.

Methods used for the laboratory control of oral anticoagulant treatment

The one-stage prothrombin time of Quick is the most commonly used test. However, lack of standardization of the thromboplastin preparations used in this simple test has caused great discrepancies in the results. In addition, different methods of expressing the prothrombin time results have led to varying intensities of treatment in different parts of the world. The use of ISI, the International Sensitivity Index, to assess the sensitivity of any given thromboplastin, and the use of INR, the International Normalized Ratio, which is the prothrombin time ratio expressed in terms of a common international reference thromboplastin, should minimize these difficulties and ensure uniformity of anticoagulation and interpretation throughout the world (see later).

The Thrombotest of Owren[9] is a test popular in the Scandinavian countries. The results are expressed as a percentage which can in turn be transformed into INR.

The partial thromboplastin time with kaolin is occasionally used to assess the effects of long-term anticoagulant treatment especially before a surgical procedure. It cannot be used alone for safe anticoagulant control; it remains an additional test to be used in special circumstances only.

Chromogenic substrates have been used for the control of anticoagulant treatment in factor X, VII or II assays. Athough it is possible to use such a single factor measurement, it must be remembered that the one-stage prothrombin time and the Thrombotest measure three vitamin-K-dependent factors (factors VII, X and II) and are also affected by the presence of PIVKAs or the acarboxy forms of vitamin-K-dependent factors. This makes them safer and more sensitive tests in the control of this potentially dangerous treatment. Amidolytic versions of the prothrombin time using thromboplastin, calcium and a chromogenic substrate for thrombin have been introduced recently and may prove a viable alternative.

The prothrombin and proconvertin (P & P) method or Owren and Aas[10] was introduced in an attempt to make the prothrombin time more sensitive to vitamin-K-dependent factors. It was described in previous editions of this book.

CONTROL OF ORAL ANTICOAGULANT TREATMENT BY THE ONE-STAGE PROTHROMBIN TIME

Principle. The test is carried out as described in Chapter 18, p. 281. It is, however, essential to use a thromboplastin standardized by the commercial supplier or according to a local, regional or national procedure. To ensure safety and uniformity of anticoagulation, the results should be reported in INR either alone or in parallel with the locally accepted method of reporting.

Reporting the results

Reporting varies from laboratory to laboratory. In its simplest form the result can be reported as patient's time in seconds and control time in seconds, e.g. patient 24 s, control 12 s. This is usually reported as a *ratio* which is the result with the test plasma divided by the result with the control plasma, e.g. in this case 2.0. Many laboratories are using *INR (the International Normalized Ratio)* for reporting the results, i.e. the prothrombin time ratio which would have been obtained with the patient's plasma, had the primary reference thromboplastin been used to perform the test. For details see p. 337.

Some laboratories report the results as a *percentage of normal clotting activity* derived from a graph prepared by the manufacturer or locally. This graph is prepared by plotting dilutions of the normal plasma against the clotting times. There are serious drawbacks to this method because the diluted normal plasma does not reflect the anticoagulant defect in the anticoagulated plasma and its use may lead to either bleeding or thrombotic complications in patients whose treatment is controlled in this way. Finally, in a few laboratories, *the prothrombin time index* remains in use: this is a reciprocal of the ratio reported as percentage. In the case mentioned above it would be 50%. It is cumbersome and may be confused with the percentage activity. The definition and the use of the INR is described on p. 339. The relationship between the ratio, index, per cent activity and INR for a thromboplastin with a known ISI is shown in Table 21.1.[8]

Standardization of thromboplastin[7]

There are a number of commercial thromboplastins of animal origin. Human brain thromboplastin is no longer used for the prothrombin time because of the potential danger of the transmission of retroviruses. Each thromboplastin gives a different ratio or percentage on the same test and control plasma; even different batches of the same thromboplastin behave differently. It is not possible to define the therapeutic range unless the thromboplastin used is also specified or calibrated in terms of the International Sensitivity Index (ISI).

Table 21.1 Comparison of different ways of reporting the prothrombin time using a thromboplastin with ISI of 2.3 (Modified from Lewis[8])

PT time, s	PT ratio	PT index	% activity	INR
12	1.0	100	100	1.0
13.2	1.1	91	74	1.2
14.4	1.2	83	57	1.5
15.6	1.3	77	48	1.8
16.8	1.4	71	41	2.2
18	1.5	67	35	2.7
19.2	1.6	62	31	2.9
20.5	1.7	59	28	3.4
21.6	1.8	56	25	3.9
22.9	1.9	53	23	4.4
24	2.0	50	21	4.9
25.5	2.1	48	20	5.5
26.5	2.2	45	18.5	6.1
27.6	2.3	43	17.4	6.8
28.8	2.4	42	16.4	7.5
30	2.5	40	15.4	8.2
36	3.0	33	12	12.5

PT: prothrombin time. The therapeutic range lies between INR 2.0 and 4.0.
ISI: International Sensitivity Index. INR: International Normalized Ratio.

The calibration of thromboplastins is achieved by comparing the results from the test thromboplastin with those given by a reference thromboplastin calibrated in accordance with the method recommended by the WHO Expert Committee on Biological Standardization.

Reference thromboplastins may be the WHO Reference Preparations or certified reference materials from the European Community Bureau of Reference. The first are obtained from the National Institute for Biological Standards and Control, and are usually only issued for the calibration and standardization of national or secondary WHO standards. The European reference materials are available to manufacturers and individual laboratories from the European Community Bureau of Reference. All the reference preparations have been calibrated in terms of a primary WHO human brain thromboplastin established in 1967 which is no longer available. Rabbit and bovine reference preparations are also available from both sources.

The following terms are employed in the calibration procedure which is described below:
International Sensitivity Index (ISI).[7] This is the slope of the calibration line obtained when the logarithms of the prothrombin times obtained with the reference preparation are plotted on the vertical axis of log-log paper and the logarithms of the prothrombin times obtained by the test thromboplastin are plotted on the horizontal axis. The same normal and anticoagulated patient's plasma samples are used.

International Normalized Ratio (INR). This is the prothrombin time ratio which would have been obtained had the original primary, human reference thromboplastin been used to perform the prothrombin time.

CALIBRATION OF THROMBOPLASTINS

Principle. The test thromboplastin must be calibrated against a reference thromboplastin of the same species (rabbit *v* rabbit, bovine *v* bovine). All reference preparations are calibrated in terms of the primary material of human origin and have an ISI which is assigned after a collaborative trial involving many laboratories from different countries.

Reagents

Normal citrated plasma. From 4–6 healthy donors.

Anticoagulated plasma. From 12–18 patients stabilized on oral anticoagulant treatment for at least 6 weeks.

The tests need not all be done at the same time but may be carried out on freshly collected samples on successive days.

Reference and test thromboplastin.

$CaCl_2$. 0.025 mol/l.

Method

Carry out prothrombin time (PT) tests as described in Chapter 18, p. 281. Allow the plasma and thromboplastin to warm up to 37°C for at least 2 min before adding $CaCl_2$. Test each plasma in duplicate with each of the two thromboplastins in the following order with minimum delay between tests:

	Reference thromboplastin	Test thromboplastin
Plasma 1	Test 1	Test 2
	Test 4	Test 3
Plasma 2	Test 5	Test 6
	Test 8	Test 7 etc

Record the mean time for each plasma. If there is a discrepancy of more than 10% in the clotting times between duplicates, repeat the test on that plasma.

Calibration

Plot the prothrombin times (PTs) on log-log graph paper, with results using the reference preparation (y) on the vertical axis and results with the test thromboplastin (x) on the horizontal axis (Fig. 21.1). On arithmetic graph paper it is necessary to plot the logarithms of the PTs (Fig. 21.2). The relationship between the two thromboplastins is determined by the slope of the line (b).

A rough estimate of the slope can be obtained as shown in Figs 21.1 and 21.2; this can then be used to obtain an approximation of the ISI of the test thromboplastin.

Whenever possible however, to obtain a reliable

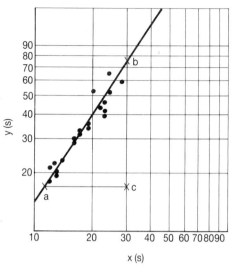

Fig. 21.1   Calibration of Thromboplastin.
The PTs (in seconds) with the test thromboplastin are plotted on the horizontal axis (x) and with the reference thromboplastin on the vertical axis (y) on double log graph paper. The best fit line is drawn by eye, and the slope is obtained as follows: – Points **a**–**b** are marked on the line just below the lowest recorded PT and just above the longest recorded PT, respectively. **c** is a point where a horizontal line through **a** and a vertical through **b** meet. The distance between **b** and **c** are measured accurately in mm. The slope

(b) = $\dfrac{b-c}{a-c}$. In this example **b**–**c** = 55 mm, **a**–**c** = 35 mm,

b = 55/35 = 1.57. The ISI of the reference thromboplastin was 1.11. Therefore, the ISI of the test thromboplastin = 1.11 × 1.57 = 1.74.

measurement, the following more complicated calculation should be used instead.

Calculation of ISI

Calculate the slope of the line (l) as follows:

1. Convert all measurements of PTs into their logarithms; thus, x = log PT with test thromboplastin and y = log PT with reference thromboplastin.

2. $\Sigma x = A$; $\Sigma x^2 = B$; $\Sigma y = C$; $\Sigma y^2 = D$; $\Sigma xy = E$.

3. $F = \dfrac{D - C^2}{n}$, $G = \dfrac{B - A^2}{n}$ and $H = \dfrac{E - AC}{n}$

   where n = no. of PTs with each thromboplastin.

4. $m = \dfrac{F - G}{2H}$

5. Slope (b) = $m + \sqrt{m^2 + 1}$

6. ISI of test thromboplastin = ISI of reference thromboplastin × slope.

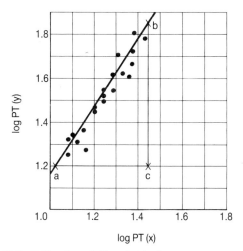

Fig. 21.2   Calibration of Thromboplastin.
The PTs (in seconds) are converted to their logarithms which are plotted on arithmetic graph paper. The slope is calculated as in Fig. 21.1. In this example, **a–c** = 42 mm, **b–c** = 65 mm, b = 65/42 = 1.54. Therefore, ISI = 1.11 × 1.54 = 1.71.

STANDARDIZATION OF COMMERCIAL THROMBOPLASTINS

A more complex procedure has been recommended for the standardization of commercial thromboplastins. A total of 20 normal plasma samples and 60 samples from patients stabilized on long-term anticoagulant treatment should be tested in batches over a 10-day period. The ISI is then calculated as described above.

Calculation of the INR[7,11,13]

This is the prothrombin ratio which would have been obtained on the particular plasma had the original primary human reference material been used to perform the prothrombin time. If the ISI of the thromboplastin used is known the INR can be calculated from the following formula:

INR = Prothrombin time ratio obtained using the test thromboplastin to the power of the ISI of the test reagent.

For example a ratio of 2.5 using a thromboplastin with ISI of 1.4 can be calculated from the formula to be:

$$2.5^{1.4} = 3.61,$$

which is either read from a logarithmic table or calculated on an electronic calculator.

In this way the level of anticoagulation in all plasma samples regardless of the thromboplastin used can be compared and a meaningful therapeutic range established.

Therapeutic range

The recommended therapeutic range using the INR is between 2.0 and 4.0. INRs of over 4.0 are not always a reliable measure of the degree of hypocoagulability. This may be particularly dangerous with thromboplastins with ISI values over 1.6, where a small prolongation of the prothrombin time and prothrombin time ratio may denote a large change in the blood hypocoagulability. This is illustrated in Fig. 21.3 and Tables 21.1 and 21.2.

THROMBOTEST

Principle. The Thrombotest reagent* is a commercial preparation containing absorbed bovine plasma, bovine thromboplastin and cephalin. It is a lyophilized material, stored under vacuum in glass ampoules. The Thrombotest can be used to test capillary blood, in which case the reagent is dissolved in water, or venous blood, when it is dissolved in the calcium chloride solution provided by the manufacturer.

The Thrombotest measures the overall clotting activity and is sensitive to deficiency of factors II, VII, IX and X, as well as to the PIVKA effect (the effect of the acarboxy forms of vitamin-K-dependent factors on the coagulation reactions). Bovine thromboplastin is sensitive to factor VII deficiency and has an ISI of just over 1 (1.0 to 1.05 for different batches).

The actual technique of the test varies according to whether venous or capillary blood is used. Only the technique for venous blood is described here.

Reagents

Thrombotest reagent. The ampoule must be opened carefully in order to prevent the sudden

---

*Nyegaard & Co, Oslo.

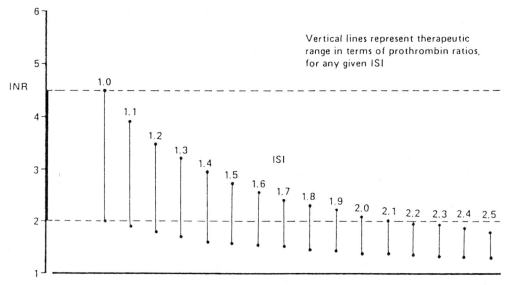

Fig. 21.3 The ratios obtained with thromboplastins with given ISI values equivalent to INR therapeutic range of 2.0–4.5. (Slightly modified, from Poller.[11] With the permission of publisher and editors.)

rush of air into the vacuum-sealed ampoule which may lead to the dispersion of the contents.

$CaCl_2$, 3.21 mol/l. Provided by the manufacturer.

Citrated venous blood. From the patient to be tested.

Method

Dissolve the reagent powder in the calcium chloride provided according to the manufacturer's instructions. Pipette 0.25 ml volumes into glass tubes. Unused tubes may be capped and stored at $-20°C$ for up to 2 months. Place the tube containing 0.25 ml of reagent in the water-bath at 37°C or the heating block of the coagulometer. Allow it to warm for a few minutes. Then add 0.05 ml of venous

blood. The mixture may be left undisturbed for 30s for normal blood and 50s for blood obtained from anticoagulated patients if a manual technique is used. Thereafter record the clotting time in the usual way.

Normal range

35–45 s.

Table 21.3 INR equivalents of percentage activities and clotting times of a batch of Thrombotest, ISI = 1.01 (Modified from Tomenson and Thomson[13])

	Thrombotest	INR
s	% activity	
38.5	100	1.0
40.5	80	1.1
44.5	55	1.2
49.5	40	1.3
52.5	35	1.4
55.5	30	1.5
61	25	1.6
68	20	1.8
72	18	1.9
81	16	2.1
84	14	2.2
93	12	2.5
99	11	2.6
106	10	2.8
114	9	3.3
138	7	3.6
157	6	4.2
182	5	4.8
220	4	5.9

Table 21.2 Therapeutic ranges equivalent to an INR of 2.0–4.0 using different commercial thromboplastins (Modified from Poller[11])

Thromboplastin	ISI	Ratios equivalent to INR 2.0–4.0
Thrombotest	1.03	2.0–3.8
Thromborel	1.23	1.7–3.1
Dade FS	1.35	1.65–2.8
Simplastin	2.0	1.3–2.0
Boehringer	2.1	1.35–1.9
Ortho	2.3	1.3–1.8

ISI: International Sensitivity Index. INR: International Normalized Ratio.

Table 21.4 Investigation of bleeding in a patient receiving an oral anticoagulant

Test	Result	Comment
PT or TT	INR 2.0–4.0, Fibrinogen and platelets normal	Non-haemostatic cause of bleeding
PT or TT	INR over 4.0, Fibrinogen and platelets normal	Overanticoagulated. Stop or reduce oral anticoagulant
PT or TT	INR over 4.0, Fibrinogen and/or platelets low	DIC? Liver or renal disease? Stop or reduce oral anticoagulant

PT = prothrombin time. TT = Thrombotest. INR = International Normalized Ratio.

Calculation of the results

Read the percentage activity from the graph supplied by the manufacturers for each batch. Correction for an abnormal PCV is occasionally required and is carried out from the graph also supplied by the manufacturers.

Therapeutic range

Between 6 and 12% or between INR 2.5 and 4.2, as shown on Table 21.3.

Investigation of a patient who bleeds

The tests commonly used when investigating bleeding by a patient on oral anticoagulants, and their interpretation are shown on Table 21.4.

HEPARIN TREATMENT

The anticoagulant action of heparin is primarily due to its ability to bind to antithrombin III, thereby accelerating and enhancing the latter's rate of inhibition of the major coagulation enzymes, i.e. thrombin, factor Xa, and to a lesser extent factors IXa, XIa and XIIa. The two main effects of heparin, the anti-thrombin and the anti-Xa effect, are separate and specific: fractionated, low molecular weight heparins have a strong anti-Xa activity with little or no anti-thrombin activity, whereas conventional, unfractionated, higher molecular weight heparin has both anti-thrombin and anti-Xa activity.[12] Heparin also has other effects: interaction with the histidine-rich glycoprotein in plasma and an effect on the plasma lipases, as well as various interactions with platelets and the products of platelet activation, such as PF4. In an attempt to potentiate the anticoagulant effect of heparin without increasing the risk of bleeding, new preparations of heparin have been developed for therapeutic use. These are: low molecular weight or fractionated heparins and heparin analogues or heparinoids (sulphated polysaccharides of plant or animal origin such as pentosan polysulphate).

Heparin may be used to treat a thrombo-embolic event, such as venous thrombosis or pulmonary embolism, or to prevent it. If heparin is used to treat an established event, a plasma concentration of between 0.2 and 0.6 iu/ml is desirable. For prophylaxis, a lower concentration, between 0.05 and 0.2 iu/ml, is sufficient.

Selection of patients

Treatment with heparin carries a high risk of bleeding even in haemostatically normal people and it is advisable to perform the first-line tests of haemostasis as described in Chapter 18 before starting treatment. In the presence of a reduced platelet count or deranged coagulation, heparin may be contra-indicated or if used the dose must be reduced.

LABORATORY CONTROL OF HEPARIN TREATMENT

The laboratory control of heparin treatment will be considered under two headings: curative and prophylactic.

Curative heparin treatment

For treating an established thrombotic or embolic event heparin can be administered intravenously (i.v.), preferably as a continuous infusion, or on occasions as intermittent intravenous injections. Patients also may be treated by subcutaneous (s.c.) injection, usually twice daily. The half-life of intravenously administered unfractionated heparin is about 1.5 h; after s.c. injection, heparin is slowly released into the circulation and is present in plasma for on average 12 h. Thus the timing of the blood sample in relation to the heparin injection is important if heparin is not given by continuous infusion. For those receiving intermittent i.v. or s.c. heparin, the blood should be collected 30 min before the next dose is due to assess the effectiveness of the treatment. Heparin is a powerful anticoagulant and its use carries a high risk of bleeding. To minimize this risk, its effect on the coagulation should be monitored every 24 hours while the patient is on treatment.

The following tests are available for the control of heparinization: whole-blood clotting time, thrombin time, partial thromboplastin time with kaolin (PTTK) on plasma or whole blood, anti-Xa assays using either coagulation or amidolytic methodology, and the protamine neutralization test. The advantages and disadvantages of the various tests are shown in Table 21.5. Measurement of the whole-blood coagulation time, as described in the 5th edition of this book (p. 328), was widely used in the past in the control of heparin therapy. The test is time-consuming, must be performed at the bedside one test at a time, and is also relatively insensitive to the lower concentrations of heparin. The PTTK, anti-Xa assay and the protamine neutralization test are described here.

Table 21.5 Tests used in the laboratory control of heparin treatment

Test	Advantages	Disadvantages
Whole blood clotting time	Simple, inexpensive, no equipment needed	Time consuming, can only be carried out at the bedside, one at a time, insensitive to <0.4 iu, and to LMW heparins
PTTK	Simple, many tests can be carried out in parallel	Not all reagents sensitive to heparin, insensitive to <0.2 iu and to LMW heparins, affected by variables other than heparin
Thrombin time	Simple, many tests can be carried out in parallel	Insensitive to <0.2 iu and to LMW heparins.
Protamine neutralization	Sensitive to all concentrations	Time consuming and insensitive to LMW heparins
Anti-Xa assays	Sensitive to all concentrations and to LMWT heparins	Expensive if commercial kits used; time consuming if home-made reagents used

PTTK: partial thromboplastin time with kaolin. LMW: low molecular weight.

PARTIAL THROMBOPLASTIN TIME WITH KAOLIN (PPTK)

Principle. This test can be performed on citrated plasma or on whole citrated blood. The test on plasma is currently the most widely used test for monitoring heparin therapy.[4] It is very sensitive to heparin but has a number of shortcomings which must be kept in mind: firstly, different commercial phospholipids (platelet substitutes) have different sensitivities to heparin and with some there is no linear relationship between clotting times and heparin concentration in the therapeutic range (0.2–0.6 iu/ml). Such reagents are not suitable for the control of heparinization.

If a phospholipid reagent carries no manufacturer's information on its sensitivity to heparin, or is home-made, it is necessary to establish whether it is reliable guide to plasma heparin concentration. A crude test for linearity can be made by adding known concentrations of heparin to a normal plasma pool and measuring the PTTK immediately after the addition. The PTTK is expressed as a ratio

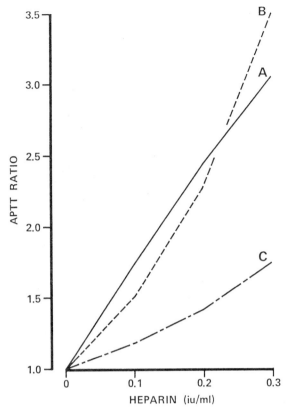

Fig. 21.4 PTTK response to heparin added to plasma in vitro. PTTK response expressed as APTT ratio (PTTK of heparinized plasma/PTTK of plasma without heparin). Three different reagents and methods shown. (Slightly modified, from Tomenson & Thomson.[13] With the permission of publisher and editor.)

of the time obtained with the normal pool containing no heparin. An example of different responses is shown in Fig. 21.4.

The second shortcoming of the PTTK in the control of heparin treatment is that the PTTK is affected by a number of variables not related to heparin (see p. 283). The most important of those are fibrinogen and factor VIII:C concentration and the presence of FDP. In patients with DIC, liver disease or renal disease,[5] heparinization should be controlled using one of the other tests described below.

Reagents and method

The reagents and method are described on p. 282.

Therapeutic range

0.2 – 0.6 iu/ml.

The prolongation of the PTTK achieved with these concentrations varies between reagents according to the sensitivity of the phospholipid used. The results may be expressed as clotting time in seconds or as a ratio. For the majority of sensitive reagents ratios of 1.5–3.0 cover the therapeutic range.

THROMBIN TIME

This test is simple and popular, since it can be performed on batches of plasma in the laboratory. The therapeutic range depends on the strength of the thrombin solution used for the test. When using a concentration of 10 NHS units with a control time of c 15 s, the therapeutic range lies between 25 and 100 s. For details of the test see p. 289.

ANTI-Xa ASSAY FOR HEPARIN

Principle. Plasma anti-Xa activity is enhanced by the addition of heparin, and a coagulation or amidolytic (chromogenic) assay of anti-Xa activity can be adapted to measure heparin. The anti-Xa assays are generally used to measure the low concentrations of heparin obtained after the prophylactic administration of low dose or low molecular weight heparins. However, the anti-Xa assay can also be used to measure the higher concentrations of heparin in plasma if a different standard curve is constructed. A number of commercial kits such as Heptest and Hepaclot, as well as various kits based on chromogenic substrates, are in use and give linear and reproducible responses.

A coagulation anti-Xa assay is described under the section on *prophylactic heparin treatment* (p. 345).

Therapeutic range

0.2–0.6 iu/ml.

The concentration of heparin is read off a standard curve constructed according to the manufacturer's instructions.

PROTAMINE NEUTRALIZATION TEST[1]

Principle. This test is an extension of the thrombin time, various amounts of protamine sulphate being added to the plasma before the addition of thrombin. When all the heparin present in plasma has been neutralized, the clotting time should become normal. From the amount of protamine sulphate required to produce this effect, the concentration of heparin in the plasma can be calculated. The protamine neutralization test is used mainly to calculate the dose of protamine sulphate needed to neutralize circulating heparin after cardiopulmonary surgery and haemodialysis, but it is also used to control treatment or to calculate the dose of protamine to be administered if the patient needs quick reversal of heparinization.

Reagents

Protamine sulphate. Prepare dilutions (0–50 mg/ml) in barbitone buffer, pH 7.4. Dilute 5 ml of protamine sulphate (10 g/l) 1 in 20 with buffer to give 1 dl of a stock solution containing 50 mg/ml. Then make working solutions to cover the range of 0 to 50 mg in 5 mg steps from the stock solution by dilution with buffer. The solutions keep indefinitely at 4°C.

Thrombin. Dilute thrombin in barbitone buffer to a concentration of about 20 NIH units/ml. Adjust the concentration so that 0.1 ml of thrombin clots 0.2 ml of normal plasma at 37°C in 10 ±1 s. Keep the thrombin in a plastic tube in melting ice during the assay.

Plasma. Citrated platelet-poor plasma from the patient.

Method

Place 0.2 ml of test plasma and 20 μl of barbitone buffer in a glass tube kept in a water bath at 37°C. Allow the mixture to warm and then blow in 0.1 ml of thrombin. Record the clotting time. If this is *c* 10 s there is no demonstrable heparin in the plasma. If the thrombin time is prolonged, repeat the test using 20 μl of the 50 mg/ml protamine solution instead of buffer. Repeat the test if necessary, until a concentration of protamine is found which gives a clotting time of *c* 10s.

Calculation

If 20 μl of 15 mg/ml protamine sulphate produce a normal thrombin time (whereas the clotting time is prolonged with 10 mg/ml protamine), then the concentration of 15 μg of protamine is sufficient to neutralize the heparin in 1 ml of plasma. Assuming weight for weight neutralization, the patient's plasma contains 15 μg of heparin per ml or 1.5 iu, assuming that 1 mg of heparin is equivalent to 100 iu. This figure can be further converted to concentration of heparin per ml of whole blood by multiplying by 1 − PCV.

In the above example, for in-vivo neutralization of heparin by protamine sulphate, assuming a total blood volume of 75 ml per kg body weight, the required dose of protamine would be:

$$\frac{15 \times \text{total blood volume}}{1 \div (1 - \text{PCV})}\, \text{mg}$$
$$= \frac{15 \times 75 \times \text{body weight} \times (1 - \text{PCV})}{1000}\, \text{mg}.$$

Prophylactic heparin treatment

Heparin is administered prophylactically in a much lower dosage than that used therapeutically, usually as a subcutaneous (s.c.) injection. The low concentrations achieved (0.05 to 0.2 iu/ml) are sufficient to increase the anti-Xa activity of the plasma and prevent the onset of thrombosis. The derangement of haemostasis is minimal and in most instances monitoring is not required. However, in patients on long-term s.c. heparin, such as pregnant women, and those about to undergo major surgery, as well as in some special cases (i.e. patients undergoing hip replacement, the elderly, those with splenomegaly and/or a marginally reduced platelet count, etc) it may be necessary to confirm that the heparin concentration is sufficient to prevent thrombosis yet not so high as to cause haemorrhage. The heparin concentration and its effect must also be monitored if one of the newer low molecular weight heparins with improved bio-availability is used. The peak plasma concentration after a s.c. injection of conventional unfractionated heparin occurs approximately 2 h later and an estimation at this time indicates the probable maximum effectiveness of the treatment. With low molecular weight heparins the plasma concentration reaches a peak within 1–2 h and remains at this level for up to 24 h.

An anti-Xa assay is the method of choice for measuring the effect of low dose or low molecular weight heparin. The PTTK test can also be used but only to assess whether the concentration of heparin is unacceptably high. The majority of commercial PTTK reagents are not sensitive to heparin concentrations below 0.15 iu/ml and it is generally accepted that the patient's PTTK should be within 8 s of the control time. If the clotting time is longer, the plasma heparin concentration is in excess of 0.2 iu/ml and the patient may bleed if haemostatically challenged.

ANTI-Xa ASSAY FOR MONITORING LOW-DOSE SUBCUTANEOUS HEPARIN[2]

Principle. The anti-Xa activity of antithrombin III is enhanced by the addition of heparin. A standard curve is constructed by adding varying amounts of heparin to a normal plasma pool which provides the source of the antithrombin III. The inhibition of factor Xa by heparin is measured in a modified factor-X assay.

Reagents

Pooled normal plasma. From 20 normal donors, see p. 301.

Patient's plasma. Citrated platelet-poor plasma should be collected between 2 and 4 h after the injection of heparin; it should be tested as soon as possible after the collection and kept at + 4°C or on crushed ice until tested.

Buffer. Trisodium citrate 30 volumes, glyoxaline buffer (p. 281) 150 volumes, and 20% bovine albumin 1 volume.

Commercially prepared artificial factor-X-deficient plasma.★ Reconstitute according to instructions.

Platelet substitute.

Mix equal volumes of factor-X-deficient plasma and platelet substitute.★ This is the working reagent and is kept at 37°C.

★Diagen, Diagnostic Reagents Ltd, Thame, Oxon.

Factor Xa. Reconstitute as instructed by the manufacturer. Dilute further in the buffer to give a 1 in 100 dilution. Keep on crushed ice until used.

Heparin. 1000 iu/ml. Dilute in saline to 10 iu/ml. Ideally, the same batch of heparin as the patient is receiving should be used.

CaCl₂. 0.025 mol/l.

Method

A standard curve is constructed as shown in Table 21.6. Add 0.05 of each dilution to 0.45 ml of the normal plasma pool. This will give final concentrations of heparin from 0.05 to 0.30 iu/ml in 0.05 iu steps.

Pipette 0.3 ml of diluted factor Xa into a large glass tube at 37°C.

Add 0.1 ml of the first standard dilution. Start the stop-watch. At 1 min and 30 s exactly transfer duplicate 0.1 ml volumes of the mixture into two tubes each containing 0.1 ml of pre-warmed CaCl₂.

At 2 min after sub-sampling add 0.2 ml of the mixture of factor-X-deficient plasma and platelet substitute, start the stop-watch, mix and record the clotting time.

Repeat for each dilution of standard. The patient's sample is tested undiluted in pooled normal plasma if the clotting time is longer than the times used to construct the standard curve.

Calculation

Plot the clotting times against the heparin concentration on log-linear paper, with the clotting times on the linear axis. The concentration of heparin in the patient's sample can be read directly from the standard curve. It is multiplied by the dilution factor if necessary.

Table 21.6 Preparation of a standard curve for an anti-Xa assay

Reagent	Tube 1	2	3	4	5	6
Heparin (10 iu/ml)	0.05	0.10	0.15	0.20	0.25	0.30
Saline (ml)	0.95	0.90	0.85	0.80	0.75	0.70
Concentration of heparin (iu/ml)	0.5	1.0	1.5	2.0	2.5	3.0
Final conc. of heparin after addition to normal plasma pool	0.05	0.10	0.15	0.20	0.25	0.30

Comment

Anti-Xa assay for measuring low concentrations of heparin can be carried out using commercial kits based on the coagulation of plasma or on chromogenic substrates. Such assays are technically simple and give reliable results.

INVESTIGATION OF A PATIENT WHO BLEEDS WHILE RECEIVING HEPARIN

Minor bleeding (microscopic haematuria, bruising, bleeding from venepuncture sites, etc) is common during treatment with heparin and may herald a more serious haemorrhagic episode. A potentially serious side effect to the use of heparin, heparin–associated thrombocytopenia, also presents with bleeding. For this reason every episode of bleeding

Table 21.7 Investigation of a patient who is bleeding while on heparin treatment

Test	Result	Comment
PTTK	2–3 × Normal	Excessive heparin dose.
Platelets	Normal	Reduce or stop heparin.
Fibrinogen	Normal	
PTTK	Within range or long	Heparin-associated
Platelets	Low	thrombocytopenia.
Fibrinogen	Normal	Stop heparin.
PTTK	Very long	DIC, liver or renal
Platelets	Low	disease. If heparin is to
Fibrinogen	Low	be continued, determine conc. using protamine neutralization or anti-Xa assay. Modify dose.

should be investigated. A suggested plan of investigation is shown in Table 21.7.

THROMBOLYTIC THERAPY

The thrombolytic agents currently in use are: urokinase, streptokinase, streptokinase-plasminogen complex and acylated compounds (APSAC), and the tissue type plasminogen activator (t-PA) obtained by recombinant technology or from tissue culture. Single chain urokinase and various activator molecules modified through recombinant techniques are also being developed and studied.

Urokinase. This is a trypsin-like protease found in urine. Urokinase directly converts plasminogen into plasmin by cleaving a single Arg-Val bond. The active enzyme is isolated in either a two-chain or a one-chain form. Both forms have been cloned and can be used therapeutically; they are administered intravenously in doses between 2500 and 4450 units per kg body weight.

Streptokinase. This is a purified fraction of the filtrate from cultures of *Str. haemolyticus*. Streptokinase interacts with plasminogen or plasmin to form a plasminogen activator; the activator complex in turn cleaves a bond in the plasminogen molecule to give rise to plasmin. Streptokinase is a foreign protein and induces antibody production in man. It also cross-reacts with anti-streptococcal antibodies

and this may cause a resistance to therapy. Streptokinase treatment is often started with a loading dose of between 250 000 and 500 000 units and continued at 100 000 units per h for up to 72 h. A single very high dose (usually over 1 000 000 u) is administered to achieve thrombolysis in myocardial infarction.

Biochemical manipulations have resulted in the preparation of a number of forms of the streptokinase-plasminogen complex, including complexes with the acylated forms of plasmin and plasminogen which have strong fibrin-binding characteristics. These complexes are used for coronary thrombolysis.

The fibrinolytic state induced by urokinase and streptokinase is short-lived once the infusion has been stopped. While the infusion lasts there is fibrinolysis at the site of thrombosis as well as systemic fibrinolysis. The fibrinogen and plasminogen concentration in plasma fall and the FDP concentration rises.

Tissue-type plasminogen activator (t-PA). This is a single- or double-chain polypeptide obtained by recombinant techniques or from tissue cultures. It is a potent activator of plasminogen and induces a thrombolytic state of a longer duration then either streptokinase or urokinase infusion. t-PA has a strong affinity for fibrin-bound plasminogen and causes less fibrinogenolysis than any of the previously mentioned agents.

Selection of patients

Thrombolytic treatment carries a serious risk of bleeding and thrombolytic agents should not be given to individuals suffering from a variety of illnesses where there is a high risk of bleeding. In addition, each patient should have his haemostatic function assessed (PT, PTTK and thrombin time or fibrinogen estimation, platelet count) before treatment is started.

Determining the initial dose of streptokinase

Streptokinase cross-reacts with anti-streptococcal antibodies and in some individuals who have experienced streptococcal infections in the past it is important to determine the dose which is required to saturate the neutralizing antibodies and yet achieve therapeutic lysis. Titration is pointless in patients undergoing coronary thrombolysis because the doses used are much higher and invariably exceed the capacity of cross-reacting antibodies to neutralize them.

TITRATION OF THE INITIAL DOSE OF STREPTOKINASE

Principle. Different amounts of streptokinase are added to patient's plasma in vitro and the samples clotted with thrombin. The smallest amount of streptokinase which causes the clot to lyse within 10 min is multiplied by the presumed plasma volume to give the titrated dose of streptokinase.

Reagents

Patient's plasma. Citrated platelet-poor plasma (see p. 280).

Streptokinase. Vials containing the freeze-dried material to be given to the patient are suitable. Open the vial and add sufficient 9 g/l NaCl to make a solution containing 2000 iu/ml. From this initial solution, make further dilutions containing 1500, 1000 and 500 iu/ml.

Thrombin. A solution containing c 50 NIH units per ml of 9 g/l NaCl.

Method

Place four glass tubes in the water-bath at 37°C. Pipette 1 ml of plasma into each tube followed by 0.1 ml of the four streptokinase dilutions and add 0.1 ml of thrombin. Mix the contents of the tubes by inversion and start the stop-watch when clotting has taken place. Lysis will commence first in the tube with 2000 iu/ml of streptokinase. Note the tube containing the smallest amount of streptokinase which will cause clot lysis in 10 min.

Calculation of the dose

Suppose that the clot lysed in the three tubes containing 1000, 1500 and 2000 iu/ml. The least amount of streptokinase able to induce lysis in 1 ml of plasma was 100 iu. If the patient is an adult with a presumed plasma volume of 50 ml per kg body weight and if he weighs 60 kg, the presumed total plasma volume is 3000 ml. The necessary initial dose of streptokinase would be 100 × 3000 = 300000 iu.

LABORATORY CONTROL OF THROMBOLYTIC THERAPY

Many laboratory tests are abnormal during thrombolytic therapy, but the perfect and specific procedure for monitoring is not available. All screening tests of coagulation are prolonged reflecting the hyperplasminaemic state with the reduction in the fibrinogen concentration and the presence of FDP. The prolongation is most marked with streptokinase and streptokinase-plasminogen complex; it is less marked with urokinase and least with t-PA. The fibrinogen concentration commonly falls to below 0.05 g/l and the FDP concentration may rise to over 1000 ng/l.

Monitoring in venous thrombosis. The thrombin time is commonly used to monitor therapy. A few hours after the start of the infusion, the thrombin time is prolonged to 40 s or more (control 10 ± 1 s); it then settles to approximately 20–30 s. Very long thrombin times carry a high risk of bleeding and are indicative of severe hyperplasminaemia. Many centres use a standard streptokinase and urokinase regime without any laboratory control and carry out laboratory tests only if the patient bleeds.

Monitoring in coronary thrombolysis. This is carried out to ensure that the patient is not at risk of bleeding or to establish that the thrombolysis is proceeding satisfactorily. In the first case, the PTTK or thrombin time are sometimes carried out;

Table 21.8 Investigation of a patient who is bleeding while on thrombolytic treatment

Timing	Test	Result	Comment
During infusion	TT or PTTK	Very long	Hyperplasminaemia.
	Fibrinogen	Low	Stop infusion, transfuse (FFP).
Before heparin	TT or PTTK	Very long	Hypofibrinogenaemia.
	Fibrinogen	Very low	DO NOT give heparin, transfuse if necessary.
While on heparin	PTTK	Very long	
	a. Fibrinogen	Normal	Excess heparin, reduce
	Platelets	Normal	dose.
	b. Fibrinogen	Low	Heparin given too
	Platelets	Normal	soon.*
	c. Fibrinogen	Low	DIC, liver or renal
	Platelets	Low	disease.* Investigate.

PTTK = partial thromboplastin time with kaolin. TT = thrombin time.
*Use anti-Xa assay to measure heparin concentration.

in the second, one of the tests for the lysis of fibrin (as distinct from fibrinogen) is performed. The two commonest tests are the measurement of cross-linked D-dimer using a monoclonal antibody and the measurement of a fibrin-specific early FDP called Bβ 15–42. Both tests are available as commercial kits and are usually performed as a part of pharmacological studies or therapeutic trials.

Timing the start of anticoagulant therapy. Heparin and oral anticoagulants are started within hours of stopping the infusion of the thrombolytic agent. The timing of anticoagulation is crucial: if it is given too soon, while the fibrinogen concentration is very low, the risk of bleeding is substantial. It is usually considered safe to start anticoagulants when the fibrinogen concentration exceeds 0.05 g/l of plasma. If the fibrinogen concentration is 0.05 g/l and the prolongation of PTTK does not exceed twice the base line clotting time, heparin treatment can be safely given and monitored. This usually occurs 4–6 hours after streptokinase and urokinase infusion and sooner after t-PA. However, after streptokinase infusion occasional patients may show persistent hypofibrinogenaemia for up to 24 h. Such individuals must be monitored at 4 h intervals and not given heparin and warfarin until their PTTK is at least twice the base line clotting time time.

INVESTIGATION OF A PATIENT WHO BLEEDS WHILE ON THROMBOLYTIC AGENTS OR IMMEDIATELY AFTERWARDS

The tests, the timing and the likely mechanism of bleeding are shown in Table 21.8.

ANTI-PLATELET THERAPY

Many drugs inhibit platelet function in vitro but only a few have anti-platelet activity in acceptable doses. Each category of drugs has a different pharmacological action and requires different methods to demonstrate its effect on platelets. Anti-platelet agents are used in primary and secondary prevention of coronary heart disease, in unstable angina, in certain forms of cerebrovascular disease, to prevent thrombo-embolism associated with val-

vular disease and prosthetic heart valves, and to prevent thrombosis in arteriovenous shunts. Haematologists are only exceptionally asked to monitor these aspects of anti-platelet therapy.

A proportion of patients with thrombocytosis or thrombocythaemia experience episodes of arterial thrombosis. Such patients are often given anti-platelet drugs and the effect of these drugs is sometimes monitored. Three techniques are available for monitoring: prolongation of the bleeding time (see p. 285), inhibition of platelet aggregation response to standard agonists (see p. 293) and normalization of platelet survival using [111]Indium-labelled platelets. Such monitoring is usually tailored to the individual patient and the choice of test depends on the drug used, on the abnormalities

detectable in the patient, and on the laboratory facilities available. Thus aspirin affects both bleeding time and platelet aggregation, whereas the effect of dipyridamole on platelet aggregation is unpredictable, and can only be reliably shown by measuring platelet survival.

REFERENCES

[1] DACIE, J. V. and LEWIS, S. M. (1975). *Practical Haematology*, 5th edn, p. 413. Churchill Livingstone, Edinburgh.

[2] DENSON, K. W. E. and BONNAR, J. (1973). The measurement of heparin. A method based on the potentiation of antifactor Xa. *Thrombosis et Diathesis Haemorrhagica*, **30**, 471.

[3] Commission of European Communities (1982). *BCR information: Certification of three reference materials for thromboplastins*. EEC, Brussels

[4] FENNERTY, A. G, RENOWDEN, S., SCOLDING, N., BENTLEY, D. P., CAMPBELL, I. A. and ROUTLEDGE, P. A. (1986). Guidelines to control heparin treatment. *British Medical Journal*, **292**, 579.

[5] FEY, M. F., LANG, M., FURLAN, M. and BECK, E. A. (1987). Monitoring heparin therapy with the activated partial thromboplastin time and chromogenic substrate assays. *Thrombosis and Haemostasis*, **58**, 853.

[6] HAWKEY, C. and HOWELL, M. (1964). The laboratory control of thrombolytic therapy. *Journal of Clinical Pathology*, **17**, 287.

[7] KIRKWOOD, T. B. L. (1983). Calibration of reference thromboplastins and standardization of the prothrombin ratio. *Thrombosis and Haemostasis*, **49**, 238.

[8] LEWIS, S. M. (1985). ICSH/ICHT recommendations for reporting prothrombin time in oral anticoagulant control. *Journal of Clinical Pathology*, **38**, 133.

[9] OWREN, P. A. (1959). Thrombotest: a new method for controlling anticoagulant therapy. *Lancet*, **ii**, 754.

[10] OWREN, P. A. and AAS, K. (1951). The control of dicumarol therapy and the quantitative determination of prothrombin and proconvertin. *Scandinavian Journal of Clinical and Laboratory Investigation*, **3**, 201.

[11] POLLER, L. (1987). Oral anticoagulant therapy. In *Haemostasis and Thrombosis*. Eds. Bloom, A. L. and Thomas, D. P., 2nd edn, p. 870. Churchill Livingstone, Edinburgh.

[12] THOMAS, D. P. (1986). Current status of low molecular weight heparin. *Thrombosis and Haemostasis*, **56**, 241.

[13] TOMENSON, J. A. and THOMSON, J. M. (1985). Standardization of the prothrombin time. In *Blood Coagulation and Haemostasis. A Practical Guide*. Ed. Thomson, J. M., p. 370. Churchill Livingstone, Edinburgh.

22. Use of radionuclides in haematology

In this chapter a brief general account will be given of the methods of using radionuclides in haematological diagnosis. For a more complete account of the theory and practice of nuclear medicine techniques the reader is referred to recent reviews by Sorenson and Phelps,[9] Bowring[1] and Lewis and Bayly.[6] The main properties of the radionuclides useful in diagnostic haematology are summarized in Tables 22.1 and 22.2. Specific instructions for their use are given in Chapters 23–25.

FORMS OF RADIATION

Radioactivity results from the spontaneous decay of unstable atomic nuclei; this is accompanied by the emission of charged particles (α, β^+ and β^- rays) or electromagnetic radiation (γ or X-rays). Radioactive isotopes which emit γ rays are particularly useful as they have the advantage that their emissions penetrate tissues well so that they can be detected at the surface of the body when they have originated within organs. The radiation from α- and β-ray emitters has little tissue penetration; these are less useful for certain clinical purposes and are potentially more harmful than γ-ray emitters. The different types of radiation can be detected and distinguished by their ionization effect, by chemical and photochemical effects and by the production of scintillations in certain materials. The systems used for measuring radioactivity are described on p. 354.

Table 22.1 Radionuclides used in haematological diagnosis

Element	Physical half-life	Principal radiations	Energies (MeV)	Availability
^{57}Co	270d	γ	0.122, 0.136	**
^{58}Co	71.3d	β^+ γ	0.48 0.811, 0.511	**
^{51}Cr	27.8d	γ X-rays	0.320	**
^{52}Fe*	8.2h	β^+ γ	0.804 0.511, 0.165	Cyclotron
^{59}Fe	45d	β^- γ	0.475, 0.273 1.09, 1.29	**
^{3}H	12.3yr	β^-	0.0186	**
^{125}I	60d	γ	0.035	**
^{131}I	8.05d	β^- γ	0.606, 0.33 0.364, 0.637	**
^{111}In	2.81d	γ	0.247, 0.173	**
^{113m}In	1.67h	γ	0.393	**
^{32}P	14.3d	β^-	1.71	**
^{99m}Tc	6h	γ	0.140	**

* Decays to ^{52}Mn ($T_{1/2}$ 21 min).
**Commercial suppliers, e.g. Amersham International.

RADIATION DOSAGE

When using radionuclides, account must be taken of their potential risk both for the recipient and the laboratory worker. The extent of radiation hazard in relation to the small amount of isotope employed in

351

Table 22.2 Application of radionuclides in haematological diagnosis

Element	Radiopharmaceutical	Application	Usual dose (MBq)	Approximate Equivalent (µCi)*
^{57}Co	Vitamin B$_{12}$	Investigation of megaloblastic	0.02–0.04	0.5–1
^{58}Co		anaemias	0.02–0.04	0.5–1
^{51}Cr	Sodium chromate	Red cell volume	0.4–0.8	10–20
	Sodium chromate	Red cell life-span	1–2	30–50
	Sodium chromate	Sites of red cell destruction	3.5	100
	Sodium chromate	Measurement of gastro-intestinal bleeding	3.5	100
	Sodium chromate	Platelet life-span	1–2	25–50
	Sodium chromate	Spleen scan	3.5–5.5	100–150
	Sodium chromate	Spleen pool	9	250
^{52}Fe	Ferric chloride or citrate	Ferrokinetics	3.5	100
^{59}Fe	Ferric chloride or citrate	Absorption of iron	0.2–0.8	5–20
		Ferrokinetics and erythropoiesis	0.2–0.4	5–10
^{3}H	Folic acid	Folic acid metabolism	0.8–1.5	20–40
	DFP	Red cell life-span	18	500
^{125}I	Iodinated human	Plasma volume	0.08–0.2	2–5
^{131}I	serum albumin		0.08–0.2	2–5
^{111}In	Indium chloride	Platelet life-span	7.5	200
	(→ oxine or	Red cell volume	1–2	25–50
	acetylacetone)	Spleen scan	7.5	200
^{113m}In	Indium chloride	Red cell volume	2–4	50–100
	(→ oxine or	Spleen scan	9	250
	acetylacetone)	Spleen pool	18	500
^{32}P	DFP	Red cell life-span	2–2.5	50–70
		Platelet life-span	2–2.5	50–70
^{99m}Tc	Pertechnetate	Red cell volume	2–4	50–100
		Spleen scan	35	1000
		Spleen pool	75	2000

* 1 µCi = 3.7×10^4 Bq.

diagnostic work depends on a number of factors: e.g. the energy and range of the radiations; whether the isotope is widely distributed in the body or becomes localized in specific organs; the physical half-life of the isotope and its biological half-time in the body. The isotope should, as a rule, have as short a half-life as is compatible with the duration of the test. An isotope with a very short half-life can be administered in much higher amounts than isotopes which are likely to remain active in the body for a considerably longer time.

Formerly radioactivity was expressed in curies (Ci); 10^{-3} Ci = 1 mCi and 10^{-6} Ci = 1 µCi. The basic SI unit of radioactivity is the bequerel (Bq). 1 Bq corresponds to one disintegration per second, so that 1 Ci = 3.7×10^{10} Bq. 1 millicurie (mCi) = 3.7×10^7 Bq or 37 megabequerels (MBq), and 1 microcurie (µCi) = 3.7×10^4 Bq or 0.037 MBq; 10^3 MBq = 1 GBq.

The effect of radiation depends, essentially, on the amount of energy deposited in the body. This is expressed in grays (Gy). 1 Gy is the amount of radiation which deposits 1 joule of energy per kg of tissue. In the past this has been expressed in rads (1 rad = 0.01 Gy). The reaction of the body to the radiation is also affected by the type of the particular ionizing ray, and the biological effect of the radiation is calculated from the amount in Gy (or rad) multiplied by an ionization quality factor; this factor varies with the type of ray and is 20 times more for α rays than for β and γ rays. The unit for describing the biological effect of radiation, i.e. the radiation dose, is the Sievert (sv) or the rem (1 rem = 0.01 sv). The maximum total whole body dose limit for somebody working with radioisotopes is 50 msv, with a smaller amount for individual organs. Lower dose limits apply to members of the public. Radioisotopes should not be given to pregnant women, especially after the first two months and, because of possible genetic effects, only minimal doses should be given to persons of reproductive age.

RADIATION PROTECTION

The quantity of radioactivity used in diagnostic work is usually small and good laboratory practice is all that is necessary for safe working. However, before using isotopes, workers should familiarize themselves with the problem of radiation protection for themselves, their fellow workers and patients. In Britain there is a code of practice which describes the procedures which must be followed in medical and dental practice.[3,7] An important recommendation is that radioactive isotopes should be handled only in approved laboratories. They must be used under the direction of an authorized person and the doses administered must not exceed the limits laid down by the Administration of Radioactive Substances Advisory Committee.[2,3]

The greatest danger to individuals in handling diagnostic radioisotopes is from ingestion, inhalation or by skin contact, while contamination of apparatus and working area will affect the validity of tests. Working with radionuclides requires the same order of technical competence, experience, discipline and precautions as are needed in handling infective materials. To monitor radiation, each designated radiation worker must wear a personal monitor which records the radiation dose it receives. This is usually in the form of a photographic film badge or a thermo-luminescent dose-meter (TLD) badge.* The laboratory should be equipped with a monitoring device to detect contamination in the working area, including sinks and drains. In general, the radioactive waste from isotopes used in haematological diagnostic procedures may be poured down a single designated laboratory sink. It should be washed down with a large quantity of running water. If the waste material exceeds the

---

*The National Radiological Protection Board, Harwell, Didcot, provides a film badge service; the TLD system is available from Pitman Instruments, Weybridge, Surrey.

amount allowed for disposal in this way, it should be stored in a suitable place until its radioactivity has decayed sufficiently for it to be disposed of via the refuse system. All working and storage areas and disposal sinks should be clearly labelled with the internationally recognized trefoil symbol.

Decontamination of working surfaces, walls and floors can usually be achieved by washing with a detergent such as Decon 90 (Decon Laboratories Ltd). Glassware can be decontaminated by soaking in Decon 90 and plastic laboratory ware by washing in dilute (e.g. 1%) nitric acid.

Protective gloves must always be worn when handling isotopes; any activity which does get on to the hands can usually be removed by washing with soap and water, or if that fails, with a detergent solution. For each laboratory in which isotopes are used, a radiological safety officer should be nominated to supervise protection procedures.

A good account of the general procedures to be followed in handling radioactive materials is given in a monograph published by the International Atomic Energy Agency.[4]

SOURCES OF RADIONUCLIDES

The long-lived isotopes which are used for haematological investigations are generally available from commercial suppliers. The usual way of obtaining certain short-lived isotopes is by means of a radionuclide generator, in which a moderately long-lived parent isotope decays to produce the required short-lived isotope. The parent isotope is adsorbed onto a support material such as an ion exchange resin, surrounded by an aqueous buffer. The daughter nuclide appears in the buffer as it forms, and may be obtained by elution of the generator column. In this way ^{99m}Tc ($T_{1/2}$ 6 h) can be derived from ^{99}Mo ($T_{1/2}$ 66 h); and ^{113m}In ($T_{1/2}$ 100 min) from ^{113}Sn ($T_{1/2}$ 120 days).

Radioactive elements are often mixed with a proportion of a non-radioactive but chemically identical element which is known as 'carrier'. The specific activity is a measure of the radioactivity per unit mass of total material. A compound which is carrier-free offers the highest attainable specific activity. As an isotope decays, its specific activity decreases. The activity of the isotope which is administered is chosen in order to have sufficient radioactivity for the subsequent sample measurements; it is important to ensure that the concentration of the chemical element is not so great as to be non-physiological or even toxic.

APPARATUS FOR MEASURING RADIOACTIVITY

Scintillation detectors

These are widely used for the detection and measurement of radiation. Detection is based on the fact that certain crystals (phosphors) have the property of emitting a flash of light (a scintillation) when energetic photons enter them. Sodium iodide activated with thallium is used in nearly all detectors. The scintillations produced are too weak to be detected except as emitted electrons. The light is detected by the photocathode of a photomultiplier tube which produces a response to this light. The electrons are accelerated towards a series of metal grids ('dynodes') each held at a higher positive voltage than the previous dynode. For each electron striking this dynode several electrons are emitted. The number of electrons is progressively increased at each dynode; they accumulate at the anode where they constitute a small pulse, the size of which is proportional to the total energy absorbed by the crystal. The pulses are amplified and are counted in a scaler or ratemeter (see below).

The magnitude of the pulses from the scintillation detector is proportional to the energy of the rays which give rise to the scintillations. In a gamma-ray spectrometer the pulses are analysed by an analyser with respect to their height (Fig. 22.1). The number of pulses within a selected channel are counted. By selecting a part of the spectrum in which energies produced by other isotopes are either not counted or are minimized, a selected isotope can be counted when present in a mixture. Pulse selection also enables background noise to be minimized in instruments set to count with a high degree of sensitivity. Care must be taken in in-vivo counting to exclude components of a spectrum which result from scattered activity arising from activity not within the required field of view.

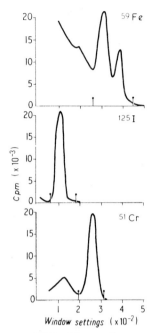

Fig. 22.1 Spectra of ^{59}Fe, ^{125}I and ^{51}Cr obtained on a scintillation spectrometer. The isotopes should be counted with the window set at the limits indicated by the vertical lines.

Thallium-activated sodium iodide crystals are available in various shapes and sizes. A 'well-type' crystal contains a cavity into which is inserted a small container or test-tube holding up to 5 ml of fluid; since the sample is almost surrounded by the crystal, counting is achieved with high efficiency. As the geometric efficiency of a well-counter depends on the position of the sample in relation to the crystal, it is important to use the same volume for each sample in a series. Another form is a solid circular cylinder, 2.5–10 cm in diameter. In this form it is used for in-vivo measurements on patients and occasionally for the measurement of bulky samples, e.g. 24 h urine specimens.

Ionization chambers

A known volume of air or other gas is subjected to irradiation by a radioactive material. Ions produced in the gas are collected on a pair of electrodes and this collection of ions results in the flow of a very small current in an external circuit. This current, which is proportional to the intensity of radiation passing through the chamber, is measured by an electrometer. This type of apparatus is used for the measurement of comparatively large quantities of radioactivity (>37 MBq or 1 mCi); its main use is for the measurement of the activity of a stock isotope.

Geiger-Müller counters (GM tubes)

GM counters are used mostly in survey meters for radiation protection and to detect contamination. The detector is of an end-window type. The window is a thin layer of mica which is sufficiently thin to permit the passage of α and β particles into the counter. If intended for detecting γ rays the window will be thicker, and made of aluminium or stainless steel, and the inner walls will be coated with lead to induce secondary emission of electrons.

Liquid scintillation counters

Low-energy β-emitters can be counted with high efficiency in a liquid scintillator in which the radioactive material is mixed with an organic scintillator in a solvent, and the scintillation activity is then measured between a pair of photomultiplier tubes. The apparatus is usually operated in a refrigerated unit at 4°C to reduce spurious electrical signals. Liquid scintillation solutions have three components:

1. A solvent (e.g. xylene or toluene).
2. A primary solute such as p-terphenyl, 1-phenyl, 4-phenyloxazole (PPO), and various conjugated phenyls.
3. A secondary solute such as 1,4-di-(2-5-phenyloxazole) benzene ('POPOP'), which traps the excitation energy from the primary solute, emitting photons of a longer wavelength which are measured more efficiently.

A problem of liquid scintillation which is particularly pertinent to haematological work is that a quenching effect with a decrease in counting efficiency is caused by material which is coloured or contains proteins or insoluble substances. To count such material accurately requires careful preparation and the adoption of special procedures to correct for the quenching effect.

Measurement of radioactivity in bulky material

By using two detectors in a single counting system, it is possible to measure, with relative precision, the radioactivity in a sample of faeces or an organ without the necessity for homogenization. Similarly, the radioactivity in a large volume of urine or other fluid can be measured without the necessity of concentrating to a smaller volume. The sample is contained in a 450 ml waxed cardboard carton with a screw-top lid, and positioned between two counters, placed above and below it, respectively. It is separated from the lower counter by a plastic ring to ensure that the specimen in the carton is approximately equidistant from both crystals. The counting system is surrounded by lead and the responses of both crystals are counted together. If a single detector system is used it is essential to homogenize the samples.

Another large-volume counting system, which is available commercially, consists of a counting chamber surrounded by a scintillation fluid and linked to a series of photomultiplier tubes.

Scalers, timers and ratemeters

These instruments record the output signals from radiation detection after the pulse-height analysis of the signals. A device that only counts pulses is called a scaler. An auxiliary device that controls the scaler counting time is called a timer and an instrument that incorporates both functions in a single unit is called a scaler-timer. Ratemeters record the mean rate of arrival of pulses from the analyser where extraneous pulses are excluded. A recorder may be fitted in place of the meter, with an inked pointer, tracing a line on to a moving paper chart on which is a calibrated scale. This instrument is useful for observing changes in count rates over periods of time.

Associated with the scaler or ratemeter is a high voltage unit. Its function is to supply the high voltage necessary to operate the radiation detector. In addition, each counter has a pulse amplifier, the function of which is to increase the voltage of the pulse produced to a size suitable for operating the scaler or ratemeter.

Dead-time

After each pulse there is a short period during which the apparatus cannot respond to a further stimulus. This is the 'dead-time', during which any signal entering the counter will not be registered. Dead-time losses also occur in pulse-height analysers and scalers. In modern instruments the dead-time is short and correction is unnecessary in clinical investigations unless the count is more than about 3×10^5 counts/min.

IN-VIVO MEASUREMENT OF RADIOACTIVITY

Surface counting

This depends on shielding the crystals by means of a lead collimator to exclude as far as possible the radiation from outside a well defined area of the body.[5] It is thus possible to measure the radioactivity in individual organs. Positioning of the counter in relation to the patient is critical, and if the collimation is sufficiently narrow it is possible by counting over individual organs to detect sites of concentration of radioactivity. For most purposes a crystal with a diameter of 5–7 cm is suitable, and increased sensitivity, as well as more reliable positioning, can be achieved by using a dual counting system, with two opposed counters positioned above and below the patient.

Imaging

Radionuclide imaging has become an important application of radioactivity in clinical medicine. Its purpose is to obtain a picture of the distribution of a labelled substance within the body after it has been administered. This requires an isotope which emits γ rays, the energies of which are sufficient for the rays to penetrate body tissues and allow deep-lying organs to be imaged. The most widely used method for imaging is by the gamma camera. This consists of a large diameter (usually about 40 cm), 5–10 mm thick, thallium-activated sodium iodide detector crystal, an array of photomultiplier tubes, electronics for positioning the scintillations and for pulse-height analysis, a collimator (usually with multiple parallel holes), a cathode ray tube for image display and a film recording system.

Scanning camera

The gamma camera will normally visualize a circumscribed area of the body. To obtain a whole-body image on a single sheet of film a modification of the gamma camera, called the scanning camera, is used. The detector passes linearly head to foot over the patient's body, recording and displaying the image on a computer screen. The image moves on the display in synchrony with the movement of the detector head, so that the whole-body image is built up and recorded.

The gamma camera can be used not only to obtain the image but also to measure the quantity of the isotope in various parts of the body. This requires computerized calibration of the scanner by means of a calibration factor which relates the intensity of the image or the number of dots in the scan area to the activity obtained from a phantom containing a known amount of the isotope.[8]

Whole-body counting

It is possible by means of a whole-body counter consisting of a thallium-activated sodium iodide scintillator to measure the fraction of an administered isotope still present in the body with the passing of time. The technique is particularly useful in studying retention and turnover, as it overcomes the problems of collecting and measuring excreta. As the distribution of an isotope in the patient's body may vary during the course of an investigation, it is necessary to use several large crystals encompassing the entire body area and to apply careful calibration procedures. Extensive shielding around the detector ('shadow shield') is required to reduce background counts, or if very long-term studies are envisaged, a shielded low background room.

MEASUREMENT OF RADIOACTIVITY BY MEANS OF A SCINTILLATION COUNTER

Standardization of working conditions

Four controls require adjustment:

1. High voltage applied to the photomultiplier.
2. Amplifier gain applied to the incoming pulses before they reach the pulse-height analyser.
3. Analyser threshold.
4. Window.

The pulse-height analyser threshold and window are arbitrary settings and for simplification it is convenient to make the analyser setting correspond to the energy of the γ rays. Thus, a threshold scale of 0–100 can be made to correspond to a range of 0–1000 keV.★

The procedure is as follows: a radionuclide of known γ emission, peferrably one with a single energy such as ^{99m}Tc (0.140 MeV) or ^{51}Cr (0.320 MeV) is placed in front of the detector. The high voltage is fixed at a convenient level (e.g. 1000 V). The threshold scale is then set to correspond to the photo-peak of the isotope (i.e. the energy at which the maximum number of pulses in the pulse-height spectrum are emitted) and the window is set at about 10% of the threshold reading. The amplifier gain is varied until the spectrometer's ratemeter shows a definite peak. It should be established that the peak corresponds to the photopeak of the isotope and is not a scattered peak by starting with a high analyser setting and then gradually reducing it. The settings may be checked by means of another isotope of different energy when the analyser threshold should yield a maximum ratemeter deflection at a scale reading corresponding to the new energy. Examples of spectra and selected settings are illustrated in Fig. 22.1.

The setting of the apparatus, once determined, should remain constant for many months. The threshold and sensitivity of the equipment should be checked from time to time using a known standard. Ideally, this should be a sample of the isotope that is being measured. With a short-lived isotope this is not practical, and, instead, an isotope

★eV = electron volt, 10^3 keV = 1 MeV

with a long half-life and comparable emission, e.g. ^{57}Co (270 day half-life), can be used. A further standard of sensitivity is the background itself, as this tends to vary little from day to day.

Counting technique

Measurement of radioactivity

Measurements are usually carried out for a fixed period of time, the results being recorded as counts per s (cps) or counts per min (cpm). Radioactivity is subject to random but statistically predictable variation. The accuracy of the count depends upon the total number of the counts recorded (see p. 47). The variance of a radioactive count = $\sqrt{\text{total count}}$ and the count CV is given by

$$\frac{\text{SD}}{\text{Count}} \times 100\%.$$

Thus, on a count of 100 the inherent error is 10%; it is 1% on a count of 10 000. Any measured activity represents the difference between the sample count and the background count, in which the errors of both counts are cumulative. Other errors include those related to the calibration of the apparatus and those related to techniques, so that in-vivo radioactive measurements rarely have a CV <5% unless the count-rate is very high or the counting time unusually prolonged. In practice, a net count of 2500 over background is adequate for the accuracy required in in-vivo clinical studies.

Background counts should be measured alongside that of the radioactive material. If the count-rate of the sample is not much above background, then the background should be counted for as long a time as the sample. If the sample-count rate is less than the background, accurate measurement requires extremely long counting times.

Correction for physical decay

As physical decay is a continuous process which proceeds at an exponential rate and is specific for each particular radionuclide it is possible to correct mathematically for the loss of radioactivity with time and so convert any measurement back to that on Day 0. This is necessary when successive observations made at different times after the administration of an isotope to a patient are compared. An alternative method is to prepare a standard from an accurately measured sample of the originally administered material and to compare the sample measurements with the measurements of the standard at the same time. The loss of radioactivity due to physical decay can then be ignored as both are decaying at identical rates.

Correction for dead-time

If the count rate is so high that the interval between counts is shorter than the dead-time, some counts will not be recorded. The extent of dead-time error can be estimated and a calibrated chart prepared from the expected and corresponding measured counts on samples in various known dilutions or by counting a high activity radioisotope at various times as it decays. When the solution being measured has a count-rate near to the instrument limit it should be diluted or allowed to decay until the count-rate decreases to a level where loss due to dead-time becomes negligible.

DOUBLE ISOTOPE MEASUREMENTS

If more than one isotope is present in a sample, it is possible to measure the radioactivity of each isotope separately by one of several techniques:

Mechanical separation

When plasma is labelled with ^{131}I and red cells with ^{51}Cr, the separation of the two components is simple. For example:

(a) counts per ml whole blood
  = activity of ^{131}I + ^{51}Cr per ml of blood;
(b) counts per ml plasma × (1 − PCV)
  = activity of ^{131}I per ml of blood;
  (a) − (b) = activity of ^{51}Cr per ml of blood.

Differential decay

This is of value especially when one of the isotopes has a very short half-life (e.g. ^{99m}Tc, half-life 6 h). The method is to count the activity in the mixture twice, with the time interval between the counts chosen to allow for the decay of three or more half-lives of the short-lived isotope.

Physical separation

When the two isotopes produce γ rays of widely different energies they can be counted separately at different settings in a γ-ray spectrometer, as determined by pulse-height analysis. If there is interference of one isotope by the other because of overlap of the spectra a correction can be applied by establishing a ratio of counts from a standard of the particular isotope measured at the setting for the other isotope. For example, to separate ^{99m}Tc and ^{51}Cr in a mixture, a ^{51}Cr source is counted in window 1 (optimal for Tc) and window 2 (optimal for Cr). The ^{51}Cr ratio (R) is calculated as counts of ^{51}Cr source in window 1 divided by counts of ^{51}Cr source in window 2. Then, when the mixture is measured, the counts due to ^{51}Cr interference in window 1 (N_1) = R × ^{51}Cr counts in window 2, and the true ^{99m}Tc count in window 1 = total count in window 1 − N_1 ^{51}Cr.

REFERENCES

[1] BOWRING, C. S. (1981). *Radionuclide Tracer Techniques in Haematology*. Butterworth, London.
[2] Department of health and social security (1979). *Health service management: administration of radioactive substances to persons* HC(79)17. DHSS, London.
[3] Health and Safety Commission (1985). *Approved Code of Practice: The protection of persons against ionising radiation arising from any work activity. The ionising radiations regulations 1985*. HMSO, London.
[4] International Atomic Energy Agency (1973). *Safe handling of radionuclides*. IAEA Safety Series No. 1. IAEA, Vienna.
[5] International Committee for Standardization in Haematology (1975). Recommended methods for surface counting to determine sites of red-cell destruction. *British Journal of Haematology*, **30**, 249.
[6] LEWIS, S. M. and BAYLY, R. J. (Ed) (1986). *Radionuclides in Haematology*. Churchill Livingstone, Edinburgh.
[7] National Radiological Protection Board (1988). *Guidance*

notes for the protection of persons against ionising radiations arising from medical and dental use. HMSO, London.

[8] SHORT, M. D., RICHARDS, A. R. and GLASS, H. I. (1972). The use of a gamma camera as a whole-body counter. *British Journal of Radiology,* **45,** 289.

[9] SORENSON, J. A. and PHELPS, M. E. (1986). *Physics in Nuclear Medicine,* 2nd edn. Grune & Stratton, New York.

23. Blood volume

The haemoglobin content, total red cell count and PCV do not invariably reflect the total red cell volume. Whilst in most cases for practical purposes there is adequate correlation between peripheral-blood values and (total) red cell volume,[2] there will be a discrepancy if the plasma volume is reduced or increased disproportionately. Plasma volume is influenced by bed rest, exercise, change in posture, food and ambient temperature. Fluctuation in plasma volume may result in haemodilution or conversely in haemoconcentration, giving rise to pseudoanaemia or pseudopolycythaemia respectively. In contrast to the fluctuations in plasma volume, red cell volume does not fluctuate to any extent if erythropoiesis is in a steady state. Some of the causes of variations are given in Table 23.1.

Blood volume should be measured whenever the PCV is persistently higher than normal; demonstration of an absolute increase in red cell volume is necessary to diagnose polycythaemia and to assess its severity. The component parts of the blood volume (i.e. red cell and plasma volume) should also be measured, separately, in the elucidation of obscure anaemias when the possibility of an increase in plasma volume cannot be excluded.

METHODS OF MEASUREMENT OF BLOOD VOLUME

Principle. The principle is that of dilution analysis. A small volume of a readily identifiable radionuclide is injected intravenously either bound to the red cells or to a plasma component and its dilution is measured after time has been allowed for the injected material to become thoroughly mixed in the circulation, but before significant quantities have left the circulation. The most practical method now available is to use a small volume of the patient's red cells labelled with radioactive chromium (^{51}Cr), technetium (pertechnetate) (^{99m}Tc) or indium (^{113m}In or ^{111}In). The relative advantages and disadvantages of each radionuclide are discussed later.

The labelled red cells are diluted in the whole blood of the patient and from their dilution the total blood volume can be calculated; the red cell volume, too, can be deduced from knowledge of the PCV. The plasma volume can be measured directly by injecting human albumin labelled with radioactive iodine (^{125}I or ^{131}I): the albumin is diluted in the plasma compartment only and thus gives a value for plasma volume only.

Table 23.1 Clinical effect of variable relationship between red cell volume and plasma volume

Red cell volume	Plasma volume	Cause	Effect
Normal* (or low)	High	Pregnancy Cirrhosis Nephritis Congestive cardiac failure Myelomatosis Macroglobulinaemia	Pseudoanaemia or anaemia less severe than indicated by red-cell count
Normal	Low	Stress Peripheral circulatory failure Essential hypertension Diuretic drugs Dehydration Oedema Prolonged bed rest High altitude (1st 2 weeks)	Pseudopolycythaemia
Low	Normal	Anaemia	Accurate reflection of degree of anaemia
Low	High	Anaemia	Anaemia less severe than indicated by red cell count
Low	Low	Haemorrhage Severe anaemia (when PCV below 0.2)	Anaemia more severe than indicated by red cell count
High	Normal to Low	Polycythaemia	Accurate reflection of polycythaemia or polycythaemia less severe than apparent
High	High	Polycythaemia	Polycythaemia more severe than apparent
Normal (or even high)	High	Marked splenomegaly	Pseudoanaemia

In contrast to measurement of red cell volume, plasma-volume measurements are only approximations as the labelled albumin undergoes continuous slow interchange between the plasma and extracellular fluids and part of it also probably exchanges with a small rapidly exchanging pool, even during the mixing period. For these reasons it is undesirable to attempt to calculate red cell volume from plasma volume, on the basis of the observed PCV. On the other hand, as the red cell volume is generally more stable, calculation of total blood volume from red cell volume is usually more reliable, provided that the difference between whole body and venous PCV is appreciated and allowed for (see p. 365). Measurement of red cell and plasma volumes separately by direct methods is to be preferred. As the γ rays from ^{51}Cr can easily be distinguished from those of ^{125}I, red cell and plasma volumes can be measured simultaneously.

The subject of blood volume and its measurements has a large literature. The reviews of Mollison,[20] Mayerson[17] and Najean and Cacchione[24] include extensive bibliographies; practical information is provided in the recommendations on standard techniques of the International Committee for Standardization in Haematology.[13]

DETERMINATION OF RED CELL VOLUME

RADIOACTIVE CHROMIUM METHOD

Add approximately 10 ml of blood to 1.5 ml of sterile NIH-A acid-citrate dextrose (ACD) solution (see p. 535), in a 30 ml bottle with a screw cap. Centrifuge at 1200–1500 g for 5 min. Discard the supernatant plasma and buffy coat and slowly add to the cells, with continous mixing, 4–8 × 10^3 Bq (0.1–0.2 μCi) of $Na_2^{51}CrO_4$ per kg of body weight.

The sodium chromate should be in a volume of at least 0.2 ml, being diluted in 9 g/l NaCl (saline). Allow the blood to stand for 15 min at 37°C for labelling to take place. Wash the red cells twice in 4–5 volumes of sterile saline.* Finally, resuspend the cells in a volume of sterile saline sufficient for an injection of about 10 ml and the preparation of a standard. Take up the appropriate volume to the mark in a precalibrated syringe or into a syringe which is weighed before and after the injection. In the latter case the volume injected is calculated from the following formula:

volume injected (ml)

$$= \frac{\text{weight of suspension injected (g)}}{\text{density of suspension (g/ml)}}$$

where density of suspension =

$$1.0 + \frac{\text{Hb conc. of suspension (g/l)} \times 0.097}{340}.$$

(This assumes that packed red cells have a MCHC of 340 g/l and a density of 1.097).

Accurate and aseptic filling of the syringe and exclusion of air bubbles are facilitated by drawing up the solution beyond the required volume and then returning the excess to the original bottle by means of a U-shaped needle or a length of plastic tubing attached to the nozzle of the syringe.

Inject the suspension intravenously without delay and note the time, and 10, 20 and 30 min later, collect 5–10 ml of the patient's blood and add it to the appropriate amount of a solid anticoagulant (e.g. K_2 EDTA). This blood should preferably be withdrawn from a vein other than that used for the injection. However, it is often convenient to insert a self-retaining (e.g. butterfly) needle; in this case care must be taken to ensure that the isotope is well dispersed into the blood stream when injected by flushing through with 10 ml of sterile saline. When the mixing time is likely to be prolonged as in splenomegaly, cardiac failure or shock, another sample should be taken 60 min after the injection.

Measure the PCV of each sample. Deliver 1 ml volumes into counting tubes and lyse with saponin; a convenient method is to add 2 drops of Saponin (Coulter). Measure their radioactivity in a scintilla-

tion counter. Then dilute the residue of the original suspension which was not injected 1 in 500 in water (for use as a standard) and determine the radio-activity of a 1 ml volume. Then red cell volume (RCV) (ml) =

$$\frac{\begin{array}{c}\text{radioactivity of standard (cpm/ml)}\\ \times \text{ diln. of standard}\\ \times \text{ volume injected (ml)}\end{array}}{\text{radioactivity of post-injection sample (cpm/ml)}} \times \text{PCV}\star$$

The total blood volume (BV) can be calculated by multiplying the value for RCV by 1/(whole-body PCV) (see p. 365). Plasma volume can be calculated by subtracting RCV from BV.

If a sample has been taken at 60 min in cases where delayed mixing is suspected and there is a significant difference between the measurements at 10–30 min and 60 min, the 60 min measurement should be used for calculating the red cell volume.

TECHNETIUM METHOD

^{99m}Tc is prepared as sodium pertechnetate. This passes freely through the red cell membrane and will become attached to the cells only if it is present in a reduced form as it enters the cells when it binds firmly to β-chains of haemoglobin. For this to occur, the red cells require to be treated with a stannous (tin) compound. This may be carried out either in vitro[14] or in vivo,[26] followed by in-vitro labelling. The in-vivo method of pre-treatment is recommended.

Dissolve a vial of Pyrolite (New England Nuclear)** or Amerscan Stannous agent (Amersham International)*** in 8 ml of sterile saline and inject 4 ml intravenously. After 15 min, collect 10 ml of blood into a sterile container to which has been added 200 iu of liquid heparin. Centrifuge and wash twice with sterile saline to remove the extra-cellular tin. Then add 2 MBq (c 50 μCi) of freshly generated ^{99m}Tc in approximately 0.2 ml of saline or 75 MBq (c 2 mCi) if measurement of splenic red cell pool and scanning are also required. Allow to

---

* 12 g/l NaCl should be used when red cell osmotic fragility is greatly increased, e.g. in cases of hereditary spherocytosis.

*As measured on the blood sample by an electronic counting system or by microhaematocrit (see p. 48).
**Sodium pyrophosphate, sodium trimetaphosphate and stannous chloride
***Stannous fluoride and sodium medronate

stand at room temperature for 5 min. Centrifuge; wash twice in cold sterile saline and resuspend in a sufficient volume of cold sterile saline for an injection of 10 ml and preparation of a standard. Reinject and carry out subsequent procedures as for the chromium method. Because of the short half-life of ^{99m}Tc, radioactivity must be measured on the day of the test. Because 5–10% of the radioactivity is eluted from the red cells within 1 h,[7] the method is less suitable than are the chromium and indium methods when there is splenomegaly or another cause of delayed mixing is suspected.

Indium is available as ^{111}In chloride or it can be produced as ^{113}In in a generator by elution from ^{113}Sn. The labelling procedure is simpler than with ^{99m}Tc and there is less elution during the first hour. It is thus particularly suitable for delayed sampling. For labelling blood cells, the indium is complexed with oxine,[9] acetylacetone[31] or tropolone.[5,25] The latter two are easier to prepare, and their use is described below.

INDIUM METHOD

1. Preparation of acetylacetone complex

Take approximately 5 ml of blood into a sterile bottle or tube containing 100 iu of liquid heparin. Wash once in sterile saline. To the packed cells, add 10 ml of 1.9 g/l acetylacetone (Sigma or E. Merck) in HEPES or tris buffer, pH 7.6 (p. 538). The acetylacetone should be stored at 4°C but brought to room temperature before use. Mix gently for 1 min, then add 2–3.5 MBq (c 50–100 µCi) of freshly generated ^{113}In or ^{111}In. Mix on a roller mixer for 5 min, then wash twice in saline. Resuspend in a sufficient volume of saline for an injection of 10 ml and preparation of a standard.

2. Preparation of tropolone complex

Prepare a solution of 2.5 mg/ml of tropolone* in HEPES saline buffer pH 7.6 (p. 538). Filter through a 0.22 µm Millipore filter. This solution can be used for up to 3 months if kept at 4°C. Take approximately 5 ml of blood into a sterile container containing 100 iu of liquid heparin. Add c 50 µg

---

* 2 hydroxy-2, 4, 6 -cycloheptatrien-1-one (Fluorchem Ltd, Gossop; Sigma)

(20 µl) of the tropolone solution per ml of blood. Mix gently for 1 min, then add 2–3.5 MBq (c 50–100 µCi) of freshly generated ^{113m}In or ^{111}In chloride. Mix on a roller mix for 5 min, then wash twice in saline. Resuspend in a sufficient volume of saline for an injection of 10 ml and preparation of a standard.

Repeated blood-volume measurements

When repeated blood-volume measurements are required within a few days, the ^{51}Cr method can be used if the residual radioactivity is measured in the blood immediately before each test. However, the residual radioactivity increases the counting error and it may be necessary to increase the amount of tracer injected. The short-lived isotopes (^{99m}Tc, ^{113m}In) have the advantage that they can be used for repeated tests without this problem and also that the patient will be subjected to lower doses of radioactivity. The isotopes are slowly eluted in vivo and in vitro. With ^{99m}Tc, elution is slight within the first 10–20 minutes; it gives results which compare closely with those of ^{51}Cr but because of progressively increasing elution the method is less satisfactory when delayed mixing necessitates sampling at 60 min post-injection.

The labelling procedure using indium is much simpler than with technetium and, as elution is less than with ^{99m}Tc during the first hour, it is particularly suitable for delayed sampling.[30]

DETERMINATION OF PLASMA VOLUME

^{125}I- OR ^{131}I-HUMAN SERUM ALBUMIN (HSA) METHOD[13]

Human serum albumin (HSA) labelled with ^{125}I or ^{131}I is available commercially.* The albumin concentration should not be less than 20 g/l. The user must be reassured that only HIV antibody and hepatitis antigen-negative donors are used as the source of albumin. ^{125}I has the advantage over ^{131}I that it is readily distinguished from ^{51}Cr, ^{99m}Tc and ^{113m}In, and this makes possible the simultaneous direct determination of red cell volume and plasma volume (see p. 365).

---

* e.g. Amersham International

Withdraw *c* 20 ml of blood into a syringe containing a few drops of sterile heparin solution and transfer to a 30 ml sterile bottle with a screw cap. After centrifuging at 1200–1500 *g* for 5–10 min, transfer *c* 7 ml of plasma to a second sterile bottle and add 2×10^3 MBq (*c* 0.05 µCi) of the radionuclide-labelled HSA per kg body weight. Inject a measured amount (e.g. 5 ml) and retain the residue for preparation of a standard.

^{125}I-HSA is also available commercially prepacked in 1 ml volumes containing 0.1–0.2 MBq (*c* 3–5 µCi). The contents of an ampoule can be injected intravenously and a similar ampoule should then be used to prepare a standard. After 10, 20 and 30 min, withdraw blood samples from a vein other than that used for the original injection (or after flushing through with 10 ml of sterile 9 g/l NaCl (saline) if a butterfly needle has been used) and deliver into bottles containing EDTA or heparin.

Measure the PCV, centrifuge the sample and separate the plasma. Prepare a standard by diluting part of the residue of the uninjected HSA 1 in 100 in saline.

Measure the radioactivity of the plasma samples in a scintillation counter, and by extrapolation on semilogarithmic graph paper calculate the radioactivity of the plasma at zero time. If only a single sample is collected 10 min after the injection, the radioactivity at zero time may be obtained approximately by multiplying by 1.015. Reliance on a single 10 min sample will lead to error if the mixing of the albumin in the plasma is delayed.[15] After measuring the radioactivity of the standard, the plasma volume (ml) is calculated as follows:

$$\frac{\text{radioactivity of standard (cpm/ml)} \times \text{diln. of standard} \times \text{vol. injected (ml)}}{\text{radioactivity of post-injection sample (cpm/ml, adjusted to zero time)}}.$$

Other radionuclide methods for determination of plasma volume

[132]I has the very short half-life of 2.26 h and, like ^{131}I and ^{125}I, it can be combined with human serum albumin,[34] but the advantage of the radionuclide—its short half-life—is outweighed by the necessity of labelling the albumin shortly before it is used.

[99m]Tc has also been used in combination with human serum albumin[3] and [113m]In with transferrin.[35]

DETERMINATION OF TOTAL BLOOD VOLUME

As has already been indicated, the total blood volume is frequently calculated from the red cell volume and PCV. But before this can be done the observed PCV has to be corrected for the difference between the whole-body and venous PCV. The reason for this difference is described below.

Whole-body and venous PCV ratio

It is well known that the PCV measured on venous blood is not identical with the average PCV of all the blood in the body. This is mainly because the red cell : plasma ratio is less in small blood vessels (capillaries, arterioles and venules) than in large vessels. The ratio between the whole-body PCV and venous-blood PCV is normally about 0.9[13] and it is thus necessary in the calculation of total blood volume from measurements of red cell volume to multiply the observed PCV by 0.9. Thus total blood volume is given by:

$$\text{red-cell volume} \times \frac{1}{\text{PCV} \times 0.9}.$$

Unfortunately, the ratio varies from 0.85 to 0.95 in normal subjects and may even fall outside this range in some pathological states.[15] Thus, the ratio is often notably raised in splenomegaly because of the increased volume of splenic blood of relatively high PCV, while in oedema or cardiac failure it may be lower than normal. The ratio is increased in pregnancy[4] and at high altitudes.[18] In such cases it is better to estimate red cell volume and plasma volume by separate measurements rather than to attempt to calculate one of these from an estimate of the other. Nevertheless, in many diseases the ratio is not far from 0.9 and total blood volumes can be calculated from red cell volume measurements with reasonable accuracy.

Simultaneous measurement of red cell volume and plasma volume

When ^{99m}Tc is used, it is first necessary to inject the stannous complex (p. 363). Then collect *c* 10 ml of blood into a sterile container with 200 iu of liquid heparin. Wash twice in sterile 9 g/l NaCl (saline). Then label the red cells with ^{99m}Tc (see p. 363), wash twice in the saline and resuspend to a volume of c 12 ml.

When ^{51}Cr is used, collect the blood into ACD and label the red cells as described on p. 362. When ^{113m}In is used, collect blood into a heparinized container and label the red cells as described on p. 364. Add ^{125}I-HSA (see p. 365) and mix it with the labelled red cell suspension. Inject an accurately measured amount and dilute the remainder 1 in 500 in water for use as a standard. Collect three blood samples at 10, 20 and 30 min, respectively, after the administration of the labelled blood and estimate the radioactivity of a measured volume of each sample and a similar volume of the standard.

When ^{99m}Tc or ^{113m}In has been used in combination with ^{125}I, count on the same day; then leave for 2 days to allow the ^{99m}Tc or ^{113m}In to decay and count again for ^{125}I activity. Subtract the ^{125}I counts (corrected for decay) from the original counts to obtain a measurement of the counts due to the ^{99m}Tc or ^{113m}In.

When ^{51}Cr has been used in combination with ^{125}I, and a multi-channel counter is available, measure the radioactivity due to the ^{51}Cr and ^{125}I at the appropriate settings for ^{51}Cr and ^{125}I. Whereas the ^{51}Cr counts are obtained free from ^{125}I counts, some ^{51}Cr radioactivity will be counted in the ^{125}I channel. A correction factor for this can be calculated by measuring a standard of ^{51}Cr in the ^{125}I channel.

Calculate the radioactivity due to ^{51}Cr, ^{99m}Tc or ^{113}In in the blood from the mean of the 10, 20 and 30 min samples, and obtain that due to ^{125}I from the value extrapolated to zero time. Calculate red cell volume as described on p. 363.

Plasma volume is calculated from the formula:

$$\frac{\text{radioactivity of standard (cpm/ml)} \times \text{dil. of standard} \times \text{vol.}^\star \text{ injected (ml)}}{\text{radioactivity of post-injection sample (cpm/ml, corrected to zero time)}} \times (1 - \text{PCV}).$$

Total blood volume = red cell volume + plasma volume

Expression of results of blood-volume estimations

Red cell volume, plasma volume and total blood volume are usually expressed in ml/kg of body weight. Because fat is relatively avascular, low values are obtained in obese subjects and the relation between blood volume and body weight varies according to body composition. Blood volume is more closely correlated with lean body mass.[12,22] Earlier methods for determination of lean body mass were not practical as a routine procedure, but there are now available instruments that are simple to use for estimating body composition by the different response of fat and other tissues to electrical impedance* or to a near infra red light beam.**[36]

An alternative is to discount excess fat by using an estimate of so-called 'ideal weight' by reference to standard tables which are based on height, age, build and sex.[6] These methods are somewhat arbitrary and tend to overcorrect for the avascularity of fat.

More complicated formulae have been proposed for predicting the normal blood volume. These are slightly more reliable than those based on weight alone. But the 95% confidence limits are at least $\pm 10\%$ of the mean values given by the formulae.[13] The table given by Hurley[11] which relates both red cell and plasma volume to surface area is derived from a relatively large series of measurements (Table 23.2). In practice the diagnosis of absolute polycythaemia can be made with confidence from Hurley's table if the red cell volume is >125% of the predicted normal value, and the plasma volume is abnormally reduced if it is <80% of the predicted normal value[15] Approximately similar figures are obtained using Nadler's formula.[27]

Range in health

Red cell volume: men, 30 ml/kg (2 SD $\pm$ 5 ml); women, 25 ml/kg (2 SD $\pm$ 5 ml).

---

*See p. 363.

* Holt body composition analyser, Holtain Ltd, Crosswell, Dyfed, Wales.
** Futrex-5000, Self-care Products Ltd, Amersham, Bucks.

Table 23.2 Mean values for red cell mass (RCM) and plasma volume (PV) (in ml) related to body surface area (SA in m^2) for men and women

SA	Men RCM	Men PV	Women RCM	Women PV	SA	Men RCM	Men PV	Women RCM	Women PV
1.39	–	–	1136	1964	1.77	1907	2922	1588	2666
1.40	–	–	1148	1982	1.78	1917	2940	1599	2682
1.41	–	–	1162	2000	1.79	1927	2958	1610	2702
1.42	–	–	1172	2018	1.80	1938	2976	1622	2720
1.43	–	–	1184	2039	1.81	1951	2994	1634	2740
1.44	–	–	1196	2058	1.82	1964	3013	1645	2760
1.45	–	–	1208	2076	1.83	1977	3031	1657	2778
1.46	–	–	1220	2094	1.84	1990	3050	1670	2796
1.47	–	–	1232	2112	1.85	2003	3069	1681	2815
1.48	–	–	1242	2132	1.86	2016	3087	1692	2838
1.49	–	–	1254	2148	1.87	2029	3106	1704	2854
1.50	1684	2498	1268	2168	1.88	2042	3125	–	–
1.51	1692	2513	1280	2184	1.89	2055	3144	–	–
1.52	1699	2529	1291	2204	1.90	2070	3164	–	–
1.53	1707	2544	1302	2222	1.91	2087	3183	–	–
1.54	1715	2560	1315	2252	1.92	2104	3202	–	–
1.55	1722	2575	1326	2258	1.93	2112	3222	–	–
1.56	1730	2591	1338	2278	1.94	2138	3242	–	–
1.57	1737	2606	1349	2296	1.95	2156	3261	–	–
1.58	1745	2621	1362	2314	1.96	2173	3280	–	–
1.59	1752	2637	1376	2336	1.97	2191	3299	–	–
1.60	1760	2652	1386	2354	1.98	2208	3318	–	–
1.61	1768	2667	1398	2374	1.99	2226	3337	–	–
1.62	1776	2682	1408	2392	2.00	2244	3358	–	–
1.63	1784	2697	1421	2410	2.01	2266	3390	–	–
1.64	1792	2712	1434	2428	2.02	2288	3402	–	–
1.65	1800	2727	1445	2444	2.03	2310	3424	–	–
1.66	1809	2742	1458	2462	2.04	2332	3446	–	–
1.67	1817	2757	1468	2480	2.05	2354	3468	–	–
1.68	1826	2772	1480	2500	2.06	2375	3490	–	–
1.69	1834	2787	1492	2520	2.07	2397	3513	–	–
1.70	1842	2802	1504	2538	2.08	2419	3536	–	–
1.71	1851	2819	1516	2558	2.09	2441	3558	–	–
1.72	1861	2837	1527	2576	2.10	2463	3580	–	–
1.73	1870	2854	1540	2592	2.11	2486	3604	–	–
1.74	1880	2871	1552	2612	2.12	2510	3628	–	–
1.75	1889	2888	1563	2630	2.13	2535	3653	–	–
1.76	1898	2905	1576	2648	2.14	2560	3679	–	–
					2.15	2586	3704	–	–

Reproduced with permission from Hurley[11].

Plasma volume: 40–50 ml/kg.

Total blood volume: 60–80 ml/kg.

In newborn infants, at comparable levels of PCV, the red cell volume and plasma volume are the same, relative to body weight, as in adults.[21] The total blood volume is thus c 250–350 ml at birth. After infancy the volume increases gradually until adult life. As a rule, the blood volume remains remarkably constant in an individual and rapid adjustments take place within a few hours after blood transfusion or intravenous infusion.

In pregnancy both the plasma volume and total blood volume increase. The plasma volume increases especially in the first trimester, the total volume later,[16] and by full term the plasma volume will have increased by c 40% and total blood volume by c 32% or even more. The blood volume returns to normal within a week post partum.

Bed rest causes a reduction in plasma volume[32] and muscular exercise and changes in posture cause transient fluctuations. In practice, the patient should always be allowed to rest in a recumbent position for 15 min prior to measuring the blood volume.

SPLENIC RED CELL VOLUME

The red cell content of the normal spleen (the red cell 'pool') is less than 5% of the total red cell volume (i.e. <100–120 ml in an adult). In spleno-megaly the pool is increased, e.g. by as much as 5–10 times in myelofibrosis, polycythaemia, hairy cell leukaemia and lympho-proliferative disorders.[28] Increase in the volume of the splenic red cell pool may by itself be a cause of anaemia; measurement of the pool is thus useful in the investigation of anaemia in these conditions. It is also useful in determining the cause of erythrocytosis, as the expanded pool in polycythaemia vera contrasts with that in secondary polycythaemia in which it is normal.[1]

An approximate estimate of the splenic red cell volume can be obtained from the difference between the apparent red cell volume, as measured immediately after the injection of radionuclide-labelled cells, and that measured after mixing has been completed, i.e. after a delay of c 20 min,[29] or from the difference in surface counts over the spleen before and after mixing has been completed.[33] The splenic red cell volume can be estimated more accurately by quantitative scanning, after injecting viable red cells labelled with ^{99m}Tc or ^{113m}In (p. 356).[10] The blood volume is measured in the usual way using c 2 mCi (74 MBq) of ^{99m}Tc or 1 mCi (37 MBq) of ^{113m}I. The splenic area is scanned 20 min after the injection or after 60 min when there is splenomegaly. To delineate the spleen more precisely, it may be necessary to carry out a second scan after an injection of heat-damaged labelled red cells (see p. 391). From the radioactivity in the spleen, relative to that in a standard, and knowledge of the total red cell volume, the proportion of the total red cell volume contained in the spleen can be calculated. This technique is also useful for demonstrating localized accumulation of blood in haemangiomas in the liver,[19] telangiectasia and other vascular abnormalities.[8]

REFERENCES

[1] BATEMAN, S., LEWIS, S. M., NICHOLAS, A. and ZAAFRAN, A. (1978). Splenic red cell pooling: a diagnostic feature in polycythaemia. *British Journal of Haematology,* **40,** 389.

[2] BENTLEY, S. A. and LEWIS, S. M. (1976). The relationship between total red cell volume, plasma volume and venous haematocrit. *British Journal of Haematology,* **33,** 301.

[3] CALLAHAN, R. J., MCKUSICK, K. A., LAMSON, M., CASTRONOVO, F. P. and POTSAID, M. S. (1976). Technetium-99m-human serum albumin: evaluation of a commercially produced kit. *Journal of Nuclear Medicine,* **17,** 47.

[4] CATION, W. L., ROBY, C. C., REID, D. E. et al (1951). The circulating red cell volume and body hematocrit in normal pregnancy and the puerperium by direct measurement using radioactive red cells. *American Journal of Obstetrics and Gynecology,* **61,** 1207.

[5] DANPURE, H. J., OSMAN, S. and BRADY, F. (1982). The labelling of blood cells in plasma with ^{111}In-tropolonate. *British Journal of Radiology,* **55,** 247.

[6] Documenta Geigy (1970). *Scientific Tables* (Eds. K. Diem and C. Lentner) 7th edn., p. 712. J. R. Geigy, Basel.

[7] FERRANT, A., LEWIS, S. M. and SZUR, L. (1974). The elution of ^{99m}Tc from red cells and its effect on red cell volume measurement. *Journal of Clinical Pathology,* **27,** 983.

[8] FRONT, D. and ISRAEL, O. (1981). Tc-99m-labelled red blood cells in the evaluation of vascular abnormalities. *Journal of Nuclear Medicine,* **22,** 149.

[9] GOODWIN, D. A. (1978). Cell labelling with oxine chelates of radioactive metal ions: techniques and clinical implications. *Journal of Nuclear Medicine,* **19,** 557.

[10] HEGDE, U. M., WILLIAMS, E. D., LEWIS, S. M., SZUR, L., GLASS, H. I. and PETTIT, J. E. (1973). Measurement of splenic red cell volume and visualization of the spleen with ^{99m}Tc. *Journal of Nuclear Medicine,* **14,** 769.

[11] HURLEY, P. J. (1975). Red cell and plasma volumes in normal adults. *Journal of Nuclear Medicine,* **16,** 46.

[12] HUFF, R. L. and FELLER, D. D. (1956). Relation of circulating red cell volume to body density and obesity. *Journal of Clinical Investigation,* **35,** 1.

[13] International Committee for Standardization in Haematology (1980). Recommended methods for measurements of red-cell and plasma volume. *Journal of Nuclear Medicine,* **21,** 793.

[14] JONES, J. and MOLLISON, P. L. (1978). Simple and efficient method of labelling red cells with ^{99m}Tc for determination of red cell volume. *British Journal of Haematology,* **38,** 141.

[15] LEWIS, S. M. and LIU YIN, J. A. (1986). Blood volume studies. *Methods in Hematology,* **14,** 198.

[16] LUND, C. J. and SISSON, T. R. C. (1958). Blood volume and anemia of mother and baby. *American Journal of Obstetrics and Gynecology,* **76,** 1013.

[17] MAYERSON, H. S. (1965). Blood volume and its regulation. *Annual Review of Physiology,* **27,** 307.

[18] METZ, J., LEVIN, N. W. and HART, D. (1962). Effect of altitude on the body/venous haematocrit ratio. *Nature* (London), **194,** 483.

[19] MILLER, J. H. (1987). Technetium-99m-labelled red blood cells in the evaluation of the liver in infants and children. *Journal of Nuclear Medicine,* **28,** 1412.

[20] MOLLISON, P. L., ENGELFRIET, C. P. and CONTRERAS, M. (1987). *Blood Transfusion in Clinical Medicine,* 8th edn., Ch. 3. Blackwell Scientific Publications, Oxford.

[21] MOLLISON, P. L., VEALL, N. and CUTBUSH, M. (1950). Red cell and plasma volume in newborn infants. *Archives of Disease in Childhood,* **25,** 242.

[22] MULDOWNEY, F. P. (1957). The relationship of total red cell mass to lean body mass in man. *Clinical Science,* **16,** 163.

[23] NADLER, S. B., HIDALGO, J. U. and BLOCH, T. (1962). Prediction of blood volume in normal human adults. *Surgery,* **51,** 224.

[24] NAJEAN, Y. and CACCHIONE, R. (1977). Blood volume in health and disease. *Clinics in Haematology,* **6,** 543.

[25] OSMAN, S. and DANPURE, H. J. (1987). A simple in vitro method of radiolabelling human erythrocytes in whole blood with ^{113m}In-tropolonate. *European Journal of Haematology,* **39,** 125.

[26] PAVEL, D. G., ZIMMER, A. M. and PATTERSON, V. N. (1977). In vivo labelling of red blood with ^{99m}Tc: a new approach to blood pool visualization. *Journal of Nuclear Medicine,* **18,** 305.

[27] PEARSON, T. C. and GUTHRIE, D. L. (1984). The interpretation of measured red cell mass and plasma volume in patients with elevated PCV values. *Clinical and Laboratory Haematology,* **6,** 207.

[28] PETTIT, J. (1977). Spleen function. *Clinics in Haematology,* **6,** 639.

[29] PRYOR D. S. (1967). The mechanism of anaemia in tropical splenomegaly. *Quarterly Journal of Medicine,* **36,** 337.

[30] RADIA, R., PETERS, A. M., DEENMAMODE, M., FITZPATRICK, M. L. and LEWIS, S. M. (1981). Measurement of red cell volume and splenic red cell pool using ^{113m}indium. *British Journal of Haematology,* **49,** 587.

[31] SINN, H. and SILVESTER, D. J. (1979). Simplified cell labelling with indium-111-acetylacetone. *British Journal of Radiology,* **52,** 758.

[32] TAYLOR, H. L., ERICKSON, L., HENSCHEL, A. and KEYS, A. (1945). The effect of bed rest on the blood volume of normal young men. *American Journal of Physiology,* **144,** 227.

[33] TOGHILL, P. J. (1964). Red-cell pooling in enlarged spleens. *British Journal of Haematology,* **10,** 347.

[34] VEALL, N., PEARSON, J. D. and HANLEY, T. (1955). The preparation of ^{132}I and ^{131}I labelled human serum albumin for clinical tracer studies. *British Journal of Radiology,* **28,** 633.

[35] WOCHNER, R. D., ADATEPE, M., van AMBURG, A. and POTCHEN, E. J. (1970). New method for estimation of plasma volume with the use of the distribution space of transferrin-113m indium. *Journal of Laboratory and Clinical Medicine,* **75,** 711.

[36] LUKASKI, H. C. (1987). Methods for the assessment of human body composition: traditional and new. *American Journal of Clinical Nutrition,* **46,** 537.

24. Erythrokinetics and platelet kinetics

Whilst much can be learnt about the rate and efficiency of erythropoiesis from the red cell count, reticulocyte count, blood film and bone marrow, studies of iron metabolism and measurement of red cell life-span with radioactive isotopes may provide useful additional information.

RADIOACTIVE IRON

Three isotopes of iron, ^{59}Fe, ^{55}Fe and ^{52}Fe have been used in clinical investigations to measure:

1. The absorption of iron following an oral dose
2. The distribution of radioactivity after an intravenous injection
3. Imaging of radio-iron uptake.

^{59}Fe

This isotope has a moderately short half-life, 45 days, and labels haemoglobin after ingestion or injection. If injected intravenously, it labels, too, the plasma iron pool and this allows the measurement of iron clearance and calculation of plasma-iron turnover. Its subsequent appearance in haemoglobin permits the assessment of the rate of haemoglobin synthesis and the completeness of the utili-

zation of iron. Since it is a γ-ray emitter, radioactivity can be measured in vivo by surface counting, and the sites of distribution of the administered iron and the probable sites of erythropoiesis can thus be determined.

^{52}Fe

This isotope has a short half-life, 8.2 h, and this has advantages as well as disadvantages. Because of its very short half-life, it cannot be kept in stock, and has to be freshly prepared shortly before it is administered to the patient. On the other hand, it can be administered successively, if required, at short intervals, and, because of its physical characteristics and the fact that it can be given in a relatively large dose, it can be used for identifying the sites and rate of the absorption of iron in the intestine[28] and for tracing the extent of active marrow in the bones and elsewhere,[31,59] neither of which can be accomplished as satisfactorily using ^{59}Fe in permissible dosages. However, its very short half-life prevents it from being used to study the utilization of iron by red cells.

[55]Fe

Because of its long half-life (2.16 yr), this isotope is now not used in studies in man because of the radiation hazard. It had, however, been used in double-isotope investigations, e.g. for measuring iron absorption.[13c]

IRON ABSORPTION

Principle. A small amount of isotope-labelled inorganic iron is administered by mouth and the amount of radioactivity subsequently eliminated in the faeces is measured. The difference between the radioactivity administered and that excreted is taken as the amount absorbed. Alternatively, the absorption of iron can be estimated by measuring the radioactivity retained in the body after ingestion of the iron, using a whole-body counter.[13c]

Method

Prepare the test dose no longer than 30 min prior to administration. Add 18 mg of ascorbic acid to 15 mg of iron sulphate ($FeSO_4.7H_2O$) in a beaker containing 10 ml of 1 mmol/l HCl. Add 0.1–0.2 MBq (c 3–5 µCi) of ^{59}Fe in the form of ferric chloride in 10 mmol/l HCl. Make up the solution to c 25 ml with water. Keep 1 ml as a standard. Measure an exact volume of the remainder. The patient takes this by mouth, in the early morning after an overnight fast, and is not allowed to eat for a further 3 h. The faeces passed during the following 5–7 days (see below) are collected in plastic or cardboard cartons.

Count each sample in a large-volume scintillation counter against 1 ml of the standard diluted in c 100 ml of water in a similar carton.

Calculation

% excreted

$$= \frac{cpm/ml \ of \ sample}{cpm/ml \ of \ standard} \times 100.$$
$$\times \ volume \ administered \ (ml)$$

Stool collections are continued until <1% of the administered dose is excreted in a 24 h collection.

If a whole-body counter is used, measurements should be made immediately after ingestion of the test dose, and continued at intervals for about 7–10 days. Then:

$$\% \ excreted = \frac{cpm \ after \ 7–10 \ days}{original \ cpm \ after \ dose} \times 100.$$

% absorbed = 100 − total % excreted.

Interpretation of results

Iron absorption is a complex process (for reviews, see Bothwell et al[13a], Cook and Lipschitz[20]), and a test based on the absorption of a small dose of a soluble iron salt is not a reliable indicator of the ability of the gastro-intestinal tract to absorb less available forms of iron from different foods. The situation is further complicated by the role of ascorbic acid and chelators in the diet, the presence or absence of achlorhydria, dietary food interactions and the fact that iron may be absorbed but retained in the epithelial cells of the intestine and lost subsequently by the normal process of desquamation. An iron absorption test is, thus, of very limited value.

In normal subjects the absorption averages about 15–30% of a test dose of a soluble iron salt, but it varies enormously; in iron-deficiency anaemia, absorption depends on the degree of iron deficiency and transferrin saturation, but it is usually in the range 50–80%. Absorption is decreased in the malabsorption syndromes (e.g. in sprue and 'idiopathic' steatorrhoea).

Because of the variation in normal subjects it is difficult to conclude from a single test dose that absorption is impaired. The test is of more use in demonstrating normal absorption (i.e. >10% of the test dose absorbed) in a patient suspected of having an absorption defect. However, the validity of the result depends on the completeness of the faecal collection.

In iron deficiency, in which absorption of iron from a test dose is generally greater than normal, almost all of the administered radioactivity may be expected to appear in the peripheral blood if the patient is absorbing iron normally. Blood radioactivity figures can thus be used in such cases as a simple test of iron absorption obviating the necessity of stool collection. In other cases, if an oral dose of $^{131}BaSO_4$ is given with the ^{59}Fe, this will serve as a marker of the passage of the iron through the intestinal tract, and thus distinguish between absorbed iron and iron which is retained but not absorbed. This has some value in distinguishing between primary and secondary iron overload.[12]

IRON DISTRIBUTION

Principle. Iron for incorporation into erythroblasts is transported to the bone marrow bound to transferrin. At the surface of the erythroblasts the complex releases its iron which enters the cell to be incorporated into haem, leaving the transferrin free for recycling. Iron not bound to transferrin finds its way to the liver and to other organs rather than to the bone marrow, whilst colloidal particles of iron are rapidly removed by phagocytic cells.

The ferrokinetic studies with ^{59}Fe which provide information on erythropoiesis include the rate of clearance of the radioiron from the plasma, plasma-iron turnover, iron incorporation into circulating red cells (iron utilization) and surface counting to measure the uptake and turnover of iron by organs. These are relatively simple procedures which provide clinically useful information. They do not, however, take account of the recirculation of iron which returns to the plasma from tissues, nor of iron turnover resulting from dyserythropoiesis or haemolysis. To take account of these factors requires much more detailed analysis of the iron kinetics with multiple sampling over an extended period.[7,15,16,60] These more complex and time-consuming procedures are essential for quantitative measurement of effective and ineffective erythropoiesis and to provide data on non-erythroid iron turnover. Even so, their interpretation depends on a model which does not necessarily correspond to reality.

In ferrokinetic studies it is important to ensure that any iron administered is bound to transferrin. As a rule, normal (or patient's) plasma has an adequate amount of transferrin. The unsaturated iron-binding capacity (UIBC) or transferrin concentration of the patient's plasma should be measured before the test is carried out and, if the UIBC is <1 mg/l (20 μmol/l) or the transferrin concentration is <0.6 g/l, normal donor plasma (HIV antibody and hepatitis antigen (HB$_s$)-negative) should be used instead of that of the patient for the subsequent labelling procedure. Some workers, e.g. Cavill,[14] recommend passing the labelled plasma through an exchange resin to ensure removal of non-transferrin-bound iron prior to injection.

The subject of ferrokinetics in health and disease was extensively reviewed in an early monograph by Finch et al[30] and has been more recently dealt with by Bothwell et al.[13]

Method

Under sterile conditions, obtain 5–10 ml of plasma from freshly collected heparinized blood. Add 0.3–0.4 MBq (c 7–10 μCi) of ^{59}Fe ferric citrate (sp activity >0.2 MBq/μg). Incubate at 37°C for 30 min. Fill a syringe with all but 1 ml of the mixture. Weigh the syringe to the nearest 10 mg. Inject its content intravenously into the patient, starting a stop-watch at the mid-point of the injection. Re-weigh the empty syringe and calculate the volume injected:

$$\text{volume of plasma (ml)} = \text{wt of plasma (g)} \times \frac{1}{1.015}.$$

Dilute the residual portion of the dose (1 ml) 1 in 100 in 0.1 mol/l HCl, and use as a measure of the total amount of radioactivity and as a standard in subsequent measurements.

PLASMA-IRON CLEARANCE

Commencing 10 min after injection, take four or five blood samples over a period of 1–2 h, collecting them into heparin or EDTA. Retain a portion of one sample for measurement of plasma iron. Measure the radioactivity in unit volumes of plasma from the samples and plot the values obtained on log-linear graph paper. A straight line will usually

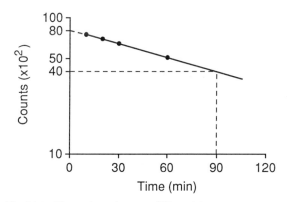

Fig. 24.1 Plasma iron clearance. ^{59}Fe activity in plasma at 10, 20, 30 and 60 min extrapolated to the vertical axis to obtain activity at To. The $T_{1/2}$ was 90 min.

be obtained for the initial slope. The radioactivity at the moment of injection is inferred by extrapolation back to zero time and the time taken for the plasma radioactivity to decrease to half its initial value ($T_{1/2}$-plasma clearance) is read off the graph (Fig. 24.1).

Range of $T_{1/2}$-plasma clearance in health.
60–140 min.

The clearance rate is influenced by the intensity of erythropoiesis and also by the activity of the macrophages of the reticulo-endothelial system, especially in the liver, spleen and bone marrow, where the iron is retained as storage iron. Also, to a lesser extent, circulating reticulocytes may take up some of the iron. A rapid clearance indicates hyperactivity of one or more of these mechanisms, as for instance in iron-deficiency anaemias, haemorrhagic anaemias, haemolytic anaemias and polycythaemia vera. The clearance rate is decreased in aplastic anaemia. In leukaemia and in myelosclerosis the results are variable, depending upon the amount of erythropoietic marrow and the extent of extramedullary erythropoiesis; in myelosclerosis, however, rapid clearance is by far the more common finding. In dyserythropoiesis the clearance may be normal or accelerated.

PLASMA-IRON TURNOVER (PIT)

When the plasma-iron clearance is related to the iron content of the plasma, a value can be obtained for plasma-iron turnover in mg/l or μmol/l of blood per day.

PIT (mg/l/day) is calculated from the formula:

plasma iron (mg/l)$\star$ × 0.693$\star\star$

$$\frac{\times\ (60 \times 24)}{T_{1/2}\ (\text{min})} \times (1 - \text{PCV}).$$

which may be simplified to:

$$\frac{\text{plasma iron (mg/l)} \times 10^3}{T_{1/2}\ (\text{min})} \times (1 - \text{PCV}).$$

PIT (μmol/l/day) is calculated from the formula:

$$\frac{\text{plasma iron (μmol/l)} \times 10^3}{T_{1/2}\ (\text{min})} \times (1 - \text{PCV}).$$

The range in normal subjects is 4–8 mg/l/day or 70–140 μmol/l/day.

The PIT is increased in iron-deficiency anaemia, haemolytic anaemias and myelosclerosis. It is increased also in ineffective erythropoiesis, particularly so in thalassaemia. In aplastic anaemia the PIT is normal or decreased, but when the plasma iron is raised, the PIT may be above normal. The calculation of PIT assumes a constant rate of iron transport and, while it is an indicator of total erythropoiesis, it does not distinguish between effective and ineffective erythropoiesis. For the reasons discussed earlier and because the findings in health and disease overlap, measurement of the PIT has only limited clinical usefulness.

IRON UTILIZATION

Collect blood samples daily or at least on alternate days for a period of about 2 weeks after the administration of the ^{59}Fe. Measure the radioactivity per ml of whole blood and calculate the percentage utilization on each day from the formula:

$$\frac{\text{cpm/ml daily whole blood sample}}{\text{cpm/ml whole blood sample at zero time}} \times 100\% \times f$$

where f is a PCV correction factor, i.e.

$$f = \frac{0.9\ \text{PCV}}{1 - 0.9\ \text{PCV}}.$$

$\star$ Because of marked diurnal variation, the plasma iron should be measured on a sample of blood collected during the plasma clearance study.
$\star\star$ Natural log of 2.

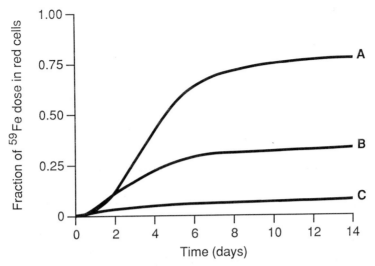

Fig. 24.2 Iron utilization. Red-cell uptake of ^{59}Fe in a normal subject (A), in dyserythropoiesis (B) and in severe aplastic anaemia (C) .

When there is reason to suspect that the body:venous PCV ratio is not 0.9 (see p. 365), measure the red cell volume by a direct method (p. 362)* and calculate the percentage utilization on each day from the formula:

Percentage utilization =

$$\frac{\text{red cell volume (ml)} \times \text{cpm/ml red cells} \times 100}{\text{total radioactivity injected (cpm)**}} .$$

Plot the daily measured percentages against time on arithmetic graph paper. Record the maximum utilization (Fig. 24.2).

The calculation gives a measure of effective erythropoiesis. In normal subjects red cell radio-activity rises steadily from 24 h, and reaches a maximum of 70–80% utilization on the 10–14th day.

A rapid plasma clearance is usually associated with early and relatively complete utilization and the converse also applies. The results are inconsistent in megaloblastic anaemias and in haemoglobinopathies in which there is ineffective erythropoiesis; and also in myelosclerosis and polycythaemia vera, depending on the extent of extramedullary erythropoiesis

*Calculation of plasma volume from extrapolation of the ^{59}Fe disappearance curve is often unreliable and the figure for plasma volume should not be used as the basis for the calculation of red cell volume.
**The radioactivity is adjusted for physical decay up to the day of measurement.

and whether the red cell life-span is reduced. If there is rapid haemolysis, the utilization curve will be distorted by destruction of some of the labelled red cells; this may be recognized if frequent (daily) samples are measured. In aplastic anaemia the utilization is usually 10–15%; in ineffective erythropoiesis it is as a rule 30–50%.

If the iron utilization is known, it is possible to determine the red cell iron turnover expressed as mg/l blood per day (PIT) × % maximum utilization). This provides a measure of effective erythropoiesis. In normal subjects it is about 5 mg/l, but it gives an underestimate if there is increased haemolysis. In normal subjects the ratio of plasma iron turnover to red cell iron turnover is 1.2–1.3:1.0.[30]

The ferrokinetic patterns in various diseases are shown in Table 24.1.

Marrow transit time

This can be determined from the red cell utilization data and is the time taken to reach one-half the maximum red cell uptake of the radioiron. It is normally about 80 h. It is thought, to some extent, to reflect the effectiveness of erythropoiesis.[42]

SURFACE COUNTING OF ^{59}Fe

The technique of surface counting is similar to that of ^{51}Cr, as described on p. 388. In addition to

Table 24.1 Ferrokinetic patterns in various diseases

	Plasma clearance $T_{1/2}$	Plasma iron turnover	Red cell utilization
Normal	60–140 min	70–140 μmol/l/d	70–80%
Iron deficiency	↓	N	↑
Aplastic anaemia	↑	N	↓
Secondary anaemia	Slightly ↓	N	N
Dyserythropoiesis	Slightly ↓	↑	↓
Myelofibrosis	↓	↑	↓
Haemolytic anaemia	↓	↑	↑

↓ = Shortened/ decreased   ↑ = Prolonged/increased

measurements over the heart, liver and spleen, the ^{59}Fe activity in the marrow can be measured by placing a collimated counter over the upper portion of the sacrum with the patient lying prone. In order to obtain a pattern of the distribution of the radioactive iron, count the sites mentioned as soon as possible after the intravenous administration of the isotope, as described on p. 373. Count again after 5, 20, 40 and 60 min, and hourly for 6–10 h. Then make measurements daily or on alternate days for the next 10 days or so. In order to compare the pattern in different patients express the initial counts at each site as 100% and convert subsequent counts proportionately after correction for the physical decay of the isotope. The results obtained in a normal subject are illustrated in Fig. 24.3.

Surface counting after the administration of ^{59}Fe is laborious, but the technique has a place in the investigation of patients thought to be suffering from aplastic anaemia, myelosclerosis or 'refractory' anaemia. It may be helpful to know the sites and extent of extramedullary erythropoiesis, especially if splenectomy is contemplated. The patterns of surface counts in disease are illustrated in Figs. 24.3–24.5.

WHOLE-BODY SCANNING

When [52]Fe is available it can be used to visualize iron distribution and erythropoiesis. The isotope is prepared and administered in the same way as [59]Fe. A dose of 3.5 MBq (*c* 100 μCi) is usually suitable.

Obtain blood samples for measurement of plasma clearance. At 3 h after administration, and again at about 20–24 h, scan the body by a gamma camera. The extent of erythopoiesis in the bony skeleton and in the liver and spleen can be readily identified (Fig. 24.6).

In aplastic anaemia, characteristically, the radio-iron accumulates in the liver. [52]Fe disintegrates to [52m]Mn, which also accumulates in the liver. This isotope decays very rapidly (half-life 21 min) and should not cause interference, especially in scans taken at 20–24 h.[44]

[59]Fe is less suitable for whole-body scanning than is [52]Fe because the long half-life of ^{59}Fe limits the amount which can be administered; however, using suitable collimation and appropriate instrument settings it is possible to obtain fairly reasonable images with a gamma camera when a dose of 0.4 MBq (*c* 10 μCi) is given.[6,17] As [111]In (indium) chloride also binds to transferrin it has been suggested that this isotope could be used as a convenient, and more readily available, substitute for [52]Fe. However, this is not recommended as results with this isotope are inconsistent and its distribution in the body does not always parallel that of iron.[18,32,45]

MEASUREMENT OF BLOOD LOSS FROM THE GASTRO-INTESTINAL TRACT USING [51]Cr

The ^{51}Cr method of red cell labelling can be used to measure quantitatively blood lost into the gastro-intestinal tract, as ^{51}Cr is neither excreted nor more than minimally reabsorbed.[62] Accordingly, when the blood contains ^{51}Cr-labelled red cells faecal radioactivity is at a very low level unless bleeding has taken place somewhere within the gastro-intestinal tract. Measurement of the faecal radio-activity then gives a reliable indication of the extent of the blood loss.

Method

Label the patient's own blood with approximately 3.5 MBq (*c*100 μCi) of ^{51}Cr, as described on p.362. On each day of the test collect the faeces in plastic or waxed cardboard cartons. Prepare a standard by adding a measured volume (3–5 ml) of the patient's blood, collected on each day, to approximately

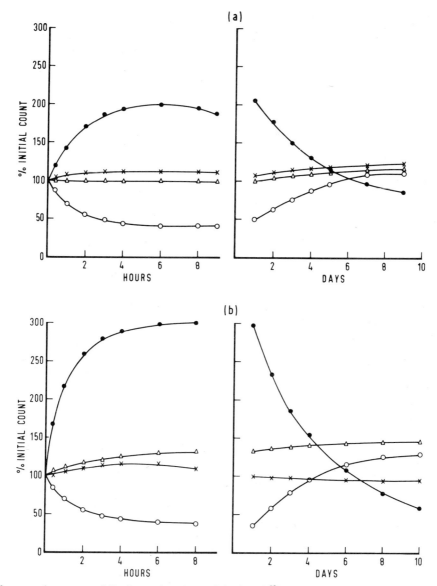

Fig. 24.3 Surface-counting patterns following an intravenous injection of ^{59}Fe. (a) Normal subject and (b) a subject suffering from iron-deficiency anaemia. Radioactivity was measured over the heart (O), sacrum (●), spleen (△) and liver (×). The patient with the iron-deficiency anaemia showed an excessive uptake of ^{59}Fe by the bone marrow.

100 ml of water in a similar cartoon. Compare the radioactivity of the faecal samples and the corresponding daily standard in a large-volume counting system (see p. 355). Then, volume of blood in faeces (in ml) =

$$\frac{\text{cpm/24 h faeces collection}}{\text{cpm/ml standard}}.$$

Blood loss from any other source, e.g. surgical operation or menstruation, can be measured in a similar way by counting swabs, dressings etc, placed in a carton. It is not, however, possible to measure blood or haemoglobin loss in the urine (haematuria or haemoglobinuria) by this method as free ^{51}Cr is normally excreted in the urine.

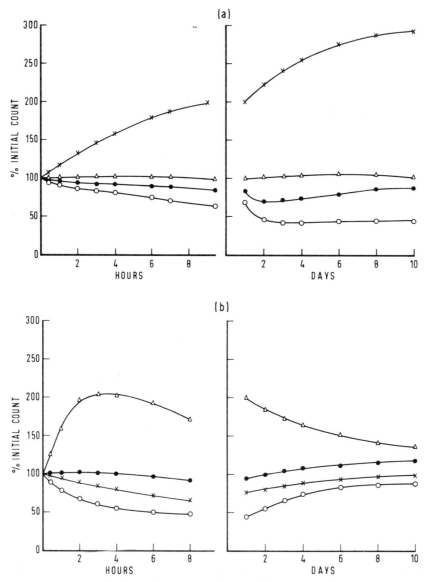

Fig. 24.4 Surface-counting patterns following an intravenous injection of ^{59}Fe. (a) Aplastic anaemia and (b) myelosclerosis. Radioactivity was measured over the heart (O), sacrum (●), spleen (△) and liver (×). In aplastic anaemia the rate of clearance of the ^{59}Fe from the blood (heart counts) is unusually slow and the bulk of the ^{59}Fe is taken up by the liver. In myelosclerosis there is little or no uptake of ^{59}Fe by the bone marrow but a clear excess uptake by the spleen. The subsequent decrease in radioactivity over the spleen is an indication that the iron is being used for erythropoiesis and is not merely being stored in the organ. (cf. the liver in aplastic anaemia.)

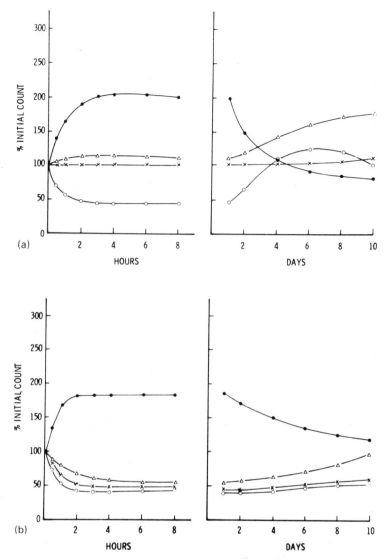

Fig. 24.5 Surface-counting patterns following an intravenous injection of ^{59}Fe. (a) Haemolytic anaemia and (b) dyserythropoiesis. Radioactivity was measured over the heart (O), sacrum (●), spleen (△) and liver (×). In the haemolytic anaemia there is a delayed excess uptake of ^{59}Fe by the spleen which was the main site of red cell sequestration. In dyserythropoiesis there is active uptake of ^{59}Fe by the bone marrow. The subsequent retention of most of the radioactivity in the marrow is an indication of ineffective erythropoiesis.

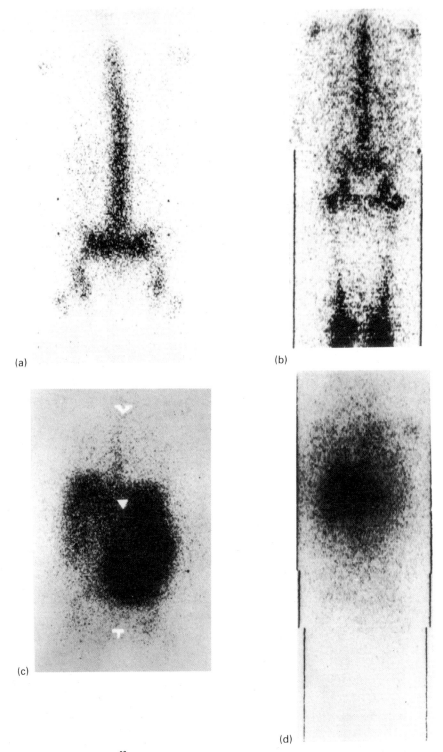

(a)

(b)

(c)

(d)

Fig. 24.6   Scan showing distribution of ^{52}Fe. (a) Normal subject, (b) polycythaemia vera, (c) myelofibrosis and (d) aplastic anaemia. In myelofibrosis there is extramedullary erythropoiesis in the liver and spleen; in aplastic anaemia the iron accumulated slowly in the liver.

ESTIMATION OF THE LIFE-SPAN OF RED CELLS IN VIVO

There have been extensive studies of, and a vast literature on, the survival of red cells in haemolytic anaemias (see review by Bentley & Miller[9]). Although now undertaken less frequently than in the past, measurement of red cell survival can still provide important data in cases of anaemia in which increased haemolysis is suspected but not clearly demonstrated by other tests. The majority of studies are carried out using the patient's own red cells. Donor red cells are, however, sometimes used to distinguish between an intrinsic and an extrinsic red cell defect.

The differential agglutination method of Ashby

This was the first practical method of estimating red cell life-span. Although comparatively easy to carry out, and an elegant method, it suffered from a major defect: it was only possible to estimate the survival of normal red cells transfused to the patient being investigated, or perhaps that of the patient's red cells in a normal recipient. The survival of the patient's red cells could *not* be estimated in his own circulation.

Principle. The recipient is transfused with red cells of a different but compatible blood group; the resulting mixture of cells is separated in vitro by means of a potent agglutinating serum which agglutinates the recipient's red cells but not those of the donor, and the unagglutinated cells are counted by a standard method of red cell counting.

It was essential to have available a highly avid agglutinating serum, and this usually restricted the method to tracing the survival of group-O red cells in a group-A or -B, or -AB recipient, using an anti-A or anti-B serum. In practice it was necessary to transfuse a major amount of blood, e.g. in an adult the red cells from 1 litre of blood, in order to obtain a substantial number of donor cells to count. With the advent of ^{51}Cr, the Ashby method became outmoded, but it is still sometimes used, for instance, when the survival of normal cells is to be compared with that of the patient's own cells (labelled by ^{51}Cr) in the patient's circulation or

when it is undesirable to expose the patient to a radioactive isotope. The technique that can be used is essentially that described by Dacie and Mollison,[47] with the exception that an electronic cell counter can be used to count the unagglutinated cells and a low ionic strength medium can be used to enhance agglutination.[63]

ISOTOPIC METHODS

There are two ways in which red cells can be labelled by an isotope:

1. Cohort labelling in which an isotope is incorporated into haemoglobin during its synthesis by erythroblasts and the radioactivity in red cells produced over a restricted period of time is measured.
2. Random labelling in which a population of circulating red cells, of all ages, is labelled.

Cohort labelling

Cohort labelling has the potential advantage that it provides information about the relative importance of red cell senescence and random destruction. The isotope labels the red cells at the time of their formation, and the labelled cells appear in the circulation as a cohort of cells of closely similar age. The total radioactivity of the blood increases steeply and eventually reaches a plateau which is maintained until the labelled cell population reaches the end of its life-span, provided that there is no intervening random destruction. Average life-span is determined by the time which elapses between corresponding points on the rising and falling parts of the curve. The exact form of the curve varies according to the technique used, the rate of incorporation of the label and the extent of its reutilization. The mathematical interpretation of the data is complex.[11] The most satisfactory label is [^{14}C] glycine which labels both the haem and globin components of haemoglobin.[10]

Red cell life-span can also be calculated from measurements of red cell iron turnover obtained with ^{59}Fe.[61] But the results have to be interpreted with caution because of the major reutilization for haem synthesis of iron derived from red cells at the end of their life-span.

Random labelling

Random labelling is a much more practical method than is cohort labelling. Either radioactive chromium (^{51}Cr) or radioactive phosphorus (^{32}P) can be used. ^{51}Cr is used as a label for anionic hexavalent sodium chromate ($Na_2^{51}CrO_4$) and ^{32}P as a label for di-isopropyl phosphofluoridate (DF^{32}P). While ^{51}Cr can only be used as an in-vitro label, DF^{32}P is normally used as an in-vivo label. DF^{32}P inhibits cholinesterase, to which it becomes irreversibly bound, and it thus labels red cell membranes. However, in the amount required for labelling it does not damage the red cells. Neither ^{51}Cr nor DF^{32}P is reutilised or transferred to other cells in the circulation. The choice of ^{51}Cr or DF^{32}P depends on a number of circumstances. ^{51}Cr is a γ-ray emitter and its radioactivity can be counted in blood after withdrawal and in vivo over the liver and spleen; and it is also practicable to combine a study of red cell survival with measurement of blood volume. The main disadvantage of ^{51}Cr is that it gradually elutes from red cells as they circulate; there may be, too, an increased loss over the first 1–3 days, and thus the uncertainty as to how much has been lost may make it impossible to estimate red cell life-span accurately.

DF^{32}P has the advantage over ^{51}Cr in that the isotope is not lost by elution. Whilst there is some early loss of radioactivity this can be minimized and confined to the first 24 h or so by the use of high-specific-activity material. The radioactivity curves are thus relatively easy to interpret. A disadvantage of DF^{32}P is that surface counting is not possible because the ^{32}P is a β-emitter.

RADIOACTIVE CHROMIUM (^{51}Cr) METHOD

^{51}Cr has a half-life of 27.8 days. After passing through the surface membrane of the red cells, the labelled chromium in the form of sodium chromate is reduced to the trivalent form which binds to protein, preferentially to the β-polypeptide chains of haemoglobin.[51] Chromium, whether radioactive or non-radioactive, is toxic to red cells, probably by its oxidizing actions; it inhibits glycolysis in red cells when present at a concentration of 10 μg/ml or more[39] and blocks glutathione reductase activity at a concentration exceeding 5 μg/ml.[40,41] Blood should thus not be exposed to more than 2 μg of chromium per ml of packed red cells.

$Na_2^{51}CrO_4$ is available commercially at a specific activity of 13–22 GBq/mg Cr (350–600 mCi/mg); it is usually dissolved in 9 g/l NaCl (saline). It is convenient to dilute the stock in saline and to dispense 2–5.5 MBq (50–150 μCi) amounts in ampoules which can then be sterilized by autoclaving. ACD must not be used as a diluent as this reduces the chromate to the cationic chromic form.

Care must be taken to avoid lysis when the red cells are washed; and it may be necessary, especially if the blood contains spherocytes, to use a slightly hypertonic solution, e.g. 12 g/l NaCl. This should certainly be used if an osmotic-fragility test has demonstrated lysis in 9 g/l NaCl. In patients whose plasma contains high-titre, high-thermal-amplitude cold agglutinins the blood must be collected in a warmed syringe, delivered into ACD solution previously warmed to 37°C and the labelling and washing in saline carried out in a 'warm room' at 37°C.

Method

The technique of labelling red cells is the same as for blood-volume measurement (see p. 362). To ensure as little damage to red cells as possible, with subsequent minimal early loss and later elution, it is important to maintain the blood at optimal pH. This can be achieved by adding 10 volumes of blood to 1.5 volumes of the recommended (NIH-A) ACD solution[36] (see p. 535), or CPD solution (see p. 535).

For a red cell survival study 0.02 MBq (c 0.5 μCi) of $Na_2^{51}CrO_4$ per kg body weight is recommended. But if surface counting is to be carried out also, a higher dose (e.g. 0.04 MBq or 1 μCi/kg) should be used, bearing in mind that <2 μg of chromium should be added per ml of packed red cells.

After injection, allow the labelled cells to circulate in the recipient for 10 min (or for 60 min in patients with cardiac failure or splenomegaly in whom mixing may be delayed). Then collect a sample of blood from a vein other than that used for the injection (or after washing the needle through with saline if a butterfly needle is used) and mix with EDTA anticoagulant. The radioactivity in this sample provides a base line for subsequent observations. Retain part of the labelled cell suspension which was not injected into the patient to serve as a standard. This enables the blood volume to be calculated if required.

Take further 4–5 ml blood samples from the patient 24 h later (Day 1) and subsequently at intervals, the frequency of the samples depending on the rate of red cell destruction. The recommended produre is to take three specimens between Day 2 and Day 7, and then two specimens per week for the duration of the study.[36] Measurements should be continued until at least half the radioactivity has disappeared from the circulation.

Measure the haemoglobin or PCV in a part of each sample; then lyse the samples with saponin, mix well and deliver 1 ml into counting tubes, if possible in duplicate.

Measurement of radioactivity

Estimate the percentage survival (of ^{51}Cr) on any Day (t) by comparing the radioactivity of the sample taken on that day with that of the Day 0 sample, i.e. the sample withdrawn 10 (or 60) min after the injection of the labelled cells. Thus ^{51}Cr survival on Day t (%) =

$$\frac{\text{cpm/ml of blood on Day t}}{\text{cpm/ml of blood on Day 0}} \times 100.$$

No adjustment is necessary for the physical decay of the isotope, provided that the standard is counted within a few minutes of the Day t sample.

Carry out the measurements in any high quality scintillation counter, at least 2500 counts being recorded in order to achieve an accuracy of $\pm 2\%$.

Processing of radioactivity measurements

Before the data can be analysed and interpreted, factors, other than physical decay, which are involved in the disappearance of radioactivity from the circulation have to be considered. There are two processes: ^{51}Cr-labelled cells are lost from the circulation by lysis, phagocytosis or haemorrhage and, in addition, ^{51}Cr is eluted from intact red cells.

The rate of elution differs to a small extent from one individual to another. It is thought to vary to a greater extent between different diseases,[19] especially when the red cell life-span is considerably reduced. However, in such cases elution and variation in the rate of elution become unimportant. The rate of elution is also influenced by technique, especially by the anticoagulant solution into which the blood is collected prior to labelling. With the NIH-A ACD and CPD solutions the rate of elution is c 1% per day.[36] It is about the same rate with CPD.

Sometimes, in addition to the elution that occurs continuously and at a relatively low and constant rate, up to 10% of the ^{51}Cr may be lost within the first 24 h. The cause of this major early loss is obscure and several components may be involved. If this major loss does not continue beyond the first 2 days, it is often looked upon as an artefact, in the sense that it does not denote an increased rate of lysis in vivo, and it can be and usually is ignored by replotting the figures as described on p. 385. This procedure is acceptable, at least for clinical studies, but it does not take into account the possibility that a small proportion of red cells are present that are unusually prone to lysis and the rate of elimination of the rest of the labelled cells is not representative of the entire cell population. Even when the ^{51}Cr data are corrected for elution the survival curve may not be strictly comparable with an Ashby survival curve. This is, however, not of great importance provided the findings are compared with ^{51}Cr survival curves obtained in strictly normal subjects by an identical technique (see Table 24.2 and Fig. 24.7). It is common practice to calculate the $T_{50}Cr$,* i.e. the time taken for the concentration of ^{51}Cr in the blood to fall to 50% of its initial value, after correcting the data for physical decay but not for elution. The chief objection to the use of $T_{50}Cr$ is that it may be misleading without additional information on the pattern of the survival curve. Moreover, the mean red cell life-span cannot be directly derived from it. With the technique described above, the mean value of T_{50} in normal subjects is c 30 days, range 25-33 days.

---

*T_{50} is used rather than $T_{1/2}$ when the fractional rate of elimination is not constant.

Table 24.2 Normal range for ⁵¹Cr survival curves with correction for elution[36]

Day	% ⁵¹Cr (corrected for decay; *not* corrected for elution)	Elution correction* factors
1	93–98	1.03
2	89–97	1.05
3	86–95	1.06
4	83–93	1.07
5	80–92	1.08
6	78–90	1.10
7	77–88	1.11
8	76–86	1.12
9	74–84	1.13
10	72–83	1.14
11	70–81	1.16
12	68–79	1.17
13	67–78	1.18
14	65–77	1.19
15	64–75	1.20
16	62–74	1.22
17	59–73	1.23
18	58–71	1.25
19	57–69	1.26
20	56–67	1.27
21	55–66	1.29
22	53–65	1.31
23	52–63	1.32
24	51–60	1.34
25	50–59	1.36
30	44–52	1.47
35	39–47	1.53
40	34–42	1.60

*To correct for elution, multiply the measured survival by the elution factor for the particular day.

Correction for elution

When haemolysis is marked, elution is of minor importance and can be ignored. When haemolysis is not greatly increased, it is essential to correct for elution. This can be done by multiplying the measured survival by the factors given in Table 24.2.

Drawing survival curves and deriving the mean red cell life-span

Plot the % radioactivity figures or count-rates per ml of whole blood (corrected for physical decay and for elution) on arithmetic and semi-logarithmic graph paper and attempt to fit straight lines to the data. Then:

1. If a straight line *can* be fitted to the arithmetic plot, the mean red cell life-span is given by the point in time at which the line or its extension cuts the abscissa (Fig. 24.8).

2. If a straight line *can* be fitted to the semi-logarithmic plot, the mean red cell life-span can be read as the exponential e^{-1}; i.e. the time when 37% of the cells are still surviving (Fig 24.9), or calculated by multiplying the half-time of the fitted line by the reciprocal of the natural log of 2 (0.693), i.e. multiplying by 1.44.

3. If a straight line *cannot* be fitted satisfactorily as in (1) or (2), the mean cell life-span can be deduced approximately by extrapolation to the abscissa of a tangent drawn to the initial slope of the data plotted on arithmetic paper (Fig. 24.10).

Using a small computer the mathematical analysis can be readily automated. With the aid of a

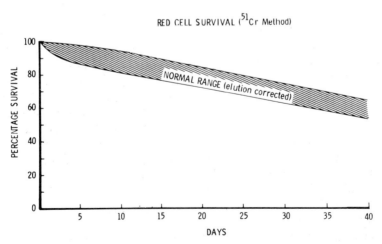

Fig. 24.7   ⁵¹Cr red cell survival. The hatched area shows the normal range.

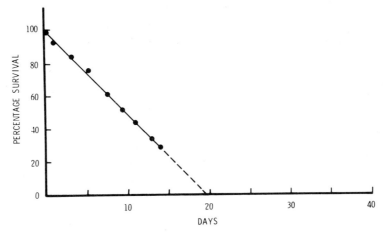

Fig. 24.8 **^{51}Cr red cell survival curves.** Patient with hereditary spherocytosis. The results give a straight line when plotted on arithmetic graph paper. The mean cell life-span is indicated by the point at which its extension cuts the abscissa (20 days).

computer program more complex mathematical formulae can also be used in order to fit the curves more precisely;[8,36] the more complex procedure may have value in physiological investigations but it is not likely to improve overall accuracy of the results for clinical purposes.

Interpretation of survival curves

In the auto-immune haemolytic anaemias, the slope of elimination is usually markedly curvilinear when the data are plotted on arithmetic graph paper. Red cell destruction is typically random and the curve of elimination is thus exponential, and the data give a straight line when plotted on semi-logarithmic graph paper.

In some cases of haemolytic anaemia (? only when there are intracorpuscular defects) the survival curve appears to consist of two components, an initial steep slope being followed by a much less steeply falling slope. This suggests the presence of cells of widely varying life-span. This type of 'double population' curve is seen in paroxysmal nocturnal haemoglobinuria and in sickle-cell anaemia, and in some cases of hereditary enzyme-deficiency haemolytic anaemias, and when the labelled cells consists of a mixture of transfused normal cells and short-lived patient's cells. The mean cell life-span of the entire cell population can be deduced by extrapolation of the initial steep slope to the abscissa. The proportion of cells

belonging to the longer-lived population can be estimated by extrapolating the less steep slope, if linear, back to the ordinate, and the life-span of this population can be estimated by extending the same slope to the abscissa (Fig. 24.10). The life-span of the short-lived cells can be deduced from the formula:

$$MCL_S = \frac{\%S}{\dfrac{100}{MCL_T} - \dfrac{\%L}{MCL_L}}$$

where S = short-lived population, L = longer-lived population, T = entire cell population and MCL = mean cell life.

Correction for early loss

The simplest method is to ignore the early loss by taking as 100% the radioactivity still present at the end of 24–48 h. Alternatively, the following method can be employed; it has the advantage that the slope of the survival curve is not altered. The data are plotted on arithmetical graph paper, the line of the slope beyond the initial steep part is extrapolated back to the ordinate and the point of intersection is taken as 100% and the ordinate scale recalibrated accordingly.

Blood-volume changes

There is no need to correct the measurements of radioactivity per ml of whole blood for alterations in

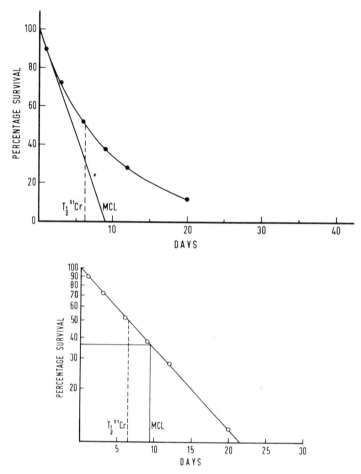

Fig. 24.9 ^{51}**Cr red cell survival curves.** Patient with auto-immune haemolytic anaemia. In the upper chart the results have been plotted on arithmetic graph paper and the mean cell life-span was deduced by extrapolation of a tangent at the initial slope to the abscissa (9 days). In the lower chart the results have been plotted on semilogarithmic graph paper and the mean cell life-span was read as the time when 37% of the cells were still surviving (9–10 days). The T_{50}Cr was 6–7 days. MCL = mean cell life-span.

PCV provided that the total blood volume remains constant throughout the study. However, if it is suspected that the blood volume may be changing, e.g. in patients with renal failure, suffering from haemorrhage or being transfused, serial determinations of blood volume should be carried out, and the observed radioactivity should be multiplied by the observed blood volume and divided by the initial blood volume. In practice, if a patient receives a blood transfusion during a survival study, it can, as a general rule, be assumed that the blood volume will have returned to its pre-transfusion level within 24–48 h.

Correction of survival data for blood loss

When there is a relatively constant loss of blood during a red cell survival study, the true mean red cell life-span can be obtained by the following equation:

$$\text{true MCL} = Ta \times \frac{\text{RCV}}{\text{RCV} - (Ta \times \text{L})},$$

where Ta = apparant time of MCL (days), RCV = red cell volume (ml), and L = mean rate of loss of red cells (ml/day).

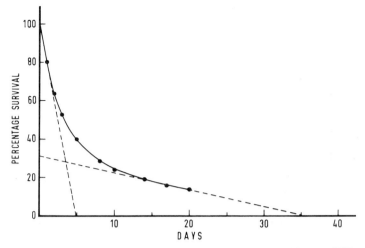

Fig. 24.10 ^{51}Cr **red cell survival curve showing a 'double population'.** The mean cell life-span (MCL) of the entire cell population was deduced by extrapolation of a tangent at the initial slope to the abscissa (5 days). By extrapolation of the less steep slope to the ordinate it was deduced that approximately 30% of the red cells belonged to one population, and by extrapolation of the same slope to the abscissa the MCL of this population was deduced as 35 days. The life-span of the remaining 70% of cells was calculated to be 3.6 days (see formula on p. 385). The T_{50}Cr was 3–4 days.

COMPATIBILITY TEST

The behaviour of ^{51}Cr-(or ^{113m}In-)labelled donor cells in a recipient will provide important information on the compatibility or otherwise of the donor blood:

1. When serological tests suggest that all normal donors are incompatible.
2. When in the presence of an allo-antibody no non-reacting donor can be found.
3. When the recipient has had an unexplained haemolytic transfusion reaction.
4. When the viability of the donor cells may possibly have been affected by suboptimal storage conditions.

Method[36]

Remove 1–2 ml of blood from the donor bag using a sterile technique. Label 0.5 ml of the red cells with 0.8 MBq (c 2 µCi) of ^{51}Cr, ^{111}In, ^{113m}In or ^{99m}Tc in the standard way (p. 362) and administer to the recipient. Collect 5–10 ml of blood into EDTA or heparin at 3, 10 and 60 min after the injection from a vein other than that used for the injection. Prepare 1 ml samples in counting vials. Centrifuge the remainder of the specimens and pipette 1 ml of the plasma into counting vials.

Measure the radioactivity in the usual way. Calculate the activity in the blood and plasma samples as a percentage of the 3 min blood sample.

Interpretation

With compatible blood the radioactivity in the 60 min sample is, on average, 99% of that of the 3 min sample, but it may vary between 94% and 104%. If the blood radioactivity at 60 min is not less than 70% and the plasma activity is not more than 3%, the donor cells may be transfused with minimal hazard.[36]

RADIOACTIVE PHOSPHORUS (DF^{32}P) METHOD

DFP binds within the red cells to acetylcholinesterase. It inhibits the enzyme irreversibly but this does not affect the survival of the cells.

Labelling with DF^{32}P in vivo is carried out by injecting intravenously. Dilute a stock solution, if necessary, in sterile 9 g/l NaCl (saline) immediately before injection so as to obtain a dose of 0.03 MBq (c 0.7 µCi)/kg body weight. The specific activity must be high enough to ensure that the amount of DFP does not exceed 20 µg/kg body weight. Inject the solution slowly (over a period of 10–15 min) through a butterfly needle inserted into one of the patient's veins.

Collect the first blood sample 60 min after the injection, and a second sample at 24 h; collect three further samples between Day 2 and Day 7 and subsequently at least three further samples each week for the duration of the study. Estimate the PCV of each sample and pipette a measured volume of the blood into a tube marked at 10 ml. Centrifuge the blood, remove the plasma carefully and wash the red cells three times with saline. Care must be taken that no red cells are lost during this procedure. Then lyse the cells by adding a small amount of saponin; add saline to the 10 ml mark and measure the radioactivity of the lysate in a liquid scintillation counting system after appropriate treatment of the samples (see p. 355).

Plotting the radioactivity data

Express the radioactivity as counts per min per ml of whole blood and plot the figures on graph paper as for ^{51}Cr. Do not use the 60 min sample as 100%, but obtain a value for 100% by extrapolating a line fitted to the data back to the ordinate.

Normal red cell life-span

The mean red cell life-span in health is usually taken as 120 days, and the SD 15 days.[36]

DETERMINATION OF SITES OF RED CELL DESTRUCTION USING ^{51}Cr

The sites of destruction of red cells, with special reference to the spleen and liver, can be determined by in-vivo surface counting using a shielded scintillation counter placed, respectively, over the heart, spleen and liver.

A collimated scintillation detector with a crystal of not less than 7.5 cm diameter and not less than 3.75 cm thickness is required.[35] The collimator should exclude radiation from extraneous sources and should be capable of surveying a representative area of the organ being studied. A cylindrical-hole collimator about 7 cm deep, 5 cm internal hole diameter and 10 cm external diameter is suitable. However, more reliable results are probably obtained by using two counters, 25–30 cm apart,

positioned above and below the counting couch. It is essential when counting on successive days to make the measurements over the chosen points under standardized conditions. Thus, the patient should always be supine in the same position.

Mark the following selected points with marking ink and cover by a layer of transparent dressing:

Heart: third interspace at left sternal border.
Liver: halfway between mid-clavicular and anterior axillary lines on the right side of the body, 3–4 cm above the costal margin.
Spleen: select the site of maximum activity on the first occasion by means of a preliminary count for a few seconds over each of several adjacent sites; then mark this position as the point for subsequent counting.

To ensure that the scanned area consists of the spleen some workers recommend that the spleen should first be visualized by injecting ^{99m}Tc-labelled heat-damaged red cells (see p. 391); this will not interfere with subsequent surface counting if 24 h are allowed to elapse.

If a single detector is used, this should be placed directly over the liver, heart and splenic counting points, just touching the skin. Dual counters, if used, should be placed above and below the selected point in the same vertical axis, and at a fixed distance from each other.

In haemolytic anaemias the first measurements are normally made 30–60 min after injection of the ^{51}Cr-labelled red cells and they are usually made thereafter daily or on alternate days depending on the rate of haemolysis. At least 2500 counts should be recorded at each site, and it is convenient to count at each site for two periods of 1 min and to average the counts. The measurements should be repeated if there is a difference of more than 2% between the counts. After Day 0, the counts have to be corrected for physical decay of the isotope by reference to a standard counted on each occasion under conditions of constant geometry.

In order to compare the results in different patients irrespective of the amount of isotope administered, the initial count over the heart is taken as the base-line. This is recorded as '1000 counts', irrespective of the actual number of counts recorded, and all the other counts at every site are adjusted ('normalized') proportionately. The fall in heart counts parallels the loss of the labelled red cells from the circulation, although the actual counts usually fall off more slowly than the radio-activity of the blood measured in vitro, probably because ^{51}Cr is deposited in all tissues before it is excreted. Alternatively, the changes in blood radio-activity as measured in vitro can be used to 'normalize' the observed count-rate over liver and spleen. This may at times give more consistent results. Theoretically, the counts over the spleen and the liver should fall at the same rate as the heart and blood counts unless lysis or sequestration of red cells is taking place within the organ(s) or unless ^{51}Cr eluted from red cells in the blood stream accumulates in the organ(s). When the counts over the liver or spleen exceed the calculated amount (based on the fall in heart or blood count), the excess radioactivity is recorded by subtracting the expected counts from the counts actually obtained. The counts recorded in a patient suffering from haemolytic anaemia are illustrated in Table 24.3.

It is useful to calculate an index, the Spleen:Liver Ratio, which reflects the relative accumulation of ^{51}Cr in the spleen and liver. The ratio between the counts on Day 0 is recorded as 1.00 and all subsequent ratios are related to this.

Normal surface-counting patterns are illustrated in Fig. 24.11. The interrupted lines indicate the limits of accumulation observed in normal subjects.

In haemolytic anaemias the results differ from case to case. Four patterns can be distinguished[43] (Fig. 24.12)

1. Excess accumulation in the spleen, as in hereditary spherocytosis (HS) and hereditary ellip-tocytosis and some cases of auto-immune hae-molytic anaemia (AIHA).

2. Excess accumulation chiefly in the liver; seen only in sickle-cell anaemia, especially in older patients.

3. Little or no excess accumulation in either spleen or liver, as in some hereditary enzyme-deficiency haemolytic anaemias and in paroxysmal nocturnal haemoglobinuria.

4. Excess accumulation in both liver and spleen, as in some cases of AIHA.

Clinical experience has shown that splenectomy usually benefits patients giving pattern (1) and to a more limited degree, in parallel with the Spleen:Liver Ratio, patients giving the pattern (4). The degree of improvement is not, however, closely correlated with the magnitude of the ^{51}Cr accumu-lation in the spleen.[2]

Surface-counting studies have their limitations. Even minor alterations in the conditions of count-ing and positioning of the patient may produce significant changes. Isolated readings may, there-fore, be misleading. Amongst the variables which affect the count-rate are the volume of the organ

Table 24.3   Example of method for calculation of surface counting data

Day	0	1	2	5	8	10	12	14
Heart	1000	850	780	720	670	600	500	370
Liver								
Actual counts	670	670	660	560	640	630	550	530
Expected counts		570	522	482	449	402	335	248
Excess		100	138	78	191	228	215	282
Spleen								
Actual counts	970	1265	1490	1800	2130	2370	2210	2020
Expected counts		825	756	698	650	582	485	359
Excess		440	734	1102	1480	1788	1725	1661
Spleen:Liver ratio								
Actual*	1.45	1.89	2.26	3.21	3.33	3.76	4.02	3.81
Adjusted	1.00	1.30	1.56	2.21	2.30	2.59	2.77	2.62

The actual count rate over the heart on Day 0 was 7500 counts per min. This was recorded as 1000 and all other counts were adjusted proportionately.
* Obtained from the actual counts of the organs. The ratio on Day 0 was recorded as 1.00 and the results on subsequent days were adjusted proportionately.

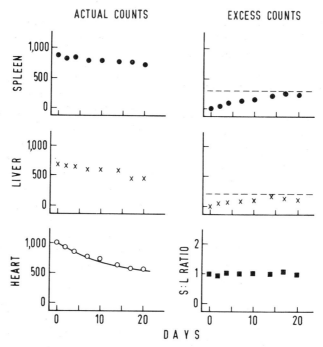

Fig. 24.11 **Surface-counting pattern in a normal subject following labelling of his red cells with** ^{51}**Cr.** The interrupted lines indicate the limits of accumulation in normal subjects.

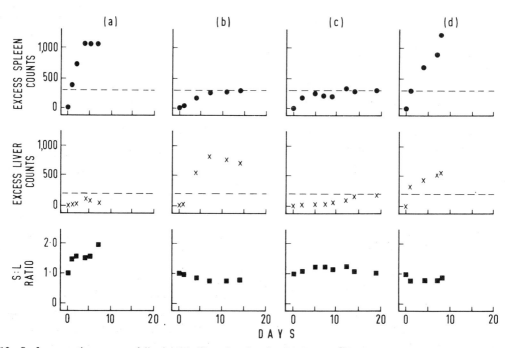

Fig. 24.12 **Surface-counting patterns following labelling of patients' red cells with** ^{51}**Cr in various haemolytic anaemias.** The interrupted lines indicate the limits of accumulation in normal subjects. Only excess counts and the spleen:liver ratio are shown. (a) Hereditary spherocytosis; (b) sickle-cell disease; (c) pyruvate-kinase deficiency; (d) auto-immune haemolytic anaemia. See text.

counted in relation to its total volume, the distance of the organ from the surface of the body, the absorption of radiation by the overlying tissues and the rate of loss of deposited ^{51}Cr from the organ. Nevertheless, despite these difficulties, surface counting has proved to be of value in the management of patients with some types of haemolytic anaemia when used in conjunction with other clinical and laboratory investigations.[2,29]

Methods have been developed by which the counts over the spleen can be related quantitatively to red cell destruction within the spleen.[65] In HS up to 95% or more of the loss of the labelled cells from the circulation can, in some cases, been accounted for by sequestration in the spleen; in other haemolytic anaemias the contribution of the spleen to haemolysis can be shown to be far less than this, e.g. 1–2% in hexokinase deficiency, 15–50% in AIHA, but up to 80% in thalassaemia major.[29,65] In severe haemolysis splenic uptake can also be measured directly during the first two to three days by quantitative gamma camera imaging of ^{111}In-labelled red cells.[33]

Simultaneous measurements of ^{51}Cr and ^{59}Fe

It is possible to study simultaneously the rate and sites of both erythropoiesis and haemolysis using ^{59}Fe and ^{51}Cr. However, although the separate measurement of the radioactivity due to each isotope in blood and plasma is theoretically simple (see p. 358), in practice the reliability of the ^{51}Cr measurement may be invalidated by the presence of ^{59}Fe and if possible the procedures should not be performed together.

VISUALIZATION OF THE SPLEEN BY SCINTILLATION SCANNING

This procedure is a development and extension of the techniques of surface counting described above. It has been used:

1. To demonstrate enlargement or abnormal position of the spleen or accessory splenic tissue.
2. To identify the nature of a mass in the left hypochondrium.
3. To demonstrate the presence of space-occupying lesions within the spleen.
4. To assess splenic function.

It is especially useful for demonstrating splenic atrophy in conditions such as thrombocythaemia and idiopathic steatorrhoea. Mention has been made of the value of delineating the spleen for surface counting (p. 388) and for estimating the splenic blood pool (p. 368).

Methods which have been used to alter red cells in vitro to ensure that after re-injection they are selectively removed from the circulation by the spleen include heat-damage, antibody sensitization and exposure to chemicals such as N-ethyl maleimide (NEM), mercuri-hydroxypropane (MHP) and paramercuribenzoate (PMB) (for review of the literature, see Pettit[58]).

By appropriate isotope labelling of these altered cells the accumulation of radioactivity within the organ provides a means of demonstrating its size and position. The heat-damage method is recommended; ^{51}Cr, ^{99m}Tc or ^{111}In are equally suitable as the label. Scintillation scanning is usually started about 1 h after the injection of the damaged cells, but it can be performed up to 3–4 h later; satisfactory scans can also be obtained with ^{51}Cr and ^{111}In up to 24 h after the injection.

Methods using heat damage

With ^{51}Cr as the label[45]

Deliver approximately 10 ml of the patient's blood into 1.5 ml of sterile ACD solution. Centrifuge the sample at 1200–1500 g for 5–10 min. Keep the plasma in a sterile container. Label the red cells with Na$_2$^{51}CrO$_4$, using 0.06–0.08 MBq (c 1.5–2.0 μCi) per kg body weight. Wash the labelled cells three times in sterile 9 g/l NaCl (saline). Place the packed cells in a sterile 30 ml glass bottle with a screw cap. Heat the bottle in a water-bath at a constant temperature of 49.5–50°C for exactly 20 min with occasional gentle mixing. Resuspend the cells in their own plasma and inject intravenously as soon as possible. Follow a standardized technique meticulously. It is important to use a glass bottle as some plastic containers take considerably longer than glass to reach the required temperature.

With ^{99m}Tc as the label

Carry out pretinning in vivo by an injection of a stannous compound as described on p. 363. Then collect 5–10 ml of blood into a sterile bottle containing 100 iu of heparin. Wash twice in sterile 9 g/l NaCl (saline), centrifuging at 1200–1500 g for 5–10 min. Transfer 2 ml of the packed red cells to a 30 ml glass bottle with a screw cap; heat the bottle in a water-bath at a constant temperature of 49.5–50°C for exactly 20 min with occasional gentle mixing. Wash the cells in saline until the supernatant is free from haemoglobin and discard the final supernatant. Label with 35 MBq (c 1 mCi) of ^{99m}Tc by the method as described on p. 363. After standing for 5 min, wash twice in saline. Resuspend in about 10 ml of saline and inject as soon as possible.

With ^{111}In or ^{113}In as the label

Prepare 2 ml of heat-damaged red cells as for the ^{99m}Tc method. Wash twice in sterile 9 g/l NaCl (saline). Add 9 MBq (c 250 µCi) of ^{111}In or ^{113}In, as described on p. 364. Then wash twice in saline. Resuspend in about 10 ml of saline and inject as soon as possible.

RATE OF CLEARANCE OF DAMAGED RED CELLS

Information on splenic activity may be obtained by measuring the rate of clearance of heat-damaged labelled red cells from the circulation. A blood sample is taken exactly 3 min after the mid-point of the injection and further samples are collected at 5 min intervals for 30 min and a final sample at 60 min. The radioactivity in each sample is measured and expressed as a percentage of the radioactivity in the 3 min sample. The results are plotted on semi-logarithmic graph paper, the 3 min sample being taken as 100% radioactivity.

For constant results a carefully standardized technique is necessary to ensure that the red cells are damaged to the same extent.

The disappearance curve is, as a rule, exponential. The initial slope reflects the splenic blood flow; the rate of blood flow is calculated as the reciprocal of the time taken for the radioactivity to fall to half the 3 min value, i.e. $0.693/t_{1/2}$, where 0.693 is the natural log of 2.

When the spleen is functioning normally the $t_{1/2}$ is 5–15 min and fractional splenic blood flow is 0.05–0.14/min, i.e. 5–14% of the circulating blood per min. The clearance rate is considerably prolonged in thrombocythaemia and in conditions associated with splenic atrophy such as sickle-cell anaemia, coeliac disease and dermatitis herpetiformis.[58] It thus provides some indication of spleen function. However, the disappearance curve is a complex of at least two components. The first (mentioned above) reflects the splenic blood flow, and the second component mainly measures cell trapping, the consequence of both transient sequestration and phagocytosis with irreversible extraction of the cells from circulation.[53,54] Measurement of phagocytosis is obtained more reliably with IgG (anti-D) coated red cells.[52,57]

ASSAY OF ERYTHROPOIETIN

Erythropoietin is a heat-stable glycoprotein hormone which regulates red cell production. It is produced mainly in the kidney. Only a small quantity is demonstrable in normal human plasma or urine.

The original method for measuring erythropoietin was an in-vivo biological assay, based on the uptake of ^{59}Fe by laboratory animals (usually rats) following the injection of test plasma or extract.[25,26] It was, unfortunately, not sufficiently sensitive to demonstrate small but significant overproduction of erythropoietin unless the plasma or urine was first concentrated by a fairly laborious procedure.[27] It is thus not practical for routine clinical purposes but it still serves as a reference method.[49] Subsequently in-vitro methods were developed, e.g. a fetal mouse liver-cell culture,[48,64] haemagglutination inhibition[50] or radio-immune assay.[21,23] The haemagglutination-inhibition method does not appear to be sufficiently reliable and the results are poorly correlated with those obtained by bioassay method,[50] whilst the liver-cell culture method gives results which are not specific for human erythropoietin.[22] The radio-immune assay, which is based on pure human erythropoietin as the labelled antigen, appears to be the most practical and reliable method. The results are expressed in international units by reference to an international (WHO) reference preparation with a potency of 10 iu per ampoule.[5]

Normal range

The normal range in plasma or serum has varied considerably according to the method of assay. By radio-immune assay the range is $18–35 \times 10^{-3}$ iu/ml (mean 25×10^{-3} iu/ml).[24]

Significance

Increased amounts of erythropoietin are found in the plasma in various anaemias and considerable amounts occur in secondary polycythaemia due to respiratory and cardiac diseases, in the presence of abnormal haemoglobins with high oxygen affinity, in association with hypernephroma and other renal lesions, and with erythropoietin-secreting tumours such as hepatoma, uterine fibroma, ovarian carcinoma and some other rare tumours.[4]

In polycythaemia vera the values are often lower than normal but in some cases they may be within the normal range.[24,27] Assay is particularly useful in patients with erythrocytosis of undetermined cause. However, in such cases there may be an intermittent abnormality in erythropoietin secretion. Thus, determining the erythropoietin level in a single sample of plasma may be misleading.[24]

In normal subjects diurnal variation and a sex difference have been reported.[1,3]

MEASUREMENT OF PLATELET LIFE-SPAN

Principle. The procedure for measuring platelet life-span is broadly similar to that for red cell survival (see p. 381). A method using ^{51}Cr-labelled platelets, recommended by the International Committee for Standardization in Haematology,[37] was described in the 5th edition of the book. More recently ^{111}In has been used as an alternative label. It has several advantages over ^{51}Cr: a shorter half-life, higher photon emissions and a greater affinity for platelets. It is thus possible to carry out a survival study on patients with low platelet counts and to combine this with measurement of platelet pooling and identification of sites of platelet destruction. It is now the recommended method.

METHOD USING ^{111}In[38]

Collect *c* 43 ml of blood into a 50 ml syringe containing 7 ml of ACD (p. 535). If the platelet count is low, it will be necessary to collect the blood into more than one syringe: 100–150 ml of blood is required when the platelet count is $20–30 \times 10^9$/l.

Deliver all but 9 ml of the citrated blood into one or more sterile plastic conical centrifuge tubes (A). Deliver the remaining 9 ml into a similar tube containing 1 ml of trisodium citrate (p. 536) (B). Centrifuge tubes A at 200 *g* for 12 min. Separate the supernatant (platelet-rich plasma) into another set of tubes (C); add an equal volume of buffered ACD★ warmed to 37°C; centrifuge at 640 *g* for 10 min and then decant the supernatant into containers (D). Wash the residual platelet deposit (without resuspension) in tubes C with *c* 5 ml of buffered ACD, resuspend in 4 ml of the buffer, pool into a single tube (E) and keep at 37°C in a water-bath. Centrifuge tube B at 800 *g* for 10 min. Transfer the supernatant platelet-poor plasma into tube F. Gently resuspend the platelets in tube E. Add 5 MBq (*c* 150 µCi) of ^{111}In-oxine (p. 364) and leave in a water-bath at 37°C. After 1 min add 5 ml of an equal volume of plasma from tube D and buffered ACD.

★1 volume of ACD, 7 volumes of 90 g/l NaCl; adjust pH to 6.5 with 1 mol/l NaOH.

Mix by inversion and leave in the water-bath for 5 min. Centrifuge at 640 *g* for 10 min.

Decant supernatant. Resuspend platelet button in 5 ml of platelet-poor plasma (F). Centrifuge the labelled platelet suspension in tube E at 100 *g* for 3 min, remove any contaminating red cells and then take up the platelet suspension into a 10 ml plastic syringe.

Add 0.5 ml of the platelet suspension to 100 ml of water in a volumetric flask as a standard. Weigh the syringe, inject the platelets through a butterfly needle and reweigh.

$$\text{Volume injected} = \text{wt (g)} \times \frac{1}{1.015},$$

where 1.015 = sp gr of plasma.

Collect blood samples in EDTA at 20 min, 2 h, 3 h and 4 h after injection and thereafter daily for up to 10 days.

Lyse the samples with saponin (p. 363) and measure the radioactivity of 1–2 ml volumes of each and a similar volume of the diluted standard.

Calculation

% Platelets surviving at each sampling time =

$$\frac{\text{cpm/ml blood sample}}{\text{total radioactivity *injected}} \times \text{blood volume (ml)}.$$

Analysis of data

Plot the % survival against time on arithmetic graph paper and estimate the survival time as for red cell survival (see p. 384). Normal mean platelet life-span: 8–10 days

The validity of the analysis is based on the assumption that the blood volume is constant and the pattern of disappearance of each cohort of platelets from the circulation remains constant during the course of the study.

This analysis is adequate when the platelet life-span is markedly shortened, as in most of the

---

* cpm/ml std × diln. of std × vol injected

clinical situations in which the survival study is likely to be undertaken. When more precise assessment and analysis of the shape of the survival curve is required, more complex procedures have to be carried out. The International Committee for Standardization in Haematology has published computer programs for obtaining estimates of mean platelet survival based on a 'multiple hit'.[38]

Platelet survival in disease

In idiopathic thrombocytopenia purpura (ITP) platelet life-span is considerably reduced, and the measurement may have diagnostic and prognostic importance. The platelet life-span is shortened, too, in consumption coagulopathies, and in thrombotic thrombocytopenia purpura. In thrombocytopenia due to defective production of platelets the life-span should be normal provided that platelets are not being lost by bleeding during the course of the study. In thrombocytopenia associated with splenomegaly the recovery of injected labelled platelets is low, but their survival is usually almost normal. Surface counting of radioactivity over the spleen and liver in ^{51}Cr studies has given inconsistent results and has not proved helpful in ITP in determining which patients will benefit from splenectomy. By quantitative scanning with ^{111}In, it is possible to measure the splenic platelet pool and to distinguish the relative importance of pooling and destruction of platelets in the spleen.[55,56] It must be recognized, however, that platelet kinetic studies are often difficult to interpret, and are only occasionally helpful in the management of patients with thrombocytopenia.

The splenic platelet pool is normally about 30% of the total platelet population, and it is thought that each platelet spends a third of its life-span in the spleen.[56] The size of its pool is increased in splenomegaly, resulting in thrombocytopenia but not necessarily in a reduced mean platelet life-span. In immune thrombocytopenias antibody-coated platelets may be destroyed in the liver (whilst only the normal pool is present in the spleen) or they may be destroyed in the liver and in the spleen.

REFERENCES

[1] ADAMSON, J. W., ALEXANIAN, R., MARTINEZ, C. and FINCH, C. A. (1966). Erythropoietin excretion in normal man. *Blood*, **28**, 354.

[2] AHUJA, S., LEWIS, S. M. and SZUR, L. (1972). Value of surface counting in predicting response to splenectomy in haemolytic anaemia. *Journal of Clinical Pathology*, **25**, 467.

[3] ALEXANIAN, R. (1966). Urinary excretion of erythropoietin in normal men and women. *Blood*, **28**, 344.

[4] ALEXANIAN, R. (1977). Increased erythropoietin production in man. In *Kidney Hormones, Vol. II: Erythropoietin*. Ed. J. W. Fisher, p. 531. Academic Press, London.

[5] ANNABLE, L., COTES, P. M. and MUSSETT, M. V. (1972). The second international reference preparation of erythropoietin, human, urinary, for bioassay. *Bulletin of the World Health Organization*, **47**, 99.

[6] AUBERT, B., KAHN, E., PARMENTIER, C. and DI PAOLA, R. (1983). Physical requirements of a ^{59}Fe bone marrow distribution digital scanning survey. *European Journal of Nuclear Medicine*, **8**, 162.

[7] BAROSI, G., BERZVINI, C., CAZZOLA, M., COLLI FRANZONE, P., MORANDI, S., STEFANELLI, M., VIGANOTTI, C. and PERUGINI, S. (1976). An approach by means of mathematical models to the analysis of ferrokinetic data obtained by liquid scintillation counting of ^{59}Fe. *Journal of Nuclear Biology and Medicine*, **20**, 8.

[8] BENTLEY, S. A. (1977). Red cell survival studies reinterpreted. *Clinics in Haematology*, **6**, 601.

[9] BENTLEY, S. A. and MILLER, D. T. (1986). Radionuclide blood cell survival studies. *Methods in Hematology*, **14**, 245.

[10] BERLIN, N. I., LAWRENCE, J. H. and LEE, H. C. (1954). The pathogenesis of the anemia of chronic leukemia: measurement of the life-span of the red blood cell with glycine-2-^{14}C. *Journal of Laboratory and Clinical Medicine*, **44**, 860.

[11] BERLIN, N. I., WALDMANN, T. A. and WEISSMAN, S. M. (1959). Life span of red blood cell. *Physiological Reviews*, **39**, 577.

[12] BOENDER, C. A. and VERLOOP, M. C. (1969). Iron absorption, iron loss and iron retention in man: studies after oral administration of a tracer dose of ^{59}FeSO$_4$ and ^{131}BaSO$_4$. *British Journal of Haematology*, **17**, 45.

[13] BOTHWELL, T. H., CHARLTON, R. W., COOK, J. D. and FINCH, C. A. (1979). *Iron Metabolism in Man*, (a) Ch. 12, (b) Ch. 20, (c) Ch. 21. Blackwell Scientific Publications, Oxford.

[14] CAVILL, I. (1971). The preparation of ^{59}Fe-labelled transferrin for ferrokinetic studies. *Journal of Clinical Pathology*, **24**, 472.

[15] CAVILL, I. (1986). Plasma clearance studies. *Methods in Hematology*, **14**; 214.

[16] CAZZOLA, M., BAROSI, G., ORLANDI, E. and STEFANELLI, M. (1980). The plasma ^{59}Fe clearance curve in man; an evaluation of methods of measurement and analysis. *Blut*, **40**, 325.

[17] CHAUDHURI, T. K., EHRHARDT, J. C., DE GOWIN, R. L. and CHRISTIE, J. H. (1974). ^{59}Fe whole-body scanning. *Journal of Nuclear Medicine*, **15**, 667.

[18] CHIPPING, P., KLONIZAKIS, I. and LEWIS, S. M. (1980). Indium chloride scanning: a comparison with iron as a tracer for erythropoiesis. *Clinical and Laboratory Haematology*, **2**, 255.

[19] CLINE, M. J. and BERLIN, N. I. (1963). The red cell chromium elution rate in patients with some hematologic diseases. *Blood*, **21**, 63.

[20] COOK, J. D. and LIPSCHITZ, D. A. (1977). Clinical measurement of iron absorption. *Clinics in Haematology*, **6**, 567.

[21] COTES, P. M. (1982). Immunoreactive erythropoietin in serum I. Evidence for the validity of the assay method and the physiological relevance of estimates. *British Journal of Haematology*, **50**, 427.

[22] COTES, P. M. (1983). Erythropoietin. In *Hormones in Blood*. Ed. C. H. Gray and V. H. T. James, Vol. 4, 3rd edn., p. 195. Academic Press, London.

[23] COTES, P. M., CANNING, C. E. and GAINES DAS R. E. (1983). Modification of a radioimmunoassay for human serum erythropoietin to provide increased sensitivity and investigate non-specific serum responses. In *Immunoassays for Clinical Chemistry*. Eds. W. M. Hunter and J. E. T. Corrie, p. 106. Churchill Livingstone, Edinburgh.

[24] COTES, P. M., DORÉ, C. J., LIU YIN, J. A., LEWIS, S. M., MESSINEZY, M., PEARSON, T. C. and REID, C. (1986). Determination of serum immunoreactive erythropoietin in the investigation of erythrocytosis. *New England Journal of Medicine*, **315**, 283.

[25] ERSLEV, A. (1977). Erythropoietin assay. In *Hematology*. Ed. W. J. Williams, E. Beutler, A. J. Erslev and R. W. Rundles, 2nd edn., p. 1616. McGraw Hill, New York.

[26] ERSLEV, A. J. and CARO, J. (1984). Pure erythrocytosis classified according to erythropoietin titers. *American Journal of Medicine*, **76**, 57.

[27] ERSLEV, A. J., CARO, J., KANSU, E., MILLER, O. and COBBS, E. (1979). Plasma erythropoietin in polycythemia. *American Journal of Medicine*, **66**, 243.

[28] FAWWAZ, R. A., WINCHELL, H. S., POLLYCOVE, M., SARGENT, T., ANGER, H. and LAWRENCE, J. H. (1966). Intestinal iron absorption studies using iron-52 and Anger positron camera. *Journal of Nuclear Medicine*, **7**, 569.

[29] FERRANT, A., CAUWE, J. L., MICHAUX, C., BECKERS, C., VERWILGHEN, R. and SOKAL, G. (1982). Assessment of the sites of red-cell destruction using quantitative measurement of splenic and hepatic red-cell destruction. *British Journal of Haematology*, **50**, 591.

[30] FINCH, C. A., DEUBELBEISS, K., COOK, J. D., ESCHBACH, J. W., HARKER, L. A., FUNK, D. D., MARSAGLIA, G., HILLMAN, R. S., SLICHTER, S., ADAMSON, J. W., GANZONI, A and GILBERT, E. R. (1970). Ferrokinetics in man. *Medicine*, **49**, 17.

[31] FRANCOIS, P. E. and SZUR, L. (1958). Use of iron-52 as a radioactive tracer. *Nature* (London), **182**, 1665.

[32] HARNSBERGER, H. R., DATZ, F. L., KNOCHEL, J. Q. and TAYLOR, A. T. (1982). Failure to detect extramedullary hematopoiesis during bone-marrow imaging with indium-111 or technetium-99m sulfur colloid. *Journal of Nuclear Medicine*, **23**, 589.

[33] HEYNS, A. DU. P., LÖTTER, M. G., KOTZE, H. F., WESSELS, P., PIETERS, H. and BADENHORST, P. N. (1985). Kinetics, distribution and sites of destruction of ^{111}In-oxine labelled red cells in haemolytic anaemia. *Journal of Clinical Pathology*, **38**, 128.

[34] International Committee for Standardization in Haematology (1971). Recommended methods for radioisotope red-cell survival studies. *British Journal of Haematology*, **21**, 241.

[35] International Committee for Standardization in Haematology (1975). Recommended methods for surface counting to determine sites of red-cell destruction. *British Journal of Haematology*, **30**, 249.

[36] International Committee for Standardization in Haematology (1977). Recommended methods for radioisotope survival studies. *Blood*, **50**, 1137.

[37] International Committee for Standardization in Haematology (1980). Recommended methods for radioisotope red-cell survival studies. *British Journal of Haematology*, **45**, 659.

[38] International Committee for Standardization in Haematology (1988). Recommended method for ^{111}In platelet survival studies. *Journal of Nuclear Medicine*, **29**, 564.

[39] JANDI, J. H., GREENBERG, M. S., YONEMOTO, R. H. and CASTLE, W. B. (1956). Clinical determination of the sites of red cell sequestration in hemolytic anemias. *Journal of Clinical Investigation*, **35**, 842.

[40] KOUTRAS, G. A., HATTORI, M., SCHNEIDER, A. S., EBAUGH, F. G. and VALENTINE, W. N. (1964). Studies of chromated erythrocytes. Effect of sodium chromate on erythrocyte glutathione reductase. *Journal of Clinical Investigation*, **43**, 323.

[41] KOUTRAS, G. A., SCHNEIDER, A. S., HATTORI, M. and VALENTINE, W. N. (1965). Studies of chromated erythrocytes. Mechanisms of chromate inhibition of glutathione reductase. *British Journal of Haematology*, **11**, 360.

[42] LABARDINI, J., PAPAYANNOPOULOU, T., COOK, J. D., ADAMSON, J. W., WOODSON, R. D., ESCHBACH, J. W., HILLMAN, R. S. and FINCH, C. A. (1973). Marrow radioiron kinetics. *Haematologia*, **7**, 301.

[43] LEWIS, S. M., SZUR, L. and DACIE, J. V. (1960). The pattern of erythrocyte destruction in haemolytic anaemia, as studied with radioactive chromium. *British Journal of Haematology*, **6**, 122.

[44] LILICRAP, S. C., STEERE, H. and CLINK, H. M. (1976). Distribution of dosimetry of ^{52}Fe in bone marrow and other organs. *Radioaktive Isotope in Klinik und Forschung*, **12**, 79.

[45] McINTYRE, P. A., LARSON, S., EIKMAN, E. A., COLMAN, M., SCHEFFER, V. and HODKINSON, B. A. (1974). Comparison of the metabolism of iron labelled transferrin and indium labelled transferrin by the erythropoietic marrow. *Journal of Nuclear Medicine*, **15**, 856.

[46] MARSH, G. W., LEWIS, S. M. and SZUR, L. (1966). The use of ^{51}Cr-labelled heat-damaged red cells to study splenic function. I. Evaluation of method. *British Journal of Haematology*, **12**, 161.

[47] MOLLISON, P. L., ENGELFRIET, C. P. and CONTRERAS, M. (1987). *Blood Transfusion in Clinical Medicine*, 8th edn., p. 810. Blackwell Scientific Publications, Oxford.

[48] NAPIER, J. A. F. and EVANS, J. (1980). Erythropoietin assay using fetal mouse liver cultures; a modified technique using semi-automated harvesting of ^{125}I deoxyuridine labelled erythroblasts. *Clinical and Laboratory Haematology*, **2**, 13.

[49] National Committee for Clinical Laboratory Standards (1979). Standard assay for the determination of erythropoietin activity in body fluids. NCCLS, Villanova, Pa., USA.

[50] OMRAN, N. and NEUMANN, E. (1979). A haemagglutination inhibition test kit for routine analysis of erythropoietin. *Blut*, **39**, 225.

[51] PEARSON, H. A. (1963). The binding of ^{51}Cr to hemoglobin. I. In vitro studies. *Blood*, **22**, 218.

[52] PETERS, A. M. (1983). Splenic blood flow and blood cell kinetics. *Clinics in Haematology*, **12**, 421.

[53] PETERS, A. M., RYAN, P. F. J., KLONIZAKIS, I., ELKON, K. B., LEWIS, S. M. and HUGHES, G. R. V. (1981). Analysis of heat-damaged erythrocyte clearance curves. *British Journal of Haematology*, **49**, 581.

[54] PETERS, A. M., RYAN, P. F. J., KLONIZAKIS, I., ELKON, K. B., LEWIS, S. M., HUGHES, G. R. V. and LAVENDER, J. P. (1982). Kinetics of heat damaged autologous red blood cells. *Scandinavian Journal of Haematology*, **28**, 5.

[55] PETERS, A. M., SAVERYMUTTU, S. H., BELL, R. N. and LAVENDER, J. P. (1985). The kinetics of short-lived indium-111 radiolabelled platelets. *Scandinavian Journal of Haematology*, **34**, 137.

[56] PETERS, A. M., SAVERYMUTTU, S. H. WONKE, B., LEWIS, S. M. and LAVENDER, J. P. (1984). The interpretation of platelet kinetic studies for the identification of site of abnormal platelet destruction. *British Journal of Haematology*, **57**, 637.

[57] PETERS, A. M., WALPORT, M. J., ELKON, K. B., REAVY, H. J., FERJENCIK, P. P., LAVENDER, J. P. and HUGHES, G. R. V. (1984). The comparative blood clearance kinetics of modified radiolabelled erythrocytes. *Clinical Science*, **66**, 55.

[58] PETTIT, J. E. (1977). Spleen function. *Clinics in Haematology*, **6**, 639.

[59] PETTIT, J. E., LEWIS, S. M., WILLIAMS, E. D., GRAFTON, C. A., BOWRING, C. S. and GLASS, H. I. (1976). Quantitative studies of splenic erythropoiesis in polycythaemia vera and myelofibrosis. *British Journal of Haematology*, **34**, 465.

[60] RICKETTS, C., JACOBS, A. and CAVILL, I. (1975). Ferrokinetics and erythropoiesis, ineffective erythropoiesis, and red cell lifespan using ^{59}Fe. *British Journal of Haematology*, **31**, 65.

[61] RICKETTS, C., CAVILL, I. and NAPIER, J. A. F. (1977). The measurement of red cell lifespan using ^{59}Fe. *British Journal of Haematology*, **37**, 403.

[62] ROCHE, M. and PÉREZ-GIMÉNEZ, M. E. (1959). Intestinal loss and reabsorption of iron in hookworm infection. *Journal of Laboratory and Clinical Medicine*, **54**, 49.

[63] VALERI, C. R., LANDROCK, R. D., PIVACEK, L. E., GRAY, A. D., FINK, J. G. and SZYMANSKI, I. O. (1985). Quantitative differential agglutination method using the Coulter counter to measure survival of compatible but identifiable red blood cells. *Vox Sanguinis*, **49**, 195.

[64] WARDLE, D. F. H., BAKER, I., MALPAS, J. S. and WRIGLEY, P. F. M. (1973). Bioassay of erythropoietin using foetal mouse liver cells. *British Journal of Haematology*, **24**, 49.

[65] WILLIAMS, E. D., SZUR, L., GLASS, H. I., LEWIS, S. M., PETTIT, J. E. and AHUJA, S. (1974). Measurement of red cell destruction in the spleen. *Journal of Laboratory and Clinical Medicine*, **84**, 134.

25. Investigation of megaloblastic and iron-deficiency anaemias

(By D. W. Dawson, A. V. Hoffbrand and M. Worwood)

MEGALOBLASTIC ANAEMIA

Megaloblastic anaemia can be suspected from the presence in a blood film of macrocytes, oval red cells, pear-shaped poikilocytes and polymorphonuclear neutrophils with hypersegmented nuclei (see Chapter 8). The first indication in many cases is the finding of a raised MCV, often without anaemia. The diagnosis may be confirmed by finding megaloblasts and giant metamyelocytes in the marrow. Assay of serum cobalamin (B_{12}) and serum and red cell folate can provide the additional evidence for a firm diagnosis to be made. Serum B_{12} assay is particularly important in the diagnosis of B_{12} neuropathy, as this is often associated with little haematological abnormality.

B_{12} in serum is predominantly methylcobalamin bound to carrier proteins, transcobalamins (TCs). A fall in the serum B_{12} is an early sign of deficiency, found before the cellular changes in the marrow and blood. A low serum level is not, however, specific for B_{12} deficiency and may be found in folate deficiency (perhaps due to a failure in methylation), normal pregnancy, multiple myeloma, TC I deficiency and sometimes for no apparent reason.

On the other hand, megaloblastic anaemia due to B_{12} deficiency or failure in metabolism can occur in the presence of a normal serum level with TC II deficiency, with elevated TC I levels, as in chronic granulocytic leukaemia, and with nitrous oxide anaesthesia. Depletion of B_{12} bound to TC II occurs early in B_{12} deficiency[48] and its assay may help to clarify equivocal serum B_{12} levels, but its estimation demands precise assays. Assay of serum methylmalonic acid and homocysteine may reveal minimal B_{12} deficiency[63] but their estimation is not suitable for general laboratory use and will not be described here.

Serum folate (methyltetrahydrofolate) shows an early fall with changes in folate intake or balance and may be low without significant deficiency.[15e] The red cell folate (largely folate polyglutamate) concentration shows better correlation with megaloblastic change,[50] though it is not a specific sign of folate deficiency. It is also low in about half the patients with B_{12} deficiency[15f] due to the requirement for B_{12} in the provision of tetrahydrofolate which is needed rather than methyltetrahydrofolate as substrate for folate polyglutamate synthesis.[18, 61] The red cell folate may be normal despite folate deficiency when there is a reticulocytosis,[50] following a recent blood transfusion or when anaemia is absent.[50] Vitamin assays should not therefore be interpreted in isolation.

The deoxyuridine suppression test is a sensitive and specific test of both B_{12} and folate deficiency[96] and may be abnormal before obvious morphological changes develop.[13]

The elucidation of the cause of deficiency of B_{12} and folate depends both on the clinical diagnosis and on laboratory tests. The latter include measurement of the absorption of B_{12}, other intestinal absorption tests, demonstration of antibodies to intrinsic factor or gastric parietal cells, and measurement of gastric secretion of intrinsic factor. The estimation of serum B_{12}-binding capacity and transcobalamins are of occasional help.

In this chapter we shall first consider microbiological assays followed by the more widely used radioisotope assays for B_{12} and folate. The deoxyuridine suppression test is given next and finally tests to determine the cause of either deficiency.

MICROBIOLOGICAL ASSAY OF VITAMIN B_{12} IN SERUM

Several methods are available, using *Euglena gracilis*, *Lactobacillus leichmannii*, *Eschericha coli* and *Ochromonas malhamensis*. *E. gracilis* is sensitive, accurate and especially suitable for the assay of a large number of specimens though it has been largely confined to use in centres with a particular interest in B_{12} metabolism. It was the assay method chosen to assign a potency value to the British Standard for human serum B_{12}[22] and is described in detail in the 6th edition of this book. Assay with *L. leichmannii* is used with decreasing frequency because of its poor precision and the greater convenience of radioisotopic methods for routine work.

MICROBIOLOGICAL ASSAY OF SERUM AND RED CELL FOLATE

The folate activity of serum is due mainly to the presence of a folic acid co-enzyme, 5-methyltetrahydrofolic acid. Because this compound is a growth requirement for *Lactobacillus casei*, this organism is used for the assay of naturally-occurring folates in serum and in red cells.

The material necessary for the growth of *L. casei* is extremely labile, but it can be protected during assay with ascorbic acid.[94] When this precaution is taken the serum folate levels of patients with megaloblastic anaemia due to folate deficiency are lower than in normal subjects and in patients with pernicious anaemia.[94]

Serum to which 5 mg/ml of ascorbic acid has been added can be stored at $-20°C$ for up to 2 months. For assay of red cell folate, whole blood anticoagulated with EDTA can be stored for up to 1 week at 4°C. A lysate is prepared by adding 0.2 ml of whole blood (of known PCV) to 1.8 ml of 10 g/l freshly prepared aqueous ascorbic acid, with incubation for at least 10 min at room temperature before assay. The lysate may be stored for up to 5 months at $-20°C$.

A protein-free extract was originally used for serum and red cell assays.[50, 94] An aseptic technique without protein precipitation[44] simplified the assay and the use of a *L. casei* strain resistant to chloramphenicol now permits automated and semi-automated methods.[23, 69]

CHLORAMPHENICOL-RESISTANT *L. CASEI* METHOD[23,69]

Reagents and materials

Glassware. Carry out the assays in 100 × 16 mm (disposable) glass tubes.

Water. Use glass-distilled water throughout.

Organism. Chloramphenicol-resistant *Lactobacillus casei* NCIB 10463.* Maintain the organism in dried gelatin discs by the method of Stamp.[91] Store in a desiccator over phosphorus pentoxide at 18–25°C.

Chloramphenicol solutions.

A. 1 g/l. Dissolve 100 mg of chloramphenicol base B.P. in 1 ml of absolute ethanol and make up to 100 ml with water.

B. 3 g/l. Dissolve 300 mg of chloramphenicol base B.P. in 1 ml absolute ethanol and make up to 100 ml with water.

---

*National Collection of Industrial Bacteria, Torrey Research Station, Aberdeen, Scotland AB9 9DG

Table 25.1 Preparation of standard solutions for the *L. Casei* method for assay of serum and red cell folate

*Folic acid solution C 100 µg/l (ml)	0	0.1	0.2	0.4	0.6	0.8	1.0	1.2	1.4
Water (ml)		5	4.9	4.8	4.6	4.4	4.2	4.0	3.8	3.6
Concentration of standard (µg/l)	0	2.0	4.0	8.0	12.0	16.0	20.0	24.0	28.0

* Store at − 20°C; use a fresh set for each assay.

Maintenance medium. Bacto Lactobacillus Broth AOAC (Difco 0901-15-3). Suspend 19 g of dehydrated medium in 450 ml of water and dissolve by boiling for 2 min, protected from light. To 180 ml of broth add 20 ml of chloramphenicol solution B and to 270 ml of broth add 30 ml of chloramphenicol solution A. Distribute 10-ml volumes into screw-capped glass bottles and autoclave at 121°C for 15 min. Store in the dark at 4°C. Use the stronger chloramphenicol broth for the stock culture and subculture the organism for assay in the weaker chloramphenicol broth.

Propagation and storage of organism

Transfer a disc of dried culture to 10 ml of maintenance medium containing chloramphenicol solution B and incubate at 37°C for 24 h. Wash the organism four times with water and adjust the absorbence of the suspension to read 0.2 at 530nm (total volume 200–300 ml). Distribute 2 ml volumes into freezing vials and store enough vials for 1 year's assays in liquid nitrogen. Washing in bulk saves time and improves precision between assays.

Assay medium

Prepare Folic Acid Medium* according to instructions. Protect it from light during heating and use, to avoid destruction of riboflavin.[3] Dilute the medium to single strength(1:1) with water. Add 10 ml of chloramphenicol solution A, a few drops of Tween 80 and 1 g ascorbic acid to each litre of single strength medium, and if necessary adjust the pH to 6.4 with 3 mol/l KOH.

Preparation of standards

Dry pteroylglutamic acid powder** at 100°C for 2 h.

---

*Difco 0822; Dano (Hopkins and Williams) or Merck 532012L(BDH)
**Sigma or Halewood Chemicals Ltd

Stock solution A. Prepare an aqueous folic acid solution (1 g/l) by bringing the folic acid into solution with a few drops of 0.2 mol/l NaOH. Store at − 20°C in 1.5 ml volumes.

Solution B. Dilute the stock solution A 1 in 100 in 20% ethanol to give a solution of 0.1 g/l. Store in a dark bottle at 4°C.

Solution C. Dilute solution B 1 in 100 with water to give a solution of 100 µg/l.

Standard curve. Dilute solution C in water according to Table 25.1.

Inoculum

Take one vial of frozen organism, thaw and add to 2 litres of assay medium. Stir continuously with a magnetic stirrer.

Method

Rinse out automatic diluter with dilute bleach, and then with water followed by assay medium. Set up 0.05 ml volumes of sera and lysates in duplicate and standards in triplicate. Add 4.95 ml assay medium to each tube. Cover the tubes with cling film and incubate at 37° C for 20–24 h.

Reading the assay

Remove the tubes from the water-bath and cool at 4°C for 30 min. Mix in a vortex mixer and read the turbidity at 620 nm in a spectrophotometer, preferably with a flow-through cell and recorder, first setting the instrument to zero with the standard tubes containing no folic acid.

Calculation

Plot the absorbence against the folic acid concentration in µg/l on arithmetic paper to prepare a standard curve. Read the serum and haemolysate folates directly from the curve. Correct the lysate for the dilution factor of 20 and divide by the haematocrit to obtain the red cell folate. It is not usually necessary to correct the lysate for the small amount of serum folate present, though the following formula can be used:

red cell folate μg/l =

$$\frac{[(\text{whole blood folate} \times 20) - \text{serum folate}] \times (1 - \text{PCV})}{\text{PCV}}$$

Normal reference range

Serum folate. 3–20 μg/l (7–46 nmol/l); mean 10 μg/l (23 nmol/l)

Red cell folate. 160–640 μg/l (365–1460 nmol/l); mean 316 μg/l (720 nmol/l).

In the series reported by Waters and Mollin,[94] patients with megaloblastic anaemia due to folate deficiency had serum folate levels of <4.0 μg/l and patients with pernicious anaemia had levels of 4.0–27 μg/l (mean 16.6 μg/l). In patients with megaloblastic anaemia due to folate deficiency the red cell folate was 8–143 μg/l, mean 79 μg/l, and in pernicious anaemia 26–395 μg/l, mean 146 μg/l.[50] Variations in results relate to the assay medium used and to its pH.

Effect of drugs on the serum folate (L. casei) assay[15d]

The growth of *L. casei* is inhibited by penicillins, tetracycline, erythromycin, streptomycin, lincomycin, rifampicin, trimethoprim and sulphonamides. Methotrexate and pyrimethamine also inhibit the assay. Alkylating agents do not usually inhibit the assay at conventional dosage whereas some antimetabolites do. Drug inhibition will depend on the dosage given as well as on the nature of the drug. Serious inhibition is evident if the growth of the organism is less in the test serum than in the blank (zero folic acid) standard tube and inhibition can also be detected by assay of a mixture of the patient's serum and a normal serum, or of a higher dilution of the patient's serum. Inhibition is rarely observed with haemolysate assays because of their higher dilution.

Quality control materials for B₁₂ and folate assays

Sera and haemolysates of known B_{12} and folate content must be included in each assay. It is usual to collect pools of low, intermediate and normal values, to store these in 1 ml volumes at $-20°C$ and to thaw one for each assay. Their vitamin content is determined by assay alongside samples of known concentration from another laboratory or samples from previous external quality assessment surveys. The British Standard for human serum B_{12} is available to workers developing or researching an assay.* Recovery experiments with the addition of B_{12} and folic acid to normal samples (to increase the concentration by about one quarter of the reference interval) are of some value though they do not assess the extraction stage in B_{12} assays or the haemolysate preparation in folate assays. The repeat assay of three to five sera from the previous batch and plotting the mean or median of each batch (providing the samples come from an unchanging population) help to assure reproducibility of the assay.

MEASUREMENT OF SERUM VITAMIN B₁₂ BY RADIOASSAY

Assay of serum B_{12} by radioisotope dilution (competitive binding) was first described nearly 30 years ago.[7] Many variations have since been reported and commercial kits have extended the use of the test. Radioimmunoassay has been developed[85] and is more sensitive but anti-sera are not generally available. Radioisotope dilution (RID) only will be considered here. Isotope methods have the advantage over microbiological assays in that they are simpler and more rapid and the results are unaffected by antibiotics and other drugs which may affect the living organism.

Principle of radioisotope dilution assay. A known amount of radioactive 'hot' B_{12} is diluted with the non-radioactive 'cold' B_{12} in the test serum which is released from the serum binders by heat or chemical means. A measured volume of the mixture of hot and cold cobalamin is bound to a

---

*From National Institute for Biological Standards and Control, South Mimms, EN6 3QG.

binding protein which is added in an amount insufficient to bind all the 'hot' B_{12}. The bound cobalamin is separated from the free and its radioactivity counted. This count will be inversely proportional to the cobalamin concentration in the test serum as the higher the serum cobalamin the greater will be the dilution of the radioactive cobalamin and thus less radioactivity will be attached to the binding protein. By comparison with standards of known B_{12} content, the B_{12} content of the serum can be calculated. Variations at each assay step that can affect the results include:

1. Extraction of B_{12} from serum transcobalamins.

Boiling or autoclaving at an acid pH with removal of the protein precipitate by filtration or centrifugation, as for *L. leichmannii*, was first used and is the most satisfactory method of extraction.[19,32] The pH of the extract does not require adjustment for a subsequent binding stage by intrinsic factor (IF). Denaturation of the binders by boiling at a pH of 9.2–11.7 or at room temperature at pH 12.9–13.0, without removal of the protein products, is used in many commercial methods but in both the residue gives a varying amount of non-specific binding (NSB) which may be excessive with certain sera (e.g. those with high transcobalamin levels as in chronic granulocytic leukaemia). Dithiothreitol (DTT) reduces NSB.[62] The effect of NSB on the apparent serum levels depends on the separation stage (see below). Alkaline extraction will require subsequent adjustment of the pH to that optimal for the binding stage. Intrinsic factor antibodies do not appear to affect the assays.[32] In many assays only 200 µl of test material are required and it could be advantageous to use EDTA plasma; however, another reference range may be required.

2. Binding agent.

IF of human or porcine origin is commonly used. The IF may be purified (e.g. by affinity chromatography), contaminating R binder may be rendered inactive (blocked) by the addition of excess analogue (e.g. cobinamide)[4] or the IF may be coupled to a solid phase carrier, prior to the assay, at a pH inimical to R binder uptake.[90] Carriers used include polyacrylamide beads, glass particles, microcrystalline cellulose and magnetizable particles. The specificity of pure and blocked IF can be demonstrated by the addition of 10 µg/l

cobinamide dicyanide (Sigma) to sera; crossreactivity should be minimal with no significant increase in the assay value.

Other binders used include normal human serum,[77] essentially transcobalamin II, and unsaturated TC I[84] and the R binders of saliva[12] and of chicken serum[41] which give higher results, estimating both B_{12} and the microbiological inert analogues, i.e. total corrinoids.* The first commercial kits used crude IF preparations and sometimes gave falsely normal results,[20,60] attributed to such analogues. The use of binders which are not specific for B_{12} is acceptable, providing a reference range is determined for each one.[46,55] However in some situations, e.g. following partial gastrectomy and in folate deficiency,[80] the analogue level may not fall *pari passu* with the B_{12} level and may maintain the total corrinoid level within the normal range.

3. B_{12} standards.

For non-commercial methods, the pharmaceutical preparation of cyanocobalamin (Duncan, Flockhart), 250 µg/ml, is satisfactory. The cobalamins of the sera are converted to the cyano form during the extraction. The standards usually range from 50 or 100 to 2000 µg/l. With heat extraction, aqueous standards are usually satisfactory, but a protein matrix, to 'balance' that of the test serum, is required for alkaline extracts. The *Biorad* standards containing B_{12} and folic acid in human serum albumin are suitable.

4. Radioisotope tracer.

^{57}Co-labelled cyanocobalamin is used in all methods. $CN(^{57}Co)$ cobalamin, 0.05 µg in 1 ml with activity 370–740 kBq, is available from Amersham International (product number CT2). The best precision is required at the lower end of the reference range and the amount of tracer added should be such that 40–50% is bound at this level.[82]

5. Separation of free from bound B_{12}.

Charcoal coated with albumin or haemoglobin is most commonly used though it is messy and invariably takes

---

*Vitamin B_{12} (cobalamin) contains a nucleotide, 5–6 dimethylbenzimidazole, attached to the corrin ring through a ribose group and directly to the central cobalt atom. Corrinoids are compounds containing the corrin ring with either altered side chains and/or lacking the specific B_{12} nucleotide. They are commonly called B_{12} analogues and are essentially microbiologically inactive. Pure IF binds only cobalamins whereas other binding proteins may bind analogues.

up some bound B_{12}.[1] Alternative agents are Sephadex gel and DEAE-cellulose.[34, 93] Following centrifugation, the supernatant containing the bound B_{12} is decanted into counting tubes without disturbing the deposit. Centrifugation in solid phase methods leaves the free B_{12} in the supernatant; the deposit in the assay tube is counted, sometimes after washing.[72] The removal of the supernatant calls for care and a standard technique. Tween 20 may enhance the pelleting of the deposit.[72] Bound $^{57}Co\text{-}B_{12}$ gives the higher counts at the lower B_{12} concentrations. B_{12} bound non-specifically remains in the supernatant in the liquid systems, adds to the counts of that specifically bound and gives apparently lower serum B_{12} levels, whereas in solid phase systems the NSB-B_{12} is discarded, giving apparently higher serum B_{12} levels. The zero standard will allow correction for NSB only when the protein content of the standards is the same as in the test material.

6. Calculation of results. The bound B_{12} in the standards and sera are counted in a gamma counter, a curve relating counts to B_{12} concentration in the standards is drawn and the unknowns are read from this. However, with the usual workload this needs to be done automatically or semi-automatically. Computerized programs are available with modern counters. The choice of methods for expressing results has been reviewed by Ekins;[28] the most popular is the percentage binding (B/B_o × 100, where B is the count of the test and B_o the count of the zero standard) on the log ordinate axis and the B_{12} concentration on the log abscissa axis. Adjustment of the data in a computer program usually contributes little to the total imprecision of the assay.

MEASUREMENT OF SERUM FOLATE BY RADIOASSAY

The development of commercial radioisotope dilution (RID) kits followed upon the discovery of suitable folate binders and the production of γ-emitting iodinated folate compounds. The principle of the assay is the same as for serum B_{12} assay and the procedures are similar.

1. Extraction of folate from the serum binder. In contrast to microbiological assay the folate has to be released by heat or alkaline denaturation of the endogenous binder. Ascorbic acid must not be added to sera for preservation of folate during extraction (and storage) if the sample is also to be used for B_{12} assay because it destroys B_{12}. Dithiothreitol (DTT) is used in most combined B_{12} and folate assays to keep the folate in the reduced, stable form. Without it, stored sera may give low results.[24]

2. Binding agent. Beta-lactoglobulin isolated from cow's milk[36] is commonly used. At pH 9.3 ± 0.1 the binding affinities of the serum methylfolate and the folic acid of the standards are similar. It is essential that the pH at this stage is strictly maintained.[39] Porcine serum is a less satisfactory binder. There is cross-reactivity with methotrexate and folinic acid.

3. Folate standards. Methylfolate is unstable and the majority of assay methods use folic acid standards, which may cause under-estimation of serum folate.

4. Radioactive tracer. ^{125}I-labelled folic acid is generally used.

5. Separation of free from bound folate. The liquid and solid phase methods used for B_{12} are satisfactory for folate assays.

MEASUREMENT OF RED CELL FOLATE BY RADIOASSAY

Whereas *L. casei* responds equally to both tri- and mono-glutamates, the affinity of the binder for folates varies with the number of glutamate residues. Reproducible assays can only be obtained by release and conversion of the protein-bound polyglutamates, mainly $5\text{-}CH_3H_4Pte_5$ and $5\text{-}CH_3H_4Pte_6$, to a monoglutamate. Adequate dilution of the red cells,[5] a pH between 3 and 6,[75] plasma conjugase (deconjugase), and ascorbic acid to preserve the reduced form,[50] are required. Sodium ascorbate does not lyse the red cells completely. Inadequate lysis and deconjugation give falsely high results.[73,89]

To prepare the lysate dilute 100 μl of whole blood (of known PCV) in 1.9 ml of *freshly* prepared aqueous ascorbic acid. Incubate for 90 min at room temperature before assay or storage at − 20°C.

Which Method?

The choice should be based upon technical performance, clinical value and compatibility with current laboratory procedures and with the user.

A laboratory setting up B_{12} assays would not now introduce a microbiological method since radioassays are generally satisfactory and more convenient. ELISA techniques are still in the developmental stage. The accuracy of a B_{12} assay can be judged by assay of reference sera and by its performance in external quality assessment schemes, in which the mean from a large number of participants appears to be the true value.[24] The accuracy of most RID kits is acceptable. A satisfactory assay gives CVs of 5% or less with within-batch duplicates and of 10% or less with between-batch assays. All manufacturers claim that these levels can be reached. A laboratory carrying out other in-house B_{12} investigations may wish to establish its own method. The solid phase boil technique of Muir and Chanarin[72] (though the bead preparation is both time-consuming and not inexpensive) and the boil technique with charcoal separation of Gutcho and Mansbach[42] are recommended.

The lack of reference preparations limits a technical assessment of folate assays. Serum and red cell folates show considerable variation in relative accuracy though the correlation between them is reasonable.[38] The precision of serum assays at normal concentrations is similar to that of B_{12} assays but that of red cell assays is worse.[5] Some laboratories may wish to measure only a serum or red cell folate, but because of the limitations of both (see p. 397) it is advisable to assay both, or to do the red cell assay whenever the serum folate is low. A laboratory should continue with *L. casei* assays until the variations between different radioassay kits have been resolved.

Table 25.2 lists the kits in use in the UK. Kits using solid phase binders for B_{12} and folate assays are preferable since they reduce the number of assay steps and are as satisfactory as charcoal separation. A boil technique with a solid phase binder is probably the best for detecting B_{12} deficiency.[19] The features mentioned previously which affect radioassays and the references to their performance should help in the choice of an appropriate kit. The protocol should be studied before a trial kit is obtained. A new kit requires full evaluation including the assay of sera of low B_{12} content.

SOLID PHASE SERUM VITAMIN B_{12} RADIOASSAY

Method of Muir and Chanarin.[72]

Principle. Boil-extraction at pH 4.6 is followed by solid phase binding with IF coupled to polyacrylamide beads at the same pH.

Reagents

Sodium acetate (2.5 mol/l). Sodium acetate trihydrate, 340.2 g in 1 litre water; add 0.2 g of sodium azide and store at 4°C.

Acetic acid (5.0 mol/l). Glacial acetic acid, 286 ml, in 1 litre water. Add 0.2 g of sodium azide and store at 4°C.

Acetate buffer (0.5 mol/l, pH 4.65). Add 200 ml of sodium acetate solution to 1 litre water (A). Make up 100 ml acetic acid to 1 litre in water (B). To 1 litre of A add approximately 800 ml of B until pH is 4.65. Make up fresh for each assay.

Acetate buffer (5 mmol/l, pH 5.3). Two ml of sodium acetate in 1 litre (C). One ml of acetic acid in 1 litre water (D). Adjust pH of C with D to 5.3.

Sodium cyanide (0.5 mol/l). Dissolve 2.5 g in 100 ml water.

Acetate cyanide buffer. Add 1 ml of sodium cyanide solution to 1 litre of 0.5 mol/l acetate buffer.

Acetate tween 20 buffer. Add 10 ml of Tween 20 (Sigma) to 1 litre of 0.5 mol/l acetate buffer.

Acetate cyanide Tween buffer (AC 20). Mix equal volumes of acetate cyanide and AC20 buffers.

Phosphate-buffered saline (PBS) (pH 7.4). Make up NaCl 8 g, KCl 0.2 g, Na_2HPO_4 (anhydrous) 1.15 g and KH_2PO_4 0.2 g to 1 litre.

Polyacrylamide beads (Immunobeads, Biorad). 200 mg vial of lyophilized beads.

Carbodimide hydrochloride (EDAC) (Sigma). Use fresh for each coupling.

Bovine serum albumin (BSA) (BDH, Sigma). Dialyse a 24% solution against 5 mmol/l acetate buffer overnight and store at 4°C.

Table 25.2 Commercial kits for B_{12} and folate radioassays

Manufacturer	Kit		Extraction pH	Binding pH	Separator	Relative accuracy[24] (microbiological assay = 100%)			Selected references
						B_{12}	Folate Serum	Red cell	
Amersham International plc	B_{12}/folate [+]	A	12.9	9.5	charcoal	90		155	19,24,37,38
Becton-Dickinson	B_{12}	B	9.3	9.3	charcoal				4,76,81
	Simultrac B_{12}/folate	B	9.3	9.3	charcoal	93	80	115	16,19,24,32,37
	Simultrac-S " "	B	9.3	9.3		99	82	85	24
	Simultrac-SNB " "	A	12–13	9.3		94	96	104	24
	Folic acid	B	9.3	9.3					5
Biorad	Quantaphase B_{12}/folate [+]	B	11.7	9.2	polymer beads	100	98	73	24,37,38,76,81
Ciba-Corning	Immophase B_{12}	B	9.3		glass particles	95	104	90	19,24,32,37,76
	Immophase folate	B	9.3		glass particles				24
	Magic B_{12}/folate	B			{ paramagnetic				38
	Magic B_{12}/folate	A	12–13	9.3	{ particles				
Diagnostics Products Corporation	Dualcount SP	A	13.0	9.3	{ cellulose	92	96	135	24,76,81
	Dualcount SP	B	9.4		{ particles				16,76,81
Micromedic Systems	Combostat	A	12–13	9.3	cellulose particles	107	87	131	24,32,38,79

A = Alkaline denaturation, B = Boil. The binder in all kits is IF, purified except in Simultrac kits when R is blocked by analogue in tracer.
[+] Reagents for a single B_{12} or folate assay are available.

Gastric juice. Processing and determination of IF concentration. (See p. 409.) Make up to 180 units in 20 ml volume.

Radioisotope tracer. $(CN^{57}CoB_{12})$. (See p. 401.) Make up freshly a dilution in AC20 to give 75 pg in 100 μl (about 1 in 60 dilution).

Coupling of IF to polyacrylamide beads (PBeIF) Add 50 ml of acetate buffer (5 mmol/l) to vial of beads, transfer to glass universal containers, wash twice with 50 ml buffer and pellets by centrifugation. Add the gastric juice and 20 mg of BSA to the pellets. Adjust the pH to 5.3 with 1.0 mol/l HCl. Leave 30 min at room temperature and recheck pH. Add 20 mg EDAC. Leave 2 h, monitoring the pH during the first hour. Transfer to 4 plastic centrifuge tubes and make up the volumes in each to 20 ml with PBS. Centrifuge at 1000 *g* for 20 min. Wash pellets twice with PBS, suspend in cold PBS containing 1.4 mol/l NaCl and centrifuge. Wash twice with cold PBS and leave overnight at 4°C. Wash pellets with PBS containing 1% BSA, then twice with PBS containing 0.1% sodium azide. Pool, centrifuge and resuspend the pellet in 20 ml PBS sodium azide and store at 4°C. The beads are stable for about 3 months.

Titration of PBeIF

Wash 100 μl of suspension with 10 ml AC20 and resuspend in 5 ml AC20. Pipette volumes in duplicate ranging from 50 μl to 1 ml (equivalent to 1 to 20 μl stock PBeIF suspension) into 4-ml polystyrene tubes and make up all volumes to 2.1 ml with AC20. Add 75 pg $^{57}CoB_{12}$ to all tubes, mix and leave 3 h. Centrifuge at 1000 *g* for 15 min, wash the pellets with 3.8 ml AC20, centrifuge and count the radioactivity of the pellets. The volume of PBeIF binding 30–40% of the added tracer is used in the assay.

Preparation of serum extract

Add 1 ml to 4 ml of acetate cyanide buffer in a screw-capped container and heat in a boiling waterbath for 30 min. Centrifuge at 1000 *g* for 20 min. Use the supernatant.

Cyanocobalamin standards

Dilute 0.2 ml of 250 μg/ml solution in 25% ethanol in water (v/v) to give 200 ng/ml. Keep in the dark at 4°C. This is the working solution.

The assay

Wash an appropriate volume of PBeIF once with AC20 and resuspend in AC20 so that 100 μl binds about 40% of the radio tracer.

Dispense with a micropipette duplicate volumes of working cyanocobalamin solution to give 0, 4, 10, 20, 50, 100, 150 and 200 pg in 2 ml volumes of AC20 (0 to 1000 ng/l B_{12}).

Set up the assay as follows:

Incubate all the tubes at room temperature for 4 h, centrifuge all the tubes except 1 and 2 at 1000 g for 5 min, wash the pellets once with 3.8 ml AC20 and centrifuge again. After each centrifugation decant the supernatant at once by one smooth inversion, touching the mouth of the tube against absorbent paper to remove the last traces of supernatant.

Count the radioactivity of all the tubes. Draw a standard curve from the average of counts of the paired tubes 5 to 16 on log scale against the B_{12} concentration on arithmetic scale. Read off averages of the test and control counts.

In this assay there is no protein in the standards and no correction is made for NSB. Tubes 1 and 2 (the total counts) and tubes 3 and 4 (B_0 binding of tracer by PBeIF) are used to check that the appropriate amount of binder has been used. Tubes 3 and 4 are used if the percentage binding ($B/B_0 \times 100$, see p. 402) is plotted against B_{12} concentration.

Normal Reference range

160–760 ng/l (118–561 pmol/l), mean 318 ng/l (235 pmol/l).

DEOXYURIDINE SUPPRESSION TEST[96]

Priniciple. Pre-incubation of normal bone marrow with an appropriate concentration of deoxyuridine (du) suppresses the subsequent incorporation of tritiated thymidine (^{3}H-TdR) into DNA. This suppression is less in patients with B_{12} or folate deficiency, but normal when the cause of the megoloblastic anaemia is neither B_{12} nor folate deficiency, nor any other defect in thymidylate synthesis.

Materials

Bone marrow. 10–50 $\times$ 10^6 nucleated cells or 0.5–2.0 ml aspirated marrow, in EDTA. It is preferable to test the marrow freshly but it can be left overnight at 18–25°C without affecting the results significantly.

Blood. 10 ml heparinized blood.

Reagents

Hanks balanced salt solution (GIBCO Cat. No. 041–4020) ready for use.

KCl, 0.6 mol/l. 4.473 g in 100 ml water.

Phosphate buffered saline, pH 7.4. Add 90 ml of 0.15 mol/l $NaH_2PO_4.2H_2O$ (23.4 g/l) and 410 ml of 0.15 mol/l Na_2HPO_4 (21.3 g/l) to 500 ml of saline.

Perchloric acid, 0.5 mol/l. Make up 20.8 ml of concentrated perchloric acid to 500 ml with water.

Hydroxocobalamin, 1000 μg/ml.

Folinic acid (calcium leucovorin) (Lederle), 3 mg/ml.

5-methyltetrahydrofolic acid (Sigma), 1 mg. Reconstitute with 33 μl saline immediately before use.

Tritiated thymidine TRA 120 (Amersham), 185 GBq/mmol. Dilute 0.1 ml in 10 ml of saline.

Deoxyuridine (Sigma), 100 mmol/l. Prepare a working solution of 11.4 mg in 0.5 ml of saline. This is stable at 4°C.

Scintillation fluid. e.g. Packard emulsifier scintillator 299™ Cat. No. 6013079.

Method

Whenever possible, except when stated, carry out all procedures at 4°C.

Wash marrow once in buffered Hanks solution, centrifuging at 4°C at 1000 g for 5 min.

Lyse the red cells by adding 3 ml of cold water; mix for 30 s; add 1.0 ml of 0.6 mol/l KCl; add 1–2 ml of buffered Hanks solution to maintain the pH, and then centrifuge at 1000 g for 5 min.

Wash the deposit with buffered Hanks solution, centrifuging at 1000 g for 5 min. Discard the supernatant. Repeat the lysing process if a visible button of red cells remains.

Suspend the pellets in 1 ml of Hanks solution, checking that there are no clumps in the final suspension. If necessary, pass the suspension through a 19-gauge needle attached to a 1 ml syringe.

Count the number of cells present and express the number as $\times 10^6$/ml.

Add 1 volume of autologous plasma to 4 volumes of Hanks solution and dilute the cells with this solution to obtain $1–3 \times 10^6$ cells/ml.

Set up the plastic centrifuge tubes as shown in Table 25.3.

Transfer the tubes into an ice-bath.

Centrifuge at 1000 *g* for 5 min and discard the supernatant.

Vortex-mix and wash the pellets once with 2.0 ml of cold phosphate buffered saline. Discard the supernatant.

Mix and add 2 ml of the perchloric acid to each pellet.

Mix and stand in the ice-bath for 10 min. Centrifuge and discard the supernatant. If necessary, the pellets can be left overnight at this stage.

Mix, add 0.5 ml of the perchloric acid, mix and place the tubes in a water-bath at 80°C for 20 min.

Centrifuge at 18–25°C at 1000 *g* for 5 min.

Transfer 100 μl of the supernatant into counting vials. Add 10 ml of scintillation fluid, allow to equilibrate for 30 min and count for 200 s.

Calculate % counts per min using the counts of ^{3}H-TdR alone as 100%.

Interpretation

Deoxyuridine suppression in normal marrow <8%. Deoxyuridine suppression in megaloblastic marrow >8%.

Correction, partial or complete, with added B_{12} in B_{12} deficiency.

Correction with added folinic acid to <5%, in both B_{12} and folate deficiencies.

Correction, partial, with added 5-methyl-tetrahydrofolic acid in folate deficiency.

There may be partial correction with both B_{12} and 5-methyltetrahydrofolic acid in a mixed B_{12} and folate deficiency.

A microtitre plate method is reported to be less cumbersome and more economic in sample requirement, thus allowing more replicate tests.[66] The use of peripheral blood lymphocytes has been criticised since the cultured cells develop folate deficiency.[96]

INVESTIGATION OF THE ABSORPTION OF VITAMIN B_{12}

An important step in the study of a patient suffering from B_{12} deficiency is to establish whether or not he or she has the capacity to absorb the vitamin normally. This is best accomplished with the aid of B_{12} labelled by a radioactive isotope of cobalt. Originally, ^{60}Co was employed, but the shorter-lived isotopes, ^{58}Co (half-life 71 days) and ^{57}Co (half-life 270 days), are more suitable. ^{57}Co emits one gamma ray and no particulate energy; it can be used in larger tracer doses than ^{58}Co and is the isotope of choice when a well-type scintillation counter is used. ^{58}Co can be used with all counting methods, but its counting efficiency is low and relatively large amounts must be given to obtain adequate count-rates, especially for measuring blood radioactivity. Labelled cyanocobalamin (B_{12}) is used routinely.

Method

Give an oral dose of 1 μg (37 kBq) of ^{57}Co or ^{58}Co-B_{12} in about 200 ml of water to a subject who has fasted overnight; he or she takes no further food for a further 2 h. Prepare a standard from a similar dose of radioactive B_{12} suitably diluted in water.

One (or more) of the procedures outlined below is then adopted to assess the absorption of the test dose.[21] The urinary-excretion test has been recommended by the International Committee for Stan-

Table 25.3 Preparation of assay tubes for the deoxyuridine suppression test

Tubes	Saline	Vitamin B_{12}	Folinic acid	5-methyl-THF	Cells		dU		^{3}H-TdR	
1 & 2	100 μl	—	—	—	1 ml		—		100 μl	
3 & 4	100 μl	—	—	—	1 ml	Mix–incubate	10 μl	Mix–incubate	100 μl	Mix–incubate
5 & 6	—	100 μl	—	—	1 ml	at 37°C	10 μl	at 37°C	100 μl	at 37°C
7 & 8	90 μl	—	10 μl	—	1 ml	15 min with	10 μl	1 h with	100 μl	1 h with
9 & 10	90 μl	—	—	10 μl	1 ml	shaking	10 μl	shaking	100 μl	shaking
11 & 12	90 μl	—	—	—	1 ml		10 μl		100 μl	

dardization in Haematology as being the most convenient and reliable in practice.[54].

If absorption is found to be subnormal, the test can be repeated with the simultaneous administration of a source of intrinsic factor. Intrinsic Factor Concentrate capsules are available* in a dose of 10 mg blended with lactose. Capsules should be opened and their contents mixed with the liquid dose.[64]

Urinary excretion (Schilling) test[86]

Give 1.0 µg of radioactive B_{12} (^{57}Co or ^{58}Co) by mouth to the fasting patient and at the same time give 1 mg of non-radioactive hydroxocobalamin intramuscularly (a flushing dose). Collect the urine for 24 h. Measure the radioactivity of this urine and of a standard. Calculate the percentage dose excreted in the urine as follows:

$$\frac{\text{total cpm in 24 h urine}}{\text{cpm in standard} (\equiv \text{test dose})} \times 100.$$

It is, however, both more convenient and cheaper to prepare 10 test doses at one time. Vial CT3P* contains c 10 µg of B_{12} with activity c 0.37 MBq (10 µCi). Using sterile containers, dilute the contents to 100 ml in water. Take 100 µl for the standard. Dispense the remainder in 10 ml volumes. Dilute the 100 µl standard to 100 ml in water. Store doses and standard at 4°C. This standard is a 1 in 10 000 dilution of the test dose.

Mix the 24 h urine collection well and measure equal volumes of urine and standard. Calculate the percentage of the test dose excreted as follows:

$$\frac{\text{Urine cpm} \times \text{urine volume (ml)}}{\text{Standard cpm} \times \text{dilution of standard}} \times 100.$$

A dual isotope *(Dicopac)* kit of free ^{58}Co-B_{12} and ^{57}Co-B_{12} bound to intrinsic factor is available.* The dual test can be used with whole-body counting.

Interpretation of results

The normal urinary excretion is >10% of the test dose in the first 24 h; in patients with pernicious anaemia or with B_{12} deficiency associated with

___
*Amersham International plc.

intestinal malabsorption, the excretion is usually <5%. This can be increased in pernicious anaemia by the simultaneous administration of intrinsic factor, whereas absorption remains subnormal if the malabsorption is due to an intestinal defect. The second test dose, with intrinsic factor, can be given 48 h after the first, provided that an additional flushing injection is given 24 h after the first oral dose. Low results may be found in patients with renal disease, when exretion may be delayed. In such cases urine should be collected for 48 h.

The method is generally reliable (except in renal disease); the results are clear-cut and the technique is simple. The need for large flushing doses of B_{12} is a disadvantage in that they may interfere with other studies, and the tests depend on a complete collection of urine.

Deficiency of B_{12} and of folate may cause temporary malabsorption of B_{12}.[45] It is advisable to repeat tests which have given discrepant results after replacement therapy for 2 months.

With the *Dicopac* test the results differ from those of separately performed tests,[29] partly because of the difference in size of oral doses and partly because some exchange of isotopes occurs in the combined test. In normal subjects the quoted figures are: ^{58}Co 11–28%, ^{57}Co 12–30%; in pernicious anaemia ^{58}Co 0–5.5%, ^{57}Co 5–14%. A ratio of % ^{57}Co excreted/^{58}Co excreted may be calculated and this may be of value if the urine collection is incomplete.[15c] Normal subjects and patients with intestinal malabsorption give a ratio of 0.7–1.5, whereas patients with pernicious anaemia usually give ratios >1.8.

Achlorhydria due to atrophic gastritis and following partial gastrectomy may be associated with normal absorption of aqueous B_{12} but malabsorption of protein-bound B_{12}.[26] Tests with B_{12} attached to binders in egg yolk[27] and in chicken serum[25] have been described.

Faecal excretion method[71]

Give 1 µg of radioactive B_{12} by mouth as described above. Collect all faeces passed in 450 ml waxed cardboard cartons and measure their radioactivity in a GM ring counter or other large-sample counting system. Continue the collection until less than 2% of the dose appears in a 24 h sample (usually 4–6 days). Calculate the percentage of the dose which has been absorbed as follows:

$$\frac{\text{cpm standard } (\equiv \text{test dose}) - \text{cpm faeces}}{\text{cpm standard}} \times 100.$$

Interpretation of results

Normal subjects absorb >0.45 µg of a 1 µg dose. Patients with pernicious anaemia or with B_{12} deficiency associated with intestinal malabsorption absorb <0.30 µg, usually <0.2 µg. As in the Schilling test, these causes of B_{12} deficiency can be distinguished from each other if the test is repeated, adding intrinsic factor to the test dose. Under these conditions patients with pernicious anaemia absorb normal amounts of the test dose, whereas absorption remains subnormal if the malabsorption is due to an intestinal defect.

The test has the advantage that it is one in which the absorption of B_{12} is measured directly; it has the disadvantage that it entails collection of faeces and that incomplete collection may lead to erroneous conclusions. Moreover, the test takes some days to complete. It is less practical as a routine diagnostic procedure than the Schilling test.

A 'spot' faeces test[49] has been devised to overcome these drawbacks. In this the radioactive B_{12} is administered with non-absorbable $^{51}CrCl_3$ and carmine red. When the faeces become red a sample is counted for ^{51}Cr radioactivity. The fraction of the $^{51}CrCl_3$ dose in the sample is calculated from a standard. The ^{57}Co counts are adjusted to give the total ^{57}Co excretion. The test correlates well with the faecal excretion test but assumes similar intestinal transport rates, which may not be the case in the presence of diarrhoea.[59]

Plasma radioactivity method[31,65]

In normal subjects the plasma radioactivity due to absorbed labelled B_{12} increases 3 h after an oral dose and subsequently reaches a peak between 8 h and 12 h. As the amount of radioactivity in the plasma will be small, it is essential to use B_{12} labelled with ^{57}Co.

Measurement of plasma radioactivity is suitable as a rapid screening test for the detection of absorption but it is not possible to measure absorption quantitatively with any degree of accuracy, and discrepancies have been reported between the results of this test and the Schilling test in patients with malabsorption.[31,65] Both methods can be combined in a single test with advantage.

Carry out the urinary excretion test as above and at 8 h collect 20 ml of heparinized blood. Separate the plasma and measure its radioactivity. Record the result as the percentage of the dose given per litre of plasma.

Results

Normal, usually >0.5% dose per litre plasma; PA usually <0.2% dose per litre plasma.

Whole-body counting

The advantage of this method is that a 'flushing' dose of B_{12} is not given so that the patient's B_{12} metabolism is not affected, though the necessity to withhold treatment may sometimes be a disadvantage. It requires specialized equipment and, normally, a low-background room. Initial counting (100% value) is performed 1 h after swallowing the dose. Repeat counting is done after 7 days to establish how much has been retained. A system has been described which can be used in the absence of a low-background room and fairly accurate measurements of ^{58}Co absorption have been reported.[10] $^{57}Co\text{-}B_{12}$ can also be used[92] and a double isotope test has been described.[9]

Results

Normal subjects absorb >30% and usually >50% of a 1 µg dose. Patients with PA absorb <20%.

ESTIMATION OF INTRINSIC FACTOR (IF) IN GASTRIC JUICE[8]

Direct estimation of the IF content of gastric juice is useful in the diagnosis of PA, particularly when there is associated small intestinal disease which complicates the interpretation of B_{12} absorption studies.

Principle. B_{12} binding by the gastric juice is due to its content of IF and R proteins (salivary and gastric). Normally more than 90% is due to IF. Estimation of this may be done by determining the difference in the binding capacity of the gastric juice with and without neutralization of the IF by serum IF antibody (IFA).[40] An assay in which the non-IF binding is neutralized by the addition of B_{12} analogue (e.g. cobinamide) gives comparable results, does not depend upon the availability of IFA of certain potency and is simpler.

This technique is described here.

Reagents

Buffer. 0.01 mol/l tris-HCl, pH 8.0 containing 0.15 mol/l NaCl and 50 µg/ml 22% bovine albumin.

Activated albumin-coated charcoal (25 g/l). Heat 2.5 g of charcoal (Norit A*) at 110°C overnight. Suspend in 50 ml water. Add 6.8 ml of 22% bovine albumin in 50 ml water and mix well for 10 s. Activated charcoal is stable for several months and the coating is done immediately before use.

Vitamin B_{12}. Dilute ^{57}Co-B_{12}, 45–85 ng B_{12}, 370–740 kBq (10–20 µCi)/ml,** with water to 1 ng/l. Store in the dark at 4°C. This is stable for 3 months. For the assay add non-radioactive cyanocobalamin to give a solution containing 200 ng/l.

Cobinamide. Make up a stock solution of 10 mg/l. Store at 4°C. For use dilute to give 50 ng in 100 µl.

Collection of gastric juice. Collect into an ice-cooled container the basal secretion for 1 h followed by a further hour collection after subcutaneous administration of pentagastrin as a stimulus (8 µg/kg body weight). Centrifuge at $1000\,g$ for 15 min to separate the mucus. Record the pH. Take clear juice, add sufficient 5 mol/l NaOH to obtain a pH of 11.0, stand for 20 min at room temperature to inactivate peptidases and then neutralize to pH 7.0 with 1 mol/l HCl. Measure the volume. It may be stored for some months at − 20°C without loss of activity.

Method

Set up controls and samples, in duplicate, as shown in Table 25.4. Mix and incubate at c 20°C for 30 min. Add 100 µl ^{57}Co-B_{12} to each tube. After mixing, again incubate at c 20°C for 10 min. Add

---

* Sigma.
** Amersham International plc. Product code CT2.

Table 25.4 Preparation of control and sample tubes for the estimation of intrinsic factor in gastric juice

Tube	Buffer (ml)	Gastric juice (µl)	Cobinamide (µl)
A Untreated	3.7	0	0
B Charcoal control	2.2	0	0
C Standard	2.0	100	100
D Test	2.0	100	100

1.5 ml of coated charcoal suspension to all tubes except A. Mix and incubate for 10 min. Centrifuge the tubes and deliver 2 ml into counting vials. Measure the radioactivity and average the counts.

Calculation

By definition 1 unit of IF binds 1 ng of B_{12}.

$$\text{Units IF/ml gastric juice} = \frac{D - B}{A} \times 10 \times 20.$$

The total binding capacity of a gastric juice may be determined by omitting the cobinamide in the assay.

Interpretation

The normal range varies widely from 15 to 115 u/ml with a total secretion per hour of 500 to several thousand units.[15b] In females the concentration is the same as in males, but because of a smaller volume of gastric juice there is only half the total secretion. The concentration in PA is usually zero and never more than 10 u/ml, with a total secretion of less than 250 u in 1 h.

INTRINSIC FACTOR ANTIBODIES[15g]

Two types of antibody to IF have been detected in the sera of patients with PA. Type I (blocking antibody) prevents the attachment of B_{12} to IF, while type II (precipitating antibody) prevents the attachment of IF or the IF-B_{12} complex to the ileal receptors. Type I antibody is present in over two-thirds of cases of PA; type II probably occurs with equal frequency.[17] The presence of antibodies in a patient under investigation for PA confirms the diagnosis and renders an absorption test unnecessary. The antibodies occur only rarely in conditions other than PA, e.g. they have been described in a few patients with thyroid disorders, diabetes mellitus and the Eaton-Lambert myasthenic syndrome. The gastric juice in PA usually contains IF antibodies, but tests for these are not carried out routinely and will not be described here.

DETECTION OF TYPE I ANTIBODY

Reagents

Normal gastric juice. Determine the IF content (p. 409). Dilute in 0.154 mol/l NaCl to give a solution containing 25 u/ml. Store at −20°C in volumes suitable for a batch of tests.

Normal serum. Pool the sera from six or more normal subjects.

$^{57}Co\text{-}B_{12}$. 50 μg/l (p. 401).

Albumin-coated charcoal. 25 g/l (p. 409).

Method

Set out a series of tubes, in duplicate, as shown in Table 25.5. Mix and incubate at room temperature for 30 min with periodic mixing. Add 5 ng $^{57}Co\text{-}B_{12}$ in 100 μl volumes to all tubes. Incubate at room temperature for 10 min. Add 1.5 ml of charcoal suspension to tube B onwards. Mix and incubate at room temperature for 5 min. Centrifuge at 1500 *g* for 15 min and transfer 2 ml of the supernatant to counting vials. Measure the radioactivity and calculate ratio of normal to test serum counts.

Interpretation

Negative sera, ratio <1.02; *positive sera*, ratio >1.10. Ratios between these figures are termed indeterminate and the test should be repeated using 500 μl volumes of the test and normal sera. These ratios are given as guidelines, and each laboratory should determine its own normal range.

In this method the proportion of ng IF to ml serum is 4:1.[88] The sensitivity of the test can be enhanced by reducing this proportion but preliminary treatment of the sera is required to neutralize the effect of their transcobalamins.[74]

ESTIMATION OF TYPE II (PRECIPITATING OR CO-PRECIPITATING) INTRINSIC FACTOR ANTIBODY

Reagents

Barbitone buffer, pH 8.3. 0.04 mol/l sodium diethyl barbitone 100 ml; 0.2 mol/l HCl 6.21 ml. Make up the solution freshly every 4 weeks, and keep at 4°C.

Anhydrous sodium sulphate. 300 g/l and 150 g/l.

Albumin-coated charcoal. (See p. 409.)

Gastric intrinsic factor/$^{57}Co\text{-}B_{12}$ complex. For every 1 ml of normal gastric juice add an excess of $^{57}Co\text{-}B_{12}$, e.g. 200 ng. Leave at *c* 20°C for 30 min, and then remove excess (free) B_{12} by adding 1 ml of charcoal suspension. After a further 10 min at *c* 20°C, centrifuge the suspension for 15 min at 1500 *g*; dispense the supernatant in 2 ml volumes and store at −20°C.

Method

Place 0.3 ml of serum, including negative and positive control sera, in 10 ml centrifuge tubes. Add 0.5 ml of barbitone buffer and 1.0 ml of IF/$^{57}Co\text{-}B_{12}$ complex, diluted 1 to 5 with saline. Incubate at 37°C for 30 min. Add 2 ml of 300 g/l sodium sulphate, warmed to 37°C. After mixing, incubate for a further 10 min, and then centrifuge the suspensions at 1500 *g* for 15–20 min. Discard the supernatant and add 1 ml of 150 g/l sodium sulphate and centrifuge twice. After discarding the supernatant, add 3.5 ml of saline to each tube to dissolve the precipitate. Place 3 ml volumes from each tube in counting vials and count the radioactivity. A radioactive control containing 1.0 ml of the diluted IF/$^{57}Co\text{-}B_{12}$ complex and 2.0 ml of water is also set up and counted.

Table 25.5 Estimation of Type I intrinsic factor antibody. Preparation of control and sample tubes

Tube	0.154 mol/l NaCl (ml)	Gastric juice (μl)	Normal serum (μl)	Test serum (μl)
A Radioactive control	3.7	0	0	0
B Charcoal control	2.2	0	0	0
C Normal serum pool	1.85	50	300	0
D Positive serum	1.85	50	0	300
E etc Test sera	1.85	50	0	300

Interpretation

Precipitating antibodies are indicated by a high count in the precipitate, usually ten times higher than that of the negative controls.

A sensitive radio-immune assay using [17]I-labelled IF[17] and an ELISA technique[95] for the simultaneous detection of types I and II antibodies have been reported recently.

PARIETAL CELL ANTIBODIES

These are present in the sera of about 90% of patients with PA but also occur in other conditions and with increasing frequency with age so that about 15% of elderly individuals may exhibit them. They are usually detected by an immunofluorescent technique, using human or rat stomach.

PLASMA VITAMIN B_{12} BINDING CAPACITY[15a,40]

The total binding capacity (TBBC) of plasma comprises the sum total of the serum B_{12} concentration and the plasma unsaturated binding capacity (UBBC). 80% or more of the serum B_{12} is bound to transcobalamin I (TC I). A small fraction is bound to TC II, and TC III is virtually unsaturated. TC I and TC III (R binders) are both gylcosolated proteins and differ only in their sugar moiety. B_{12} bound to R proteins may be a circulating part of the storage pool. Congenital absence of R binders results in a very low serum B_{12} level, normal TBBC, no evidence of B_{12} deficiency and no adverse effects. It is suggested that some 'idiopathic' low B_{12} levels may be due to a decrease in R binder concentration.[11]

TC II delivers B_{12} to the tissues. Rare congenital absence results in a fulminating pancytopenia and megaloblastosis within 2 months of birth. The serum B_{12} is normal, the UBBC reduced and the deoxyuridine suppression test is abnormal.

Estimation of the unsaturated binding capacity of the individual TCs requires a separation technique; the absorption of TC II to silica powder[57] is a suitable procedure. Estimation of the UBBC and of its components needs care in the collection of the sample. To minimize release of TC I and TC III from granulocytes blood should be added to an anticoagulant mixture of 1 mg EDTA and 2 mg sodium fluoride per ml blood.[87] If serum is used, this should be separated within 2 h of collection.

Table 25.6 Preparation of tubes for the estimation of plasma B_{12} binding capacity

Tube	Saline (ml)	Plasma (ml)
A Standard	2.5	0
B Supernatant control	0.5	0
C Test	0	0.5

ESTIMATION OF UBBC

Reagents

$^{57}Co\text{-}B_{12}$, Dilute a volume of $^{57}Co\text{-}B_{12}$, specific activity *c* 6.6–8.1 MBq (180–220 µCi)/µg,* in non-radioactive cyanocobalamin to give a concentration of 2 µg/l.

Albumin-coated charcoal. (See p. 409.)

Method

Set up a series of conical centrifuge tubes containing plasma or 9 g/l NaCl as shown in Table 25.6. Add 1 ml of $^{57}Co\text{-}B_{12}$ to each tube. After mixing and incubating at *c* 20°C for 30 min, add 2 ml of charcoal suspension to each tube except A. After standing for 10 min, centrifuge the tubes at 1500 *g* for 10 min. Pipette 3 ml volumes of the supernatant into counting vials. Measure the radioactivity and correct for background counts.

Calculation

$$\text{UBBC (ng/l)} = \frac{C - B}{A} \times \text{ng/l}\,^{57}Co\text{-}B_{12} \times \text{plasma dilution.}$$

If the UBBC is equal to or greater than the amount of $^{57}Co\text{-}B_{12}$ added, the test should be repeated after appropriately diluting the plasma with saline.

---

*Amersham International plc. Product Code CT2.

Normal range

The normal range for serum UBBC is 670–1200 ng/l; that of plasma collected into EDTA-sodium fluoride is 505–1208 ng/l[87].

RESPONSE TO TREATMENT AS AN AID TO DIAGNOSIS

Assessment of response to treatment should be an integral part of the diagnosis of a megaloblastic anaemia. An optimum response is shown by the red cell count rising, depending upon the severity of the anaemia, to $3.0 \times 10^{12}/l$ and by at least $1.0 \times 10^{12}/l$, or to be normal by the 15th day after the start of therapy. In patients with little or no anaemia, therapeutic doses of the deficient vitamin should normalize the MCV within 3 months. This response confirms former deficiency but is not specific for either vitamin and depends upon other causes for macrocytosis, especially alcohol intake and smoking, and also iron status, remaining unaltered.

Deficiency of B_{12} or folate can be distinguished in a patient with megaloblastic anaemia by administering daily physiological doses of one or the other vitamin and observing whether there is an appropriate haematological response. To do this trial successfully the patient must be in a clinically satisfactory state with a haemoglobin between 60 and 100 g/l. A preliminary period of observation, e.g. 3–4 days, should be allowed to ensure that the patient is not responding to a previously administered haematinic. The megaloblastic anaemia must be uncomplicated and a diet low in B_{12} and folate must be given. In practice, this entails omitting liver and large quantities of fresh vegetables or yeast from the diet. A dose of 1 µg B_{12} or of 200 µg folic acid is given daily parenterally. Orally administered vitamins may also produce a satisfactory response if the deficiency is of nutritional origin. The trial should be continued for 10 days with one vitamin and daily reticulocyte counts carried out. A response is indicated by a peak reticulocyte count before the 8th day.

IRON-DEFICIENCY ANAEMIA

ESTIMATION OF SERUM IRON

The method below is a modification[101] of that recommended by the International Committee for Standardization in Haematology (ICSH) and is based on the development of a coloured complex when ferrous iron is treated with a chromagen solution.[52]

Reagents and materials

All reagents must be of analytical grade with the lowest obtainable iron content.

Protein precipitant. 100 g/l trichloracetic acid and 30 ml/l thioglycollic acid in 1 mol/l HCl. This solution may be stored in a dark brown bottle for 2 months.

Chromagen solution. 1.5 mol/l sodium acetate containing 0.025% ferrozine [3-(2-pyridil)-5,6-bis-(4-phenylsulphonic acid)-1,2,4-triazine]. Store in a dark brown bottle wrapped in aluminium foil for up to 2 weeks.

Iron standard; stock. Dissolve 100 mg of freshly cleaned pure iron wire in 4 ml of 7 mol/l HCl (overnight) and make up the volume to 1 litre with water.

Iron standard; working. Dilute 2 ml of the stock iron standard in 100 ml with water (= 2 mg/l).

Preparation of glassware. It is essential to avoid contamination by iron. Wash all glassware, including reagent bottles, in a detergent solution; soak in 2 mol/l HCl for 24 h and finally rinse in iron-free water. If possible use plastic test-tubes.

Iron-free water. Use de-ionized, double-distilled water for the preparation of all solutions and for rinsing glassware.

Method

Place 0.5 ml of serum (free of haemolysis), 0.5 ml of working iron standard and 1 ml of iron-free water (as a blank), respectively, in three separate iron-free test tubes. Add 0.5 ml of protein precipitant to each. Mix the contents vigorously, e.g. with a vortex mixer, and allow to stand for 5 min. Centrifuge the tube containing the serum at 1500 g for 15 min to obtain an optically clear supernatant. To 0.5 ml of this supernatant, and to 0.5 ml of each of the other mixtures, add 0.5 ml of the chromagen solution with thorough mixing. After standing for 10 min, measure the absorbence in a spectrophotometer against water at 562 nm.

Calculation

Serum iron (μmol/l) =

$$\frac{A^{562} \text{ test} - A^{562} \text{ blank}}{A^{562} \text{ standard} - A^{562} \text{ blank}} \times 35.8.$$

A similar procedure can be used in a micromethod in which only 0.1 ml of serum is required when measurement is carried out by automated analysis.

Normal range of serum iron[30]

13–32 μmol/l (70–180 μg/dl).

The serum iron is slightly lower in women than in men. Diurnal variation of up to 30%, with the level lower at night than during the day, has been described. Characteristically, the serum iron is very low in iron-deficiency anaemia and in infections; it is high in idiopathic haemochromatosis, following multiple transfusions and when the flow of iron from plasma to erythroid cells is decreased as in hypoplastic and aplastic anaemias. High concentrations are also found when haemoglobin breakdown is increased as in sideroblastic and megaloblastic anaemia with ineffective erythropoiesis or in haemolytic anaemia.

IRON-BINDING CAPACITY

In the plasma, iron is bound to a β-globulin (transferrin) and the total iron-binding capacity depends on the concentration of this protein. The transferrin to which iron is not actually bound is known as the 'unsaturated iron-binding capacity'. The serum-iron concentration plus the unsaturated iron-binding capacity together give the total iron-binding capacity.

Iron-binding capacity is usually measured by adding an excess of iron and measuring the iron retained after the action of a suitable reagent such as light magnesium carbonate, an ion-exchange resin, haemoglobin-coated charcoal or Sephadex G-25. All methods are empirical, and none is completely satisfactory. That described below is fairly reliable.[53]

ESTIMATION OF TOTAL IRON-BINDING CAPACITY (TIBC)

Principle. Excess iron as ferric chloride is added to serum. Any iron which does not bind to transferrin is removed with excess magnesium carbonate. The iron concentration of the iron-saturated serum is then measured.

Reagents

Basic magnesium carbonate, $MgCO_3$, 'light grade'. *Ferric chloride*, $FeCl_3.6H_2O$. A stock iron solution is made by placing 300 mg of ferric chloride and 4 ml of concentrated HCl in a volumetric flask and making up to 1 litre with water. Make a 1 in 10 dilution with iron-free water on the day of each assay. The 'saturating iron solution' contains 6 μg Fe/ml.

Method

Place 1 ml of plasma or serum in an iron-free tube and add 1 ml of saturating iron solution. Mix carefully by hand and leave at room temperature for 15 min. Use a plastic scoop or tube to add 200 mg ($\pm$ 25 mg) light magnesium carbonate and cap the tube with a rubber stopper covered with Parafilm. Shake vigorously and allow to stand for 30 min with occasional mixing. Centrifuge at 1500 g for 30 min. If the supernatant contains traces of magnesium carbonate remove the supernatant and recentrifuge. Carefully remove 1 ml of the supernatant and treat as serum for the iron estimation described above. Multiply the final result by two.

ESTIMATION OF SERUM TRANSFERRIN BY IMMUNOLOGICAL METHODS

The measurements of iron-binding capacity described above require relatively large amounts of serum and may also include non-transferrin iron[51] when the transferrin is saturated. There are numerous immunological methods which are available commercially for measuring transferrin concentrations directly by radial-immunodiffusion, turbidimetry and nephelometry. They have been adapted to most types of automated analyzers. These methods are sensitive and specific but suffer from lack of standardization. There is at present no suitable preparation of transferrin solution because of the variable amounts of residual water and other contaminants in the lyophilized material available.[51]

A study in 1985 showed that the results obtained by six immunochemical methods (five radial-immunodiffusion and one nephelometry) were not interchangeable for diagnostic purposes.[6]

Normal range of transferrin and total iron-binding capacity

In health the serum transferrin is c 2.0–3.0 g/l, and 1 mg of transferrin binds 1.4 µg of iron. The normal serum total iron-binding capacity is 45–70 µmol/l (250–400 µg/dl), with about 33% saturation.

The iron-binding capacity is raised in iron-deficiency anaemia, when saturation may be as low as 5% and in pregnancy; it is lower than normal in infections, malignant disease and renal disease. In pathological iron overload the iron-binding capacity of the serum is reduced and the serum is completely saturated with iron.

ASSAY OF SERUM FERRITIN

With the recognition that the small quantity of ferritin in human serum (normal 15–300 µg/l in men) reflects body iron stores, measurement of serum ferritin has been widely adopted as a test for iron deficiency and iron overload.

The first reliable method to be introduced was an immunoradiometric assay[2] in which excess radiolabelled antibody is reacted with ferritin and the excess antibody removed with an immunoadsorbent. This assay was supplanted by the two-site immunoradiometric assay[68] which is sensitive and convenient but suffers from the 'high-dose hook' effect (see later). This means that at high concentrations of ferritin the amount of labelled antibody bound to the tube or bead begins to decrease instead

of continuing to increase. Since then the principle of the two-site immunoradiometric assay has been extended to labelling with enzymes (ELISA methods) and the method described below is of this type. These assays do not appear to suffer from 'high-dose hook' effect.

ENZYME IMMUNOASSAY FOR FERRITIN

The technique is based on well-known principles and is one developed by the International Committee for Standardization in Haematology (Expert Panel on Iron). Further details may be found in reference 33.

Reagents and materials

Ferritin may be prepared from human liver or spleen, either normal or iron-loaded and obtained at operation (spleen) or post mortem. The permission of the patient or the patient's relatives should be obtained before the tissue is removed. Tissue should be obtained as soon as possible after death and may be stored at − 20°C for 1 year. Remember the risk of infection when handling tissues and extracts. Ferritin is purified by methods which exploit its stability at 75°C. Further purification is obtained by chromatography and either by ultracentrifugation[98] or by precipitation from cadmium sulphate solution.[56] Purity should be assessed by polyacrylamide gel electrophoresis[98] and the protein content determined by the method of Lowry et al as decribed in reference 98. Human ferritin may be stored in solution at 4°C, at 1–4 mg protein/ml, in the presence of sodium azide as a preservative, for up to 3 years.

Antibodies to human ferritin. High affinity antibodies to human liver or spleen ferritin are suitable. Polyclonal antibodies may be raised in rabbits or sheep by conventional methods[47] and the titre checked by precipitation with human ferritin.[98] An IgG enriched fraction of antiserum is required for labelling with enzyme in the assay. The simplest method is to precipitate IgG with sodium sulphate.[43] Monoclonal antibodies which are specific for 'L' subunit rich ferritin (liver or spleen ferritin) are also suitable. Ascitic fluid preparations should be purified by sodium sulphate precipitation to obtain an IgG fraction for labelling with enzyme and for coating plates. Store in water at 10 mg protein/ml at −20°C.*

Conjugation of antiferritin IgG preparation to horseradish peroxidase[97]

1. Dissolve 4 mg of horseradish peroxidase (Sigma Type VI P-8375) in 1 ml of water and add 200 µl of freshly prepared 0.1 mol/l sodium periodate solution. The solution should turn greenish brown. Mix gently by inverting and leave for 20 min at room temperature, mixing gently every 5 min. Dialyse overnight against 1 mmol/l sodium acetate buffer, pH 4.4.

2. Add 20 µl of 0.2 mol/l sodium carbonate buffer pH 9.5 to a solution of antiferritin IgG fraction (8 mg in 1 ml). Add 20 µl of 0.2 mol/l sodium carbonate buffer pH 9.5 to the horseradish peroxidase solution to raise the pH to 9.9–9.5 and immediately mix the two solutions. Leave at room temperature for 2 h and mix by inversion every 30 min.

3. Add 100 µl of freshly prepared sodium borohydride solution (4 mg/ml in distilled water) and stand at 4°C for 2 h. Dialyse overnight against 0.1 mol/l borate buffer pH 7.4.

4. Add an equal volume of 60% glycerol in borate buffer to the conjugate solution and store at 4°C.

Assay reagents

Buffer A. Phosphate buffered saline, pH 7.2, containing 0.05% Tween 20. Prepare a 10 times concentrated (1.5 mol/l) stock solution by dissolving sodium chloride, 80 g; potassium chloride, 2 g; anhydrous disodium phosphate, 11.5 g and anhydrous potassium phosphate (KH_2PO_4) in 1 litre of water. Store at room temperature. Prepare Buffer A by diluting 100 ml of stock solution to 1 litre with water and adding 0.5 ml of Tween 20. Store at 4°C for up to 2 weeks.

Buffer B. Prepare by dissolving 5 g of BSA in 1 litre of buffer A. Store at 4°C for up to 2 weeks.

Buffer C. Carbonate buffer, 0.05 mol/l, pH 9.6. Dissolve sodium carbonate, 1.59 g and sodium

bicarbonate, 2.93 g in 1 litre of water and store at room temperature.

Buffer D. Citrate phosphate buffer, 0.15 mol/l pH 5.0. Dissolve 21 g of citric acid monohydrate in 1 litre of water and store at 4°C. Dissolve 28.4 g of anhydrous disodium phosphate in 1 litre of water and store at room temperature. Prepare fresh buffer on the day of assay by mixing 49 ml of citric acid solution with 51 ml of phosphate solution.

Substrate solution. Prepare immediately before use by adding 33 µl of hydrogen peroxide, 30%, to 100 ml of buffer and mixing well. Add 34 mg of *o*-phenylenediamine dihydrochloride (Sigma) and mix. Take care in weighing this carcinogen.

Preparation and storage of a standard ferritin solution. Dilute a solution of human ferritin to approximately 200 µg/ml in water. Measure the protein concentration by the method of Lowry after diluting further to 20–50 µg/ml.[98] Then dilute the ferritin solution (approx. 200 µg/ml) to a concentration of 10 µg/ml in 0.05 mol/l sodium barbitone solution containing 0.1 mol/l NaCl, 0.02% NaN_3, bovine serum albumin (5 g/l) and adjusted to pH 8.0 with 5 mol/l HCl. Deliver 200 µl into small plastic tubes, cap tightly and store at 4°C for up to 1 yr. For use, dilute in Buffer B to 1000 µg/l, then prepare a range of standard solutions between 0.2 and 25 µg/l. Calibrate this working standard against the WHO standard for the assay of serum ferritin (reagent 80/602, human liver ferritin).*

Coating of plates. 96-well microtitre plates for immunoassay are required.** Do not use the outer wells until you have established the assay procedure and can check that all wells give consistent results. Coat the plates by adding to each well 200 µl of antiferritin IgG preparation diluted to 2 µg/ml in Buffer C. Cover the plate with 'parafilm' or 'clingfilm' and leave overnight at 4°C. On the day of the assay empty the wells by sharply inverting the plate and dry by tapping briefly on paper towels. Block unreacted sites by adding 200 µl of 0.5% (w/v) bovine serum albumin (Sigma, A-7030) in Buffer C. After 30 min at room temperature wash each plate three times by filling each well with Buffer A (using

---

*Suitable antibodies (including a preparation labelled with horseradish peroxidase) may also be obtained from Dako Ltd, High Wycombe, Bucks.

*Available from National Institute for Biological Standards and Control (NIBSC), South Mimms, Herts EN6 3QG.
**e.g. Immuno Plate 11, Nunc or Immulon-11, Dynatech Laboratories.

a syringe and needle) and emptying and draining as decribed above.

Preparation of test sera. Collect venous blood and separate the serum. Samples may be stored at 4°C for 1 week or for 2 yr at −20°C. Plasma obtained from heparinized blood is also suitable. For assay, dilute 50 µl of serum to 1 ml with Buffer B. Further dilutions may be made in the same buffer if required.

Assay procedure

The use of a multi-channel pipette for rapid addition of solutions is recommended. Standards and sera, in duplicate, should be added to each plate within 20 min.

Add 200 µl of standard solution or diluted serum to each well. Cover the plate and leave at room temperature on a draught-free bench away from direct sunlight for 2 h. Empty the wells by sharply inverting the plate and dry by draining on paper towels. Wash three times by filling each well with Buffer A, leaving for 2 min at room temperature and draining as described above. Dilute the conjugate in 1% bovine serum albumin in Buffer A. The optimal dilution (of the order of 10^3–10^4 times) must be ascertained by experiment.

Add 200 µl of diluted horseradish peroxidase conjugate to each well and leave the covered plate for a further 2 h at room temperature. Wash three times with Buffer A. Add 200 µl of substrate solution to each well. Incubate the plate for 30 min in the dark. Stop the reaction by adding 50 µl of 25% (v/v) sulphuric acid to each well. (Dilute the acid by carefully adding concentrated acid to water.) Read the absorbence at 492 nm within 30 min using an automatic plate tender. Alternatively, transfer 200 µl from each well to a tube containing 800 µl of water and read the absorbence in a spectrophotometer.

Calculation of results

Calculate the mean absorbence for each point on the standard curve and plot against ferritin concentration using semilogarithmic paper. Read concentrations for the serum from this curve. For serum ferritin concentrations >200 µg/l reassay at a dilution of 100 times or greater. Control sera should be included in each assay.

Selecting an assay method

The following notes may be of use for those considering introducing the ferritin assay into a clinical laboratory by purchasing a commercially available kit.

1. Limit of detection. Two-site immunoradiometric assays are intrinsically more sensitive than radioimmunoassays. For example, concentrations of ferritin in buffer solution as low as 0.01 µg/l may be detected. Avoidance of serum effects (see below) requires dilution of samples, however, and, for practical purposes, the lower limit of detection is of the order of 1 µg/l. For some radioimmunoassays the limits of detection may approach 10 µg/l and this may cause difficulties in using the assay for detection of iron deficiency. This point should be examined carefully. The detection limits for enzyme-linked assays are gradually improving.

2. The 'high-dose hook'. This is a problem peculiar to labelled antibody assays, particularly two-site immunoradiometric assays.[78,83] Two causes have been suggested: (a) heterogeneity of the solid phase antiserum and (b) incomplete washing after the first reaction (binding) of ferritin to the solid phase). Exhaustive washing may move the 'hook' to higher ferritin concentrations but does not usually eliminate it. The only safe method is to assay all serum samples at two dilutions to ensure that both dilutions are on the 'ascending' part of the dose response curve. In view of the wide range of serum ferritin concentrations which may be encountered in hospital patients (0–40 000 µg/l) this is, in any case, a good practice.

3. Serum effects. These may be found with any method but particularly with labelled antibody assays. It is usually found that the serum proteins inhibit the binding of ferritin to the solid phase when compared with the binding in buffer solutions alone. Serum effects may be avoided by diluting the standards in a buffer containing a suitable serum and by diluting serum samples as much as possible. For example, for two-site immunoradiometric assays, the sample may be diluted 20 times with buffer while the standards are prepared in 5% normal rabbit serum in buffer. Further dilutions of the sera are carried out with this solution.

4. Reproducibility. Most assays are satisfactory, but this must always be established for any method introduced into the laboratory. Particular problems (different readings in the outer wells for example) may be encountered with enzyme-linked assays which have microtitre plates as the solid phase.

5. Dilution of serum samples. It should be established that both standard and serum samples dilute in parallel over at least a 10-fold range.

6. Accuracy. The use of a reference ferritin preparation is recommended (see above).

Interpretation of results

The use of serum ferritin for the assessment of iron stores has become well-established.[99] In most normal adults serum ferritin concentrations lie within the range 15–300 µg/l. During the first months of life mean serum ferritin concentrations change considerably, reflecting changes in storage iron concentration. Concentrations are lower in children than in adults and from puberty to middle life are higher in men than in women. In adults concentrations of <15 µg/l indicate an absence of storage iron but in children the lower limit of normal is lower and the assay is less valuable for detecting iron deficiency.

The interpretation of serum ferritin concentration in many pathological conditions is less straightforward. Concentrations of less than 15 µg/l indicate depletion of storage iron, but many patients with acute or chronic diseases have serum ferritin concentrations up to about 50 µg/l despite an absence of stainable iron in the bone marrow.

Iron overload causes high concentrations of serum ferritin but these may also be found in patients with liver disease, infection, inflammation or malignant disease. Careful consideration of the clinical evidence is required before it is concluded that a high serum ferritin concentration is primarily the result of iron overload and not due to tissue damage or enhanced synthesis of ferritin. However, a normal ferritin concentration provides good evidence against iron overload.

Serum ferritin concentrations are high in patients with advanced haemochromatosis but the serum ferritin estimation should not be used alone to screen the relatives of patients or for assessing re-accumulation of storage iron after phlebotomy. This is because in many patients the early stages of iron accumulation (when total iron stores are not much elevated) are detected by an increased serum iron concentration and transferrin saturation even when the serum ferritin concentration is within the normal range. This is one of the few instances where the measurement of serum iron and total iron-binding capacity provides useful information not given by the ferritin assay.

Immunologically, plasma ferritin resembles the 'L'-rich ferritins of liver and spleen and only low concentrations are detected with antibodies to heart or HeLa cell ferritin, ferritins rich in 'H' subunits. The heterogeneity of serum ferritin on isoelectric focusing is largely due to glycolysation and the presence of variable numbers of sialic acid residues and not variation in the ratio of H to L subunits.[100] Attempts to assay for 'acidic' (or 'H'-rich) isoferritins in serum as tumour markers have not been successful.[14,58]

REFERENCES

[1] ADAMS, J. F. and MCEWAN, F. C. (1974). The separation of free and bound vitamin B_{12}. *British Journal of Haematology,* 26, 581.

[2] ADDISON, G. M., BEAMISH, M. R., HALES, C. N., HODGKINS, M., JACOBS, A. and LLEWLLIN, P. (1972). An immunoradiometric assay for ferritin in the serum of normal subjects and patients with iron deficiency and iron overload. *Journal of Clinical Pathology,* 25, 326.

[3] ANDERSON, B. and COWAN, J. D. (1968). Effect of light on the *Lactobacillus casei* microbiological assay. *Journal of Clinical Pathology,* 21, 85.

[4] BAIN, B., BROOM, G. W., WOODSIDE, J., LITWINCZUK, R. A. and WICKRAMASINGHE, S. N. (1982). An assessment of a radioisotopic assay for vitamin B_{12} using an intrinsic factor preparation with R protein blocked by cobinamide. *Journal of Clinical Pathology,* 35, 1110.

[5] BAIN, B. J., WICKRAMASINGHE, S. N., BROOM, G. W., LITWINCZUK, R. A. and SIMS, J. (1984). Assessment of the value of a competitive protein binding radioassay of folic acid in the detection of folic acid deficiency. *Journal of Clinical Pathology,* 37, 888.

[6] BANDI, Z. L., SCHOEN, I. and BEE, D. E. (1985).

Immunochemical methods for measurement of transferrin in serum: effects of analytical errors and inappropriate reference intervals on diagnostic utility. *Clinical Chemistry*, **31**, 1601.

[7] BARAKAT, R. M. and EKINS, R. P. (1961). Assay of vitamin B_{12} in blood. *Lancet*, **ii** 25.

[8] BEGLEY, J. A. and TRACHTENBERG, A. (1979). An assay for intrinsic factor based on blocking of the R binder of gastric juice by cobinamide. *Blood*, **53**, 788.

[9] BRIEDIS, D., McINTYRE, P. A., JUDISCH, J. and WAGNER, H.N. (1973). An evaluation of a dual-isotope method for the measurement of vitamin B_{12} absorption. *Journal of Nuclear Medicine*, **14**, 135.

[10] CALLENDER, S. T., WITTS, L. J., WARNER, G. T. and OLIVER, R. (1966). The use of a simple whole-body counter for haematological investigations. *British Journal of Haematology*, **12**, 276.

[11] CARMEL, R. (1983). R-binder deficiency. A clinically benign cause of cobalamin deficiency. *Journal of the American Medical Association*, **250**, 1886.

[12] CARMEL, R. and COLTMAN, C. A. (1969). Radioassay for serum vitamin B_{12} with the use of saliva as the vitamin B_{12} binder. *Journal of Laboratory and Clinical Medicine*, **74**, 967.

[13] CARMEL, R. and KARNAZE, D. S. (1985). The deoxyuridine suppression test identifies subtle cobalamin deficiency in patients without typical megaloblastic anaemia. *Journal of the American Medical Association*, **253**, 1284.

[14] CAVANNA, F., RUGGERI, G., IACOBELLO, C. et al (1983). Development of a monoclonal antibody against human heart ferritin and its application in an immunoradiometric assay. *Clinica Chimica Acta*, **134**, 347.

[15] CHANARIN, I. (1979). *The Megaloblastic Anaemias*, 2nd edn. (a) p. 59; (b) p. 87; (c) p. 121; (d) p. 190; (e) p. 193; (f) p. 194; (g) p. 362. Blackwell Scientific Publications, Oxford.

[16] CHEN, I. W., SILBERSTEIN, E. S., MAXON, H. R., SPERLING, M. and BARNES, E. (1981). Clinical significance of serum vitamin B_{12} measured by radioassay using pure intrinsic factor. *Journal of Nuclear Medicine*, **22**, 447.

[17] CONN, D. A. (1986). Detection of Type I and Type II antibodies to intrinsic factor. *Medical Laboratory Sciences*, **43**, 148.

[18] COOK, T. D., CICHOWICZ, D. J., GEORGE, S., LAWLER, A. and SHANE, B. (1987). Mammalian folylpolyglutamate synthetase. 4. In vitro and in vivo metabolism of folates and analogues and regulation of folate homeostasis. *Biochemistry*, **26**, 530.

[19] COOPER, B. A., FEHEDY, V. and BLANSHAY, P. (1986). Recognition of deficiency of vitamin B_{12} using measurement of serum concentration. *Journal of Laboratory and Clinical Medicine*, **107**, 447.

[20] COOPER, B. A. and WHITEHEAD, V. M. (1978). Evidence that some patients with pernicious anaemia are not recognized by radiodilution assay for cobalamin in serum. *New England Journal of Medicine*, **299**, 816.

[21] COTTRALL, M. F., WELLS, D. G., TROTT, N. G. and RICHARDSON, N. E. G. (1971). Radioactive vitamin B_{12} absorption studies: comparison of the whole-body retention, urinary excretion and eight-hour plasma levels of radioactive vitamin B_{12}. *Blood*, **38**, 604.

[22] CURTIS, A. D., MUSSETT, M. V. and KENNEDY, D. A. (1986). British Standard for human serum vitamin B_{12}. *Clinical and Laboratory Haematology*, **8**, 135.

[23] DAVIS, R. E., NICOL, D. J. and KELLY. A. (1970). An automated method for the measurement of folate activity. *Journal of Clinical Pathology*, **23**, 47.

[24] DAWSON, D. W., FISH, D. I., FREW, I. D. O., ROOME, T. and TILSTON, I. (1987). Laboratory diagnosis of megaloblastic anaemia: current methods assessed by external quality assurance trials. *Journal of Clinical Pathology*, **40**, 393.

[25] DAWSON, D. W., SAWERS, A. H. and SHARMA, R. K. (1984). Malabsorption of protein bound vitamin B_{12}. *British Medical Journal*, **288**, 675.

[26] DOSCHERHOLMEN, A., McMAHON, J. and RIPLEY, D. (1978). Inhibitory effect of eggs in vitamin B_{12} absorption; description of a simple ovalbumin ^{57}Co-vitamin B_{12} absorption test. *British Journal of Haematology*, **33**, 261.

[27] DOSCHERHOLMEN, A., SILVIS, S. and McMAHON, J. (1983). Dual Schilling test for measuring absorption of food-bound and free vitamin B_{12} simultaneously. *American Journal of Clinical Pathology*, **80**, 490.

[28] EKINS, R. P. (1974). Radioimmunoassay and saturation analysis. Basic principles. *British Medical Bulletin*, **30**, 3.

[29] ENGLAND, J. M., SNASHALL, E. A. and DE SILVA, P. M. (1981). Comparison of the DICOPAC with the conventional Schilling test. *Journal of Clinical Pathology*, **34**, 1191.

[30] FIELDING, J. (1980). Iron: Serum and iron binding capacity. *Methods in Hematology*, **1**, 15.

[31] FINNEY, R. D. and PAYNE, R. W. (1972). Plasma radioactivity following simultaneous oral administration of intrinsic factor-bound and free radioactive B_{12}. *Acta Haematologica*, **48**, 137.

[32] FISH, D. I. and DAWSON, D. W. (1983). Comparison of methods used in commercial kits for the assay of serum vitamin B_{12}. *Clinical and Laboratory Haematology*, **5**, 271.

[33] FLOWERS, C. A., KUIZON, M., BEARD, J. L. SKIKNE, B. S., COVELL, A. M. and COOK, J. D. (1986). A serum ferritin assay for prevalence studies of iron deficiency. *American Journal of Hematology*, **23**, 141.

[34] FRENKEL, E. P., WHITE, J. D., REISCH, J. S. and SHEENAN, R. G. (1973). Comparison of two methods for the radioassay of vitamin B_{12} in serum. *Clinical Chemistry*, **19**, 1327.

[35] GANESHAGURU, K. and HOFFBRAND, A. V. (1978). The effect of deoxyuridine, vitamin B_{12}, folate and alcohol on the uptake of thymidine and on the deoxyuridine triphosphate concentrations in normal and megaloblastic cells. *British Journal of Haematology*, **40**, 29.

[36] GHITIS, J. (1966). The labile folate of milk. *American Journal of Clinical Nutrition*, **18**, 452.

[37] GILOIS, C. R., BEATTIE, G. and MILLS, S. P. (1986). Measurement of vitamin B_{12} and serum folic acid; a comparison of methods. *Medical Laboratory Sciences*, **43**, 140.

[38] GILOIS, C. R. and DUNBAR, D. R. (1987). Measurement of low serum and red cell folate levels; a comparison of analytical methods. *Medical Laboratory Sciences*, **44**, 33.

[39] GIVAS, J. and GUTCHO, S. (1975). pH dependence of the binding of folates to milk binder in radioassay of folates. *Clinical Chemistry*, **21**, 427.

[40] GOTTLIEB, C., LAU, K-S., WASSERMAN, L. R. and HERBERT, V. (1965). Rapid charcoal assays for intrinsic factor (IF), gastric juice unsaturated B_{12} binding capacity, antibody to IF and serum unsaturated B_{12} binding capacity. *Blood*, **25**, 6.

[41] GREEN, R., NEWARK, P. A., MUSSO, A. M. and MOLLIN, D. L. (1974). The use of chicken serum for the measurement of serum vitamin B_{12} by radioisotope dilution.

Description of method and comparison with microbiological assay results. *British Journal of Haematology,* **27,** 507.

[42] GUTCHO, S. and MANSBACH, L. (1977). Simultaneous radioassay of serum vitamin B_{12} and folic acid. *Clinical Chemistry,* **23,** 1609.

[43] HEIDE, K. and SCHWICK, J. G. (1978). Salt fractionation of immunoglobulins. In *Handbook of Experimental Immunology.* Ed. D. M. Weir, Vol. I, p. 7.1–11. Blackwell Scientific Publications, Oxford.

[44] HERBERT, V (1966). Aseptic addition method for *Lactobacillus casei* assay of folate activity in human serum. *Journal of Clinical Pathology,* **19,** 12.

[45] HERBERT, V. (1969). Transient (reversible) malabsorption of vitamin B_{12}. *British Journal of Haematology,* **17,** 213.

[46] HERBERT, V., COLMAN, N., PALAT, D. et al (1984). Is there a 'gold standard' for human serum vitamin B_{12} assay? *Journal of Laboratory and Clinical Medicine,* **104,** 829.

[47] HERBERT, W. J. (1978). Laboratory animal techniques for immunology. In *Handbook of Experimental Immunology.* Ed. D. M. Weir, Vol. III, p. A.4.1–29. Blackwell Scientific Publications, Oxford.

[48] HERZLICH, B. and HERBERT, V. (1988). Depletion of serum holotranscobalamin II. An early sign of negative vitamin B_{12} balance. *Laboratory Investigation,* **58,** 332.

[49] HJELT, K., MUNCK, E., HIPPE, E. and BARENHOLT, O. (1977). Vitamin B_{12} absorption determined with a double isotope technique employing incomplete stool collection. *Acta Medica Scandinavia,* **202,** 419.

[50] HOFFBRAND, V., NEWCOMBE, B. F. A. and MOLLIN, D. L. (1966). Method of assay of red cell folate activity and the value of the assay as a test for folate deficiency. *Journal of Clinical Pathology,* **19,** 17.

[51] HUEBERS, H. A., ENG, M. J., JOSEPHSON, B. M. et al (1987). Plasma iron and transferrin iron-binding capacity evaluated by colorimetric and immunoprecipitation methods. *Clinical Chemistry,* **33,** 273.

[52] International Committee for Standardization in Haematology (1978). Recommendations for measurement of serum iron in human blood. *British Journal of Haematology,* **38,** 291.

[53] International Committee for Standardization in Haematology (1978). The measurement of total and unsaturated iron-binding capacity in serum. *British Journal of Haematology,* **38,** 281.

[54] International Committee for Standardization in Haematology. (1981). Recommended method for the measurement of vitamin B_{12} absorption. *Journal of Nuclear Medicine,* **22,** 1091.

[55] International Committee for Standardization in Haematology (1981). Proposed serum standard for human serum vitamin B_{12} assay. *British Journal of Haematology,* **64,** 809.

[56] International Committee for Standardization in Haematology (Expert Panel on Iron) (1985). Proposed international standard of human ferritin for the serum ferritin assay. *British Journal of Haematology,* **61,** 61.

[57] JACOB, E. and HERBERT, V. (1975). Measurement of unsaturated 'granulocyte-related' (TCI and TCIII) and 'liver-related' (TC II) B_{12} binders by instant batch separation using a microfine precipitate of silica (QUSO G32). *Journal of Laboratory and Clinical Medicine,* **88,** 505.

[58] JONES, B. M., WORWOOD, M. and JACOBS, A. (1980). Serum ferritin in patients with cancer: determination with antibodies to HeLa cell and spleen ferritin. *Clinica Chimica Acta,* **106,** 2003.

[59] KITTANG, E., HAMBORG, B. and SCHJONSBY, H. (1985). Absorption of food cobalamin assessed by the double isotope method in healthy volunteers and in patients with chronic diarrhoea. *Scandinavian Journal of Gastroenterology,* **20,** 500.

[60] KOLHOUSE, J. F., KONDO, H., ALLEN, N. C., PODELL, E. and ALLEN, R. H., (1978). Cobalamin analogues are present in human plasma and can mask cobalamin deficiency because current radioisotope dilution assays are not specific for true cobalamin. *New England Journal of Medicine,* **299,** 785.

[61] LAVOIE, A., TRIPP, E. and HOFFBRAND, A. V. (1974). The effect of vitamin B_{12} deficiency on methylfolate metabolism and pteryolpolyglutamate synthesis in human cells. *Clinical Science and Molecular Medicine,* **47,** 617.

[62] LEE-OWN, V., BOLTON, A. E. and CARR, P. J. (1979). Formation of a vitamin B_{12}-serum complex on heating at alkaline pH. *Clinica Chimica Acta,* **93,** 239.

[63] LINDENBAUM, J., HEALTON, E. B., SAVAGE, D. G. et al (1988). Neuropsychiatric disorders caused by cobalamin deficiency in the absence of anemia or macrocytosis. *New England Journal of Medicine,* **317,** 1720.

[64] MCDONALD, J. W. D. and BARTON, W. B. (1975). Spurious Schilling test results obtained with intrinsic factor enclosed in capsules. *Annals of Internal Medicine,* **83,** 827.

[65] MCINTYRE, P. A. and WAGNER, H. N. (1966). Comparison of the urinary excretion and 6 hour plasma tests for vitamin B_{12} absorption. *Journal of Laboratory and Clinical Medicine,* **68,** 966.

[66] MATTHEWS, J. and WICKRAMSINGHE, S. N. (1986). A method for performing deoxyuridine suppression tests on microtitre plates. *Clinical and Laboratory Haematology,* **8,** 61.

[67] METZ, J., KELLY, A., SWETT, V. C., WAXMAN, S. and HERBERT, V. (1968). Deranged DNA synthesis by bone marrow from vitamin B_{12}-deficient humans. *British Journal of Haematology,* **14,** 575.

[68] MILES, L. E. M., LIPSCHITZ, D. A., BIEBER, C. P. and COOK, J. D. (1974). Measurement of serum ferritin by a 2-side immunoradiometric assay. *Analytical Biochemistry,* **61,** 209.

[69] MILLBANK, L., DAVIS, R. E., RAWLINS, N. and WATERS, A. H. (1970). Automation of the assay of folate in serum and whole blood. *Journal of Clinical Pathology,* **23,** 54.

[70] MITCHELL, G. A., POCHRON, S. P., SMUTNY, P. V. and GUITY, R. (1976). Decreased radioassay values for folate after serum extraction when pteroylglutamic acid standards are used. *Clinical Chemistry,* **22,** 647.

[71] MOLLIN, D. L., BOOTH, C. C. and BAKER, S. H. (1970). The absorption of vitamin B_{12} in control subjects, in Addisonian pernicious anaemia and in the malabsorption syndrome. *British Journal of Haematology,* **3,** 412.

[72] MUIR, M. and CHANARIN, I. (1983). The assay of serum cobalamin by solid phase saturation analysis. In *Methods in Haematology Vol 10: The Cobalamins.* Ed. C. A. Hall, p. 85. Churchill Livingstone, Edinburgh.

[73] NETTELAND, B. and BAKKE, O. M. (1977). Inadequate sample-preparation technique as a source of error in determination of erythrocyte folate by competitive binding radioassay. *Clinical Chemistry,* **23,** 1505.

[74] NIMO, R. E. and CARMEL, R. (1987). Increased sensitivity of detection of the blocking (type 1) anti-intrinsic factor antibody. *American Journal of Clinical Pathology,* **88,** 729.

[75] OMER, A. (1969). Factors influencing the release of assayable folate from erythrocytes. *Journal of Clinical Pathology,* **22,** 217.

[76] OXLEY, D. K. (1984). Serum vitamin B_{12} assays. *Archives of Pathology Laboratory Medicine,* **108,** 277.

[77] PALTRIDGE, G., RUDZKI, Z. and RYALL, R. G. (1980). Validity of transcobalamin II-based radioassay for the determination of serum vitamin B_{12} concentrations. *Annals of Clinical Biochemistry*, **17**, 287.

[78] PERERA, P. and WORWOOD, M. (1984). Antigen binding in the two-site immunoradiometric assay for serum ferritin: the nature of the hook effect. *Annals of Clinical Biochemistry*, **21**, 393.

[79] RANIOLO, E., PHILLIPOU, G., PALTRIDGE, G. and SAGE, R. (1984). Evaluation of a commercial radioassay for the simultaneous estimation of vitamin B_{12} and folate, with subsequent derivation of the normal reference range. *Journal of Clinical Pathology*, **37**, 1327.

[80] RAVEN, J. L., ROBSON, M. B., MORGAN, J. O. and HOFFBRAND, A. V. (1972). Comparison of three methods for measuring vitamin B_{12} in serum: radioisotopic, *Euglena gracilis* and *Lactobacillus leichmannii*. *British Journal of Haematology*, **22**, 21.

[81] REYNOSO, G. and MACKENZIE, J. R. (1982). Are ligand assay methods specific for cobalamin? *American Journal of Clinical Pathology*, **78**, 621.

[82] ROBARD, D. (1978). Data processing for radioimmunoassays; an overview. In *Clinical Immunochemistry*. Eds. S. Natelson, A. Pesce, A. Dietz, p. 477. American Association for Clinical Chemistry, Washington.

[83] ROBARD, D., FELDMAN, Y., JAFFE, M. L. and MILES, L. E. M. (1978). Kinetics of two-site immunoradiometric ('sandwich') assays—II. Studies on the nature of the 'high-dose hook' effects. *Immunochemistry*, **15**, 77.

[84] ROTHENBERG, S. P. (1968). A radioassay for serum B_{12} using unsaturated transcobalamin I as the binding protein. *Blood*, **31**, 44.

[85] ROTHENBERG, S. P., MARCOULIS, G. P., SCHWARZ, S. and LADER, E. (1984). Measurement of cyanocobalamin in serum by a specific radioimmunoassay. *Journal of Laboratory and Clinical Medicine*, **103**, 959.

[86] SCHILLING, R. F. (1953). Intrinsic factor studies. II. The effect of gastric juice on the urinary excretion of radioactivity after the oral administration of radioactive vitamin B_{12}. *Journal of Laboratory and Clinical Medicine*, **42**, 860.

[87] SCOTT, J. M., BLOOMFIELD, F. J., STEBBINS, R. and HERBERT, V. (1974). Studies on derivation of transcobalamin III from granulocytes. Enhancement by lithium and elimination by fluoride of *in vitro* increments in vitamin B_{12}-binding capacity. *Journal of Clinical Investigation*, **53**, 228.

[88] SHACKLETON, P. J., FISH, D. I. and DAWSON, D. W. (1989). Intrinsic factor antibody tests. *Journal of Clinical Pathology*, **42**, 210.

[89] SHANE, B., TAMURA, T. and STOKSTAD, E. L. R. (1980). Folate assay: a comparison of radioassay and microbiological methods. *Clinica Chimica Acta*. **100**, 13.

[90] SHUM, R. Y., O'NEILL, B. J. and STREETER, A. M. (1971). Effect of pH changes on the binding of vitamin B_{12} by intrinsic factor. *Journal of Clinical Pathology*, **24**, 239.

[91] STAMP, LORD (1947). The preservation of bacteria by drying. *Journal of General Microbiology*, **1**, 251.

[92] TAIT, C. E. and HESP, R. (1976). Measurement of ^{57}Co-vitamin B_{12} uptake using a static whole-body counter. *British Journal of Radiology*, **49**, 948.

[93] TIBBLING, G. (1969). A method for determination of vitamin B_{12} in serum by radioassay. *Clinica Chimica Acta*, **23**, 209.

[94] WATERS, A. H. and MOLLIN, D. L. (1961). Studies on the folic acid activity of human serum. *Journal of Clinical Pathology*, **14**, 335.

[95] WATERS, H. M., SMITH, C., HOWARTH, J. E., DAWSON, D. W. and DELAMORE, I. W. (1989). A new enzyme immunoassay for the detection of total, type I and type II intrinsic factor antibody. *Journal of Clinical Pathology*, **42**, 307.

[96] WICKRAMASINGHE, S. N. and MATTHEWS, J. H. (1988). Deoxyuridine suppression: biochemical basis and diagnostic applications. *Blood Reviews*, **2**, 168.

[97] WILSON, M. B. and NAKANE, P. K. (1978). Recent developments in the periodate method of conjugating horseradish peroxidase (HRPO) to antibodies. In *Immunofluorescence and Related Staining Techniques*. Eds. W. Knapp, K. Holubar, G. Wick, p. 215–24. Elsevier/North-Holland, Amsterdam.

[98] WORWOOD, M. (1980). Iron: serum ferritin. *Methods in Hematology*, **1**, 59.

[99] WORWOOD, M. (1982). Ferritin in human tissues and serum. *Clinics in Haematology*, **11**, 275.

[100] WORWOOD, M. (1986). Serum ferritin (Editorial review). *Clinical Science*, **70**, 215.

[101] International Committee for Standardization in Haematology (Expert Panel on Iron) (1990). Revised recommendations for the measurement of serum iron in human blood. *British Journal of Haematology*, **75**, 613.

26. Red cell blood-group antigens and antibodies

(By A. H. Waters and E. E. Lloyd)

In one short chapter it is impossible to give a detailed survey of the human blood groups. Facts basic to an understanding of clinical blood-group serology are given together with a description of important serological techniques.

In recent years platelet and leucocyte antigens and antibodies have been extensively studied. These are discussed in Chapter 27. The present chapter deals exclusively with red cell antigens and antibodies.

RED CELL BLOOD GROUPS

Since Landsteiner's discovery in 1901 that human blood groups existed, a vast body of serological, genetic and more recently biochemical data on red cell blood-group antigens has been accumulated.

About 200 red cell antigens have been described, most of which have been assigned to well defined blood-group systems (Table 26.1). Apart from the ABO system, most of these antigens were detected by antibodies stimulated by transfusion or pregnancy.

Almost all blood-group genes are expressed as co-dominant antigens, i.e. both genes are expressed in the heterozygote. Some blood-group genes have been assigned to specific chromosomes, e.g. ABO system on chromosome 9, Rh system on chromosome 1 (Table 26.1).

The clinical importance of a blood-group antigen depends on the frequency of occurrence of the corresponding antibody and its ability to haemolyse red cells in vivo. On these criteria, the ABO and Rh systems are of major clinical importance. Anti-A and anti-B occur regularly, and are capable of causing severe intravascular haemolysis after an incompatible transfusion. The Rh D antigen is the most immunogenic red cell antigen after A and B, being capable of stimulating anti-D production after transfusion or pregnancy in the majority of Rh D-negative individuals.

Table 26.1 Major blood-group systems in historical order of discovery

Year	System	Main antigens	Chromosome location
1901	ABO	A, B	9
1927	MNSs	M, N, S, s	4
1927	P	P_1, P, P^k, p	22(?)
1939	Rh	C, c, D, (d), E, e	1
1945	Lutheran	Lu^a, Lu^b	19
1946	Kell	K, k, Kp^a, Kp^b, Js^a, Js^b	–
1946	Lewis	Le^a, Le^b	19
1950	Duffy	Fy^a, Fy^b	1
1951	Kidd	Jk^a, Jk^b	2
1952	Vel	Vel^1, Vel^2	–
1953	Wright	Wr^a, Wr^b	–
1955	Diego	Di^a, Di^b	–
1956	Cartwright	Yt^a, Yt^b	–
1956	I	Ii	–
1962	Xg	Xg^a	X
1962	Scianna	Sc^1, Sc^2	1
1965	Dombrock	Do^a, Do^b	–
1965	Colton	Co^a, Co^b	–

ABO SYSTEM

Discovery of the ABO system by Landsteiner in 1901 marked the beginning of safe blood transfusion. The ABO antigens, although most important in relation to transfusion, also have variable expression on most tissues and are important histocompatibility antigens.

Antigens (Table 26.2)

There are four main blood groups: A, B, AB and O. There is racial variation in the frequency of these groups; in the British Caucasian population the frequency of group O is 46%, A 42%, B 9% and AB 3%.[28,30]

The presence of A, B or O antigens on red cells is determined by the inheritance of the allelic genes A, B and O on chromosome 9, which are inherited in pairs as Mendelian dominants. The cellular expression of A and B antigens is determined by a further gene, the H gene, which is inherited independently: this gene codes for an enzyme that converts a carbohydrate precursor into H substance on which the A and B gene products act. The A and B genes code for specific enzymes (glycosyl transferases) which convert H substance into A and B antigens by the terminal addition of N-acetyl-D-galactosamine and D-galactose, respectively (Fig. 26.1). The O gene is a 'silent' (amorphic) allele which does not produce an active transferase, so that H substance persists unchanged in group O. In the extremely rare Oh Bombay phenotype, the H genotype is 'silent' (hh) and no H-transferase is produced; consequently no H substance is made

Table 26.2 The ABO antigens and antibodies

Blood group	Antigens	Antibodies normally present in serum	Antibodies occasionally present in serum
A_1B	$A + A_1 + B$	None	Anti-H
A_2B	A + B	None	Anti-A_1 (25–30% of sera)
A_1	$A + A_1$	Anti-B	Anti-H
A_2	A	Anti-B	Anti-A_1 (1–2% of sera)
B	B	Anti-A + Anti-A_1	Anti-H
O	None	Anti-A + Anti-A_1 + Anti-B	None

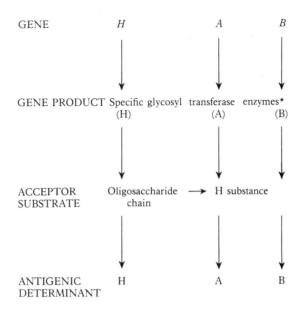

GENE	H	A	B

GENE PRODUCT Specific glycosyl transferase enzymes*
              (H)   (A)   (B)

ACCEPTOR   Oligosaccharide → H substance
SUBSTRATE   chain

ANTIGENIC DETERMINANT	H	A	B

Fig. 26.1 Pathways from *HAB* blood-group genes to antigens.
*Glycosyl transferase H transfers *L*-fucose; A transfers *N*-acetyl-D-galactosamine; B transfers *D*-galactose.

and therefore *A* and *B* genes, if present, cannot be expressed. These individuals have anti-A, anti-B and anti-H in their blood, all active at 37°C, and can only be safely transfused with other Oh blood.

Serologists have defined two common sub-groups of the A antigen: about 20% of group 'A' and group 'AB' subjects belong to group A_2 and group A_2B respectively, and the remainder belong to group A_1 and group A_1B. The distinction is most conveniently made using the lectin from *Dolichos biflorus* which only reacts with A_1 cells. When the H antigen content of red cells is assessed by agglutination reactions with anti-H, the strength of reaction tends to be graded $O > A_2 > A_2B > B > A_1 > A_1B$. Antigens weaker than A are occasionally found (called A_3, A_x etc). These serological variations in the A antigen are due to mutant forms of the glycosyl transferases produced by the *A* gene, which are less efficient at transferring N-acetyl-D-galactosamine to C-2 in the hexose ring of H substance.

The A, B and H antigens are detectable early in fetal life, but are not fully developed on the red cells at birth. The number of antigen sites reaches 'adult' levels at about 1 year of age and remains the same throughout life until old age when a slight reduction may occur.

Secretors and non-secretors (Table 26.3)

The ability to secrete A, B and H substances in water-soluble form is controlled by a dominant secretor gene *Se* (allele *se*). In a Caucasian population, about 80% are secretors (genotype *SeSe* or *Sese*) and 20% non-secretors (genotype *sese*). Secretors have H substance in the saliva and other body fluids together with A and/or B substances depending on their blood group. Only traces of these substances are present in the secretions of non-secretors, although the antigens are normally expressed on their red cells and other tissues, and the corresponding blood-group substance is present in the plasma.

An individual's secretor status can be determined by testing for ABH substance in saliva (p. 438).

Antibodies

Anti-A and anti-B. A feature of the ABO system is the regular occurrence of anti-A and anti-B in the absence of the corresponding red cell antigens (Table 26.2) This allows for reverse (serum) grouping as a means of confirming the red cell phenotype.

Table 26.3 Secretor status

	Genes	Blood group of red cells	ABH substance present in saliva	Incidence
Secretors (soluble ABH) antigens secreted)	*SeSe*	A B	A + H B + H	80%
	Sese	AB O	A + B + H H	
Non-secretors (soluble ABH antigens not secreted)	*sese*	A, B, AB or O	None	20%

The antibodies are a potential cause of dangerous haemolytic reactions if transfusions are given without regard to ABO compatibility. Anti-A and anti-B are always, to some extent, naturally occurring and of IgM class. Although they react best at low temperatures, they are nevertheless potentially haemolytic at 37°C. Hyperimmune anti-A and anti-B occur less frequently, usually in response to transfusion or pregnancy, but may also be formed following the injection of some toxoids and vaccines. They are predominantly of IgG class and are usually produced by group-O and sometimes by group-A_2 individuals. Hyperimmune IgG anti-A and/or anti-B from group-O or group-A_2 mothers may cross the placenta and cause haemolytic disease of the newborn (HDN). These antibodies react over a wide thermal range and are more effective haemolysins than the naturally occurring antibodies. Group-O donors should always be screened for hyperimmune anti-A and anti-B antibodies which may cause haemolysis when group-O whole blood is transfused to recipients with A and B phenotypes. These dangerous 'universal' donors should be reserved for group-O recipients only, or the blood should be used as packed red cells.

Anti-A_1 and anti-H. An antibody reacting only with A_1 and A_1B cells, called anti-A_1, is occasionally found in the serum of group-A_2 subjects (1–2%) and not uncommonly in the serum of group-A_2B subjects (25–30%). An antibody reacting most strongly with O and A_2 cells, probably best referred to as anti-H, is sometimes found in the serum of group-A_1, -A_1B or -B subjects (Table 26.2).

These two antibodies normally act as cold agglutinins and rarely react with the appropriate red cell antigens at temperatures over 30°C. They seldom cause haemolytic reactions in vivo, but may be a source of confusion in room temperature compatibility tests. A notable, but rare, exception is the anti-H that occurs in the Bombay phenotype Oh, which is an IgM antibody and causes lysis at 37°C.

Rh SYSTEM

The rhesus (Rh) system was so named because the original antibody that was raised by injecting red cells of rhesus monkeys into rabbits and guinea-pigs reacted with most human red cells. The clinical importance of this system is due to the fact that Rh-negative individuals are easily stimulated to form Rh antibodies if transfused with Rh-positive blood or, in the case of pregnant women, if exposed to Rh-positive fetal red cells which have crossed the placenta.

Antigens

This is a very complex system. At its simplest, it is convenient to classify individuals as Rh positive or Rh negative depending on the presence of the D antigen. This is largely a preventive measure to avoid transfusing an Rh-negative recipient with the D antigen, which is the most immunogenic red cell antigen after A and B.

At a more comprehensive level, it is convenient to consider the Rh system as a single gene complex on chromosome 1, which gives rise to various combinations of three alternative antigens C or c, D or d and E or e, as originally suggested by Fisher; the *d* gene is now known to be amorphic without any corresponding antigen on the red cell. The gene complex is named either by the component antigens (e.g. CDe, cde) or by a single shorthand symbol (e.g. R^1 = CDe; r = cde). Thus a person may inherit CDe (R^1) from one parent and cde (r) from the other, and have the genotype CDe/cde (R^1r). The Rh genes in order of frequency and the corresponding shorthand notation are given in Table 26.4. Although two other nomenclatures are also used to describe the Rh system, namely, Wiener's Rh-Hr terminology and Rosenfield's numerical notation, the CDE nomenclature, derived from Fisher's original theory, is recommended by a WHO Expert Committee[39] in the interest of simplicity and uniformity.

The Rh antigens are defined by corresponding anti-sera, with the exception of 'anti-d' which does not exist because d is amorphic. Consequently the distinction between homozygous DD and heterozygous Dd cannot be made by direct serological testing; this may be resolved by informative family studies, otherwise the genotype can only be predicted from the phenotype on the basis of probability tables for the various Rh genotypes in the population (Table 28.1).

Less common antigens, such as C^w, D^u and e^s, have been described. The D^u antigen is a weak D phenotype associated with fewer antigen sites (p. 462). Rare deletions of Rh antigens may also occur, e.g. D variants, DC^w –, – D –, Rh null. There are racial differences in the distribution of Rh antigens, e.g. Rh D negativity is a Caucasian trait (c 15%), while lower levels of negativity in other ethnic groups are thought to be due to intermingling of Caucasian genes. D^u and e^s are commoner in blacks than in Caucasians.[28]

The Rh antigens are present only on red cells and are a structural part of the cell membrane.[4]

Complete absence of Rh antigens (Rh null phenotype) may be associated with a congenital haemolytic anaemia with spherocytes and stomatocytes in the blood film.[1]

Rh antigens are well developed before birth and can be demonstrated on the red cells of very early fetuses.

Antibodies

Fisher's nomenclature is convenient when applied to Rh antibodies, and antibodies acting against all the Rh antigens, except d, have been described, namely anti-D, anti-C, anti-c, anti-E, anti-e.

Rh antigens are restricted to red cells and Rh antibodies are due to allo-immunization by previous transfusion or pregnancy, except for some naturally-occurring forms of anti-E. They are usually IgG (sometimes with an IgM component), react best at 37°C, and do not fix complement. Haemolysis, when it occurs, is therefore extravascular and predominantly in the spleen. Anti-D is the most important clinically; it may cause haemolytic transfusion reactions and was a common cause of fetal death resulting from haemolytic disease of the newborn (HDN) before the introduction of anti-D prophylaxis in 1970. The other Rh antibodies, although much less common, may nevertheless cause haemolytic transfusion reactions and HDN.

OTHER BLOOD-GROUP SYSTEMS

Routine Rh D grouping before blood transfusion and the success of anti-D prophylaxis for Rh D negative mothers bearing Rh D positive infants have greatly reduced the incidence of allo-immunization to the D antigen. At the same time, the increasing use of blood transfusion has meant that more patients are being immunized by other antigens, especially Rh (c, E) and those of the Kell (K), Duffy (Fy^a) and Kidd (Jk^a) systems.[15] These antibodies have all been associated with haemolytic transfusion reactions and HDN.

Mollison et al[26a] analysed the prevalence of transfusion-induced red cell allo-antibodies in three large reported series (Table 26.5). Rh antibodies other than anti-D (or – CD or – DE)—mainly anti-c or anti-E—accounted for 55% of the total and anti-K and anti-Fy^a for a further 40%, leaving only

Table 26.4 The Rh genes in order of frequency (Fisher nomenclature) and the corresponding short notations

Fisher	Short notations	Approximate frequency (%)
CDe	R^1	41
cde	r	39
cDE	R^2	14
cDe	R^0	3
C^wDe	R^{1w}	1
cdE	r''	1
Cde	r'	1
CDE	R^z	rare
CdE	r^y	rare

Table 26.5   Relative frequency of immune red-cell allo-antibodies*

| Patient group | No. studied | Blood group allo-antibodies (% of total) | | | | |
		Rh**	K	Fy	Jk	Others
Transfused (some pregnant)	4177	55.1	28.7	11.2	4.3	0.7
Immediate HTR†	142	42.2	30.3	18.3	8.5	0.7
Delayed HTR†	82	34.2	14.6	15.9	32.9	2.4

*Excluding antibodies of ABO, Lewis, P systems and anti-M and anti-N.
**Excluding anti-D (or -CD or -DE); almost all were anti-c or anti-E.
†Haemolytic transfusion reaction.

Reproduced with permission from Mollison et al [26a] based on published data from several sources.

about 5% (mainly anti-Jk^a) for all other immune antibodies. The same relative frequency of the different red cell antibodies was found in a smaller group of patients who experienced immediate haemolytic transfusion reactions (HTR). On the other hand, the figures for delayed HTR showed a striking increase in the relative frequency of Jk antibodies. This probably reflects two characteristics of Jk antibodies. They are difficult to detect in pretransfusion compatibility tests (p. 465), especially at low concentration, due to the tendency for the antibody to disappear after previous stimulation. However, once boosted by a further transfusion, the antibody may cause severe haemolysis due to the combined effects of both IgG and C3 (p. 427), so that delayed HTR is more readily diagnosed than when caused by some other antibodies.

For a more detailed exposition of the blood-group systems the reader is referred to the monograph of Race and Sanger[30] and Mollison et al.[26]

MECHANISMS OF IMMUNE DESTRUCTION OF BLOOD CELLS

Immune haemolysis may be used as a model to illustrate the mechanisms of immune blood-cell destruction. Immune haemolysis depends on:

1. The *Ig class* of the antibody—for all practical purposes antibodies against red cell antigens are of IgM or IgG class.
2. The ability of the antibody to activate and fix *complement*.
3. Interaction with the *mononuclear phagocyte (MP) system*. The most important phagocyte par-

ticipating in immune haemolysis is the macrophage, predominantly in the spleen.

The mechanism of immune haemolysis determines the site of haemolysis:

(a) *Intravascular haemolysis* due to complement lysis is characteristic of IgM antibodies; some IgG antibodies also act as haemolysins. Red cells are typically destroyed by intravascular complement lysis in ABO incompatible transfusion reactions (p. 470). Most other allo-immune red cell destruction is extravascular and mediated by the MP system.

Red cell auto-antibodies may also cause intravascular haemolysis, especially the IgG auto-antibody of paroxysmal cold haemoglobinuria (PCH) (p. 500) and some IgM auto-antibodies of the cold haemagglutinin syndrome (p. 479). Complement-mediated intravascular haemolysis also occurs in drug-induced immune haemolysis of the immune-complex type (p. 502).

(b) *Extravascular haemolysis* by the MP system is characteristic of IgG antibodies and occurs predominantly in the spleen. Macrophages have Fcγ receptors for cell-bound IgG, and sensitized red cells may be wholly phagocytosed or lose part of the membrane and return to the circulation as a microspherocyte. Spherocytes are less deformable and more readily trapped in the spleen than normal cells, which shortens their life-span.

In addition to Fc receptor mediated phagocytosis, *antibody-dependent cell-mediated cytotoxicity (ADCC)* may also contribute to cell damage during the phase of close contact with splenic macrophages.[9]

Complement components may enhance red cell destruction. Complement activation by some IgM and most IgG red cell antibodies is not always complete, the red cell thus escaping intravascular haemolysis. The activation sequence stops at the C3 stage, and in these circumstances complement components can be detected on the red cell by the antiglobulin test using appropriate anti-complement reagents (p. 434).

The first activation product of C3 is membrane-bound C3b, which is constantly being broken down to C3bi. Red cells with these components on their surface adhere to phagocytes (monocytes, macrophages, granulocytes) which have corresponding membrane receptors (CR1 and CR3). These sensitized cells are rapidly sequestered in the liver because of its bulk of phagocytic (Kupffer) cells and large blood flow, but no engulfment occurs. When C3bi is cleaved, leaving only C3dg on the cell surface, the cells tagged with 'inactive' C3dg return to the circulation, as in CHAD (p. 480). However, when IgG is also present on the cell surface, C3b enhances phagocytosis, and under these circumstances both liver and spleen are important sites of extravascular haemolysis.

Macrophage activity is an important component of cell destruction and further study of cellular interactions at this stage of immune haemolysis may provide an explanation for the differing severity of haemolysis in patients with apparently similar antibodies. In-vitro macrophage (monocyte) assays are being introduced to supplement conventional serological techniques in order to assess this aspect of immune haemolysis.[10]

Factors that may affect the interaction between sensitized cells and macrophages include:

1. *IgG subclass.* IgG1 and IgG3 antibodies have a higher binding affinity to mononuclear Fcγ receptors than IgG2 and IgG4 antibodies.

2. *Antigen density* affects the number of antibody molecules bound to the cell surface.

3. *Fluid-phase IgG.* Serum IgG concentration is a determinant of Fc-dependent MP function. Normal levels of IgG block the adherence of sensitized red cells to monocyte Fc receptors in vitro. Haemoconcentration in the splenic simusoids is probably a major factor in minimizing this effect in vivo, which may explain why the spleen is about 100 times more efficient at removing IgG-sensitized red cells than the liver, in spite of its greater macrophage mass and higher blood flow.[10]

The initial effect of high-dose intravenous IgG is to cause blockade of macrophage Fcγ receptors.[6,13] This reduces the immune clearance of antibody-coated cells, and has particular application in the management of auto-immune thrombocytopenia and post-transfusion purpura.

4. *Regulation of macrophage activity.* This may depend on specific cytokines which regulate expression of receptors for IgG and complement (phagocytosis) and secretion of cytotoxins (ADCC). Steroids may diminish and infection may enhance this phase of immune cell destruction.

The rate of immune cell destruction is therefore determined by antigen and antibody characteristics and MP function. The severity of the resultant cytopenia is a balance between cell destruction and the compensatory capacity of the bone marrow to increase cell production.

ANTIGEN–ANTIBODY REACTIONS

The red cell is a convenient marker for serological reactions and agglutination or lysis (due to complement action) is a visible indication (end-point) of an antigen–antibody reaction. The reaction occurs in two stages: in the first stage, the antibody binds to the red cell antigen (sensitization); the second stage involves agglutination (or lysis) of the sensitized cells.

The *first stage,* i.e. association of antibody with antigen (sensitization), is reversible and the strength of binding (equilibrium constant) depends on the 'exactness of fit' between antigen and antibody. This is influenced by:

1. *Temperature*—cold antibodies (usually IgM) generally bind best to the red cell at a low temperature, e.g. 4°C, whereas warm antibodies (usually IgG) bind most efficiently at body temperature, i.e. 37°C.

2. *pH*—there is relatively little change in antibody binding over the pH range 5.5–8.5, but to ensure comparable results it is preferable to buffer

the saline in which serum or cells are diluted to a fixed pH, usually 7.0. Some antibody elution techniques depend on altering the pH to below 4 or above 10.

3. *Ionic strength* of the suspension medium—low ionic strength increases the rate of antibody binding. This is the basis of antibody detection tests using low ionic strength saline (LISS).

The *second stage* depends on various laboratory manipulations to promote agglutination or lysis of sensitized cells. The red cell surface is negatively charged (mainly due to sialic acid residues), which keeps individual cells apart; the minimum distance between red cells suspended in saline is about 18 nm. Agglutination is brought about by antibody cross-linking between cells. The span between antigen binding sites on IgM molecules (30 nm) is sufficient to allow IgM antibodies to bridge between saline suspended red cells (after settling) and so cause agglutination. IgG molecules have a shorter span (15 nm) and are usually unable to agglutinate sensitized red cells suspended in saline; notwithstanding, heavy IgG sensitization due to high antigen density lowers intercellular repulsive forces and is able to promote agglutination in saline (e.g. IgG anti-A, anti-B). However, it is standard procedure to promote agglutination of IgG sensitized red cells by:

1. Reducing intercellular distance by the addition of albumin or pretreatment of red cells with protease enzymes, e.g. papain or bromelin (p. 430).
2. Bridging between sensitized cells with an anti-human globulin reagent in the antiglobulin test (p. 433).

Some complement-binding antibodies (especially IgM) may cause lysis in vitro (without noticeable agglutination), which can be enhanced by the addition of fresh serum as a source of complement. On the other hand, complement activation may only proceed to the C3 stage; in these circumstances cell-bound C3 can be detected by the antiglobulin test using an appropriate anti-human complement reagent (p. 434).

GENERAL POINTS OF SEROLOGICAL TECHNIQUE AND QUALITY CONTROL

Blood-group serology is passing through a transitional phase with the introduction of monoclonal antibody (Mab) reagents and microplate technology. Mab reagents are in routine use for ABO grouping and are being introduced for Rh D grouping.[25,35] The rapid evolution of microplate technology for blood grouping and antibody screening makes it difficult to recommend standard methods and optimal conditions for these tests. Basic slide and tube methods are described, and the reader is referred to BCSH guidelines on microplate technology for blood grouping and antibody screening for the current state of the art.[3]

A high standard of proficiency in blood group serology requires a series of quality control steps each designed to identify any deficiency in reagents, techniques and equipment. This should be combined with the quality control of performance by external quality assessment schemes and 'in-house' exercises. This and the following chapter emphasize the importance of quality control for careful serological work in a hospital blood transfusion laboratory. For a more detailed exposition the reader is referred to the review by Voak and Napier.[38]

Health and safety

Whenever possible use reagents that have been screened for HIV and hepatitis B infection. All high-risk samples must be handled according to the laboratory safety code.

Standard operating procedures

All procedures must be detailed in a laboratory manual which must be readily accessible and regularly reviewed.

Collection and storage of blood samples

Venous blood is desirable for blood-grouping purposes and 5–10 ml of blood should be taken and allowed to clot at room temperature in a sterile glass tube. This will provide serum and cells. If serum is required urgently, the specimen may be placed in a 37°C water-bath and centrifuged as soon as the clot can be seen to have started to retract.

If necessary, the specimen, after clotting, can be stored undisturbed at 4°C overnight. If the red cells are to be kept longer than this, it is desirable to add the blood, after withdrawal, to a one-quarter volume of sterile ACD or CPD anticoagulant. If kept sterile, the red cells will be found to react well with most antibodies even after 2–3 weeks' storage. Red cells should be washed and suspended in saline just before use.

RED CELL SUSPENSIONS

(a) Normal ionic strength saline (NISS)

A 2% suspension of washed red cells in phosphate buffered saline, pH 7.0, is generally suitable for agglutination tests in tubes. Unless otherwise specified, throughout this text 'saline' or 'buffered saline' refers to 9 g/l NaCl buffered to pH 7.0 (see Appendix, p. 538).

(b) Low ionic strength saline (LISS)

It is known that the rate of association of antibodies with red cell antigens is enhanced by lowering the ionic strength of the medium in which the reactions take place. Nevertheless, there has been some reluctance to use low ionic strength media in routine laboratory work for two reasons: first, non-specific agglutination may occur when NaCl concentrations <2 g/l (0.03 mol/l) are used, and secondly, complement components are bound to the red cells at low ionic strengths.

A number of studies have, however, demonstrated that, provided certain precautions are observed, low ionic strength solutions (LISS) may be safely used in routine laboratory work.[24,27] The LISS solution can be made up in the laboratory (see Appendix, p. 536) or purchased commercially.[8]

The major advantage of LISS is that the incubation period in the IAT (p. 436) can be shortened whilst maintaining or increasing the sensitivity of the cells to the majority of red cell antibodies. LISS can in fact be used as a substitute for saline in grouping, antibody screening and identification, and in cross-matching.

To avoid false positives, the following rules should be followed:

1. Red cells resuspended in LISS and serum should be incubated together in equal volumes: 2 volumes of cells to 2 volumes of serum are recommended.

2. The red cells should be washed in saline before suspending in LISS.

3. The working solution of LISS should be kept at room temperature.

4. Excessive centrifugation (spinning) must be avoided, if using a spin technique.

Reagent red cells

Red cells of selected phenotypes are needed for ABO and Rh D grouping, Rh phenotyping, and antibody screening and identification (see Chapter 28). Such cells are available commercially or from Blood Transfusion Centres.

STORAGE OF SERA

Great care must be taken to identify and label correctly any serum separated from the patient's original blood sample.

Patient's sera are best stored frozen at −20°C (or better still at −40°C) in 1–2 ml volumes in glass or plastic vials. Repeated thawing of a sample is harmful. If the sera are stored at −20°C or below, no precautions as to sterility are necessary. At 4°C sterility is essential; if this can be maintained, it will be found that the sera will retain their potency for months.

Complement deteriorates quickly on storage, but sera separated from blood as quickly as possible and stored at −20°C retain most of their complement activity for 1–2 weeks. For compatibility tests, samples of serum should be separated from the red cells as soon as possible and stored at −20°C until used, as the content of complement may be important for the detection of some antibodies.

USE OF ENZYME-TREATED RED CELLS

Enzyme-treated red cells have proved to be valuable reagents in the detection and investigation of auto- and allo-antibodies. Papain and bromelin are currently used for this purpose. Enzyme treatment is known to increase the avidity of both IgM and IgG antibodies. The receptors of some blood-group antigens, however, may be inactivated by enzyme-treatment, e.g. M, N, S, Fy^a, Fy^b and Pr.

The most sensitive techniques are those using washed enzyme-pretreated red cells (two-stage techniques) which should match the performance of the spin tube LISS antiglobulin test (p. 435). One-stage mixture techniques are relatively insensitive and have caused many missed incompatibilities in external proficiency trials.[17,18] A recent one-stage inhibitor papain technique[31] has been shown to be slightly less sensitive than the two-stage technique, but far superior to the traditional Löw's one-stage mixture technique.[32] As such, the papain inhibitor technique is suitable as a supportive test for antibody detection and cross-matching of small batches (e.g. 12–24 tests) in routine hospital transfusion laboratories.

A joint Working Party of the ISBT/ICSH is currently addressing the problem of standardization of enzyme techniques, in particular the selection of enzyme reference preparations, assay methods and optimum techniques. Pending the release of this report, the reader should consult the recent review of papain techniques in blood-group serology by Scott et al.[32]

Löw's method for the preparation of papain solution[23]

A 1% solution of activated papain is made as follows:

Grind 2 g of papain (Merck) in a mortar in 100 ml of Sörensen's phosphate buffer, pH 5.4 (p. 539). Centrifuge for 10 min and add 10 ml of 0.5 mol/l cysteine hydrochloride to the supernatant to activate the enzyme. Dilute the solution to 200 ml with the phosphate buffer and incubate for 1 h at 37°C. Dispense the enzyme in small volumes (e.g. 0.1–0.2 ml); it will keep satisfactorily for many months at −20°C, but once a tube is unfrozen any of the solution not immediately used should be discarded.

The level of enzyme activity should be determined using an azoalbumin assay,[33] as this will determine the incubation time for enzyme treatment of the cells.

Two-stage papain method[16,32]

Add 1 volume of 1% papain (activated as described above) to 9 volumes of Sörensen's phosphate buffer, pH 7.0 (p. 539) in a 10 × 75 mm glass tube.

Incubate at 37°C equal volumes of the freshly diluted papain and packed washed red cells for a time which must be determined for each batch of papain depending on the azoalbumin activity;[32] this is normally 15–30 min. After incubation, wash the cells in two changes of saline, pH 7.0, then dilute as required—to 3% in NISS or 1.5% in LISS. For NISS tests, add 1 drop of NISS-suspended cells to 1 drop of serum. For LISS tests add 2 drops of LISS-suspended cells to 2 drops of serum. Incubate for 15 min in a 37°C water-bath.

One-stage papain inhibitor method[31,32]

Add 1 drop of papain solution (azoalbumin activity 1.0) to 1 drop of 3% NISS-suspended red cells, or two drops of 1.5% LISS-suspended red cells, in a 10 × 75 mm glass tube. Mix by shaking and incubate for 3 min in a 37°C water-bath. Add 1 drop of a 1 in 10 dilution in PBS of 1 mmol/l E-64, a synthetic peptide papain inhibitor, shake and allow to incubate for a further 2 min for inhibition to occur. Then add 2 drops of serum, shake and incubate for 15 min, also in the 37°C water-bath.

For both methods, after incubation, centrifuge the tubes for 15 s at 500 g. Gently transfer the cells to a microscope slide by pipette and read macroscopically, then microscopically (p. 431)

Preparation of bromelin solution[29]

Prepare a 0.5% solution by dissolving the bromelin powder in a mixture of 9 volumes of saline and 1 volume of Sörensen's phosphate buffer, pH 5.4 (p. 539). Store the solution in 0.5–1.0 ml volumes at −20°C, at which temperature it will keep for months. As preservatives, add 0.1% sodium azide and 0.5% Actidione (a fungicide). Add the bromelin, as papain is added in Löw's technique, to the serum just before the addition of the red cells. There is no need to pre-treat the red cells with the enzyme. Bromelin activity can be assessed by an azoalbumin assay.

Controls are particularly important when enzyme-treated cells are being used, and it must be established without question that the altered cells are reacting appropriately with sera of known antibody content. Only in this way can the potency of the enzyme and the method of enzyme treatment be checked. Enzyme-treated cells are compared with untreated cells in reactions with a positive control (0.25 iu/ml anti-D) and a negative (inert) control (AB serum or fresh compatible serum).

AGGLUTINATION OF RED CELLS BY ANTIBODY: A BASIC METHOD

Agglutination tests are usually carried out in tubes—either sedimentation tube tests or spin tube tests. Slide tests are sometimes used for emergency ABO and Rh D grouping (p. 458, p. 462).

Add 1 volume of a 2% red cell suspension to 1 volume of serum or serum dilution in a disposable plastic tube or glass tube. Mix well and leave undisturbed for the appropriate time (see below).

Tubes. For agglutination tests use medium-sized (75 × 10 or 12 mm) disposable plastic or glass tubes. Similar tubes should be used for lysis tests when it is essential to have a relatively deep layer of serum to look through, if small amounts of lysis are to be detected. The level of the fluid must rise well above the concave bottom of the tubes.

Glass tubes should always be used if the contents are to be heated to 50°C or higher, or if organic solvents are being used. Glass tubes, however, are difficult to clean satisfactorily, particularly small bore tubes, and methods such as those given in the Appendix (p. 540) should be followed in detail.

Temperature and time of exposure of red cells to antibody

In blood-grouping work tube tests are generally done at 37°C and/or room temperature. There is some advantage in using a 20°C water-bath rather than relying on 'room temperature' which in different countries and seasons may vary from 15°C (or less) to 30°C (or more).

Agglutination reactions carried out in tubes are usually read after 1–2 h have elapsed. Strong agglutination will, however, be obvious much sooner than this. Agglutination can be read after only 5–10 min incubation if the cell-serum mixture is centrifuged.

READING RESULTS OF AGGLUTINATION TESTS

Slide tests

Because of evaporation, slide tests must be read within about 5 min. Reagents which produce strong agglutination within 1–2 min are normally used and the tests are employed for rapid ABO and Rh D grouping. Since the results are read macroscopically, strong cell suspensions (c 20%) should be used.

Tube tests

Only the strongest complete (C) grade of agglutination seems to be able to withstand a shake procedure without some degree of disruption which may downgrade the strength of reaction. The BCSH Blood Transfusion Task Force has therefore recommended the following reading procedures:[2]

(a) Microscopic reading

It is essential that a careful and standardized technique be followed. Lift the tube carefully from its rack without disturbing the button of sedimented cells. Holding the tube vertically, introduce a Pasteur pipette, with its tip cut at 90°. Carefully draw up a column of supernatant about 1 cm in length and then, without introducing an air bubble, draw up a 1–2 mm column of red cells by placing the tip of the pipette in the button of red cells. Gently expel the supernatant and cells on to a slide over an area of about 2 × 1 cm. It is important not to overload the suspension with cells, and the method described above achieves this.

The scheme of scoring the results, which is given in Table 26.6, is recommended for the UK External Quality Assessment Scheme for Blood-Group Serology.

(b) Macroscopic reading

A gentle agitation tip-and-roll 'macroscopic' method is recommended. It is possible to read agglutination tests macroscopically with the aid of a hand reading-glass or concave mirror, but it is then difficult to distinguish reactions weaker

Table 26.6   Scoring of results in red cell agglutination tests

Symbol	Agglutination score*	Description
4 + or C (complete)	12	Cell button remains in one clump, macroscopically visible
3 + or V (visual)	10	Cell button dislodges into several large clumps, macroscopically visible
2 +	8	Cell button dislodges into many small clumps, macroscopically visible
1 +	5	Cell button dislodges into finely granular clumps, macroscopically just visible
$\frac{1}{2}$(+)	3	Cell button dislodges into fine granules, only visible microscopically **
–	0	Negative result—all cells free and evenly distributed

*Titration scores are the summation of the agglutination scores at each dilution.
** May be further classified depending on the number of cells in the clumps, e.g. clumps of 12–20 cells (score 3); 8–10 cells (score 2); 4–6 cells (score 1)– this is the minimum agglutination that should be considered positive.

than + (microscopic reading) from the normal slight granular appearance of unagglutinated red cells in suspension. Macroscopic reading thus gives lower titration values than does microscopic reading. Follow the system of scoring in Table 26.6.

A good idea of the presence or absence of agglutination can often be obtained by inspection of the deposit of sedimented cells: a perfectly smooth round button suggests no agglutination whilst agglutination is shown by varying degrees of irregularity, 'graininess' or dispersion of the deposit (Fig. 26.2).

DEMONSTRATION OF LYSIS

Many blood-group antibodies lyse red cells under suitable conditions in the presence of complement.

This is particularly true of anti-A and anti-B, anti-P, anti-Lewis, anti-P + P_1 + P^k(anti-Tj^a) and certain auto-antibodies (p. 496). Lysis should be looked for at the end of the incubation period before the tubes are centrifuged, if the cells have sedimented sufficiently; it may be scored roughly quantitatively after centrifuging the suspensions and comparing the colour of the supernatant with that of the control.

If the occurrence of lysis is of interest, then the final volume of the cell-serum suspension has to be greater than is required for the reading of agglutination. 75 × 10 or 12 mm tubes should be used and the level of the cell-serum suspension must rise well above the concave bottom of the tubes.

In testing for lytic activity a high concentration of complement may be required. Therefore, in con-

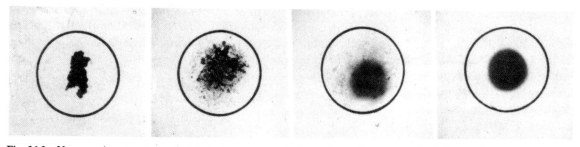

Fig. 26.2   Macroscopic appearances of agglutination in round-bottom tubes or hollow tiles. Agglutination is shown by various degrees of 'graininess'; in the absence of agglutination the sedimented cells appear as a smooth round button, as on the extreme right.

trast to tests for agglutination, it is often advantageous to use a stronger red cell suspension (c 5%).

Lysis tests are usually carried out at 37°C, but with cold antibodies a lower temperature, e.g. 20°C or 30°C, would be appropriate, depending on the upper thermal range of activity of the antibody, or, in the case of the Donath-Landsteiner antibody, 0°C followed by 37°C (p. 500).

Methods for titrating an antibody to demonstrate its lysis titre are described on p. 498. With certain antibodies, too, the pH of the cell-serum suspension affects the occurrence of lysis (p. 496).

Controls

It is necessary to be sure that any lysis observed is not artefactual, i.e. that lysis is brought about by the serum under test and not by the serum added as complement, and that the added complement is potent. A complement control (no test serum) is thus necessary and also a control using a serum known to contain a lytic antibody.

In lysis tests, great care should be taken to deliver the cell suspension directly into the serum. If the cell suspension comes into contact with the side of the tube and starts to dry, this in itself will lead to lysis.

ANTIGLOBULIN TEST

The antiglobulin test (Coombs test) was introduced by Coombs, Mourant and Race in 1945[7] as a method for detecting 'incomplete' Rh antibodies, i.e. IgG antibodies capable of sensitizing red cells, but incapable of causing agglutination of the same cells suspended in saline, as opposed to 'complete' IgM antibodies which do agglutinate saline-suspended red cells.

Direct and indirect antiglobulin tests can be carried out. In the *direct* test (DAT) the patient's cells, after careful washing, are tested for in-vivo sensitization; in the *indirect* test (IAT) normal red cells are incubated with a serum suspected of containing an antibody and subsequently tested, after washing, for in-vitro bound antibody.

The antiglobulin test is probably the most important test in the serologist's repertoire. The DAT is used to demonstrate in-vivo attachment of antibodies to red cells, as in auto-immune haemolytic anaemia (p. 487), allo-immune haemolytic disease of the newborn (p. 472), and allo-immune haemolysis following an incompatible transfusion (p. 469). The IAT has wide application in blood transfusion serology, including antibody screening and identification and cross-matching.

ANTI-HUMAN GLOBULIN (AHG) REAGENTS

(a) Polyspecific (broad-spectrum) AHG reagents

These should contain both anti-IgG and anti-complement.

The majority of red cell antibodies are non-complement-binding IgG; anti-IgG is therefore an essential component of any polyspecific reagent. Anti-IgA is not required as IgG antibodies of the same specificity always occur in the presence of IgA antibodies. Anti-IgM is also not required because clinically significant IgM allo-antibodies that do not cause agglutination in saline are much more easily detected by the complement they bind.

Antibodies to human complement components are necessary to detect clinically significant antibodies that bind complement, but which may react only weakly in anti-IgG tests.[12,33] Such antibodies include anti-Kidd, anti-Kell and anti-Lewis specificities, e.g. anti-Jk[a], which may be barely detectable by anti-IgG with heterozygous Jk(a + b +) red cells, but may be readily detected by a polyspecific reagent containing anti-complement.[36]

The question arises as to which anti-complement antibodies are best for the detection of complement binding allo-antibodies. If red cells are not lysed immediately, complement activation usually stops at the C3 stage. The first activation product of C3 is C3b which reacts with antibodies against the C3c and C3d parts of the molecule (Table 26.7). Conversion of C3b to C3bi takes place rapidly and exposes another antigenic determinant C3g[21,22] and red cells at this stage (coinciding with incubation times of 15–45 min) are agglutinated by anti-C3c, anti-C3g and anti-C3d.[2] After further inactivation C3c is split off and reactions with anti-C3g and anti-C3d remain. Conversion of C3bi to C3dg, as determined by loss of reactivity with anti-C3c, may be complete within 2 h in the presence of excess serum at 37°C.[5,34] However, with the amount of serum routinely used in the indirect antiglobulin test and the shorter incubation times which are now used, little C3c is lost.[14] Anti-C3c is therefore probably the optimal anti-complement antibody to detect cell-bound complement in polyspecific AHG; especially as it gives rise to relatively few false-positive reactions. Nevertheless, to cover the wide range of incubation times still being used in antiglobulin tests it would be safer not to rely entirely on anti-C3c, but to use a combination of anti-C3c and anti-C3g or anti-C3d. Anti-C3g would be preferable to anti-C3d as the additional antibody, as it causes fewer false-positive reactions, but it is not readily available. Unfortunately, C3d accumulates on red cells stored at 4°C (ACD, CPD or clotted samples), much more than C3c or C3g. Anti-C3d is therefore a major cause of false-positive reactions and its strength in a polyspecific AHG reagent must be carefully controlled. However, potent monoclonal anti-C3d reagents are now available (e.g. BRIC-8)[19] that cause fewer false-positive reactions at higher titres and are suitable for mixing with anti-IgG in a polyspecific reagent. The complement component C4 also accumulates on red cells stored at 4°C; for this reason the AHG reagent must contain little or no anti-C4 which is a nuisance antibody causing false-positive reactions.

(b) Monospecific AHG reagents

These can be prepared against the heavy chains of IgG, IgM and IgA and are referred to as anti-γ, anti-μ and anti-α; antibodies against IgG subclasses are also available. Specific antibodies against the complement components C4 and C3 and C3 breakdown products can be prepared as mentioned above.

The main clinical application of these monospecific AHG reagents is to define the immunochemical characteristics of antibodies. This is relevant to the mechanisms of in-vivo cell destruction and, in the case of IgG, the subclasses have different biological properties (p. 426).

QUALITY CONTROL OF AHG REAGENTS

The quality control of AHG reagents must always be carried out by the exact technique by which they are to be used. All reagents should be used according to the manufacturer's instructions, unless appropriately standardized for other methods.

The ISBT/ICSH Working Party on the Standardization of Antiglobulin Reagents has recommended the use of polyspecific AHG reagents for compatibility testing by spin tube techniques and has selected two international reference reagents:

1. Conventional polyclonal reagent (designated R3P)
2. A monoclonal anti-complement blend with a rabbit anti-IgG (designated R3M).

Table 26.7 C3 determinants in various C3 states on red cells[22]

C3 state	C3b complete →	C3bi →	C3gd(α_2D) →	C3d**
Components	c + (g −)*d +	c + g + d +	g + d +	d +
Monoclonal antibody reactions	anti-C3c anti-C3d	anti-C3c anti-C3g anti-C3d	anti-C3g anti-C3d	anti-C3d

*g is concealed in C3b.
**Red cells treated with trypsin; the final C3 fragment found on red cells in vivo is C3dg.

Both reagents are available from Professor C. P. Engelfriet, CLB, POB 9190, NL-1006 AD Amsterdam. The full specification of these reference reagents and details of the indicator systems used have been published.[12]

The quality control procedure should assess the following qualities of the reagent:

1. *Specificity.* The reagent should only agglutinate red cells sensitized with antibodies and/or coated with significant levels of complement components.

2. *Potency of anti-IgG* by serological titration.

3. *Specificity and potency of anti-complement antibodies.* A polyspecific reagent should contain anti-C3c and anti-C3d at controlled levels to avoid false-positive reactions or a suitable potent monoclonal anti-C3d (e.g. BRIC-8). It should contain little or no anti-C4. The assessment of these qualities requires red cells specifically coated with C3b, C3bi, C3d and C4. Details of the procedures recommended for the preparation of such cells have been published by the above Working Party.[36]

It is appreciated that some hospital blood banks will be unable to evaluate the specification of an AHG reagent as comprehensively as outlined above. They should, however, carry out the following minimal assessment of all new AHG reagents:

1. Test the AHG reagent for freedom from false positives by simulated cross-match tests.

(a) Test for excess anti-C3d by incubating fresh serum at 37°C by NISS and LISS tests with six ABO compatible cells from CPD-A1 donor unit segments (10–30 days old). This is a critical test for false positives due to C3d uptake by stored blood which is further augmented by incubation with fresh serum.

(b) Tests for contaminating red cell antibodies (against washed A_1, B and O cells) must be negative.

Only proceed further if the AHG reagent passes the above tests.

2. Compare the AHG reagent with the current reagent using a selection of weak antibodies. These antibodies may be selected from those encountered in routine work or can be obtained from a Regional Transfusion Centre or Reference Laboratory. Store such antibodies in small volumes at −40°C for repeated tests.

3. Dilute a weak IgG anti-D (0.8 iu, for routine AHG test controls, from undiluted (neat) to 1 in 16 and sensitize R_1r red cells with each dilution of anti-D. These sensitized cells (washed × 4) should then be tested with neat to 1 in 8 dilutions of the AHG reagents. The AHG reagent should not show prozones by immediate spin tests using 2 volumes of AHG per test. The potency of the test AHG should at least match the current AHG reagent.

One of the international AHG reference reagents can be used to calibrate an 'in-house' AHG reagent for use as a routine standard.

The quality control of Ig class and sub-class specific AHG reagents, while following the above general principles, is more complex. Details of the appropriate techniques are beyond the scope of this chapter and the reader should consult the review by Englefriet et al.[11]

RECOMMENDED ANTIGLOBULIN TEST PROCEDURE

A spin tube technique is recommended for the routine antiglobulin test and the procedure described here is based on BCSH *Guidelines for Compatibility Testing in Hospital Blood Banks.*[2] Reliable performance depends on the correct procedure at each stage of the test and appropriate quality control measures.

The test should be carried out in glass tubes (75 × 10 or 12 mm). Plastic tubes are not recommended as they may adsorb IgG which could neutralize anti-IgG of the AHG reagent.

1. Sensitize red cells (not relevant to the direct test) by using the following serum : cell ratios:

(a) For normal ionic strength saline (NISS), use 2 volumes of serum and 1 volume of a 3% suspension of red cells washed (× 3) and suspended in phosphate buffered saline (PBS) or 0.15 mol/l NaCl (Appendix, p. 538).

(b) For low ionic strength saline (LISS), use 2 volumes of serum and 2 volumes of a 1.5% suspension of red cells washed (× 2) in PBS or 0.15 mol/l NaCl and once in LISS and then suspended in 0.033 mol/l LISS (Appendix p. 534).

(c) For commercial low ionic strength additive solutions, the manufacturer's instructions must be followed.

As the volume of 'a drop' varies according to the type of pipette or dropper bottle, a measured or known drop volume should be used to ensure that appropriate serum : cell ratios are maintained.

Mix the reactants by shaking, then incubate at 37°C, preferably in a water-bath, for a minimum period of 15 min for LISS tests and 45 min for NISS tests.

2. *Wash the test cells* 4 times with a minimum of 3 ml of saline per wash. Vigorous injection of saline is necessary to resuspend the cells and achieve adequate mixing. As much of the supernatant as possible should removed after each wash to achieve maximum dilution of residual serum.

3. *Add 2 volumes of a suitable AHG reagent* to each test tube and centrifuge after thorough mixing. The combinations of centrifugal force (RCF) and time for spin-tube tests are as follows:

RCF (g)	100	200–220	500	1000
Time (seconds)	60	25–30	15	8–10

4. *Read agglutination* as previously described (p. 431).

5. *Quality control of the test* should be monitored by:

(a) An IgG anti-D diluted to give 1 + or 2 + reactions with Rh D positive (R_1r) cells as a *positive control*.

(b) An inert group AB serum with the same Rh D positive cells as a *negative control;* this is not essential as most tests are negative.

(c) *The addition of sensitized cells to all negative tests.* This is widely used to detect neutralization of the AHG reagent due to incomplete removal of serum by the wash step. The value of this test as a control depends on the strength of reaction of the sensitized cells. Appropriate control cells sensitized with IgG anti-D should give a 3 + reaction when tested directly with the AHG reagent and should still be positive (if the AHG is potent) when added to negative tests, but downgraded (1 + or 2 +) due to the 'pooled-cell' effect of the non-sensitized cells. The reaction will of course be negative if the

AHG has been neutralized by residual serum.

The production of satisfactory AHG control cells can be achieved by limiting the level of anti-D sensitization to that which gives a negative test in the presence of 1 in 1000 parts serum in saline.

The suitability of the AHG control cells can be checked as follows:

i. Prepare two tubes (10 × 75 mm) with one volume of 3% unsensitized cells; wash four times.

ii. Add two volumes of AHG to each of the tubes, mix well, spin and read the tubes to confirm the tests are negative.

iii. Add one volume of 1 in 1000 serum in saline to one tube and one volume of saline as a control to the other tube.

iv. Add one volume of AHG control cells to each tube, mix, spin and read the tests.

The test containing 1 in 1000 serum in saline should be negative and the control tube should give at least a 2 + reaction. The direct test with AHG and the AHG control cells should be 3 +, and should be 'down-graded' in a washed negative antiglobulin test to 1 + or 2 + due to the 'pooled cell' effects.

A negative reaction with this control suggests a washing deficiency and demands corrective action. If an automated cell washing centrifuge is used, the washing efficiency should be checked; see *Quality Control of Cell Washing Centrifuges.*[2]

TWO-STAGE EDTA-COMPLEMENT INDIRECT ANTIGLOBULIN TEST

Stored serum may become anticomplementary. To overcome this, a two-stage method is recommended. Antibody is taken up in the first stage and complement in the second stage.

Add 1 drop of a 3% suspension of red cells to 4 drops of EDTA-treated serum, prepared by adding 0.1 ml of neutral EDTA (i.e. 11 µmol; *c* 4 mg) (p. 536) per ml of serum, and incubate at 37°C for 1 h. Wash the cells 3 times in saline and then reincubate with 2 drops of compatible fresh normal serum for 15 min at 37°C. Finally wash the cells and treat them in the usual manner for the IAT.

ASSESSMENT OF INDIVIDUAL WORKER PERFORMANCE

It is recommended that all staff (including 'on-call' staff who do not routinely work in the blood bank) should be assessed at regular intervals. A procedure based on 'blind' replicate antiglobulin tests may be used for this purpose.[37]

The procedure, as set out in the BCSH Guidelines for Compatibility Testing in Hospital Blood Banks,[2] is as follows:

1. A local low titre (8–16) IgG anti-D, as used for the control of the AHG test, should be titrated against R_1r or pooled O Rh D-positive cells to find the dilution of anti-D that gives $1+$ or $2+$ sensitized cells (most workers use around 0.3 iu/ml).

2. A batch of sensitized cells is prepared, e.g. by incubating 16 ml of the selected anti-D dilution with 8 ml of 3–5% washed R_1r red cells.

3. Twelve tubes are labelled for blind tests by another person. One volume of 3% $1+$ or $2+$ sensitized cells and 2 volumes of group AB inert serum (to simulate the volumes of serum used in routine tests) are placed in nine random tubes, and then 1 volume of unsensitized cells + 2 volumes of group-AB inert serum are placed in the remaining tubes. The position of the various tests is recorded.

4. The cells are washed thoroughly 4 times, AHG is added and the are tests spun and read.

5. The number of false negative (and false positive) results are recorded for each worker and analysed in relation to reading and/or washing technique. It is advisable to give immediate tuition to any workers with washing or reading test faults, followed by further blind replicate trials to demonstrate improvement in procedure and to restore the confidence of the person.

TITRATION OF ANTIBODIES

Preparation of serial dilutions of patient's or other sera

When comparing the effect of different temperatures on agglutination or the different sensitivities of several types of red cells, it is important to make a set of master serial dilutions of the serum being tested and to subsample an appropriate number of small volumes from each dilution as it is made.

Doubling dilutions are usually made and can be prepared by adding an equal volume of serum to the diluent and transferring the same volume of the mixture to the next volume of diluent and so on. The dilutions may be made with a marked glass Pasteur pipette. Commercially available Pasteur pipettes are satisfactory, and provided the

Table 26.8 Comparison of titration end-points of a high-titre cold agglutinin using conventional doubling dilution techniques with those obtained by making dilutions with separate pipettes.

Final serum dilution		1 in 1024	1 in 4096	1 in 16 000	1 in 64 000	1 in 256 000	1 in 1 000 000	Control (saline)
1. in Doubling dilutions using Pasteur pipette								
(a) no mixing in stem	macro	+	+	+	[+]	–	–	–
	micro	+	+	+	+	+	[+]	–
(b) with mixing in stem	macro	+	+	+	weak	–	–	–
	micro	+	+	+	+	+	[+]	–
2. Doubling dilutions using glass automatic	macro	+	+	+	[+]	(?)	–	–
pipette	micro	+	+	+	+	+	[+]	–
3. Dilutions prepared using a separate	macro	+	+	[+]	(?)	–	–	–
pipette for each dilution	micro	+	+	+	[+]	–	–	–

The titre read macroscopically was recorded as 32,000.

Only the results of readings made on the last seven alternate tubes of the titrations are recorded. The doubling dilutions were prepared commencing with undiluted serum, and the separate dilutions (3 above) were prepared from an initial serum dilution of 1 in 256.

The titrations were carried out at room temperature (18°C) and the end-points of the titration were determined macroscopically (macro) using a concave mirror, and also microscopically (micro). The end-points are indicated [+].

The end-points determined macroscopially using the conventional doubling-dilution techniques give results which closely approximate to those is obtained when dilutions of serum are prepared using a separate pipette for each dilution and the result is read microscopically.

ends are not chipped, the pipettes, if held vertically, will deliver 30 ± 1 drops to the ml. Sometimes when the serum is in short supply it is convenient to use fine-bore '50-dropper' pipettes.

The methods of making dilutions, referred to above, suffer from 'carry over' of serum—that is to say, traces of concentrated serum remain in the pipette and tend to increase the concentration of serum in the tubes which should contain only highly diluted serum. This results in erroneously high titration figures and long drawn-out end-points. However, the titrations are easy to carry out and the results obtained have a relative value and are satisfactory for most clinical purposes. To obtain more accuracy it is necessary to use a separate accurately calibrated pipette for each dilution (Table 26.8).

Fourfold dilutions using a drop method

A method employing fourfold dilutions is economical of time and materials, and Fig. 26.3 illustrates how such a titration can be carried out using a drop technique. The master dilutions can be made by the drop method or if greater accuracy is desired by using separate pipettes for each dilution.

The diluent should be buffered saline, pH 7.0, for agglutination tests; or for lysis tests undiluted ABO-compatible fresh normal human serum acidified so that the pH of the cell-serum mixture is c 6.8. The normal serum serves as a source of complement.

Titrations which involve reading the result by the antiglobulin method should be carried out in relatively large (e.g. 75 × 10 mm) tubes so that the red cells can be washed thoroughly in the same tubes in relatively large volumes of saline.

Addition of red-cell suspensions to dilutions of serum

It is conventional to add 1 volume of red-cell suspension to 1 volume of serum or serum dilution. This means that each antibody dilution, and hence the 'final' titre, will be twice that of the original serum dilution.

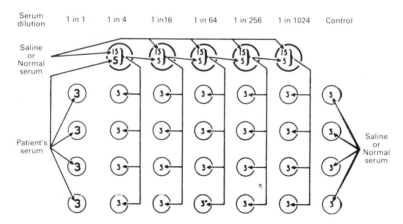

Fig. 26.3   Diagram illustrating method of preparing four sets of fourfold dilutions of a serum. The large circles at the top represent the large tubes in which the primary dilutions are made; the smaller circles the tubes in which the titrations are carried out. The figures represent drops or volumes. The patient's serum is indicated by the bold type.

TEST FOR SECRETION OF A OR B SUBSTANCES

Principle. Saliva is serially diluted, then added to anti-A or anti-B serum. The sera are tested with A$_2$ or B cells to see whether the antibodies have been neutralized. About 20% of persons are non-secretors.

Method

Dilute an anti-A or anti-B serum so that it gives good visible agglutination with A_2 or B cells at the end of 1 h at room temperature, e.g. if the titre of the serum is 128, use it at a dilution of 1 in 16.

Collect several ml of saliva in a centrifuge tube. Place the tube in boiling water for 10 min and then centrifuge. Serially dilute the clear supernatant in saline so as to give dilutions ranging from 1 in 2 to 1 in 32. Use a tube containing saline alone as a control. Add an equal volume of the diluted anti-A (or anti-B) serum to each tube and, after shaking the rack of tubes, allow it to stand for 10–15 min at room temperature. Then add an equal volume of a 2% suspension in saline of A_2 (or B) red cells to each tube. Mix the contents,

and allow to stand at room temperature for 1–2 h; then inspect for agglutination. If the saliva contains A or B substances, agglutination is usually inhibited in all the tubes except the saline-control tube. It is desirable to use saliva from a known secretor and non-secretor, respectively, as additional controls.

H substance can be demonstrated in a similar way using an extract of Ulex, eel serum or the naturally occuring 'incomplete' cold antibody as a source of anti-H.

ACKNOWLEDGEMENTS

The authors wish to thank Dr. D. Voak for advice in the preparation of Chapters 26 and 28.

REFERENCES

[1] ANSTEE, D. J. and TANNER, M. J. A. (1988). Blood group antigen deficiencies associated with abnormal red cell shape. *Blood Reviews*, **2**, 115

[2] British Committee for Standardization in Haematology (1987). Guidelines for compatibility testing in hospital blood banks. *Clinical and Laboratory Haematology*, **9**, 333.

[3] British Committee for Standards in Haematology (1990). Guidelines for microplate techniques in liquid-phase blood grouping and antibody screening. *Clinical and Laboratory Haematology*, **12**. In press.

[4] CARTRON, J. P. (1987). Recent advances in the biochemistry of blood group Rh antigens. In *Monoclonal Antibodies Against Red Blood Cell and Related Antigens*. Eds. P. Rouger and C. Salmon, p. 69–97. Arnette, Paris

[5] CHAPLIN, H., MONROE, M. C. and LACHMANN, P. J. (1982). Further studies of the C3g component of the α_2D fragments of human C3. *Clinical and Experimental Immunology*, **51**, 639.

[6] CLARKSON, S. B., BUSSEL, J. B. and KIMBERLEY, R. P. (1986). Treatment of refractory immune thrombocytopenic purpura with an anti-Fc receptor antibody. *New England Journal of Medicine*, **314**, 1236.

[7] COOMBS, R. R. A., MOURANT, A. E. and RACE, R. R. (1945). A new test for the detection of weak and 'incomplete' Rh agglutinins. *British Journal of Experimental Pathology*, **26**, 255.

[8] DYNAN, P. K. (1981). Evaluation of commercially available low ionic strength salt (LISS) solutions. *Medical Laboratory Sciences*, **38**, 13.

[9] ENGELFRIET, C. P., VON DEM BORNE, A. E. G. Kr., BECKERS, D. O. et al (1981). Immune destruction of red cells. In *A Seminar on Immune-mediated Cell Destruction*, p. 113–125. American Association of Blood Banks, Chicago.

[10] ENGELFRIET, C. P., OVERBEEKE, M. A. M. and OUWEHAND, W. H. (1988), Detection and characterisation of alloantibodies and autoantibodies. In: Blood Tranfusion. Ed. Greenwalt, T. J. *Methods in Hematology*, **17**, 106.

[11] ENGELFRIET, C. P., OVERBEEKE, M. A. M. and VOAK, D. (1987). The antiglobulin test (Coombs test) and the red cell. In *Progress in Transfusion Medicine 2*. Ed. J.D. CASH, p. 74–98. Churchill Livingstone, Edinburgh.

[12] ENGELFRIET, C. P., and VOAK, D. (1987). International reference polyspecific anti-human globulin reagents. *Vox Sanguinis*, **53**, 241.

[13] FEHR, J., HOFMANN, V. and KAPPELER, U. (1982). Transient reversal of thrombocytopenia in idiopathic thrombocytopenia by high dose intravenous gamma globulin. *New England Journal of Medicine*, **306**, 1254.

[14] GARRATTY, G. and PETZ, L. (1976). The significance of red cell bound complement components in development of standards and quality assurance for the anti-complement components in antiglobulin sera. *Transfusion*, **16**, 297.

[15] GIBLETT, E. R. (1977). Blood group alloantibodies: an assessment of some laboratory practices. *Transfusion*, **17**, 299.

[16] GOLDSMITH, K. (1955). Papain-treated red cells in the detection of incomplete antibodies. *Lancet*, **i**, 76.

[17] HOLBURN, A. M. and PRIOR, D. M. (1986). The U.K. National External Quality Assessment Scheme in Blood Group Serology. ABO and D grouping and antibody screening 1982–1983. *Clinical and Laboratory Haematology*, **8**, 243.

[18] HOLBURN, A. M. and PRIOR, D. M. (1987). The U.K. National External Quality Assessment Scheme in Blood Group Serology. Compatibility testing 1983–1984: the influence of variables in test procedures on detection of incomplete antibodies. *Clinical and Laboratory Haematology*, **9**, 33.

[19] HOLT, P. D. J., DONALDSON, C., JUDSON, P. A., JOHNSON, P., PARSONS, S. F., ANSTEE, D. J. (1985). NBTS/BRIC 8. A monoclonal anti-C3d antibody. *Transfusion*, **25**, 267.

[20] KELTON, J. G. (1985). The interaction of IgG with reticulo-endothelial cells: biological and therapeutic implications. In *Current Concepts in Transfusion Therapy*. Ed. G. Garratty, p. 51–107. American Association of Blood Banks, Arlington VA.

[21] LACHMANN, P. J., PANGBURN, H. K. and OLDROYD, R. G. (1982). Breakdown of C3bi to C3c, C3d and a new fragment C3g. *Journal of Experimental Medicine*, **156**, 205.

[22] LACHMANN, P. J., VOAK, D., OLDROYD, R. G., DOWNIE, D. M. and BEVAN, D. C. (1983). The use of monoclonal anti-C3 antibodies to characterise the fragments of C3 that are found on erythrocytes. *Vox Sanguinis*, **45**, 367.

[23] LÖW, B. (1955). A practical method using papain and incomplete Rh-antibodies in routine Rh blood-grouping. *Vox Sanguinis*, **5(OS)**, 94.

[24] LÖW, B. and MESSETER, L. (1974). Antiglobulin test in low ionic strength salt solution for rapid antibody screening and crossmatching. *Vox Sanguinis*, **26**, 53.

[25] McGOWAN, A., TOD, A., CHIRNSIDE, A. et al (1989). Stability of murine monoclonal anti-A, anti-B and anti-A, B ABO grouping reagents and a multi-centre evaluation of their performance in routine use. *Vox Sanguinis*, **56**, 122.

[26] MOLLISON, P. L., ENGELFRIET, C. P. and CONTRERAS, M. (1987). *Blood Transfusion in Clinical Medicine*, 8th edn p. 231. Blackwell Scientific Publications, Oxford.

[27] MOORE, H. C. and MOLLISON, P. L. (1976). Use of low ionic-strength medium in manual tests for antibody detection. *Transfusion*, **16**, 291.

[28] MOURANT, A. E., KOPEC, A. C. and DOMANIEWSKA-SOBCZAK, K. (1976). *The Distribution of the Human Blood Groups and Other Biochemical Polymorphisms*, 2nd. edn. Oxford University Press, Oxford.

[29] PIROFSKY, B. (1959). The use of bromelin in establishing a standard cross-match. *American Journal of Clinical Pathology*, **32**, 350.

[30] RACE, R. R. and SANGER, R.(1975). *Blood Groups in Man*, 6th edn. Blackwell Scientific Publications, Oxford.

[31] SCOTT, M. L. and PHILLIPS, P. K. (1987). A sensitive two-stage papain technique without cell washing. *Vox Sanguinis*, **52**, 67.

[32] SCOTT, M. L., VOAK, D. and DOWNIE, D. M. (1988). Optimum enzyme activity in blood grouping and a new technique for antibody detection: an explanation for the poor performance of the one-stage mix technique. *Medical Laboratory Sciences*, **45**, 7.

[33] STRATTON, F., GUNSON, H. H., and RAWLINSON, V. I. (1962). The preparation and use of antiglobulin reagents with special reference to complement-fixing blood group antibodies. *Transfusion*, **2**, 135.

[34] STRATTON, F. and RAWLINSON, V. I. (1974). Preparation of test cells for the antiglobulin test. *Journal of Clinical Pathology*, **27**, 359.

[35] VOAK, D. (1988), Monoclonal antibodies in blood grouping. *Biotest Bulletin*, **3**, 177.

[36] VOAK, D., DOWNIE, D. M., MOORE, P. B. L. and ENGELFRIET, C. P. (1986). Anti-human globulin reagent specification: the European and ISBT/ICSH view. *Biotest Bulletin*, **1**, 7.

[37] VOAK, D., DOWNIE, D. M., MOORE, P. B. L., FORD, D. S., ENGELFRIET, C. P. and CASE, J. (1986). Quality control of anti-human globulin tests: use of replicate tests to improve performance. *Biotest Bulletin*, **1**, 41.

[38] VOAK, D. and NAPIER, J. A. F. (1990). Quality assurance in the hospital transfusion laboratory: quality control in blood group serology. In *Quality Control in Haematology*. Ed. Cavill, I. *Methods in Hematology*, **22**, 129.

[39] WORLD HEALTH ORGANIZATION (1977). Twenty-eighth Report of WHO Expert Committee on Biological Standardization. Technical Report Series, 610. WHO, Geneva.

27. Platelet and granulocyte antigens and antibodies

(By A. H. Waters)

ALLO-ANTIGEN SYSTEMS

Platelet and granulocyte allo-antigens may be exclusive to each cell type (cell-specific) or shared with other cells. The currently recognized cell-specific antigen systems are shown in Tables 27.1 and 27.2. Of the shared antigens, the HLA system (Chapter 30) is the most important clinically; only class I antigens (HLA-A, -B, and to a lesser extent -C) are expressed on platelets and neutrophils. ABH antigens (Chapter 26) are also expressed on platelets (in part absorbed from the plasma), but cannot be demonstrated on neutrophils.

CLINICAL SIGNIFICANCE OF PLATELET AND GRANULOCYTE ANTIBODIES

Platelet and granulocyte antibodies may be classified on the basis of the antigenic stimulus, e.g., allo-, iso-, auto- and drug-induced antibodies.[50,58]

(a) Allo-antibodies

Allo-immunization to platelet and granulocyte antigens is most commonly due to transfusion or pregnancy. The associated clinical problems depend on the specificity of the antibody, which

Table 27.1 Platelet-specific allo-antigen systems[29]

HPA*	Antigens Traditional	Population	Phenotype frequency %	Gene frequency	GP**
HPA-la	$Pl^{A1}(Zw^a)$	Dutch	97.6	0.855	IIIa
-1b	$Pl^{A2}(Zw^b)$	Dutch	26.8	0.145	IIIa
HPA-2a	Ko^b	Dutch	99.4	0.923	Ib
-2b	Ko^a	Dutch	14.3	0.074	Ib
HPA-3a	$Bak^a(Lek^a)$	German	86.9	0.635	IIb
-3b	Bak^b	German	62.6	0.365	IIb
HPA-4a	$Yuk^b(Pen^a)$	Japanese	99.9 +	0.992	IIIa
-4b	Yuk^a	Japanese	1.7	0.008	IIIa
HPA-5a	$Br^b(Zav^b)$	German	99.2	0.888	Ia
-5b	$Br^a(Zav^a)$	German	20.5	0.112	Ia

* HPA = Human Platelet Antigen; a new nomenclature proposed by ICSH Platelet Serology Working Party. Platelet antigen systems numbered in order of discovery; allelic antigens designated alphabetically: a = high frequency; b = lower frequency.

** GP = glycoprotein localization of epitopes.

Table 27.2 Granulocyte-specific allo-antigen systems

System	Antigens	Phenotype frequency (%)	Genotype frequency
NA	NA1	61.2	0.32
	NA2	89.6	0.68
NB	NB1	90.8	0.72
NC	NC1	94.5	0.80
ND	ND1	98.5	0.88
NE	NE1	22.9	0.12
HGA-3	HGA-3a	21.5	0.11
	HGA-3b	23.9	0.13
	HGA-3c	16.1	0.08
	HGA-3d	52.6	0.31
	HGA-3e	17.2	0.09

Table 27.4 Clinical significance of granulocyte-specific allo-antibodies

1. Neonatal allo-immune neutropenia

2. Febrile reactions following transfusion (HLA antibodies also involved)

3. Pulmonary infiltrates following transfusion (passive transfer of high-titre antibody)

4. Poor survival and function of transfused granulocytes (HLA antibodies also involved)

5. Auto-immune neutropenia—some auto-antibodies have allospecificity for N system antigens.

determines the target cell involved. Cell-specific allo-antibodies are associated with well defined clinical conditions which are summarized in Tables 27.3 and 27.4. HLA allo-immunization is an important cause of refractoriness to platelet transfusion. Primary HLA immunization depends on the presence of contaminating lymphocytes in the transfused blood component; leucocyte-poor transfusions can therefore delay the onset of refractoriness due to HLA antibodies.[12,30,31] ABO incompatibility has little effect on the survival of transfused platelets, except in patients who have high titre anti-A or anti-B lytic antibodies.[4]

(b) Iso-antibodies

Occasionally, after blood transfusion or pregnancy, patients with type I Glanzmann's disease make antibodies which react with platelet glycoprotein (GP) IIb/IIIa not present on their own platelets but present on normal platelets, i.e. isotypic determinants. [3,5,36,46] Similarly, patients with Bernard-Soulier syndrome may make antibodies against isotypic determinants on GP Ib/V/IX not present

on their own platelets.[10] This may present a serious clinical problem because no compatible donor platelets can be found to treat severe bleeding episodes. Fortunately the occurrence of such antibodies is rare in these patients.

(c) Auto-antibodies

Auto-immune thrombocytopenia may be primary (idiopathic) or secondary (preceded by or associated with other conditions) (Table 27.5). Diagnosis depends on the exclusion of other causes of thrombocytopenia associated with adequate numbers of megakaryocytes in the bone marrow. Demonstration of a platelet auto-antibody is not mandatory; even with the most suitable techniques now available, platelet auto-antibodies remain elusive in a variable proportion (10–20%) of patients.[54]

Table 27.3 Clinical significance of platelet-specific allo-antibodies

1. Neonatal allo-immune thrombocytopenia
   All IgG platelet-specific antibodies

2. Post-transfusion purpura
   ? restricted to antibodies reacting with epitopes on GP IIb/IIIa, i.e. anti-P1^A(Zw), -Bak, -Pen (Yuk)

3. Refractoriness to platelet transfusion
   Usually due to HLA antibodies.

GP = glycoprotein

Table 27.5 Conditions associated with auto-immune thrombocytopenia (AIT)[49]

Post-viral infection
   Acute AIT of childhood
   Specific viral infections

Other auto-immune diseases
   Blood (e.g. Evans syndrome)
   Generalized (e.g. SLE, rheumatoid arthritis)
   Organ-specific (e.g. thyroid)

Lymphoproliferative disorders
   Chronic lymphocytic leukaemia
   Lymphoma

Cancer (solid tumours)

Immune system imbalance
   HIV infection
   Chemotherapy or radiotherapy
   Post bone-marrow graft

In the diagnosis of auto-immune thrombocytopenia it is important to consider and exclude three other immunological conditions:

1. *Post-transfusion purpura (PTP)*—a blood transfusion within 2 weeks will suggest this possibility.[57]

2. *Drug-induced immune thrombocytopenia*—a drug history is essential.[28]

3. *Pseudo-thrombocytopenia*—the patient has an EDTA-dependent platelet antibody which is active only in vitro. The antibody (IgG and/or IgM) reacts with hidden (cryptic) antigens on platelet GP IIb/IIIa, which are exposed due to conformational changes in the complex caused by the removal of Ca^{2+} by EDTA.[33] The antibody causes platelet agglutination in the EDTA blood sample associated with large platelet clumps on the blood film or platelet satellitism around neutrophils, both of which lead to a falsely low platelet count. These effects are not seen when a citrate anticoagulant is used. Similar effects, which are independent of the anticoagulant used, may be produced by a cold platelet auto-antibody.[34,47]

Failure to recognise these conditions may lead to a false diagnosis of auto-immune thrombocytopenia by the unwary, but platelet serology will help to differentiate a platelet auto-antibody from the various antibodies responsible for the above conditions.

Auto-immune neutropenia may be primary (idiopathic) or secondary (Table 27.6). Idiopathic auto-immune neutropenia is more common in infants than in adults, in whom autoimmune neutropenia is usually associated with other disorders which have in common a postulated imbalance of the immune system.[22,23,26]

Autoimmune neutropenia is the least well studied of the autoimmune cytopenias. This is partly because of the limitations of neutrophil serology, especially in the differentiation of auto-antibodies and circulating immune complexes (see below), and partly because the peripheral neutrophil count is an inadequate reflection of total granulocyte kinetics.

Neutrophil auto-antibodies (which are usually IgG) are unusual in that they often have well defined specificity for neutrophil-specific allo-antigens, especially NA[1].[22,23] However, it is not always possible to demonstrate allospecificity; such auto-antibodies may have a wider target than mature neutrophils, and are better described as granulocyte auto-antibodies. These auto-antibodies may suppress granulocyte precursors in the bone marrow and cause more severe neutropenia. The investigation of suspected auto-immune neutropenia should, when possible, include serological tests and clonal assays (e.g. CFU-GM) on bone marrow precursors as target cells, especially when antibodies to mature neutrophils are not found.

The relative importance of auto-antibodies, immune complexes and cellular mechanisms in the pathogenesis of auto-immune neutropenia has yet to be resolved and the diagnosis is therefore based on the interpretation of a combination of tests.[23,44]

Table 27.6 Auto-immune neutropenia[23,26]

1. Primary (idiopathic)
2. Secondary (a) Auto-immune conditions
       SLE
       Felty's syndrome
       AIHA ± thrombocytopenia
       (Evans syndrome)

    (b) Lymphoproliferative conditions
         ± chemotherapy and/or radiotherapy

    (c) Immune system imbalance
         Hypogammaglobulinaemia
         HIV infection
         Post bone-marrow graft

(d) Drug-induced antibodies

Drug-induced antibodies may cause selective haemolytic anaemia (p. 502), thrombocytopenia or neutropenia, or various combinations of these in the same patient.[6,15,28]

A drug may cause an immune cytopenia by stimulating production of either an *auto-antibody* (which reacts directly with the target cell independently of the drug itself) or a *drug-dependent antibody* which destroys the target cell by an immune complex mechanism or by reacting with the drug which is bound to the target cell. Laboratory tests may demonstrate both types of antibody in some patients.[14,39,41]

DEMONSTRATION OF PLATELET AND GRANULOCYTE ANTIBODIES

No single method will detect all types of platelet and neutrophil antibodies equally well. In practice it is useful to have a basic screening method that will detect most commonly occurring antibodies, both cell-bound (direct test) and in serum (indirect test), and to supplement this with other selected methods for demonstrating particular properties of an antibody and for measuring the amount of cell-bound antibody.

Labelled anti-human globulin (AHG) methods are widely used for routine platelet and granulocyte serology; fluorescent, enzyme and radioisotope-labelled AHG reagents are available. ^{125}I-labelled staphylococcal protein A(SPA) may also be used in place of labelled AHG to detect platelet and granulocyte IgG antibodies in both direct and indirect tests. There is a general trend to introduce microtechnology in order to cope with increasing work loads and to reduce the consumption of reagents. For technical details and a critical analysis of these methods, see McMillan[24] and von dem Borne.[51]

(a) Allo-antibodies

Reports of recent national and international workshops [8,56] make it possible to formulate guidelines for *platelet serology*. The basic procedure for demonstrating platelet allo-antibodies should include:

(i) A platelet test for platelet-reactive antibodies

Both fluorescent and enzyme-labelled platelet AHG methods are widely used with equal proficiency; these methods will be described in this chapter. The ISBT/ICSH Working Party on Platelet Serology [56] recommended the platelet suspension immunofluorescence test [53] as the standard for assessment of other platelet antibody techniques.

(ii) A lymphocyte test for detecting HLA antibodies

As HLA antibodies also react with platelets, a lymphocyte cytotoxicity and/or immunofluores-cence test should be included in the basic antibody screening procedure.

(iii) Tests to differentiate platelet-specific from HLA antibodies

The chloroquine-'stripping' technique is very helpful in this respect (see below). Conventional sero-logical techniques (e.g. differential reactions with a panel of normal lymphocytes and platelets; differential absorption of HLA antibodies) can also be used to differentiate cell-specific and HLA anti-bodies, but these are less suitable for rapid screening than the chloroquine-'stripping' technique.

Further characterization of platelet-specific antibodies may require referral to a reference labora-tory. Identification of allospecificity is carried out as for red cell antibodies by reaction with a selected panel of group O platelets. Allospecificity can also be confirmed by the glycoprotein localization of the corresponding epitope (Table 27.1) by immunoblotting, radioimmunoprecipitation and monoclonal antibody capture methods, which are also particularly helpful for resolving mixtures of platelet-specific antibodies.[51]

An important consideration in platelet serology is the occasional occurrence of antibodies against hidden (cryptic) antigens of the GP IIb/IIIa complex which are exposed by EDTA and paraform-aldehyde (PFA) fixation.[52] These antibodies, which are only active in vitro, are unpredicatable, but when suspected can be avoided by using unfixed test platelets from citrated blood.

Granulocyte serology is not so advanced, but the above plan for platelet serology can be used as a provisional guide.

(b) Auto-antibodies

The detection of auto-antibodies and drug-induced antibodies requires special consideration.

It can be misleading, when looking for platelet (or neutrophil) auto-antibodies, only to test the patient's serum against normal platelets (neutro-phils), as positive reactions may be due to the presence of allo-antibodies (e.g. HLA or cell-specific) induced by previous transfusion or pregnancy. It is important to show that an antibody in the patient's serum reacts with the patient's own cells. Ideally a direct antiglobulin test (e.g. platelet immunofluorescence test) should be performed before treatment is given to detect antibody bound in vivo. Where a severe cytopenia exists, it may not be possible to harvest enough cells for the test; nevertheless, serum samples should be stored at $-20°C$ and tested retrospectively against the patient's cells when the peripheral platelet (or neutrophil) count has increased in response to treatment.

A major interest in platelet auto-immunity is the quantitative measurement of platelet-associated immunoglobulins as an indication of in-vivo sensitization. A criticism of these quantitative methods is that they detect not only platelet auto-antibody, but also Ig non-specifically trapped or bound to platelets and platelet fragments,[42] and are therefore generally non-specific in the diagnosis of auto-immune thrombocytopenia.[49] On the other hand, the platelet immunofluorescence test (PIFT)[53] avoids the problem of non-specific binding by using PFA-fixed platelets which blocks the platelet Fcγ receptor so that immune complexes and IgG aggregates do not interfere with the test.[16] Moreover, PFA fixation induces platelet swelling with the expulsion of non-specific platelet-associated immunoglobulins.[55] Furthermore, as the test is read by examination of a platelet suspension using fluorescent microscopy, background fluorescence and platelet fragments can be seen and excluded. In a study of 75 patients with ITP, von dem Borne et al[54] found a weak positive ($\pm$ to $+$) direct PIFT in 60% of patients and strong reactions ($++$ to $++++$) in only 26% of patients. These results suggest that the amount of platelet-bound auto-antibody in ITP is low in most patients, and that none is present in a variable proportion of patients (10–20%). In the same study, the indirect PIFT was positive with the patient's serum in 66% of cases who had a positive direct PIFT, and positive with an ether eluate of the patient's platelets in 94% of the same cases. While these results may be a reflection of the relative insensitivity of the method, they may also be due to a low affinity antibody that is easily eluted during the assay procedure,[42] or indicate an alternative immune mechanism for thrombocytopenia in some cases.

The immunoglobulin (Ig) class of platelet auto-antibodies is similar in idiopathic and secondary autoimmune thrombocytopenia; mostly it is IgG (92%), but often (also) IgM (42%), and sometimes (also) IgA (9%).[54] All IgG subclasses occur, but IgG1 and/or IgG3 are the most frequent.

The target antigen for platelet auto-antibodies from patients with ITP appears to be the platelet glycoprotein (GP) IIb/IIIa complex. This is based on the observation that in most cases the auto-antibody does not react with platelets of patients with type I Glanzmann's disease which are deficient in GPIIb/IIIa.[35,45] Subsequent immunochemical studies with isolated platelet glycoproteins have confirmed this observation in some, but not in all cases, suggesting that the auto-antibodies may be directed against conformational determinants only present on the native GPs or that the auto-antibodies in ITP are more heterogeneous than previously thought.[2,38,49]

A major unresolved problem in *granulocyte serology* is the distinction between positive reactions due to auto-antibodies and circulating immune complexes.[13] This is particularly relevant to laboratory confirmation of the diagnosis of auto-immune neutropenia which may have to rely on other supporting evidence.[23,44]

(c) Drug-induced antibodies

The serological investigation of drug-induced immune thrombocytopenia (neutropenia) follows the same pattern as for haemolytic anaemia (p. 502), with the exception that it is not always possible to collect enough cells to test at the nadir of thrombocytopenia or neutropenia. The following blood samples are therefore necessary:

1. *Acute phase blood sample* when the cell count is at the nadir. If there are too few cells to test for cell-bound antibody and complement at this time, it is necessary to test the acute phase serum against the patient's cells during remission. These tests will demonstrate the immune basis of the cytopenia.

If the patient's acute phase serum is tested against *normal* donor cells, it is essential to take account of positive reactions due to HLA or cell-specific allo-antibody in the patient's serum. Furthermore, negative results with normal donor cells may be due to absence of the antigen for the particular drug-dependnent antibody, e.g. due to familial restriction of the antigen concerned.[7]

2. *Subsequent samples after stopping the drug.* Ideally, sampling should be done when the drug has been eliminated and the antibody is still detectable. Tests using this sample with and without the drug

in the assay system are necessary to demonstrate the part played by the drug in causing the immune cytopenia. The drug may be added directly to the assay system (and included in the wash solution) or the cells may pre-treated with the drug. For some drugs a metabolite and not the native drug is the appropriate antigen for testing; in these cases an 'ex vivo' drug antigen may be used, from urine or plasma.[40]

METHODS OF DEMONSTRATING ANTIBODIES

The basic fluorescent- and enzyme-labelled AHG methods will be described in detail. Only brief mention will be made of methods more appropriate to reference laboratories.

FLUORESCENT-LABELLED AHG METHODS

The fluorescent-labelled AHG method is based on the conventional antiglobulin technique (p. 433) and is suitable for platelet[53], granulocyte[48] and lymphocyte[9] serology. The platelet immunofluorescence test (PIFT) and granulocyte immunofluorescence test (GIFT) are described in detail in this chapter.

These tests are read by direct examination of a cell suspension using fluorescence microscopy; this enables false positive fluorescence due to debris or damaged cells to be seen and excluded.

These tests can detect allo-, auto- and drug-induced antibodies and by using appropriate monospecific AHG reagents can determine the Ig class and sub-class of the antibody and cell-bound complement components.

Both tests can be used with chloroquine-treated cells to differentiate cell-specific from HLA antibodies.[25]

Patient and screening panel cells

Platelets and granulocytes are prepared from venous blood taken into 5%(w/v) Na_2 EDTA in water (9 volumes blood : 1 volume anticoagulant).

Screening panel cells should be obtained from group O donors for platelet serology to avoid positive reactions due to anti-A and anti-B, but this is not necessary for granulocyte serology as A and B antigens cannot be demonstrated on granulocytes. If a patient's serum must be tested with ABO-incompatible platelets, anti-A and/or anti-B can be absorbed with corresponding red cells or A or B substance.

The best results are obtained with the freshest cell preparations, but some delay is tolerable. Neutrophils are more susceptible to storage damage than platelets; cells should be fixed (see below) on the day of collection, but serology may be delayed to the following day. *Platelets* are more resilient and an anticoagulated blood sample may be satisfactory for testing for up to 2 days at ambient temperature. Once fixed, platelets may be kept for up to 3–4 days at 4°C before serological testing. For longer storage, platelet-rich plasma may be kept at −40°C for at least 2 months; however, there is some membrane damage after recovery of frozen platelets, which causes increased background fluorescence that may limit the sensitivity of the test.[1,8,17] For longer-term storage a cryoprotectant, e.g. DMSO, may be used.[17]

Patients' sera

Serum from clotted venous blood should be heated at 56°C for 30 min to inactivate complement, and stored in 1–2 ml volumes (to avoid repeated thawing) at −40°C.

Control sera

Negative control serum is prepared from a pool of 10 sera from normal group AB male donors who have never been transfused. *Positive control* sera containing platelet-specific antibodies (e.g. anti-Pl[A1]), neutrophil-specific antibodies, or multispecific HLA antibodies should be obtained from reference centres.

Eluate from patient's sensitized cells

Elution is important to confirm the antibody nature of cell-bound immunoglobulin and to determine the specificity of antibodies. This applies especially when no antibody is demonstrable in the patient's serum, which often occurs in patients with auto-immune thrombocytopenia and neutropenia.

Elution by lowering the pH of the medium, by ether (or DMSO) and by heating to 56°C have been used.[18] For routine platelet serology, ether elution for platelet auto-antibodies or heating to 56°C for platelet-specific allo-antibodies is most convenient.

Heat eluate. Incubate platelets or granulocytes suspended in 0.5 ml of 0.2% bovine serum albumin (BSA) in phosphate buffered saline (PBS) for 60 minutes at 56°C. Centrifuge and remove the supernatant which contains the eluted antibody.

Ether eluate. Mix washed packed platelets from 50 ml of EDTA blood with one part of PBS-BSA (0.2%) and two parts of ether, by vigorous shaking for 2 min. Incubate the mixture for 30 min at 37°C in a water-bath with repeated shaking. After centrifugation (2800 *g*, 10 min) three layers are present, consisting of ether, stroma and the eluate. Pipette off the eluate with a Pasteur pipette and test in the indirect PIFT with normal donor platelets as described for serum.

Platelet preparation

1. Prepare platelet-rich plasma (PRP) by centrifugation of anticoagulated blood (200 *g*, 10 min).

2. Wash the platelets × 3 (2500 *g*, 5 min) in PBS/EDTA buffer (8.37 g Na_2EDTA dissolved in 2.5 1 phosphate buffered saline, pH 7.2); resuspend the platelets thoroughly each time.

3. Fix the platelets in 3 ml of 1% paraformaldehyde (PFA) solution for 5 min at room temperature.

(A stock solution of PFA is prepared by dissolving 4 g of PFA (BDH) in 100 ml of PBS by heating to 70°C with occasional mixing. Add 1 mol/l NaOH dropwise with continuous mixing until the solution clears. This 4% stock solution may be stored at 4°C protected from light for several months. Prepare a 1% PFA working solution by adding one volume of the 4% PFA stock solution to three volumes of PBS and by correcting the pH if necessary to 7.2–7.4 with 1 mol/l HCl.)

Wash the platelets twice as before and resuspend in PBS/EDTA buffer at a concentration of 250–500 × 10^9/l for use in the PIFT.

Granulocyte preparation

1. Mix anticoagulated blood or blood retained from platelet preparation after removal of PRP (and made up to its original volume with PBS) with 2 ml of Dextran solution per 10 ml of blood (Dextran 150 injection BP in 5% dextrose).* Incubate this mixture at 37°C for 30 min at an angle of about 45° to accelerate red cell sedimentation, and then remove the leucocyte-rich supernatant (LRS).

2. Granulocytes can be separated by double density sedimentation (Fig. 27.1). The LRS is underlayered with 2 ml of LSM (Lymphocyte Separating Medium = Ficoll-hypaque sp gr 1.077) which is then underlayered with 2 ml of MPRM (Mono-poly Resolving Medium = Ficoll-hypaque sp gr 1.114).** The density gradient tube is then centrifuged at 2500 *g* for 5 min. Granulocytes form an opaque layer at the LSM/MPRM interface from which they are harvested by careful pipetting (microscopic examination shows that the cells from this layer are predominantly neutrophil polymorphs). Lymphocytes can similarly be harvested from the plasma/LSM interface, e.g. for use in the lymphocyte cytotoxicity test (p. 515) or lymphocyte immunofluorescence test (LIFT).[9]

3. Wash the granulocytes three times (400 *g*, 5 min) in PBS/BSA buffer (PBS pH 7.2 with 0.2% BSA).

4. Fix the granulocytes in 3 ml of 1% PFA for 5 min at room temperature.

5. Wash the granulocytes twice as before, and

---

* Fisons Ltd, Loughborough, UK.
** Both LSM and MPRM supplied by Flow Laboratories Ltd.

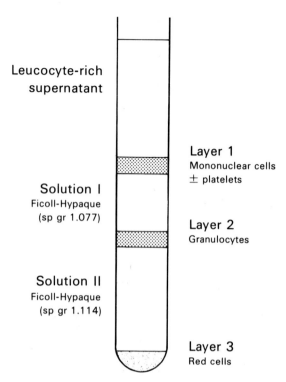

Leucocyte-rich
supernatant

Layer 1
Mononuclear cells
± platelets

Solution I
Ficoll-Hypaque
(sp gr 1.077)

Layer 2
Granulocytes

Solution II
Ficoll-Hypaque
(sp gr 1.114)

Layer 3
Red cells

Fig. 27.1 Double density separation of lymphocytes and granulocytes. A leucocyte-rich supernatant is underlayered with Ficoll-Hypaque with specific gravity of 1.077 (Solution I) and 1.114 (Solution 2) and then centrifuged at 2500 *g* for 5 min. Lymphocytes concentrate in layer 1, granulocytes in layer 2.

resuspend in PBS/BSA buffer at a concentration of about $10 \times 10^9/l$ for use in the GIFT.

PLATELET AND GRANULOCYTE IMMUNOFLUORESCENCE TESTS (PIFT AND GIFT)

The serological methods for testing platelets and granulocytes in the suspension immunofluorescence test are similar, except that platelets are washed throughout in PBS/EDTA buffer, and granulocytes in PBS/BSA buffer. A flow diagram of the PIFT is shown in Fig. 27.2.

Fluorescein-isothiocyanate (FITC) labelled anti-human globulin (AHG) reagents are used as follows: anti-Ig (polyspecific), anti-IgG, anti-IgM and anti-C3. $F(ab)_2$ fragments of these AHG reagents should be used to minimize non-specific membrane

fluorescence due to Fc receptor binding, which is a particular problem with granulocytes. The optimal dilution for each reagent should be determined by chequer-board titration. Centrifuge the FITC conjugates at 2500 *g* for 10 min before use to remove fluorescent debris and reduce background fluorescence.

Positive and negative controls (as described above) should be included with each batch of tests.

INDIRECT TEST

1. In plastic precipitin tubes (7×50 mm) mix 0.1 ml of serum and 0.1 ml of the appropriate cell suspension, as prepared above. (The method can also be adapted for use with microtitre plates which has the advantage of using smaller volumes.)

2. Incubate for 30 min at 37° C (IgG and C3 tests) and at room temperature (IgM tests). For C3 tests *only*, sediment cells (1000 *g*, 5 min), remove the supernatant and resuspend the cell button in 0.1 ml of freshly thawed human serum as a source of complement. Incubate for 30 min at 37°C.

3. Wash the cells three times (1000 *g*, 5 min) with appropriate buffer—PBS/EDTA for platelets, PBS/BSA for granulocytes; decant the final supernatant. This and subsequent steps are common for both the *indirect* test (i.e. patient's serum reacted with donor cells) and the *direct* test (i.e. patient's own cells to detect in-vivo sensitization).

4. Add the fluorescent AHG reagent (0.1 ml of the appropriate dilution determined by chequer-board titration), mix with the cell button and incubate at room temperature for 30 min in the dark.

5. Wash twice as before, and remove the supernatant.

6. Mix 0.5 ml of glycerol-PBS (3 volumes glycerol:1 volume PBS) with the cell button and mount on a glass slide under a cover-slip.

7. Examine microscopically using × 40 objective and epifluorescent UV illumination.

Scoring results

Reactions in the PIFT and GIFT may be scored on a scale from negative (−) through graded positives + to + + + + . Although subjective, this method of

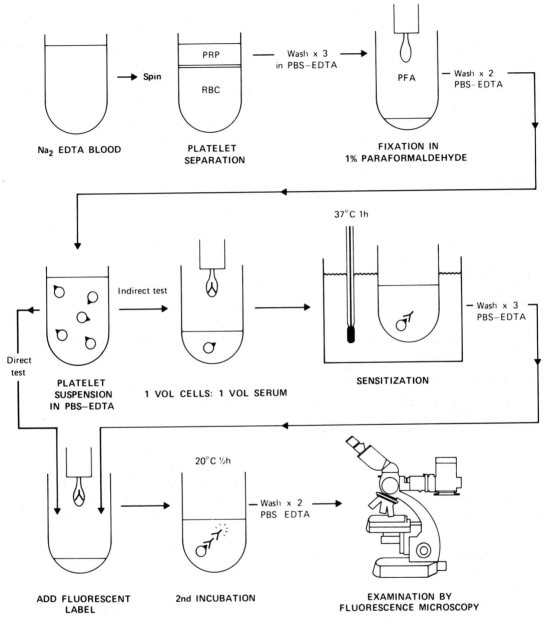

Fig. 27.2 Platelet immunofluorescence test. PRP = Platelet-rich plasma; PBS = Phosphate buffered saline; PFA = Paraformaldehyde.

scoring in experienced hands can produce semi-quantitative results in the PIFT.[55]

In general, normal platelets and granulocytes incubated with AB serum do not fluoresce after incubation with an appropriately diluted FITC AHG reagent. Sometimes the negative control may show weak fluorescence (up to two fluorescence points on some cells): in these cases the test result is classified as positive only if it is clearly stronger than the negative control (AB serum). Stronger fluorescence in the negative control should raise doubts about the performance of the test.

CHLOROQUINE TREATMENT OF PLATELETS AND GRANULOCYTES[27,32]

Platelets for chloroquine (Cq) treatment should be prepared from fresh blood or blood stored overnight at 4°C; granulocytes are suitable only if freshly prepared. An important consideration is the extent of chloroquine-induced cell membrane damage, which is minimal with fresh cells.

1. Cells are prepared as already described. Two-thirds of the cells are treated with chloroquine; the remaining one-third is not treated. After washing, and before PFA fixation, the cell button is incubated with 4–5 ml of chloroquine diphosphate (Sigma) in PBS (200 mg/ml, pH adjusted to 5.0 with 1 mol/l NaOH) for 2 h at room temperature with occasional mixing, or overnight at 4°C without mixing, if this is more convenient for the laboratory routine.

2. Wash three times in the appropriate buffer and fix in 1% PFA as previously described. Cell clumping during washing may be a problem after chloroquine treatment, especially with granulocytes; cell clumps should be dispersed by repeated gentle aspiration with a Pasteur pipette. The final cell suspension for serological testing should be prepared as previously described.

When reading the test under fluorescence microscopy, it is important to recognize and allow for any fluorescence due to chloroquine-induced cell damage, which is more likely to occur with granulocytes than platelets. Damaged cells are easily recognized by bright homogeneous fluorescence. Such cells should be excluded from assessment; only cells showing obvious punctate fluorescence should be considered positive.

Chloroquine-treated cells were tested initially in the fluorescent AHG method, but they may also be used in enzyme and radioisotope-labelled AHG methods and labelled SPA methods.

Interpretation of results with chloroquine-treated cells

Typical results with HLA and cell-specific antibodies are shown in Table 27.7. If a serum, which has been shown to contain HLA antibodies by LCT and/or LIFT, gives equal or stronger reactions with chloroquine-treated cells than with untreated cells, then a cell-specific antibody is also present. The Second Canadian Workshop on Platelet Serology[8] concluded that a weaker reaction with chloroquine-treated platelets should be interpreted with caution; this could indicate residual HLA reactivity, especially in the presence of high-titre multispecific HLA antibodies. If a platelet-specific antibody is nevertheless still suspected, other methods should be used to confirm this, e.g. immunoblotting, glycoprotein (GP) capture assays (p. 452).

Similar caution should be observed in interpreting the GIFT results with chloroquine-treated cells.

ENZYME-LABELLED AHG METHODS

The basic enzyme-labelled immunometric assay is usually referred to as ELISA—enzyme-linked immunosorbent assay.[11] ELISA is widely used to detect platelet antibodies and results are comparable to those obtained with the PIFT.[43]

In this application of ELISA, the immunosorbent is an immobilized antigen relevant to the particular antibody to be measured. After reacting the immobilized antigen with the antibody (usually in microtitre plates), the bound antibody is detected following subsequent reaction with an enzyme-labelled AHG (Fig. 27.3). The test can be used both qualitatively and quantitatively to detect in-vivo bound antibody (direct test) and platelet antibodies in serum (indirect test).

Table 27.7 Platelet and granulocyte antibody reactions using cells prepared with and without treatment with chloroquine

| Sera | Untreated cells | | Chloroquine-treated cells | |
	platelets	granulocytes	platelets	granulocytes
Negative	–	–	–	–
Multispecific HLA antibodies	+ + +	+ +	–	–
Granulocyte-specific antibody	–	+ +	–	+ + +
Platelet-specific antibody	+ + +	–	+ + +	–

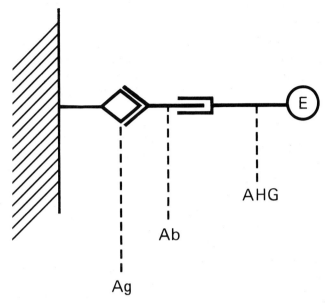

Fig. 27.3 ELISA for measuring antibodies. Platelet antibodies (Ab) bound to a solid-phase antigen (Ag) are detected by an enzyme-labelled (E) antihuman globulin (AHG).

Several ELISA methods using intact platelets and microtitre plates have been described. These are reviewed by Sintnicolaas et al[43] who describe a method which they have shown to be comparable to the standard PIFT in reproducibility and sensitivity for the detection of platelet allo-antibodies. A more complex two-stage ELISA is suitable for the quantitative measurement of platelet-associated immunoproteins.[20]

Although the ELISA is commonly used for the detection of platelet antibodies, there is little experience of its use for the detection of granulocyte antibodies. A recent report[41] suggests that a two-stage ELISA [20] can be applied for this purpose, and that this appears to have advantages over the GIFT in the investigation of drug-induced immune neutropenia.

Technical details[24,40]

ELISA involves the following steps:

1. *Platelet preparation,* as for the PIFT (p. 447), except that PFA fixation is not considered to be essential.[51]

2. *Platelet immobilization* on microtitre plates by centrifugation and incubation. Microscopic exami-

nation should reveal an even spread of platelets in the bottom of the wells.

3. *Blocking* non-specific binding of immunoproteins to the plastic microtitre plate.

4. *Platelet sensitization* (indirect test). Test and control sera (prepared as for the PIFT, p. 446) are incubated with the immobilized (solid phase) platelets.

5. *Detection of platelet-bound antibody* (both direct and indirect tests). Enzyme-labelled AHG is added to the wells. After incubation the plate is washed and an appropriate enzyme substrate is added to each well. After further incubation the reaction is stopped and the absorbence (A) read. Automated micro-ELISA readers are available.

6. *Calculation of results.* The test result is expressed as a ratio, i.e. A (test): A (negative control). The discriminating ratio between positive and negative tests should be established for the method used; the stronger the reaction, the higher the ratio above unity.

Enzyme labels include horseradish peroxidase, alkaline phosphatase and a biotin-avidin system.*
Enzyme-labelled antibodies to human immuno-

---

*Vector Laboratories.

proteins that are of interest are not always readily available. A double-antibody technique may be used to circumvent this problem by using highly specific unlabelled AHG reagents (of IgG class) as the first antibody and an appropriate enzyme-labelled secondary anti-IgG antibody.[20]

PLATELET GLYCOPROTEIN (GP) IMMUNOASSAYS

A new development in platelet serology is the application of methods to study antibody reactions at the molecular level. These include immunoblotting (Western blotting) and platelet glycoprotein (GP) assays (see ref. 51). Thus, major platelet-specific allo-antigens are located on the GP IIb/IIIa complex—Pl[A](Zw) and Yuk (Pen) on GP IIIa, and Bak (Lek) on IIb; the auto-antibody in idiopathic auto-immune thrombocytopenia usually reacts with an epitope on the GP IIb/IIIa complex.

Most of these methods are being used as research tools, but immunoblotting[19,37] and GP capture assays[21] are finding more routine applications in the confirmation of allospecificity and the resolution of mixtures of antibodies, albeit in reference laboratories.

ACKNOWLEDGEMENT

The author wishes to thank Mr. Paul Metcalfe for assistance in the preparation of this chapter.

REFERENCES

[1] ANDERSEN, E., BASHIR H. and ARCHER, G. T. (1981). Modification of the platelet suspension immunofluorescence test. *Vox Sanguinis*, **40**, 44.

[2] BEARDSLEY, D. S. (1988). Target antigens for platelet autoantibodies. *Current Studies in Hematology and Blood Transfusion*, **54**, 64. Karger, Basel

[3] BIERLING, P., FROMAT, P., ELBEZ, A., DUEDARI, N, and KIEFFER, N. (1988). Early immunization against platelet glycoprotein IIIa in a new born Glanzmann type I patient. *Vox Sanguinis*, **55**, 109.

[4] BRAND, A, SINTNICOLAAS, K., CLASS, F. H. J. and EERNISSE, J. G. (1986). ABH antibodies causing platelet transfusion refractoriness. *Transfusion*, **26**, 463.

[5] BROWN, C. H., WEISBERG, R. J., NATELSON, E. A. and ALFREY, C. P. Jr (1975). Glanzmann's thrombasthenia: assessment of the response to platelet transfusions. *Transfusion*, **15**, 124.

[6] CLAAS, F. H. J. (1987). Drug-induced immune granulocytopenia. *Bailliere's Clinical Immunology and Allergy*, **1**, 357.

[7] CLAAS, F. H. J., LANGERAK, J., DE BEER, L. L. and VAN ROOD, J. J. (1981). Drug-induced antibodies: interaction of the drug with a polymorphic platelet antigen. *Tissue Antigens*, **17**, 64.

[8] DECARY, F. (1988). Report on the second Canadian workshop on platelet serology. *Current Studies in Hematology and Blood Transfusion*, **54**, 1. Karger, Basel.

[9] DECARY, F., Vermeulen, A. and Engelfriet, C. P. (1975). A look at HLA antisera in the indirect immunofluorescence technique (IIFT). In *Histocompatibility Testing*, p. 380. Munksgaard, Copenhagen.

[10] DEGOS, L., TOBELEM, G., LETHIELLIUX, P., LEVY-TOLEDANO, S., CEAN, J. and COLOMBANI, J. (1977). A molecular defect in platelets of patients with Bernard-Soulier syndrome. *Blood*, **50**, 899.

[11] EDWARDS, R. (1985). Enzyme-labelled immunoassay methods. In Immunoassay—an introduction, p. 74. Heinemann, London.

[12] EERNESSE, J. G. and BRAND, A. (1981). Prevention of platelet refractoriness due to HLA antibodies by administration of leucocyte-poor blood components. *Experimental Haematology*, **9**, 77.

[13] ENGELFRIET, C. P., TETTEROO, P. A. T., VAN DER VEEN, J. P. W., WERNER, W. F., VAN DER PLAS-VAN DALAN, C. and VON DEM BORNE, A. E. C. Kr. (1984). Granulocyte-specific antigens and methods for their detection. In *Advances in Immunobiology: Blood cell antigens and bone marrow transplantation*, p. 121. Liss, New York.

[14] HABIBI, B. (1985). Drug induced red blood cell autoantibodies co-developed with drug specific antibodies causing haemolytic anaemias. *British Journal of Haematology*, **61**, 139.

[15] HABIBI, B. (1987). Drug-induced immune haemolytic anaemias. *Bailliere's Clinical Immunology and Allergy*, **1**, 343.

[16] HELMERHORST, F. M., SMEENK, R. J. T., HACK, C. E., ENGELFREIT, C. P. and VON DEM BORNE, A. E. G. Kr. (1983). Interference of IgG aggregates and immune complexes in tests for platelet autoantibodies. *British Journal of Haematology*, **55**, 533.

[17] HELMERHORST, F. M., TEN BOERGE, M. L., VAN DER PLAS-VAN DALEN, C. M., ENGELFRIET, C. P. and VON DEM BORNE, A. E. G. Kr (1984). Platelet freezing for serological purposes with and without a cryopreservative. *Vox Sanguinis*, **46**, 318.

[18] HELMERHORST, F. M., VAN OSS, C. J., BRUYNES, E. C. E., ENGELFRIET, C. P. and VON DEM BORNE, A. E. G. Kr. (1982). Elution of granulocyte and platelet antibodies. *Vox Sanguinis*, **43**, 196.

[19] HUISMAN, J. G. (1986). Immunoblotting: an emerging technique in immunohaematology. *Vox Sanguinis*, **50**, 129.

[20] KIEFEL, V., JAGER, S. and MUELLER-ECKHARDT, C. (1987a). Competitive enzyme-linked immunoassay for the quantitation of platelet-associated immunoglobulins (IgG, IgM, IgA) and complement (C3c, C3d) with polyclonal and

monoclonal reagents. *Vox Sanguinis*, **53**, 151.

[21] KIEFEL, V., SANTOSO, S., WEISHEIT, M. and MUELLER-ECKHARDT, C.(1987b). Monoclonal antibody specific immobilization of platelet antigens (MAIPA): a new tool for the identification of platelet-reactive antibodies. *Blood*, **70**, 1722.

[22] LALEZARI, P., KHORSHIDI, M. and PETROSOVA, M.(1986). Autoimmune neutropenia of infancy. *Journal of Pediatrics*, **109**, 764.

[23] MCCULLOUGH, J., CLAY, M. E. and THOMPSON, H. W. (1987). Autoimmune granulocytopenia. *Bailliere's Clinical Immunology and Allergy*, **1**, 303.

[24] MCMILLAN, R. (1983). Immune cytopenias. *Methods in Hematology*, **9**, 1.

[25] METCALFE, P., MINCHINTON, R. M., MURPHY, M. F. and WATERS, A. H. (1985). Use of chloroquine-treated granulocytes and platelets in the diagnosis of immune cytopenias. *Vox Sanguinis*, **49**, 340.

[26] MINCHINTON, R. M. and WATERS, A. H. (1984a). The occurrence and significance of neutrophil antibodies. *British Journal of Haematology*, **56**, 521.

[27] MINCHINTON, R. M. and WATERS, A. H. (1984b). Chloroquine stripping of HLA antigens from neutrophils without removal of neutrophil specific antigens. *British Journal of Haematology*, **57**, 703.

[28] MUELLER-ECKHARDT, C. (1987). Drug-induced immune thrombocytopenia. *Bailliere's Clinical Immunology and Allergy*, **1**, 369.

[29] MUELLER-ECKHARDT, C., KIEFEL, V. and SANTOSO, S. (1990). Review and update of platelet allo-antigen systems. *Transfusion Medicine Reviews*, **4**, 98.

[30] MURPHY, M. F., METCALFE, P., THOMAS, H. et al (1986). Use of leucocyte-poor blood components and HLA-matched platelet donors to prevent HLA alloimmunisation. *British Journal of Haematology*, **62**, 529.

[31] MURPHY, M. F. and WATERS, A. H. (1985). Immunological aspects of platelet transfusions. *British Journal of Haematology*, **60**, 409.

[32] NORDHAGEN, R. and FLAATHEN, S. T. (1985). Chloroquine removal of HLA antigens from platelets for the platelet immunofluorescence test. *Vox Sanguinis*, **48**, 156.

[33] PEGELS, J. G., BRUYNES, E. C. E., ENGELFRIET, C. P. and VON DEM BORNE, A. E. G. Kr. (1982). Pseudothrombocytopenia: an immunologic study on platelet antibodies dependent on ethylene diamine tetra-acetate. *Blood*, **59**, 157.

[34] RIBERA, A., HERNANDEZ, M., LOPEZ, R. et al (1988a). Pseudothrombocytopenia and platelet cold agglutinin. Abstracts *XX Congress International Society of Blood Transfusion in association with British Blood Transfusion Society*, p. 242.

[35] RIBERA, A., MARTIN-VEGA, C., MASSUET, L., ANGELAGUES, E., TORNOS, C. and TRIGINER, J. (1983). Autoimmune thrombocytopenia: serological behaviour of platelet antibodies. *Vox Sanguinis*, **45**, 438.

[36] RIBERA, A., MARTIN-VEGA, C., PICO M. and GONZALEZ, J. (1988b). Sensitization against platelet antigens in Glanzmann disease. Abstracts *XX Congress International Society of Blood Transfusion in association with British Blood Transfusion Society*, p. 240.

[37] ROCK, G., DECARY, F., TITTLEY, P. and FULLER, V. (1987). Electroblotting and immunochemical staining for identification of platelet antibodies. *British Journal of Haematology*, **67**, 437.

[38] ROSA, J. P., KIEFFER, N., DIDRY, D., PICARD, D., KUNICKI, T. J. and NURDEN, A. T. (1984). The human platelet membrane glycoprotein complex IIb/IIIa expresses antigenic sites not exposed on the dissociated glycoproteins. *Blood*, **64**, 1246.

[39] SALAMA, A. and MUELLER-ECKHARDT, C. (1986). Two types of nomifensine-induced immune haemolytic anaemias: drug-dependent sensitization and/or autoimmunization. *British Journal of Haematology*, **64**, 613.

[40] SALAMA, A., MUELLER-ECKHARDT, C., KISSEL, K., PRALLE, H. and SEEGER, W. (1984). Ex vivo antigen preparation for the serological detection of drug-dependent antibodies in immune haemolytic anaemias. *British Journal of Haematology*, **58**, 525.

[41] SALAMA, A., SCHUTZ, B., KIEFEL, V., BREITHAUPT, H. and MUELLER-ECKHARDT, C. (1989). Immune-mediated agranulocytosis related to drugs and their metabolites: mode of sensitization and heterogeneity of antibodies. *British Journal of Haematology*, **72**, 127.

[42] SHULMAN, N. R., LEISSINGER, C. A., HOTCHKISS, A. J. and KAUTZ, C. A. (1982). The non-specific nature of platelet associated IgG. *Transactions of Association of American Physicians*, **95**, 213.

[43] SINTNICOLAAS, K., VAN DER STEUIJT, K. J. B., VAN PUTTEN, W. L. J. and BOLHUIS, R. L. H. (1987). A microplate ELISA for the detection of platelet alloantibodies: comparison with the platelet immunofluorescence test. *British Journal of Haematology*, **66**, 363.

[44] VAN DER VEEN J. P. W., HACK, C. E., ENGELFRIET, C. P., PEGELS, J. G. and VON DEM BORNE, A. E. G. Kr. (1986). Chronic idiopathic and secondary neutropenia: clinical and serological investigations. *British Journal of Haematology*, **63**, 161.

[45] VAN LEEUWEN, E. F., VAN DER VEN, J. Th. M., ENGELFRIET, C., P. and VON DEM BORNE, A. E. G. Kr., (1982). Specificity of autoantibodies in autoimmune thrombocytopenia. *Blood*, **59**, 23.

[46] VAN LEEUWEN, E. F., VON DEM BORNE, A. E. G. Kr., VON RIESZ, L. E., NIJENHUIS, L. E. and ENGELFRIET, C. P. (1981). Absence of platelet specific alloantigens in Glanzmann's thrombasthenia. *Blood*, **57**, 49.

[47] VAN VLIET, H. H. D., KAPPERS-KLUNNE, M. C. and ABELS, J. (1986). Pseudothrombocytopenia: a cold autoantibody against platelet glycoprotein gpIIb. *British Journal of Haematology*, **62**, 501.

[48] VERHEUGT, F. W. A., VON DEM BORNE, A. E. G. Kr., DECARY, F. and ENGELFRIET, C. P. (1977). The detection of granulocyte alloantibodies with an indirect immunofluorescence test. *British Journal of Haematology*, **36**, 533.

[49] VON DEM BORNE, A. E. G. Kr. (1987). Autoimmune thrombocytopenia. *Bailliere's Clinical Immunology and Allergy*, **1**, 269.

[50] VON DEM BORNE, A. E. G. Kr. (1988a). Immunological structures of the platelet membrane. *Current Studies in Hematology and Blood Transfusion*, **55**, 32. Krager, Basel.

[51] VON DEM BORNE, A. E. G. Kr. (1988b). New technology in platelet immunology. *Current Studies in Hematology and Blood Transfusion*, **55**, 112. Karger, Basel.

[52] VON DEM BORNE, A. E. G. Kr., VAN DER LELIE, J., VOS, J. J. E. et al (1986a). Antibodies against crypt antigens of platelets. Characterisation and significance for the serologist. *Current Studies in Hematology and Blood Transfusion*, **52**, 33. Karger, Basel.

[53] VON DEM BORNE, A. E. G. Kr, VERHEUGT, F. W. A., OOSTERHOF, F., VON REISZ, E., BRUTEL DE LA RIVIERE, A. and ENGELFRIET, C. P. (1978). A simple immunofluorescence test for the detection of platelet antibodies. *British Journal of Haematology*, **39**, 195.

[54] VON DEM BORNE, A. E. G. Kr, VOS J. J. J. E., VAN DER LELIE, J., BOSSERS, B. and VAN DALEN, C. M. (1986b). Clinical significance of positive platelet immunofluorescence test in thrombocytopenia. *British Journal of Haematology*, **64**, 767.

[55] VOS, J. J. E., HUISMAN, J. G., WINKEL, I. N., RISSEEUW-BOGAERT, N. J., ENGLEFRIET, C. P.and VON DEM BORNE, A. E. G. Kr. (1987) Quantification of platelet-bound alloantibodies by radioimmunoassay: a study on some variables. *Vox Sanguinis*, **53**, 108.

[56] WATERS, A. H. (1988). Role of platelet serology workshops. Abstracts *XX Congress International Society of Blood Transfusion in association with British Blood Transfusion Society*, p.108.

[57] WATERS, A. H. (1989). Post-transfusion purpura. *Blood Reviews*, **3**, 83. Churchill Livingstone, Edinburgh.

[58] WATERS, A. H. and MINCHINTON, R.M. (1985). Immune thrombocytopenia and neutropenia. *Recent Advances in Haematology*, **4**, 309. Churchill Livingstone, Edinburgh.

28. Laboratory aspects of blood transfusion

(By A. H. Waters and E. E. Lloyd)

Safe and efficient blood transfusion practice depends on accurate documentation and the elimination of clerical errors (see BCSH *Guidelines on Hospital Blood Bank Documentation and Procedures*[5] and BCSH *Guidelines on Hospital Blood Bank Computing*[4]; consideration of the patient's clinical history, particularly with respect to previous transfusions, pregnancy and drugs; constant attention to the reliability of reagents and techniques; a satisfactory pre-transfusion testing procedure to ensure donor-recipient compatibility; and a fail-safe procedure agreed with hospital clinicians and nursing staff to ensure that compatible blood is transfused to the right patient.[27,42]

This chapter is primarily concerned with pretransfusion compatibility testing and follows the BCSH *Guidelines for Compatibility Testing in Hospital Blood Banks*.[3] It also includes sections on antenatal antibody screening and the investigation of allo-immune haemolytic disease of the newborn (HDN).

Pretransfusion Compatibility testing

A satisfactory compatibility procedure should include:

1. ABO and Rh(D) grouping of the patient
2. Antibody screening of the patient's serum to detect the presence of clinically significant antibodies and assist the selection of compatible blood
3. Cross-matching the patient's serum against donor red cells to confirm donor-recipient compatibility.

To cross-match or not to cross-match?

The BCSH *Guidelines for Compatibility Testing in Hospital Blood Banks*[3] and the AABB *Standards for Blood Banks and Transfusion Services*[1] emphasize the importance of the donor-recipient cross-match as the ultimate check of ABO compatibility. Some authorities have advocated abbreviation of the cross-match by omission of the indirect antihuman globulin (AHG) test from the compatibility procedure for patients with a negative antibody screen.[17] The technical competence of personnel is a most important factor to be considered when deciding on the compatibility procedure to meet the needs of the hospital, and the continuing unacceptable level of antibody detection failures in external proficiency trials dictates a cautious approach. However, the consultant in charge of the blood bank may, after due consideration of the technical competence of the laboratory staff, decide to delete the AHG phase of the cross-match for patients who have a negative antibody screen and no previous record of irregular antibodies. This decision should be based on periodic assessment of individual staff competence and regular monitoring of cell washing centrifuges as outlined in the BCSH *Guidelines for Compatibility Testing in Hospital Blood Banks.*[3]

Documentation

The safety of blood transfusion depends on accurate patient and sample identification at all stages, starting with taking the blood sample from the patient for compatibility testing and ending with the transfusion of compatible blood.

It is emphasized that clerical errors can be avoided in the laboratory if the worker performing the compatibility test *double checks* the identity of the patient's sample with the request form and with the compatibility label on the donor units before issuing the blood. Whenever possible, all checks should be made by two responsible persons.

Blood samples

Immediately on receipt, laboratory staff should confirm that the blood sample is appropriately labelled and that the information on the sample and request form is identical.

Great care must be taken to identify and label correctly any serum separated from the patient's original blood sample; the serum should be stored at or below $-20°C$.

ABO and Rh (D) grouping

These must be performed by an approved technique with appropriate controls. Before use, all new batches of grouping reagents should be checked for reliability by the techniques used in the laboratory. Grouping reagents should be stored according to the manufacturer's instructions.

Manual tube and slide grouping methods are described. The rapid evolution of microplate technology for blood grouping makes it difficult at this stage to recommend standard methods and optimal conditions for these tests. The reader is referred to BCSH guidelines on microplate technology for the current state of the art.[6]

ABO GROUPING

Correct interpretation of the patient's ABO group requires confirmation, whenever possible, by tests on the patient's serum (except for newborn infants up to 4 months of age in whom naturally occurring anti-A and anti-B are normally absent). Ideally, cell and serum grouping should be carried out by different workers who then check each other's results.

Reagents

Anti-A, anti-B and anti-A,B reagents are used for cell grouping tests. The anti-A,B reagent (group O serum) acts as an additional check on red cells which are agglutinated by anti-A or anti-B, and it should also detect weaker A or B antigens which might otherwise be missed. Conventional polyclonal reagents are being replaced by superior anti-A and anti-B monoclonal reagents,[24,36] each prepared from blends of two antibodies to optimize the intensity of agglutination for slide tests and their ability to detect the weaker subgroups of A (e.g. Ax) by tube techniques. Blended monoclonal anti-A,B reagents to optimize anti-A and anti-B reactions are also available. Their superior performance questions the need for the continued use of anti-A,B reagents in ABO grouping.

The monoclonal reagents should contain EDTA (0.1 mol/1 pH 7.1–7.3) to prevent haemolysis in the presence of fresh serum, as these potent IgM antibodies are strong haemolysins in the presence of complement.

Methods

ABO grouping may be carried out by tube or slide methods or in microplates. The reader is referred to the BCSH *Guidelines on Microplate Technology*[6] for the current state of the art in this rapidly changing area of serology.

Tube methods

Either spin or sedimentation tube methods can be used.

1. *Spin tube tests* may be performed in 75 × 10 or 12 mm glass or plastic tubes. Immediate spin tests may be used in an emergency, whereas routine tests are usually left for 15 min at room temperature (*c* 20°C). For details of spin force (RCF) and time see p. 436.

2. *Sedimentation tube tests* may be performed in

75 × 10 or 12 mm tubes as above, or in small glass precipitin tubes (50 × 7 mm). The tests are incubated for 1–1$^1/_2$ h at room temperature (*c* 20°C). This method is suitable for grouping large batches of tests.

Using a commercial reagent dropper or a Pasteur pipette, add 1 drop of each grouping serum to 3 tubes labelled anti-A, anti-B and anti-A,B respectively, followed by 1 drop of a 2% suspension in saline (9 g/1 NaCl) of the test red cells. In addition, add 1 volume of patient's serum to 4 tubes labelled A$_1$ cells, B cells, O cells and 'auto-agglutination control' respectively. Then add 1 volume of 2% suspensions of the control A$_1$, B and O cells, and of the test red cells to the appropriate tubes. The layout for tests and controls is shown in Fig. 28.1.

Mix the suspensions by tapping the tubes and leave them undisturbed for 15 min in the spin tube

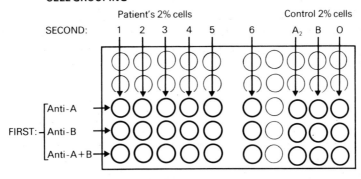

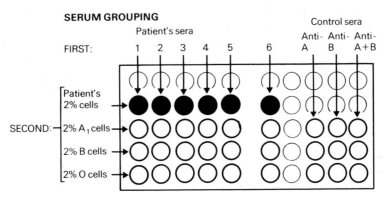

Fig. 28.1 Lay-out for tube grouping tests. The order of adding serum (first), and cells (second) is indicated. The closed circles are 'auto' controls.

method and for $1-1^1/_2$ h in the sedimentation tube method. Agglutination should be read as described in Chapter 26, p. 431.

It is essential to confirm the result of the red cell grouping by examining the patient's serum for the corresponding antibodies (Fig. 28.1). Any discrepancy between the results of the red cell grouping and the serum grouping should be investigated further.

Serum grouping is not carried out for infants under 4 months of age as the corresponding antibodies are normally absent. It is good practice to include adult group AB serum as a control when grouping the red cells of such infants to detect possible polyagglutination (p. 460), which could result in a group O baby being incorrectly grouped as AB. However, monoclonal ABO grouping reagents lack the contaminating antibody responsible for polyagglutination and should be used if available.

Controls

Each grouping test (or series of tests) must be controlled by parallel tests set up exactly as described above, using cells of known group in place of the test (patient's) cells. Group-A_2 and -B cells are used to test the potency of the grouping sera; group-O cells, which should not be agglutinated, are also included to guard against the possibility of false-positive reactions. In addition, the A_1, B and O cells used in the serum grouping test are checked against standard anti-A, anti-B and anti-A,B grouping sera, during the course of the cell grouping test.

An auto-control should also be included. Any agglutination of the A_1, B or O cells by the test subject's serum cannot be interpreted unless the auto-agglutination control gives a negative result. The possible causes of a positive auto-agglutination test are considered below.

Slide method

In an emergency, ABO grouping may be carried out rapidly on slides or tiles. The method is satisfactory if potent grouping reagents are used, but is less sensitive than tube tests for detecting weak anti-A or anti-B in reverse serum grouping. An immediate or short incubation (5 min) spin tube test is preferable.

Agglutination is rapid on flat or slightly concave surfaces, and the method is particularly useful when only one or two samples of blood are to be grouped. Controls must be set up with each test, and it is useful to have a Perspex tile permanently ruled out and labelled as shown in Fig. 28.2 as a reminder of the controls that are necessary.

Using a commercial reagent dropper, add 1 drop of each grouping serum and 1 drop of the patient's serum to each of the four squares in the horizontal rows labelled anti-A and anti-B, anti-A,B and patient's serum, respectively. Add 1 drop of a strong cell suspension (20% or more) of A cells, B cells, O cells (in normal saline) and the patient's cells (in own serum or plasma) to each of the four squares in the vertical rows under the appropriate headings. Mix the cells and serum in each square with a wooden swab-stick, breaking off the used portion after each mixing. The results may be read within 2–5 min; they are usually clear-cut and indisputable (Fig. 28.2). If doubtful, the presence or absence of agglutination may be checked by viewing the suspension under the low power of a microscope or with a hand lens ($\times 5$ or $\times 6$ magnification).

CAUSES OF DISCREPANCIES IN ABO GROUPING

Before any tests are read the controls must show that the reagents are working correctly.

(a) False positive results

(i) Rouleaux formation

Marked rouleaux formation can simulate true agglutination (Figs. 28.3 and 28.4). The two can be distinguished by repeating the test using the serum diluted 1 in 2 or 1 in 4 in saline. Rouleaux should disappear; agglutination will hardly be affected. If rouleaux are apparent in red cell grouping tests, the tests should be repeated after washing the patient's red cells thoroughly.

(ii) Cold agglutinins in the patient's serum

These will cause auto-agglutination and apparent panagglutination, if active at room temperature. If this is suspected, the serum grouping test should be

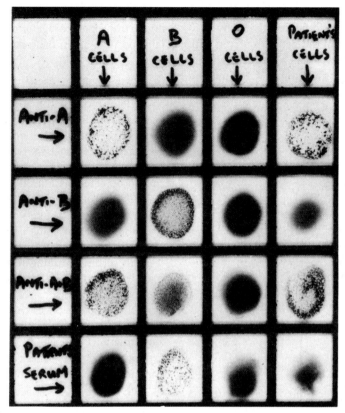

Fig. 28.2   ABO grouping on a Perspex tile.

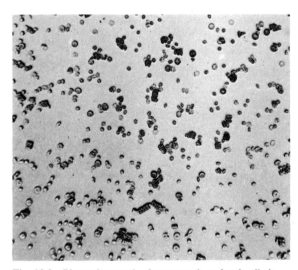

Fig. 28.3   Photomicrograph of a suspension of red cells in serum, showing a minor degree of rouleaux formation. × 300. The numerous small rouleaux are characteristically relatively evenly spaced throughout the field and do not vary greatly in size.

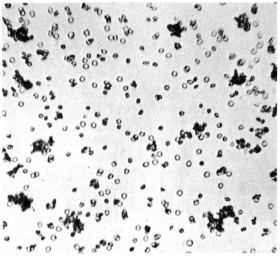

Fig. 28.4   Photomicrograph of a suspension of red cells in serum, showing weak agglutination. × 300. The small agglutinates are more irregularly distributed than rouleax and vary more in size. There are also more free cells.

repeated at 37°C, at which temperature the auto-agglutination control should be negative. Any anti-A and/or anti-B present in the patient's serum will, however, still react. The patient's red cells should be washed several times in warm (37°C) saline and the cell grouping repeated. It is advisable, too, to set up an additional test of the patient's cells in group-AB serum containing no antibodies (see below). No agglutination should result.

(iii) Warm antibodies adsorbed to the patient's red cells

When the patient's red cells are coated with antibodies and give a positive direct antiglobulin test (DAT), as in haemolytic anaemia caused by warm auto-antibodies, they may undergo auto-agglutination in normal serum; more often they agglutinate in albumin-containing media (see p. 462).

(iv) Infected red cells

Infection of a red-cell suspension by certain bacteria may cause the cells to become agglutinable by normal adult human sera. In vivo, this is thought to be the main cause of the rare phenomenon of polyagglutinability. Bacterial enzymes expose the T-receptor on red cells and polyagglutination is due to the presence of anti-T in most human sera except those of young infants. Such cells might appear to be group AB when in reality they were group O. However, polyagglutination is less obvious or does not occur at all at 37°C and the true group can usually be determined at this temperature; preferably use monoclonal grouping reagents which are free of anti-T. The special problem of polyagglutination in ABO grouping of neonates is referred to on p. 458.

Infection of blood samples in vitro can be also result in polyagglutinability of red cells. Grouping should therefore always be carried out as soon as possible after the blood has been collected or, if delay is unavoidable, the blood should be kept at 4°C. If sterility cannot be guaranteed, blood is best stored as a clot rather than in an anticoagulant. Red cells should never be stored as a suspension in saline.

Bacterial contamination of grouping reagents, due to improper storage or handling, may also cause false positive agglutination.

(b) False-negative reactions in ABO grouping

1. Failure of agglutination or weak reactions are usually due to impotent sera. Loss of potency results if sera are carelessly left at room temperature or stored frozen in large volumes so that repeated freezings and thawings are required. The controls should be carefully checked.

2. Failure to add the grouping reagents will cause false results; the standard use of coloured reagents—blue for anti-A, yellow for anti-B—is a check for this error.

3. In serum grouping tests false-negative results may be recorded if lysis is not recognized as a positive result. All serum grouping tubes should be carefully inspected for lysis and its presence recorded before attempting microscopic reading of agglutination. To avoid lysis, anti-A, and anti-B grouping reagents should contain EDTA to prevent complement activation in the presence of fresh patient sera.

(c) Mixed-field reactions

These may be due to:

1. The previous transfusion of group O cells to group A or B recipients.
2. A possible incompatible transfusion.
3. An ABO incompatible bone-marrow transplantation.
4. A permanent dual population of cells, which may be the first indication of a blood-group chimerism.

DIFFERENTIATION OF GROUP A_1 FROM GROUP A_2

Using lectins[7]

Extracts from many plants, especially from their seeds, contain substances, lectins, that will agglutinate red cells. Some lectins have a useful blood-group specificity but most react with all blood cells. A saline extract of the seeds of *Dolichos biflorus* can be diluted so that it will agglutinate A_1 and A_1B

cells preferentially, and a saline extract of the seeds of *Ulex europaeus* has anti-H specificity and will agglutinate A_2, A_2B and O cells more strongly than A_1, A_1B and B cells. *Dolichos biflorus* extract is now used routinely in sub-typing cells carrying the A antigen.

Ulex europaeus seeds can be obtained from the plant (the common gorse bush) or from a seed merchant. *Dolichos biflorus* is not indigenous to Britain, but it grows readily in India and other countries.

Using anti-A_1 sera

Group-A_1 and -A_2 cells can also be differentiated by using group-B serum absorbed with A_2 cells. Group-B serum contains anti-A and anti-A_1, and by this method the anti-A can be removed and the anti-A_1 left behind. A satisfactorily absorbed serum should react only with A_1 cells. The anti-A_1 produced in this way is often of poor quality; *Dolichos* extract is a much better reagent.

Preparation of Dolichos solution

The method of Voak et al[40] is satisfactory. The appropriate dilution of the extract has to be determined by experiment. Test serial dilutions with several examples of A_1 and A_2 cells. The dilution selected for routine use should agglutinate on a tile, within 2 min, the weakest A_1 cells and yet not agglutinate A_2 cells within the same period of time. The extract is available from commercial sources.

Rh (D) GROUPING

This is usually performed at the same time as ABO grouping to minimize clerical errors that may arise through repeated handling of patient samples. At least two different anti-D reagents should be used as a check against errors, as there is no counterpart of 'reverse serum grouping', as in ABO grouping.

Reagents

Anti-D grouping reagents of both IgM and IgG class are available. These may be polyclonal or monoclonal. The recent development of high titre monoclonal IgM anti-D reagents[34] has made it possible to use the same techniques as for ABO grouping. These reagents work equally well at room temperature (c 20°C) and at 37°C and are reliable for emergency D grouping by rapid slide or immediate spin tube techniques as described for ABO grouping. Many anti-D reagents in current use are made from polyclonal IgG anti-D which does not cause agglutination in saline unless the IgG antibody has been chemically modified or potentiating substances (e.g. albumin or protease enzymes) have been added to the diluent. These 'enhanced' IgG anti-D reagents usually require 37°C incubation and must be used strictly according to the manufacturer's instructions.

All anti-D grouping reagents should be checked by the method used in the laboratory for specificity with *positive* (OR_1r or OR_1R_2) and *negative* (Orr or Or'r) controls. Additional controls are necessary for polyclonal reagents to confirm the *absorption* of any contaminating anti-A (using A_1rr cells) and anti-B (using Brr cells). OR_1R_2 control cells would also detect any contaminating anti-C or -E. Before a new batch of reagent is introduced, it should be evaluated in parallel with the reagent in current use.

Methods

Both slide and tube methods may be used as for ABO grouping.

Working in sequence for ABO and D grouping provides for efficient batch testing.

Add 1 volume of anti-D to each tube of the anti-D row of each rack.

Then add 1 volume of the 2% red cell suspension to each tube.

The tests are mixed, incubated and read as described for ABO tests.

Controls

Controls and tests should be set up in one operation. Each batch of tests should include *positive* (O R_1r or O R_1R_2) and *negative* (Orr) controls. Each test sample must have an *auto*-control (own cells and own serum), and in tests with enhanced IgG anti-D reagents, the auto-control should also be performed with the addition of the enhancing agent, as specified by the manufacturer (*diluent* control). The diluent control is essential to demonstrate that the diluent itself does not promote agglutination of the patient's cells, as might occur with red cells already coated with immunoglobulin due to in-vivo sensitization.

EMERGENCY Rh (D) GROUPING

Spin tube method

For emergency D grouping use the spin tube method and centrifuge the tubes at 150 g for 1 min either immediately or after incubation depending on the time available. Read the results microscopically.

Slide method

Commercial anti-D reagents are available that agglutinate D-positive cells within a few minutes. The manufacturer's instructions must be followed.

For both methods it is essential to use potent anti-D reagents and to include positive, negative and absorption controls as previously described.

False positive results in Rh (D) grouping

Misclassification of a D-negative patient as D-positive could lead to the transfusion of D-positive blood. Resultant anti-D sensitization could have potentially harmful clinical consequences, especially for D-negative women of child bearing age (see also p. 465).

False positive results may occur for the following main reasons:

1. Red cells may already be coated with immunoglobulin due to in-vivo sensitization. For this reason antiglobulin and enzyme techniques should not be used for routine D grouping. Furthermore, direct agglutination tests with enhanced anti-D reagents should include an appropriate diluent control to exclude false positive results.

2. The anti-D grouping reagent may contain a contaminating antibody which has not been adequately absorbed e.g. contaminating anti-A or anti-B, or anti-C (leading to a false positive result in a D-negative C-positive patient). This type of false positive result may occur when reagents have not been adequately controlled for the method in use or when the reagent manufacturer's instructions have not been followed.

3. Bacterial contamination of reagents may also cause false positive agglutination.

Clinical significance of weak D phenotype (D^u)

Discrepant results in D grouping with different anti-D reagents may indicate a serious reagent fault (e.g. contaminating antibody as discussed above), but are usually caused by weak D phenotypes which have fewer D antigen sites than normal (called D^u).[33] The incidence of weak D (both high and low grade D^u) is *c* 0.7%, if selected by an IgM monoclonal anti-D at suitable dilution, e.g. MAD-2. If an enhanced papain IgG polyclonal anti-D is used, which reacts with high grade D^u and some low grade D^u, these will be called D-positive and not classified as D^u (D. Voak, personal communication).

In clinical practice, if the serological reactions with standard methods are equivocal, the patient should be grouped as Rh (D) negative. This 'error' will be of no clinical consequence, since the transfusion of D-negative blood will be compatible with respect to the D antigen. Similarly, a D^u pregnant woman, misclassified as D-negative, will not be harmed by prophylactic IgG anti-D. Nothing is to be gained by further testing of D-negative patients by other techniques, e.g. antiglobulin or enzyme methods, to detect possible D^u; a more important consideration is the risk of false positive results with such methods, as indicated above.

In the routine grouping of blood donors at transfusion centres only some low grade D^u samples will be misclassified as D-negative; the incidence varies, but can be reduced to as low as 0.23% by the sensitive automated methods now being used.[26a] The clinical consequences will not be serious since

D^u red cells are thought to be unlikely to undergo accelerated destruction if transfused to an immunized patient; moreover, D^u red cells are thought to be poorly immunogenic and unlikely to provoke a primary immune response in an D-negative recipient.[26b]

In addition to weak D antigens (D^u), there is a very low incidence of D variants. These are rare D-positive individuals who lack some of the epitopes of the complex D antigen. Most anti-D reagents react with the whole D antigen, but some reagents may be more specific and give negative results with D variant red cells if the antibody is directed against the missing epitopes. If such people require transfusion, they should be regarded as D-negative because they may make antibody against the epitopes which they lack if transfused with the normal (whole) D antigen. Similarly, a D variant mother may be immunized by a normal fetal D antigen, and this could cause Rh (D) haemolytic disease of the newborn.

For blood donors it is therefore important to identify D variants and classify them as D-positive, as they may immunize D-negative recipients against some of the D epitopes. All donor D-negative grouping tests should be confirmed with reagents known to detect D variants (for further details, see Mollison et al[26b]).

Rh PHENOTYPING

Determination of the Rh phenotype often has to be left to a specialist laboratory where the necessary sera are available. A brief account is given below.

The commonest reason for determining the Rh phenotype is to predict whether the partner of a D-negative woman with anti-D is homozygous or heterozygous for the D antigen. This is essential to forecast the chances of the couple having children affected by Rh (D) haemolytic disease of the newborn (HDN).

No antisera against the 'd' antigen are available as the 'd' antigen is amorphic. Because of the lack of an 'anti-d' serum, the zygosity of the D antigen is usually predicted from the results of tests with anti-C, anti-c, anti-E and anti-e sera, and from tables of the likelihood of the homo- or heterozygous association of D with the other Rh antigens. These tables have been compiled for different racial groups. It is important, therefore, to tell the specialist laboratory the racial origin of the patient.

Table 28.1 gives the results of testing samples of D-positive red cells from an English population with anti-D and four other anti-Rh antisera, and the interpretation of the data in terms of D homozygosity and heterozygosity for the common and not so common genotypes. The relative frequencies in the last column apply to a random population. They are applicable to D-positive husbands of D-negative women in general, but D-positive fathers of children who have had Rh(D) HDN are a selected rather than a random population. The chances of such a father provisionally called 'heterozygous' being in reality homozygous for the D antigen becomes more likely with every child that is affected. It may be helpful to Rh phenotype all his children and his parents.

Antisera for determining the Rh phenotype are available commercially. It is essential to follow the manufacturer's instructions in doing the tests, but the recommended quantities of serum and cells can often be reduced. The following sera are required:

Table 28.1 Interpretation of D-positive Rh genotypes in terms of homozygosity (D/D) or heterozygosity (D/d) in an English population

	Reaction with anti-				Probable genotype	% of total giving these results	Next most probable	% of total giving these results	Relative frequency of heterozygous:homozygous amongst samples giving these results
D	C	c	E	e					
+	+	+	−		$R^1r(D/d)$	94	$R^1R^0(D/D)$	6	15:1
+	+	−	−		$R^1R^1(D/D)$	96	$R^1r'(D/d)$	4	1:21
+	+	+	+		$R^1R^2(D/D)$	88	$R^1r''(D/d)$	8	1:8
+	−	+	+	+	$R^2r(D/d)$	93	$R^2R^0(D/D)$	6	15:1
+	−	+	−		$R^2R^2(D/D)$	86	$R^2r''(D/d)$	14	1:6
+	−	+	−		$R^0r(D/d)$	97	$R^0R^0(D/D)$	3	30:1
+	+	−	+		$R^1R^2(D/D)$	97	$R^zr'(D/d)$	2	1:41

anti-D, anti-C + C^w, anti-E, anti-c and anti-e. The anti-e is only necessary when the tests with anti-E are positive and anti-C + C^w are negative, i.e. to distinguish between R_2r and R_2 (provided the samples are from European Caucasian donors). In this case, it is safe to assume that if the anti-E gives a negative result the anti-e would give a positive result and that a sample giving positive results with all sera is R_1R_2 (provided the auto-agglutination test is negative). These assumptions may not be true in people of other races.

It is essential to use a panel of cells of known genotypes as controls. Cells that are heterozygous for the antigen under test are used as positive controls; cells that do not have the antigen under test (but would be agglutinated by the most common contaminants of the antibody) are used as negative controls. Absorption controls must also be

Table 28.2 Genotypes of the red cells to use as controls for Rh grouping sera

Antiserum	Negative control	Positive control	Absorption control
Anti-D	Cde/cde	CDe/cde	A_1 B cde/cde
Anti-C	cDE/cDE	CDe/cDE	A_1 B cde/cde
Anti-E	cDe/cde	CDe/cDE	A_1 B cde/cde
Anti-c	CDe/CDe	CDe/cDE	A_1 B CDe/CDe or A_1 + B, both CDe/CDe
Anti-e	cDE/cDE	cDE/cde	A_1B cDE/cDE or A_1 + B, both cDE/cDE

set up. Table 28.2 lists the most readily available red cells that may be used. In addition, appropriate patient 'auto' and reagent 'diluent' controls should be set up as previously described.

BLOOD GROUPING: SPECIAL CONSIDERATIONS

GROUPING OF RECIPIENTS

Except in the case of identical twins or when the patient's own blood is returned to him (autologous transfusion), it is impossible to obtain blood for purposes of transfusion of *exactly* the same genotype as that of the recipient. In practice, blood for transfusion is *matched only in respect of ABO and D groups*. Whilst this is usually perfectly satisfactory, allo-antibodies not infrequently develop in patients who have received many transfusions. According to Giblett's data[18] the antibodies which are most frequently found are anti-K, anti-Le^a, anti-Le^b, anti-E and anti-c. (Anti-Lewis antibodies are not uncommon in people who have not been transfused.) K, E and c are the antigens, in addition to A, B and D, which appear to be the most antigenic; Jk^a, C and S are amongst the antigens which appear to be less antigenic. In patients who are destined to receive many transfusions, therefore, a case can be made for trying to avoid transfusing them with powerful antigens such as K, E and c if they themselves lack these particular antigens.

Whilst group-O blood can be given to patients of groups A, B and AB, this practice is not recom-

mended. It is inadvisable because harmful effects can follow the transfusion of large volumes of plasma containing hyperimmune anti-A and anti-B—which can lead to a haemolytic transfusion reaction—and also because the practice leads to a relative shortage of group-O blood. If shortage of blood necessitates the transfusion of group-O blood to other groups then packed cells should be used.

When D-negative donors are in short supply and large volumes of blood are required, the problem of transfusing a D-negative patient with D-positive blood arises. This must be avoided in women in the reproductive period of life and in female children. In other cases it must be established that the recipient's serum contains no anti-D antibodies, if it is proposed to use D-positive blood.

GROUPING OF BLOOD DONORS

In grouping prospective donors it is routine practice to carry out ABO grouping and to classify donors as Rh(D)-positive or Rh(D)-negative. Rh(D)-negative donors are then tested with anti-C and anti-E sera to pick up the rare combinations Cde and cdE and

CD^{u}E and cD^{u}E. Only donors of type cde/cde (rr) are regarded as Rh-negative for the purpose of donation. The relatively more easily available mixtures of anti-D plus anti-C and anti-D plus anti-E should be used rather than pure anti-C and anti-E sera to group cells already known not to react with anti-D. However, the present restriction of the designation 'Rh-negative' to rr donors is under discussion and may be extended to include combinations including r′ and r″. It is estimated that this would provide an extra 1400 Rh-negative donors for every 100,000 donors (D. Voak, personal communication).

GROUPING IN ANTENATAL WORK

Pregnant women must be grouped for ABO and D and this should be done early in pregnancy as a routine.

Accuracy in D grouping of antenatal samples is particularly important as D-negative women erroneously grouped as D-positive carry the risk of:

1. Being transfused with D-positive blood and consequently being sensitized to the D antigen which could result in severe HDN in subsequent pregnancies.
2. Not receiving prophylactic anti-D immunoglobulin, with the same potential consequences as (1).
3. Being screened serologically less frequently during pregnancy which could result in delayed detection of significant antibodies that could compromise the management of HDN.

Ideally, the sera of all pregnant women, whether D-negative or D-positive, should be screened for antibodies other than anti-D. Although HDN due to anti-D in D-negative women is by far the most severe form of the disease, HDN can occur, although less commonly, as the result of the formation of anti-c or anti-E in D-positive mothers. Moreover, HDN has been described, albeit very rarely, as the result of incompatibilities in most of the other major blood-group systems; of these, immunization against the Kell antigen (K) is the commonest. It is best, therefore, not to confine antenatal screening to Rh(D)-negative mothers, but to screen the sera of all patients. A schedule for antenatal antibody screening is given on p. 472.

The paternal blood group phenotype should be determined in all cases where the mother has an allo-antibody. If the paternal red cells lack the corresponding antigen, the baby is not at risk. However, caution is advised, as the assumed parent may not be the biological father of the fetus!

ANTIBODY SCREENING

In parallel with determining the ABO and D groups of patients it is ideal to screen all sera for unexpected allo-antibodies, i.e. other than anti-A and anti-B. This provides an opportunity for early detection and identification of unexpected antibodies, thereby facilitating the selection of suitable blood for a patient requiring transfusion.

The patient's serum should be tested against at least two red cell suspensions, used separately and *not* pooled.

The screening cells must be group O and should encompass the common antigens of the ethnic population. In the UK the screening cells should express, as a minimum, the following antigens: C,c, D, E, e, M, N, S, s, P$_1$, K, k, Le^a, Le^b, Fy^a, Fy^b, Jk^a, Jk^b; cells with C^w should also be included if available. At least one cell must have the stronger D antigen combination R$_2$. It is also desirable, although not always possible, to have antigens in the homozygous state; particularly for Jk^a, Jk^b, S, C, Fy^a, Fy^b, because heterozygous red cells may fail to detect antibodies that would react positively with homozygous cells. Such antibodies have proved to be of clinical importance.

Screening cells taken into ACD or CPD containing a bacteriostatic will keep 3–4 weeks at 4°C. These are available commercially or from Blood Transfusion Centres.

The antibody screening procedure is designed to detect antibodies of clinical significance. No single test will detect all blood-group antibodies, but an effective compromise is as follows:

1. Direct agglutination test in normal (NISS) or low ionic strength solutions (LISS)—recommended temperature 37°C to avoid detection of insignificant cold antibodies.
2. Indirect anti-human globulin (AHG) test after incubation in NISS or LISS (p. 435).

3. Two-stage enzyme tests (p. 430) are considered useful supportive techniques, especially for Rh antibodies, although they may fail to detect some antibodies reactive in a spin tube AHG test.

A positive result in the antibody screen should be followed by antibody identification against a comprehensive cell panel. This may require referral to a Blood Transfusion Centre. As a first step it is desirable to ascertain as far as is possible the genotype of the patient whose serum is being tested. If, for instance, the patient's Rh genotype is $CDe/CDe(R^1R^1)$ the antibody might well be anti-E or anti-c; it could not be anti-C or anti-e (unless possibly associated with auto-immune haemolytic anaemia). The immuno-chemical properties of an antibody assist in the resolution of mixtures of antibodies. If the antibody is clearly cold-reacting and causing direct agglutination in saline at 20°C or 25°C, but is inactive at 37°C, it is not likely to be anti-D; but it might well be anti-P_1 or anti-Le^a. IgG antibodies are usually not active in saline tests and are best detected in enzyme or indirect antiglobulin tests (exceptions are anti-A, anti-B, anti-M, anti-N because the reactive red cells have a very high antigen density). The use of enzyme (e.g. papain)-treated washed cells is a useful test, equal in sensitivity to the spin tube AHG test for Rh antibodies. Also, as papain destroys M, N, S and Fy^a

antigens, the inclusion of an enzyme test helps to sort out these antibody specificities.

The next practical step is therefore to set up the serum against a panel of cells of known phenotype with particular reference to the antibody or antibodies which the patient appears most likely to have developed. Table 28.3 illustrates the result of a typical investigation of a patient of Rh genotype CDe/CDe, who had received many transfusions and whose serum was positive on antibody screening. The results of these tests strongly suggest a reaction with the E antigen (common to cell samples 2, 3 and 4) and also with the K antigen (present in cells 4 and 6). The positive reaction obtained with cell sample 6 cannot be due to anti-Le^b because this antigen is present in cell sample 1 which was not agglutinated. The finding of anti-E is not unexpected in a patient of genotype CDe/CDe and the patient himself was K-negative. As a further confirmatory step, the serum could be tested with several E+ K− and E− K+ cells. Without exception they should all give positive reactions.

Group, antibody screen and save procedure

This is ideal for operative procedures where blood is often not required, but where it has been

Table 28.3 Identification of unknown antibodies using a panel of red cells of known genotype

Cell sample	Genotypes and phenotypes								
1	O	CDe/CDe	MNS +	P +	Lu(a −)	K −	Le(a − b +)	Fy(a +)	Jk(a +)
2	O	CDe/cDE	MNS +	P −	Lu(a −)	K −	Le(a − b +)	Fy(a +)	Jk(a +)
3	O	cDe/cDE	NS +	P +	Lu(a +)	K −	Le(a + b −)	Fy(a −)	Jk(a +)
4	O	cde/cDE	NS −	P +	Lu(a −)	K +	Le(a + b −)	Fy(a −)	Jk(a −)
5	O	cde/cde	MNS −	P +	Lu(a −)	K −	Le(a − b −)	Fy(a +)	Jk(a +)
6	O	cde/cde	MS +	P −	Lu(a −)	K +	Le(a − b +)	Fy(a −)	Jk(a −)

	Results		
	Agglutination*		Indirect antiglobulin test
Cell sample	(20°C)	(37°C)	(37°C)
1	−	−	−
2	−	−	+
3	−	−	+ +
4	−	−	+ +
5	−	−	−
6	−	−	+

+ and + + denote agglutination; − denotes absence of agglutination.
*The cells used were not enzyme-treated.

customary to have compatible blood on standby. The patient's blood is ABO and D grouped and screened for unexpected antibodies; the serum is retained but no blood is cross-matched. When patients with a negative antibody screen require blood urgently, blood of the same ABO and D group can be given, subject only to a rapid spin cross-match (i.e. after 2–5 min incubation at room temperature) to exclude ABO incompatibility (see Emergency Blood Issue).

In order to operate an effective 'group, screen and save' policy, an understanding has to be reached with the clinical (ward and theatre) staff. This may be co-ordinated with maximum blood ordering schedules for planned surgical operations.[15]

CROSS-MATCHING

Only the 'major' cross-match between the patient's serum and the donor red cells is required. The function of the cross-match is to prevent incompatibility. This is most serious when there is ABO incompatibility and, in particular, when A or B cells are transfused into a group-O person with a high titre anti-A/anti-B.

Methods that demonstrate ABO incompatibility and other clinically significant antibodies must be used. It is important to note that in addition to agglutination, haemolysis is a sign of incompatibility.

The actual procedure followed will depend on the clinical circumstances, since in emergency situations the testing protocol may have to be modified in order to provide blood as quickly as possible for the patient.

Patient's cells and serum

Obtain blood from the patient, a day or two, if possible, before the transfusion is needed so that the pretransfusion testing may be carried out unhurriedly, with proper controls. Serum is preferred to plasma for matching purposes as strong rouleaux formation, which might be a source of confusion, is far less likely to occur. Keep the serum for 1–2 weeks at −20°C after the transfusion has been given in case there is need to investigate an unfavourable transfusion reaction.

If the patient has been transfused since the date of collection of the serum sample in hand, and if that transfusion was given more than 2 days previously, a new blood sample is required for antibody screening and cross-matching to detect the emergence of any new antibodies in pre-immunized patients.

ROUTINE CROSS-MATCHING

Select donor units for cross-matching on the basis of ABO and Rh (D) grouping and antibody identification.

Test the patient's serum against donor red cells by:

1. Direct agglutination test in NISS or LISS. Inspect for agglutination and haemolysis. The test can be read in the tube after gentle agitation over a ×5 or ×6 magnification illuminated mirror, and incorporated with (2) as one-tube procedure.

2. Indirect AHG test using a minimum incubation 15-min LISS test or a 45-min NISS test. The incubation temperature should be 37°C using a water-bath or warmed block (air incubators are not recommended).

EMERGENCY BLOOD ISSUE (WHERE TIME DOES NOT PERMIT FULL COMPATIBILITY TESTING)

An EDTA and a clotted sample should be obtained from the patient before the administration of intravenous colloids, such as Dextran and hydroxethylstarch (HES), which may cause troublesome red cell aggregation in serological testing.

Laboratories that use LISS for routine work are well placed to meet urgent compatibility requests. However, where laboratories use NISS routinely, it recommended that they change to LISS tests or emergency techniques.

Patients should be ABO and D grouped by rapid techniques and group compatible blood issued. Exclude ABO incompatibility by a rapid (2–5 min) spin cross-match and/or by group-checking the blood units before issue. For an analysis of the sensitivity and specificity of the immediate spin cross-match the reader is referred to a recent report by Meyer and Shulman.[25]

If this procedure is followed, it should seldom be necessary to have to resort to group-O D-negative blood. Should this need arise, only previously group-checked units should be issued. Furthermore, this should be changed to blood of the patient's own group as soon as possible to avoid subsequent confusion over ABO grouping.

If a massive transfusion has been given in which the number of units transfused in 24 h exceeds the recipient's blood volume, compatibility testing may be reduced to checking the ABO/D groups of the transfused units.

After the emergency has been dealt with, retrospective cross-matching should be undertaken with the pretransfusion sample.

Donor units that have not been tested, or not fully tested, against the patient's serum should be clearly labelled, e.g. 'Selected for patient. . . , but *not* cross-matched'.

SPECIAL TRANSFUSION SITUATIONS

There are some situations where the provision of compatible blood requires special consideration.

Compatibility tests in newborn infants

For infants under 4 months, both baby and maternal blood samples should be ABO and D grouped, the maternal serum screened for unexpected antibodies, and a direct AHG test done on the baby's cells.

If a negative maternal antibody screen is obtained and the baby's direct AHG test is negative, blood of the same ABO and D group as the infant may be issued without cross-matching, even after repeated transfusions, provided the ABO and D groups of the donor units are checked before issue. Recent studies indicate that infants under the age of 4 months do

not make red cell allo-antibodies even after multiple transfusions.[23]

If the infant is suffering from haemolytic disease of the newborn (HDN), or if unexpected antibodies are detected in the maternal serum, it is important to use the maternal serum for compatibility testing. This may dictate the use of group-O blood, and if the infant is not group O, care should be taken to ensure donor units have low titre anti-A and anti-B. If ABO HDN is suspected, group-O blood of low titre anti-A and anti-B should be used. An alternative to low titre group-O blood is O cells reconstituted in one-third volume of AB plasma. It should be noted that compatible red cells from adult group-A or -B donors should not be used, as adult red cells will almost certainly have more A and B antigen sites than the infant's own red cells and are likely to undergo more rapid destruction by the residual maternal anti-A or anti-B. In the event of an exchange transfusion, plasma-reduced blood is indicated.

Compatibility tests for intra-uterine transfusion

Blood for an intra-uterine transfusion should be tested for compatibility with the mother's serum. It should be group O and always D-negative (except, for example, when the mother is D-positive and has made antibodies other than anti-D or anti-D mixtures). Kell (K)-negative blood should also be used (p. 464). Compatibility tests for subsequent transfusions must be repeated every time using fresh maternal serum, for the manipulations of intra-uterine transfusions are not uncommonly followed by the escape of donor cells into the maternal circulation which could lead to the formation of antibodies of a new specificity. It is essential to test the mother's serum against a phenotyped panel of red cells between each intra-uterine transfusion to identify any new allo-antibodies formed.

Blood for intra-uterine transfusion should, preferably, be less than 24 h old. It should be negative for cytomegalovirus (CMV) antibody and for the other standard microbiological markers for HIV, hepatitis B and syphilis; it should also be γ-irradiated (1500 rads) to avoid graft-versus-host disease. Plasma-reduced blood or washed red cells suspended in saline should be used.

Compatibility tests in patients receiving transfusions at close intervals

Allo-antibodies may develop quickly following a transfusion early in a series. It is important, therefore, to obtain a fresh sample of serum from the recipient before each transfusion if they are separated by an interval of 2 days or longer; while if the patient is receiving daily transfusions, only blood that is likely to be used in the 2 days following the collection of the serum should be matched. It is advisable to do a DAT on the patient's red cells each time, as antibodies that have formed may be adsorbed to incompatible cells and not be present in the serum.

Compatibility tests in auto-immune haemolytic anaemia (AIHA)

(a) Warm-type AIHA

ABO grouping is usually straightforward, but antibody coating on the patient's red cells can cause false positive D grouping results (p. 462). Saline-reacting monoclonal IgM anti-D reagents will give reliable grouping results.

The problem here is that the auto-antibody reacts with all donor blood samples, so that no cross-match compatible blood can be found. In this situation it is essential to exclude any incompatibility due to the simultaneous presence of allo-antibodies stimulated by previous transfusion or pregnancy. Recent reports indicate that allo-antibodies may be present in up to 40% of cases, the most frequent being anti-C and anti-K.[21,41] It is therefore helpful to determine the patient's Rh phenotype and K type (at least) before transfusions are started, so that donor compatible blood can be selected. Phenotyping the patient's red cells will be made easier by removing the bound auto-antibody by various elution techniques.[20] The ABO group of any unit to be transfused should also be rechecked to avoid the possibility of ABO incompatibility being mistaken

for a reaction with the patient's auto-antibody.

Useful advice on the detection of allo-antibodies, which can be quite difficult in the presence of auto-antibody, has been given by Petz and Garratty[32] (see also p. 490). This includes:

1. Comparing the direct (DAT) and indirect (IAT) antiglobulin tests, e.g. if the IAT is significantly stronger than the DAT, the presence of allo-antibody is most likely. No conclusion can be drawn from the reverse situation when the DAT is strongly positive.

2. Testing the patient's serum with a phenotyped panel of red cells. This may show a pattern suggesting an allo-antibody.

3. Absorbing the patient's serum with the patient's own cells at 37°C to remove the auto-antibody and facilitate allo-antibody identification. This approach is possible if the patient has not been transfused during the previous 3 months. Save as many of the patient's red cells as possible and store these in ACD or CPD, or in the frozen state; these can then be used in the future for warm auto-absorption tests should repeat transfusion be necessary. While these tests will often identify a simultaneously occurring allo-antibody, the results may not always be so informative, and additional testing may be required (e.g. differential absorption of the patient's serum with red cells of different phenotypes), especially if the patient has been recently transfused.

(b) Cold-type AIHA

Cold agglutinins cause blood grouping and antibody screening problems (p. 458). Even if agglutination is avoided by performing these tests strictly at 37°C, complement binding may cause false positive results in the antiglobulin test during antibody screening and cross-matching. Useful advice on compatibility testing in the presence of cold agglutinins is given by Petz and Garratty.[32]

INVESTIGATION OF A HAEMOLYTIC TRANSFUSION REACTION

The serologist is particularly concerned with the potential immunological consequences of blood transfusion. These can be considered under two

broad headings: allo-immunization and incompatibility (Table 28.4).[43]

Donor-recipient compatibility is essential to

Table 28.4 Classification of immunological consequences of blood transfusion

Allo-immunization
i.e. the development of antibodies against:
  (i) Red cell, leucocyte and platelet antigens
  (ii) Plasma protein antigens

Incompatibility
(a) *Red cell incompatibility*
  (i) Intravascular haemolysis
      e.g. ABO incompatibility
  (ii) Extravascular haemolysis
      e.g. Rh incompatibility
      —Immediate
      —Delayed

(b) *Leucocyte and platelet incompatibility*
  (i) Febrile reaction (granulocytes, monocytes)
  (ii) Pulmonary reaction (granulocytes)
  (iii) Post-transfusion purpura (platelets)
  (iv) Poor survival of tranfused platelets and granulocytes
  (v) Graft-versus-host reaction (lymphocytes)

(c) *Plasma protein incompatibility*
      Urticarial and anaphylactic reactions

Table 28.5 Investigation of a haemolytic transfusion reaction

I. **Check for haemolysis**
  (i) Examine patient's plasma and urine for haemoglobin
  (ii) Blood film may show spherocytosis

II. **Check for incompatibility**
  (a) *Clerical causes*
      An identification error will indicate the type of incompatibility
  (b) *Serological causes*
      (i) Repeat ABO and D group of patient (pre- and post-transfusion) and donor units
      (ii) Screen for red cell antibodies
      (iii) Repeat cross-match with pre- and post-transfusion serum
      (iv) Direct antiglobulin test (pre- and post-transfusion samples)

III. **Check for DIC**
  (i) Blood film (red cell fragmentation)
  (ii) Platelet count
  (iii) Coagulation screen

IV. **Check for bacterial infection**
      Gram stain and culture donor blood

ensure normal survival of transfused red cells and to avoid the harmful effects of a haemolytic transfusion reaction. The mechanism of haemolysis depends on the Ig class of the antibody and its ability to fix complement (p. 426). This also determines the site of haemolysis. Haemolytic transfusion reactions (HTR) may be acute (intravascular or extravascular) or delayed.

(A) ACUTE INTRAVASCULAR HAEMOLYSIS

Acute intravascular haemolysis is a dreaded complication of blood transfusion. It is usually due to ABO incompatibility resulting from a misidentification error. Although an acute emergency, prompt diagnosis and treatment can be life saving. At the first suspicion of reaction the tranfusion must be stopped, as the severity of the clinical consequences depends partly on the volume of red cells transfused to the patient. The laboratory performing the pre-transfusion compatibility testing must be notified immediately.

Diagnosis depends on demonstrating haemolysis in the patient and incompatibility between the donor and the patient (Table 28.5). Patient identification and the donor unit compatibility label should be rechecked at the bedside. As clerical errors involving one patient may involve others cross-matched at the same time, it is essential to check the samples, donor units and documentation of all cross-matches done at that time. Differential diagnosis from other conditions causing a similar clinical presentation is also important, the most serious being the transfusion of infected blood (Table 28.6).

Serological investigations

Specimens required:

1. Pre-transfusion serum and red cells of the patient.

Table 28.6 *Differential diagnosis of acute haemolytic transfusion reaction*

Red cell incompatibility

Transfusion of infected blood

Other causes of haemolysis
  (i) Post-operative infection (e.g. clostridial septicaemia)
  (ii) Infusion of hypotonic solutions (including hypotonic dialysis)
  (iii) Haemolytic anaemia (e.g. PNH)

Transfusion of lysed red cells
  (i) Thermal damage (pre-transfusion heating or freezing)
  (ii) Mechanical damage (e.g. extracorporeal machines, excessive infusion pressure and/or small bore needle)

2. Post-transfusion serum and red cells of the patient.

3. The donor unit involved, together with the giving set and any other donor units transfused.

4. Urine from the patient for the first 24 hours after the reaction. This will be dark due to the presence of haemoglobin in the case of intravascular haemolysis.

Serological tests

1. Confirm the ABO and D groups of the patient's pre- and post-transfusion samples and the donor units.

2. Perform a direct antiglobulin test on the patient's pre- and post-transfusion washed red cells: a negative DAT post-transfusion does not exclude a severe haemolytic reaction.

3. Repeat the cross-match tests of donor's red cells with patient's serum, using pre- and post-transfusion samples.

4. Screen the donor plasma and the patient's pre- and post-transfusion serum samples for unexpected antibodies.

5. If the donor was group O and the patient group A or B, then titre the anti-A and anti-B levels in the donor plasma, as high titres (>128) are found in 'dangerous group- O donors'.

Haematological tests

1. Blood count—including platelet and reticulocyte counts.
2. Blood film—spherocytosis, red cell fragmentation.
3. Coagulation screen.

Disseminated intravascular coagulation (DIC) is a feature of intravascular HTR and the transfusion of infected blood; severe DIC is a bad prognostic sign.

Bacteriological tests

Inspect the donor unit(s) for any obvious haemolysis. The donor blood unit(s) and giving set should be tested by culturing the remaining blood at 4°C, 20°C and 37°C and by Gram stain and smear examination.

Biochemical tests

The patient's post-transfusion serum should be inspected for haemolysis and tested for free haemoglobin and bilirubin, and the results compared with those of the pre-transfusion sample.

If the above testing does not indicate a haemolytic transfusion reaction or infected blood, other possible causes of an adverse immunological reaction, e.g. leucocyte antibodies, allergic reactions to plasma proteins (Table 28.4), should be taken into consideration when selecting blood for further transfusions.

(B) ACUTE EXTRAVASCULAR HAEMOLYSIS

Acute extravascular haemolysis is a feature of IgG antibodies that do not cause complement lysis. This is a less severe haemolytic reaction. The main clinical features are fever, sometimes with rigors, and an inadequate haemoglobin response to the transfusion that cannot be explained by blood loss; jaundice may occur, but haemoglobinuria is not common. These reactions are not commonly seen due to improved pre-transfusion antibody screening and cross-matching procedures. Diagnosis should follow the procedure set out in Table 28.5.

(C) DELAYED HAEMOLYTIC REACTIONS

Delayed haemolytic reactions may occur in patients allo-immunized by previous pregnancy or transfusion. The antibody titre is too low to be detected in the pre-transfusion compatibility testing, but after re-exposure to the incompatible antigen, a secondary (anamnestic) immune response occurs. IgG antibodies are made and the transfused red cells are destroyed; anti-Jk^a is such an antibody (p. 426).

Haemolysis is usually extravascular, and typically the patient develops anaemia, fever, jaundice and sometimes haemoglobinuria about 1 week after transfusion. The clinical picture may resemble an auto-immune or drug-induced immune haemolytic anaemia with a positive direct antiglobulin test (in this case due to allo-antibody on the donor cells), spherocytosis and reticulocytosis. However, the history of a preceding transfusion should suggest the correct diagnosis, which should be confirmed as in Table 28.5. There is usually no need for further action in most cases as the process is self-limiting. Many delayed haemolytic transfusion reactions of this type almost certainly go undetected.

HAEMOLYTIC DISEASE OF THE NEWBORN (HDN)

HDN is an immune haemolytic anaemia affecting the fetus and newborn infant. It occurs when maternal allo-antibody to fetal red cell antigens crosses the placenta and causes haemolysis of fetal red cells. As IgG is the only immunoglobulin transferred across the placenta, only red cell antibodies of this class are a potential cause of HDN. Anti-D causes the most severe form of HDN. However, the success of anti-D prophylaxis has reduced the number of cases of Rh (D) HDN; consequently the relative proportion of cases due to other antibodies has increased, notably anti-c, anti-E and anti-K, but almost every other red cell IgG antibody has been reported as a cause of HDN. ABO-HDN is considered separately as a number of special factors combine to protect the fetus from the effects of ABO incompatibility. For a more detailed discussion of HDN the reader is referred to the review by Bowman et al[11] and the textbook by Mollison et al.[26c]

ANTENATAL SEROLOGY

Maternal ABO and D grouping and antibody screening (p. 465) is the basis of any system for the prediction and management of HDN. Protocols for antenatal screening vary in detail, but depend on the maternal D group, antibody status, transfusion history, and obstetric history of HDN. It is important to screen both D-positive and D-negative women; the D-positive woman, particularly if she has been transfused, may develop allo-antibodies that are dangerous for the fetus. A satisfactory testing schedule can be summarized as follows:[2]

Without antibodies

	Test at
D-negative and previously transfused women	Booking
	24–28 weeks
	34–36 weeks
	Delivery
Other D-positive women	Booking
	34–36 weeks

With antibodies

Mothers with antibodies or a history of HDN should be tested more frequently, e.g. monthly until 28 weeks, then at shorter intervals, e.g. every 2 weeks.

Antibody screening should be carried out as previously described (p. 465); in addition it is recommended that ABO and D grouping be repeated on each occasion to minimize the risk of error.

Antenatal assessment of severity of Rh(D) HDN

The role of the serologist is to carry out serial antibody measurements on sensitized women to determine the titre or concentration (μg/ml) of anti-D. Manual titrations are less sensitive than quantitative automated assays for detecting changes in antibody levels; a two-fold change in antibody concentration must occur before the titre is affected. Nevertheless, titration of maternal anti-D plays an important part in identifying pregnancies at risk. Individual laboratories working with local obstetricians generally establish the clinical significance of their own titration results, e.g. antiglobulin titres of the order of 8–32 suggest the need for further intervention to assess the severity of HDN.

Automated measurement of the amount of anti-D (iu or μg/ml) may define the fetal risk more accurately,[8,16] as also may the antibody-dependent cell-mediated cytotoxicity (ADCC) assay used as a model of in-vivo haemolysis in the fetus.[31,35] However, further essential information regarding management depends on amniotic fluid spectrophotometry[22] and more recently on direct fetal blood sampling by ultrasound-guided cordocentesis.[14] The last procedure provides not only direct diagnostic information,[28,29] but also a new approach to fetal therapy by direct fetal intravascular transfusion.[19,30]

The declining incidence of severe Rh (D) HDN and the increasingly specialized management of severely affected pregnancies has meant that these women are now being referred to specialist centres dealing with this condition.

TESTS ON MATERNAL AND CORD BLOOD AT DELIVERY

It should be standard practice to collect an adequate sample (e.g. 20 ml) of cord blood (both EDTA and clotted specimens) for serological studies, as subsequent (small) samples from the baby may not be enough for all the necessary tests to be carried out. There should be an agreed local procedure for labelling mother's and baby's samples to avoid misidentification errors.

The following tests should be carried out on all D-negative mothers and their babies:

(a) Tests on cord blood

1. ABO and D grouping
2. Direct antiglobulin test (if positive, test the mother's serum against a cell panel to identify the antibody)
3. Haemoglobin
4. Bilirubin (D-positive babies).

(b) Tests on maternal blood

1. Repeat ABO and D grouping
2. Repeat antibody screen (in case anti-D sensitization has occurred in a previously unsensitized woman)
3. Kleihauer test for fetomaternal red cell leakage (p. 121) if the baby is shown to be D-positive; this determines the prophylactic dose of anti-D immunoglobulin to be given to the mother to prevent sensitization (see below).

The above tests should also be carried out on the cord blood of all babies born to mothers with antibodies other than anti-D. Ideally, a direct antiglobulin test should be done on all cord blood samples, as this offers the opportunity of detecting unsuspected ABO HDN (p. 474), and other antibodies against rare or private (paternal) antigens which may be of greater clinical significance in subsequent pregnancies. Attractive as this proposal is on clinical grounds, it seems unlikely that it could be generally applied on economic grounds.

ANTI-D PROPHYLAXIS

The dose of anti-D for D-negative women at risk depends on the size of the fetomaternal red cell leakage, as determined by the Kleihauer acid elution technique (p. 121). The method depends on the Hb F of fetal red cells resisting acid elution to a greater extent than the Hb A of maternal red cells. When a treated maternal blood film is stained with eosin the fetal cells stain dark pink and the maternal cells appear as pale 'ghosts'.

Using a $\times 40$ objective and $\times 10$ eyepieces (i.e. low power), count the darkly staining fetal red cells in a single low power field (LPF). The dose of anti-D is calculated as follows:

Kleihauer count	Dose of anti-D immunoglobulin
Up to 200 cells/50 LPF	500 iu
For every 100 cells in excess of 200/50 LPF	Extra 500 iu

e.g. for a Kleihauer count of 500 cells/50 LPF the dose of anti-D would be 2000 iu.

The administration of an adequate dose of anti-D to prevent maternal sensitization is the responsibility of the clinician in charge of the patient. The following guidelines for preventing D immunization by pregnancy are based on the recommendations set out in Mollison et al.[26d]

1. Minimize the risk of misclassifying D-negative woman as D-positive by performing the D group on at least two separate occasions, i.e. (a) during pregnancy, and (b) at delivery. This presupposes accurate and unique patient identification throughout pregnancy.

2. An adequate dose of anti-D immunoglobulin should be given to *all as yet unimmunized D-negative women*. The following procedure is recommended:

(a) After delivery

1. To avoid the situation where anti-D is sometimes withheld because a report on the baby's D group has not been received, all Rh(D)-negative women should be given a *standard* dose of anti-D (500 iu) within 72 h of delivery, unless the baby is

known to be D-negative.

2. On the basis of the Kleihauer test, *extra* anti-D may be indicated to cover a larger feto-maternal leakage of red cells.

(b) During pregnancy

1. For abortion before 20 weeks a standard dose of 250 iu should be given; after 20 weeks give 500 iu or more based on the Kleihauer count.

2. Following obstetric manipulations (e.g. amniocentesis, version) and ante-partum haemorrhage (APH) give 500 iu of anti-D or more, based on the Kleihauer count.

Prophylactic anti-D is also given routinely in the third trimester in some countries,[10] but this is not current standard practice in the UK.

ABO HAEMOLYTIC DISEASE OF THE NEWBORN

This is considered separately, as a number of special factors combine to protect the fetus from the effects of ABO incompatibility. For practical purposes, only group-O individuals make high titres of IgG anti-A and anti-B. Therefore only A and B infants of group-O mothers are at risk from ABO-HDN. Although 15% of births are susceptible, only about 1% are affected; even then the condition is usually mild and very rarely severe enough to need exchange transfusion. Two mechanisms protect the fetus against anti-A and anti-B: one is the relative weakness of A and B antigens, the other is the widespread distribution of A and B glycoproteins in fetal fluids and tissues, which diverts much of the IgG antibody that crosses the placenta away from the red cell 'target'.

ABO-HDN may be seen in the first incompatible pregnancy. This is unlike anti-D HDN, where immunization usually takes place at the end of the first pregnancy, the first child thus being unaffected.

Serological investigation

ABO haemolytic disease is difficult to diagnose, especially in Caucasians, as the DAT may be negative or weak even in a case of severe haemolytic disease. Furthermore, anti-A or anti-B is normally present in the mother's serum and special tests are needed to demonstrate a high titre of IgG anti-A or anti-B in the presence of IgM anti-A or anti-B.

In cases of suspected ABO HDN the main features are:[39]

1. It is almost always confined to infants of group-O mothers as there is 16 times more IgG anti-A and anti-B in group-O than in group-A or group-B mothers.

2. As anti-A and anti-B are always present in group-O mothers, evidence for ABO-HDN depends on demonstrating a high titre of IgG anti-A or anti-B, e.g. by treating the mother's serum with 2-mercapto-ethanol (2-ME) or dithiothreitol (DTT) to distinguish between IgG and IgM antibodies (for method, see p. 501).

3. The DAT on cord blood is often weak or negative; the latter at least excludes any other serological incompatibility. This probably reflects the relative paucity of A and B antigen sites on the red cells of newborn infants.

4. The simplest evidence for the occurrence of ABO haemolytic disease is obtained by testing the serum of the cord blood sample for incompatible anti-A or anti-B by the antiglobulin test with adult A_1, B and O cells. If the baby is group A the important test is with the A_1 cells which will be positive in ABO HDN. The strong reaction with B cells will always occur with a group-A baby and is of no significance as anti-B is compatible with the baby's A cells. The test with O cells should be negative, but if positive, indicates the presence of a further antibody as a possible contributory or major cause of the disease, especially if the DAT is strongly positive. Similarly, if the baby is group-B the critical test is with adult B cells; a strong reaction will also be found with A_1 cells, but this will not harm the baby's B cells.

Note: If the blood sample from the baby is not taken until the time of crisis of the disease, usually about 2–3 days after delivery, the serological tests may be negative because most, if not all, of the maternal anti-A or anti-B will have been absorbed in the destruction of the baby's red cells.

5. The best diagnostic test of ABO HDN is to prepare a heat eluate from the baby's red cells (from the cord blood sample), and test it (together with the last wash supernatant as a control) by antiglobulin tests with adult A_1, B and O cells. In some

cases reactions occur with both A_1 and B cells due to anti-AB cross-reacting antibodies, but most severe cases of ABO HDN involve separate specific anti-A or anti-B antibodies.[37] The tests with O cells and the last wash control should be negative.

Antenatal prediction

Antenatal prediction of ABO HDN is not essential for medical management, as there is time to observe the baby after birth and to treat according to the severity of the condition. Nevertheless, a baby is likely to be more severely affected if the maternal IgG anti-A (-B) titre is greater than 128.[9]

A recent study using an ADCC assay, in which monocytes from normal donors were incubated with normal red cells sensitized with maternal anti-A or anti-B serum, suggests that a strongly positive result with this assay correlates with severe HDN.[12,13] The most severe haemolysis was associated with a maternal antibody of IgG3 subclass and a high antigen density on the fetal red cells. While the ADCC assay is not advocated as a routine screening test in group-O mothers at risk, it could be used selectively to predict the outcome of a pregnancy when there has been a previously severely affected infant.

REFERENCES

[1] AABB (1989). *Standards for Blood Banks and Transfusion Services*, 13th edn. Ed. P. V. Holland. American Association of Blood Banks, Arlington, VA.

[2] ANONYMOUS (1986) Prenatal screening for irregular blood group antibodies. *Lancet*, ii, 1369.

[3] British Committee for Standardization in Haematology (1987). Guidelines for compatibility testing in hospital blood banks. *Clinical and Laboratory Haematology*, 9, 333.

[4] British Committee for Standardization in Haematology (1986). *Guidelines for Hospital Blood Bank Computing*. British Society for Haematology, London.

[5] British Committee for Standardization in Haematology (1990). *Guidelines for Hospital Blood Bank Documentation and Procedures*. Clinical and Laboratory Haematology 12, 209.

[6] British Committee for Standards in Haematology (1990). Guidelines for microplate techniques in liquid-phase blood grouping and antibody screening. *Clinical and Laboratory Haematology* (In press).

[7] BIRD, G. W. G. (1988) Lectins in haematology and blood banking. *Methods in Hematology*, 17, 125.

[8] BOWELL, P. J., WAINSCOAT, J. S., PETO, T. E. A. and GUNSON, H. H. (1982). Maternal anti-D concentrations and outcome in rhesus haemolytic disease of the newborn. *British Medical Journal*, 285, 327.

[9] BOWLEY, C. C. and VOAK, D. (1971). What is the optimal serological analysis of haemolytic disease of the newborn due to ABO incompatibility? International Forum. *Vox Sanguinis*, 20, 183.

[10] BOWMAN, J. M. (1985). Controversies in Rh prophylaxis: who needs Rh immune globulin and when should it be given? *American Journal of Obstetrics and Gynecology*, 151, 289.

[11] BOWMAN, J. M., POLLOCK, J. M. and BIGGINS, K. R. (1988). Antenatal studies and the management of hemolytic disease of the newborn. *Methods in Hematology*, 17, 163.

[12] BROUWERS, H. A. A., OVERBEEKE, M. A. M., van ERTBRUGGEN, I. et al (1988a). What is the best prediction of the severity of ABO-haemolytic disease of the newborn? *Lancet*, ii, 641.

[13] BROUWERS, H. A. A., OVERBEEKE, M. A. M., VAN ERTBRUGGEN, I., VAN LEEUWEN, E. F., STOOP, J. W. and ENGELFRIET, C. P. (1988b). Maternal antibodies against fetal blood-group antigens A or B: lytic activity of IgG subclasses in monocyte-driven cytotoxicity and correlation with ABO-haemolytic disease of the newborn. *British Journal of Haematology*, 70, 465.

[14] DAFFOS, F., CAPELLA-PAVLOVSKY, M. and FORESTIER, F. (1985). Fetal blood sampling during pregnancy with use of a needle guided by ultrasound; a study of 606 consecutive cases. *American Journal of Obstetrics and Gynaecology*, 153, 655.

[15] DODSWORTH, H. and DUDLEY, H. A. F. (1985). Increased efficiency of transfusion practice in routine surgery using pre-operative antibody screening and selective ordering with an abbreviated cross-match. *British Journal of Surgery*, 72, 102.

[16] FRASER, I. D. and TOVEY, G. H. (1976). Observations on Rh iso-immunization: past, present and future. *Clinics in Haematology*, 5, 149.

[17] GARRATTY, G. (1982). The role of compatibility tests. *Transfusion*, 22, 169.

[18] GIBLETT, E. R. (1977). Blood group alloantibodies: an assessment of some laboratory practices. *Transfusion*, 17, 299.

[19] GRANNUM, P. A., COPEL, J. A., PLAXE, S. C., SCIOSCIA, A. L. and HOBBINS, J. C. (1986). In utero exchange transfusion by direct intravascular injection in severe erythroblastosis fetalis. *New England Journal of Medicine*, 314, 1431.

[20] JUDD, W. J. (1988). Antibody elution from red cells. *Methods in Hematology*, 17, 78.

[21] LAINE, M. L. and BEATTIE, K. M. (1985). Frequency of alloantibodies accompanying autoantibodies. *Transfusion*, 25, 545.

[22] LILEY, A. W. (1961). Liquor amnii analysis in management of pregnancy complicated by rhesus immunization. *American Journal of Obstetrics and Gynecology*, 82, 1359.

[23] LUDVIGSEN, C. W. Jr, SWANSON, J. L., THOMPSON, T. R. and McCULLOUGH, J. (1987). The failure of neonates to form red blood cell alloantibodies in response to multiple transfusions. *American Journal of Clinical Pathology*, 87, 250.

[24] McGOWAN, A., TOD, A., CHIRNSIDE, A. et al (1989). Stability of murine monoclonal anti-A, anti-B and anti-A,B

ABO grouping reagents and a multi-centre evaluation of their performance in routine use. *Vox Sanguinis*, **56**, 122.

[25] MEYER, E. A. and SHULMAN, I. A. (1989). The sensitivity and specificity of the immediate-spin crossmatch. *Transfusion*, **29**, 99.

[26] MOLLISON, P. L., ENGELFRIET, C. P. and CONTRERAS, M. (1987). *Blood Transfusion in Clinical Medicine*, 8th. edn., (a) p. 335, (b) p. 336, (c) p. 637, (d) p. 674. Blackwell Scientific Publications, Oxford.

[27] MOORE, P. B. L. (1986). Good laboratory practice before and after blood transfusion. *Haematologia*, **19**, 241.

[28] NICOLAIDES, K. H., RODECK, C. H., MILLAR, D. S. and MIBASHAN, R. S. (1985). Fetal haematology in rhesus isoimmunization. *British Medical Journal*, **290**, 661.

[29] NICOLAIDES, K. H., RODECK, C. H. MIBASHAN, R. S. and KEMP, J. R. (1986a). Have Liley charts outlived their usefulness? *American Journal of Obstetrics and Gynecology*, **155**, 90.

[30] NICOLAIDES, K. H., SOOTHILL, P. W., RODECK, C. H. and CLEWELL, W. (1986b). Rh disease: intravascular fetal blood transfusion by cordocentesis. *Fetal Therapy*, **1**, 185.

[31] OUWEHAND, W. H., MULLENS, T. E. J. M., HUISKIES, E. et al (1984). Predictive value of a monocyte-driven cytotoxicity assay for the severity of rhesus (D) haemolytic disease of the newborn; a comparison with two other techniques. In: The activity of IgG1 and IgG3 antibodies in immune-mediated destruction of red cells. Academic Thesis, Rodopi, Amsterdam, Chapter IV, pp. 87–114.

[32] PETZ, L. D. and GARRATTY, G. (1980). *Acquired Immune Hemolytic Anemias*, (a) p. 365, (b) p. 376. Churchill Livingstone, New York.

[33] SZYMANSKI, I. O. and ARASZKIEWICZ, P. (1989). Quantitative studies on the D antigen of red cells with the D^u phenotype. *Transfusion*, **29**, 103.

[34] THOMPSON, K. M., MELAMED, M. D., EAGLE, K. et al (1986). Production of human monoclonal IgG and IgM antibodies with anti-D (rhesus) specificity using heterohybridomas. *Immunology*, **58**, 157.

[35] URBANIAK, S. J., AYOUB GREISS, M., CRAWFORD, R. J. and FERGUSON, M. J. C. (1984). Prediction of the outcome of Rhesus haemolytic disease of the newborn; additional information using an ADCC assay. *Vox Sanguinis*, **46**, 323.

[36] VOAK, D. (1988). Monoclonal antibodies in blood grouping. *Biotest Bulletin*, **3**, 177.

[37] VOAK, D. (1968). The serological specificity of the sensitising antibodies in ABO hetero-specific pregnancy of the group O mother. *Vox Sanguinis*, **14**, 271.

[38] VOAK, D. (1969). The pathogenesis of ABO haemolytic disease of the newborn. *Vox Sanguinis*, **17**, 481.

[39] VOAK, D. and BOWLEY, C. C. (1969). A detailed serological study on the prediction and diagnosis of ABO haemolytic disease of the newborn (ABO HD). *Vox Sanguinis*, **17**, 321.

[40] VOAK, D., LODGE, T. W. and REED, J. V. (1969). The enhancement of *Ulex europaeus* anti-H activity by human serum. *Vox Sanguinis*, **17**, 134.

[41] WALLHERMFECHTEL, M. A., POLK, B. A. and CHAPLAIN, H. (1984). Alloimmunisation in patients with warm autoantibodies. A retrospective study employing three donor alloabsorptions to aid antibody detection. *Transfusion*, **24**, 482.

[42] WATERS, A. H. and DAVIDSON, J. F. (1988). Clinical interface of blood transfusion. *Journal of Clinical Pathology*, **41**, 601.

[43] WATERS, A. H. and MURPHY, M. F. (1986). Adverse immunological reactions to blood transfusion. *Hospital Update*, **July**, 565.

29. Serological investigation of the auto-immune and drug-induced immune haemolytic anaemias

(Written in collaboration with A. H. Waters)

In many cases of acquired haemolytic anaemia the increased haemolysis is brought about by the production of auto-antibodies directed against the patient's own red cells. These are known as the auto-immune haemolytic anaemias (AIHA). They exist as disorders of obscure origin—the 'idiopathic' type—and secondary or symptomatic types, which are mainly associated with malignant diseases of the lympho-reticular system or other auto-immune diseases, particularly systemic lupus erythematosus (SLE), or may follow atypical (Mycoplasma) pneumonia, infectious mononucleosis, or other virus infections. Paroxysmal cold haemoglobinuria (PCH) also belongs to this group of disorders.

Occasionally, drugs may give rise to a haemolytic anaemia of immunological origin which closely mimics clinically and serologically idiopathic AIHA. Thus the red cells of about 20% of patients on long-term α-methyldopa (Aldomet) treatment give a positive direct antiglobulin test (DAT) and may have auto-antibodies in their serum which will react with normal red cells, even though they often show no evidence of increased red cell destruction. Other drugs such as penicillin, phenacetin, quinidine, quinine, the sodium salt of *p*-aminosalicylic acid and salicylazosulphapyridine (see p. 502) can also in rare cases cause haemolytic anaemia by immunological mechanisms. With these drugs (with the exception of Aldomet) the antibody is directed primarily against the drug and only secondarily involves the red cells (see p. 502).

TYPES OF AUTO-ANTIBODY

The diagnosis of an auto-immune haemolytic anaemia (AIHA) depends primarily upon the demonstration of auto-antibodies adsorbed to the patient's red cells. This can be achieved by showing that the red cells are agglutinated by an anti-human globulin (AHG) serum (see p. 433)

Auto-antibodies can often be demonstrated free in the serum of a patient suffering from an AIHA. The ease with which the antibodies can be detected depends on how much antibody is being produced, its affinity for the corresponding antigen on the red cell surface and the effect that temperature has on the adsorption of the antibody, as well as on the technique used to detect it. The auto-antibodies associated with AIHA can be separated into two broad categories depending on how their interaction with antigen is affected by temperature: i.e. into warm antibodies which are able to combine with their corresponding red cell antigen readily at 37°C, and cold antibodies which cannot combine with antigen at 37°C, but form an increasingly stable combination with antigen as the temperature falls from 30–32°C to 2–4°C.

Cases of AIHA can similarly be separated into two broad categories according to the temperature characteristics of the associated auto-antibodies, i.e. into warm-type AIHA and cold-type AIHA. The relative frequency of the two categories is illustrated in Table 29.1.

WARM AUTO-ANTIBODIES

The commonest type of warm auto-antibody is an IgG immunoglobulin which behaves in vitro very similarly to an anti-Rh allo-antibody; indeed many IgG auto-antibodies have Rh specificity. IgA and IgM warm auto-antibodies are much less common, and when present they are usually formed in addition to an IgG auto-antibody (Table 29.2).

Quite frequently, patients with warm-type AIHA have complement adsorbed to their red cells, i.e. the cells are agglutinated by antisera specific for complement or a complement component, e.g. C3d

Table 29.1   Relative incidence of different types of auto-immune haemolytic anaemia*

	Males	Females	Total
Warm antibodies			
'Idiopathic'	46	65	111
Associated with drugs (mostly α-methyldopa)	1	10	11
Secondary			
Associated with:			
Lymphomas	14	23	37
SLE	1	15	16
Other possible or probable auto-immune disorders	8	13	21
Infections and miscellaneous	9	4	13
Ovarian teratoma	0	1	1
Totals	79	131	210
Cold antibodies			
'Idiopathic' (CHAD)	16	22	38
Secondary			
Associated with:			
Atypical or mycoplasma pneumonia	5	18	23
Infectious mononucleosis	1	1	2
Lymphomas	3	4	7
Paroxysmal cold haemoglobinuria			
'Idiopathic'	7	1	8
Secondary	4	3	7
Totals	36	49	85

*From Dacie and Worlledge[6]

Table 29.2 Direct antiglobulin test in warm-antibody auto-immune haemolytic anaemia: incidence of different reactions to specific antiglobulin sera[5].

Anti-IgG	Anti-IgA	Anti-IgM	Anti-C	No. of patients	%
+	–	–	–	43	36
–	+	–	–	3	2
+	+	–	–	4	3
+	–	–	+	52	43
+	–	+	+	6	5
–	–	–	+	13	11
				121	100

(Table 29.2). In these cases the complement is probably not being bound by an IgG antibody but is on the cell surface as the result of the action of small and otherwise undetected amounts of IgM auto-antibody. (IgA auto-antibodies are thought not to cause the binding on of complement.)

Sometimes patients with warm-type AIHA appear to have only complement on the red cell surface. This is more difficult to interpret, as weak reactions of this type are not uncommon in patients with a variety of disorders in whom there is little evidence of increased red cell destruction. In some patients this may be due to the binding to the red cells of circulating immune complexes.

Warm auto-antibodies free in the patient's serum are best detected by means of the indirect antiglobulin test (IAT) or by the use of enzyme-treated, e.g. trypsinized or papainized, red cells. (Antibodies that agglutinate unmodified cells directly are seldom present.) Not infrequently, antibodies that agglutinate enzyme-treated cells, sometimes at high titres, are present in the sera of patients in whom the IAT using unmodified cells is negative (Table 29.3). Occasionally, too, they are present in the sera of patients in whom the DAT is negative.

Antibodies in serum that can be shown to lyse unmodified red cells at 37°C in the presence of complement (warm haemolysins) are rarely demonstrable.[4b] If present, the patient is likely to suffer from extremely severe haemolysis. Antibodies in serum that lyse as well as agglutinate enzyme-treated cells but do not affect unmodified cells are, on the other hand, quite commonly met with. Their specificity is uncertain—they are not anti-Rh—and their presence is not necessarily associated with increased haemolysis.

COLD AUTO-ANTIBODIES

Cold auto-antibodies are nearly always IgM in type. In vivo, the antibodies can cause chronic intravascular haemolysis, the intensity of which is characteristically influenced by the ambient temperature. The resultant clinical picture is generally referred to as the cold-haemagglutinin syndrome or disease (CHAD). Haemolysis is due to destruction of the red cells by complement which is bound to the red cell surface by the antigen-antibody reaction which

Table 29.3 Results of testing for free auto-antibodies in the sera of 210 patients with warm-antibody auto-immune haemolytic anaemia*

Indirect antiglobulin test	Agglutination at 37°C of enzyme-treated red cells	Lysis at 37°C of enzyme-treated red cells	Agglutination at 20°C of normal red cells	No. and percentage of patients in group	
+	+	+	+	4	
+	+	+	–	16	
+	+	–	–	64	41%
+	–	–	–	2	
+	–	–	+	1	
–	+	+	+	16	
–	+	+	–	31	
–	+	–	–	29	40%
–	+	–	+	7	
–	–	–	–	39	19%

*From Dacie and Worlledge[6]

Notes: 1. In 41% of the patients the IAT was positive and in 80% of the patients the tests with enzyme-treated cells were positive + (in half of these patients the IAT was negative).
2. In 19% of the patients both tests were negative.
3. In 13% of the patients normal red cells were agglutinated at 20°C, probably by cold agglutinins.

Table 29.4   Main characteristics of IgG, IgM and IgA auto-antibodies

	IgG	IgM	IgA
Mol wt (daltons)	150 000	900 000*	160 000*
Sedimentation rate (s)	6.6	18	7
No. of heavy-chain subclasses	4	1	2
Cross placenta	Yes	No	No
Cause activation of complement	Yes	Yes	No
Cause monocyte/macrophage attachment	Yes	No	No
No. of antigen binding sites	2	5 or 10	2
Type of AIHA produced	Warm;PCH	Usually cold	Warm

*and multiples of this mol wt in polymers.

takes place in the blood vessels of the exposed skin where the temperature is 28–32°C or less.

The red cells of patients suffering from CHAD characteristically give positive antiglobulin reactions only with anti-complement (anti-C) sera. This is due to the presence of red cells which have irreversibly adsorbed sublytic amounts of complement; it is a sign, therefore, of an antigen-antibody reaction which has taken place at a temperature below 37°C. The complement component responsible for the reaction with anti-C sera is the C3dg derivative of C3 (see p. 427).

In vitro, a cold-type auto-antibody will often lyse normal red cells at 20–30°C in the presence of fresh human serum complement, especially if the cell-serum mixture is acidified to pH 6.5–7.0; it will usually lyse enzyme-treated red cells readily in unacidified serum, and agglutination and lysis of these cells may still be present at 37°C. Most of these cold-type auto-antibodies have anti-I specificity: i.e. they react strongly with the vast majority of adult red cells and only weakly with cord-blood red cells. A minority are anti-i and react strongly with cord-blood cells and weakly with adult red cells. Rarely, the antibodies have anti-Pr or anti-M specificity and react with antigens on the red cell surface that are destroyed by enzyme treatment.

Another quite distinct, but rarely met with, type of cold antibody is the Donath-Landsteiner (D-L) antibody. This is an IgG globulin and has anti-P specificity. The clinical syndrome the antibody produces is referred to as paroxysmal cold haemoglobinuria (PCH).

Some of the characteristics of IgG, IgM and IgA antibodies are illustrated in Table 29.4.

The clinical, haematological and serological aspects of the auto-immune haemolytic anaemias have by now an extensive literature. Relatively recent valuable reviews include those of Pirofsky,[27] Petz and Garratty,[26] Sokol, Hewitt and Stamps,[33] Issitt[16] and Sokol and Hewitt.[31]

METHODS OF INVESTIGATION

Many of the methods used in the investigation of a patient suspected of suffering from AIHA have already been described in Chapter 26. Detailed description is given here of precautions to be taken when collecting blood samples from the patient and of methods of particular value in his or her investigation.

Collection of samples of blood and serum

It is convenient in dealing with a patient suspected of having AIHA to collect venous blood using a syringe and needle already warmed to 37°C and to deliver the blood (a) into a defibrinating container warmed in a water-bath at 37°C and (b) into ACD or CPD solution (1 ml of ACD or 0.5 ml of CPD is sufficient for 4 ml of whole blood).

Defibrination has an advantage over allowing blood to clot undisturbed in that large volumes of red cells are obtained as well as serum. In the first examination of a patient, it is desirable to carry out defibrination at 37°C rather than at room temperature, so as to prevent adsorption of a cold auto-antibody should one be present. When defibrination is complete, the blood should be centrifuged to separate the serum at 37°C, e.g. in an ordinary centrifuge into the buckets of which water warmed to 37–40°C has been placed.

The red cells are available for antibody elution and the serum can be examined for free antibody or other abnormalities. The ACD or CPD sample is used for direct antiglobulin tests and other tests involving the patient's red cells. If the auto-antibody in a particular case is known to be warm in type, the blood may be defibrinated and separated at room temperature; otherwise, as already indicated, this should be carried out at 37°C. When samples are sent by post, it is best to send separately; (a) serum (separated at 37°C) and (b) whole blood added to ACD or CPD solution. Sterility must be maintained.

Storage of samples

Samples of patient's blood, while keeping quite well in ACD or CPD at 4°C, are more difficult to preserve than normal red cells. In particular, if marked spherocytosis is present considerable lysis develops on storage. However, satisfactory eluates can be made from washed red cells frozen at −20°C for weeks or months.

The patient's serum should be stored at −20°C or below in small (1–2 ml) volumes. If complement is to be titrated, the serum should be frozen as soon as practicable at −70°C or below if the titration is not performed immediately.

SCHEME FOR THE SEROLOGICAL INVESTIGATION OF A PATIENT SUSPECTED OF SUFFERING FROM A HAEMOLYTIC ANAEMIA OF IMMUNOLOGICAL ORIGIN

The problem arises as to which are the most profitable tests to carry out and the order in which they should be done. A suggested scheme covering the more important tests follows. It has been set out in the form of answers (right-hand side) to questions (left-hand side).

Question

1. Are the patient's red cells 'coated' by immunoglobulins or complement (indicating antigen–antibody reaction)? [If the DAT is negative, the diagnosis is unlikely to be an auto-immune haemolytic anaemia (AIHA), although not impossible. See DAT-negative AIHA (p. 488).

2. If the DAT is positive, are immunoglobulins or is complement adsorbed to the red cells?

3. If immunoglobulins are present on the red cells, are they auto-antibodies?

4. What is the patient's blood group?

Answer

Direct antiglobulin test (DAT) using a potent 'broad-spectrum' anti-serum at suitable dilutions (p. 484).

Repeat the DAT using serial dilutions of polyspecific and monospecific sera (p. 484), i.e. broad-spectrum, anti-IgG, anti-IgM, anti-IgA and anti-C.

Prepare eluates from the patient's red cells. Test these later (see 6a)

Determine the patient's ABO and Rh (D) and other blood-group antigens as far as possible. The Rh phenotype is particularly important in warm-type AIHA; other antigens must be determined if allo-antibodies are to be differentiated from auto-antibodies (see p. 494)

Question

5. Is there free antibody in the serum? How does it react, at what temperatures and by what methods can it be demonstrated?

6. If the antibody is a *warm* one:

(a) What is the specificity of the antibody adsorbed to the red cells?

(b) What is the specificity of any irregular (unexpected) antibody detected in the serum? Is it an auto- or allo-antibody?

(c) What is the agglutinin titre of the antibody?

(d) If the antibody is lytic, what is the lysis titre?

7. If the antibody is a *cold* one:

(a) Has the antibody any specificity? Is it an auto-antibody or an allo-antibody? What is its titre?

(b) What is the thermal range of the antibody?

(c) Has the antibody any lytic activity?

Answer

(i) Screen the serum with two or three samples of adult enzyme-treated red cells for agglutination and lysis at 20°C and 37°C and by the IAT (p. 490). The red cells chosen must be ABO-compatible and bear between them the antigens of all the common blood-group systems. If these are not available, use group-O, R_1R_2 (CDe/cDE) cells.

(ii) Determine the agglutinin titre at 4°C with ABO-compatible adult red cells, cord-blood cells and adult enzyme-treated cells (p. 497).

These tests will show whether cold or warm antibodies are present in the serum or a mixture of the two.

Test the eluate with a selected ABO-compatible panel of red cells of known blood groups by the IAT and by using enzyme-treated red cells (p. 496).

Titrate the serum by the methods that have given positive results in the screening test using the same panel of red cells (5i).

Titrate in saline and/or in albumin using normal and enzyme-treated cells and by the IAT.

Determine the lysis titre with enzyme-treated red cells (or PNH red cells) at 37°C, or with normal cells if these have been lysed in the screening test (5i).

Titrate at 4°C with ABO-compatible adult (I) cells, cord-blood (i) cells, the patient's cells, adult (i) cells (if possible) and enzyme-treated adult (I) cells (p. 497).

(i) Determine the highest temperature at which auto-agglutination of the patient's whole blood takes place (p. 498).

(ii) Titrate the patient's serum at 20°C and 30°C with the panel of cells listed under 5(i). If there was any agglutination or lysis at 37°C in the screening test (5i), titrate with the appropriate cells at this temperature.

(i) Titrate the antibody in fresh normal ABO-compatible serum with normal ABO-compatible I (or i) red cells and enzyme-treated I (or i) red cells at 20°C and (if necessary) at 37°C (p. 498).

Paroxysmal nocturnal haemoglobinuria (PNH) red cells, if available, can be used as a valuable and sensitive reagent for detecting lytic activity by both warm and cold antibodies.

Question	Answer
7. (c) Cont.	(ii) If PCH is suspected, carry out the direct and indirect Donath-Landsteiner tests (p. 500).
8. Is a drug suspected as the cause of the haemolytic anaemia?	(i) If a penicillin is suspected, test for antibodies using cells pre-incubated with the appropriate drug (p. 503). (ii) If other drugs are suspected, add the drug in solution to a mixture of the patient's serum, normal cells and fresh normal serum (p. 504). Look for agglutination of normal and enzyme-treated cells and use the IAT
9. Are there any other serological abnormalities?	Consider carrying out the following tests: quantitative estimation of serum proteins; electrophoresis and quantitative estimation of immunoglobulins; estimation of complement; tests for LE cells; tests for anti-nuclear factor (ANF); titration of heterophile (anti-sheep red-cell) antibodies; Wassermann and Kahn reactions; test for mycoplasma antibodies.

The above scheme summarizes what may be done by way of serological investigation of a patient suspected of having AIHA. It is not suggested that every patient has to be investigated in such depth. However, there are other considerations than scientific interest and curiosity. For instance, not infrequently clinical diagnosis and prognosis depend on accurate investigation; and an exact knowledge of the specificity of an antibody may be of great importance in relation to blood transfusion. In some patients, too, quantitative measurements of antibody activity or immunoglobulin may provide valuable evidence of the efficacy of treatment. As in all spheres of laboratory medicine, a close collaboration between clinician and pathologist helps in deciding what tests should be done in any particular case.

DETECTION OF INCOMPLETE ANTIBODIES BY MEANS OF THE DIRECT ANTIGLOBULIN (COOMBS) TEST (DAT)

Principle. As already described, the DAT involves testing the patient's cells without prior exposure to antibody in vitro. The anti-human-globulin serum normally used in routine screening and in the cross-match for blood transfusion is a polyspecific (broad-spectrum) one. However, for the investigation of cases of AIHA, antisera specific for IgG, IgM and IgA should be used. These reagents are available from commercial sources. Antibodies specific for the complement component C3 and breakdown product C3d can also be obtained.

Precautions

Certain precautions are necessary when investigating a patient with possible AIHA. The patient's red cells should be washed four times in a large volume of saline* warmed to 37°C. The warm saline is used as a routine in order to wash off cold antibodies and obtain a smooth suspension of cells—there is no risk of washing off adsorbed complement components.

---

*Throughout this Chapter 'saline' refers to 9 g/l NaCl buffered to pH 7.0 (see Appendix, p. 536).

However, the washing process should be accomplished as quickly as possible and the test should be set up immediately afterwards, for, occasionally, bound warm-antibody elutes off the cells when they are washed and false-negative results may be obtained. If for any reason the washing process has to be interrupted once it has begun, the cell suspension should be placed at 4°C to slow down the dissociation of the antibody. A tile method is particularly useful in the investigation of AIHA since it enables an estimation of the speed of agglutination as well as the final strength of the reaction.

QUALITATIVE DIRECT ANTIGLOBULIN TEST

A spin tube technique, as described on p. 435, is recommended.

Make a 2–5% suspension of washed red cells in saline. Add 1 volume (drop) of the cell suspension to 2 volumes (drops) of antiglobulin reagent at its recommended dilution. Centrifuge for 10–60 s (see p. 436).

Examine for agglutination after gently resuspending the button of cells. A concave mirror helps in macroscopic readings. If the result appears to be negative, confirm this microscopically.

Each DAT or batch of tests should be carefully controlled as previously described (p. 436).

Check negative results with the anti-IgG and anti-C reagents by the addition of IgG-sensitized cells and complement-coated cells.

If the qualitative DAT is positive, quantitative tests should be undertaken. The results with such tests reflect both the potency of the antiglobulin reagents and the degree to which the patients' red cells are coated with IgG and/or complement.

QUANTITATIVE DIRECT ANTIGLOBULIN TEST

A convenient method utilizing four-fold dilutions of antiglobulin serum and allowing the antiglobulin serum and cell suspension to interact on a translucent opal tile is described below. Alternatively, the reactions can be allowed to take place in 75 × 10 or 12 mm glass tubes using 2–5% suspensions of red cells, and the results read macroscopically or microscopically after the cell suspensions have spontaneously sedimented at the end of 1 h at room temperature.

Wash the cells as already described. Make four-fold dilutions of broad-spectrum, anti-IgG, and anti-C sera, ranging normally from a 1 in 4 dilution to 1 in 4096. Place 6 drops of saline in each of the master tubes to be used for preparing dilutions and add 2 drops of the appropriate undiluted anti-serum to the first tube (1 in 4 dilution), dry the pipette carefully (see below), mix the diluted serum, place

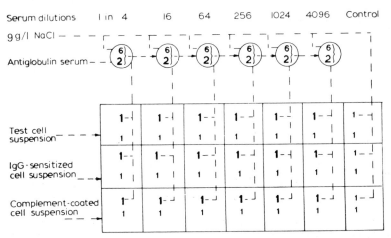

Fig. 29.1 Diagram illustrating method of dilution for the antiglobulin test. The figures represent drops. The circles indicate the tubes in which the dilutions are being made; the squares indicate the drops on a tile. The antiglobulin serum and its dilution are shown in large bold type.

1 drop on the tile and 2 drops in the next tube, and so on. The final layout is shown in Figure 29.1. Care must be taken to minimize the carry-over of more concentrated antiserum into the tubes destined to contain highly diluted serum. A simple way to minimize this is to wipe the sides and tip of the pipette with absorbent tissue between each dilution. For greater accuracy (not required for routine purposes) separate pipettes should be used for each dilution. The effect of carry-over is illustrated in Table 29.5.

Anti-IgM and anti-IgA sera should also be used if they have given a positive reaction in the qualitative test.

As soon as possible after the dilutions of antiglobulin sera have been placed on the tile, add 1 drop of a 20% suspension of the patient's cells to each drop of diluted serum, mix using a wooden swab-stick, starting for each anti-serum and cell sample with the saline control and finishing with the highest concentration of antiglobulin serum. Use a separate swab-stick for each series of serum dilutions. Rock gently and observe at 1 min intervals, assessing the results at the end of a predetermined time (e.g. 5–7 min) and scoring as illustrated in Table 26.6 (p. 432).

Normal (unsensitized) cells and normal sensitized (control) cells should be used to check the specificity and sensitivity of the antiglobulin sera.

Typical results illustrating different types of quantitative DATs are shown in Table 29.6, which includes the reactions in undiluted serum. The appearance of positive tests with cells coated with complement and IgG, respectively, are shown in Figure 29.2.

Antiglobulin test titration scores give a good indication of the degree of sensitization of the red cells with IgG and complement without the necessity of performing sophisticated quantitative measurements. However, whilst a high titre (>1000) with anti-IgG is likely to be associated with haemolysis, titration scores cannot be used to determine whether or not increased haemolysis is occurring. Titres are, however, of value in the follow-up of an individual patient; e.g. a fall in titre is often associated with remission and a rising titre with relapse. In warm-type AIHA the presence of complement on the red cell surface as well as IgG is more frequently associated with secondary than with 'idiopathic' AIHA. However, IgG without complement is typical of an α-methyldopa-induced positive DAT.

Table 29.5 Comparison of titration end-points of a high-titre cold agglutinin using conventional doubling-diluting techniques with those obtained by making dilutions with separate pipettes

Final serum dilution		1 in 1024	1 in 4096	1 in 16 000	1 in 64 000	1 in 256 000	1 in 1 000 000	Control (saline)
1. Doubling dilutions using Pasteur pipette								
(a) no mixing in stem	macro	+	+	+	[+]	–	–	–
	micro	+	+	+	+	+	[+]	–
(b) with mixing in stem	macro	+	+	+	weak*	–	–	–
	micro	+	+	+	+	+	[+]	–
2. Doubling dilutions using glass automatic pipette	macro	+	+	+	[+]	(?)	–	–
	micro	+	+	+	+	+	[+]	–
3. Dilutions prepared using a separate pipette for each dilution	macro	+	+	[+]	(?)	–	–	–
	micro	+	+	+	[+]	–	–	–

*The titre read macroscopically was recorded as 32 000.

Only the results of readings made on the last seven alternate tubes of the titrations are recorded. The doubling dilutions were prepared commencing with undiluted serum, and the separate dilutions (Series 3) were prepared from an initial serum dilution of 1 in 256.

The titrations were carried out at room temperature (18°C) and the end-points of the titrations were determined macroscopically (macro) using a concave mirror, and also microscopically (micro). The end-points are indicated thus [+].

The end-points determined *macroscopically* using the conventional doubling-diluting techniques give results which closely approximate to the truth, assuming that the correct titration figure is obtained when dilutions of serum are prepared using a separate pipette for each dilution and that the result is read microscopically.

Table 29.6   Patterns of agglutination by antiglobulin sera in the direct antiglobulin test using broad-spectrum and specific antiglobulin sera

IgG type

Reagent	Dilutions of antiglobulin sera							
	1 in 1	4	16	64	256	1024	4096	Saline
Broad-spectrum antiglobulin serum	1 +	2 +	3 +	4 +	4 +	3 +	2 +	0
Anti-IgG	1 +	2 +	3 +	4 +	4 +	3 +	2 +	0
Anti-C	0	0	0	0	0	0	0	0

IgG + C type

Reagent	Dilutions of antiglobulin sera							
	1 in 1	4	16	64	256	1024	4096	Saline
Broad-spectrum antiglobulin serum	3 +	3 +	3 +	2 +	2 +	1 +	0	0
Anti-IgG	0	1 +	1 +	2 +	2 +	1 +	0	0
Anti-C	3 +	3 +	2 +	1 +	0	0	0	0

C only type

Reagent	Dilutions of antiglobulin sera							
	1 in 1	4	16	64	256	1024	4096	Saline
Broad-spectrum antiglobulin serum	3 +	3 +	2 +	1 +	0	0	0	0
Anti-IgG	0	0	0	0	0	0	0	0
Anti-C	3 +	3 +	2 +	1 +	0	0	0	0

Reactions with antiglobulin sera against IgG subclasses

When the DAT is positive with anti-IgG, it is of interest to determine the subclass of IgG. The majority of IgG red cell auto-antibodies are IgG1, sometimes in combination with IgG2 or IgG3. The formation of IgG3 (either alone or with IgG1) appears to be associated with active disease and marked haemolysis. Patients with IgG1 only on the red cell surface may or may not have marked haemolysis, whilst IgG2 and IgG4 do not appear to be associated with any increased haemolysis.[7] Thus it is of value to know whether IgG3 is present since its presence indicates the likelihood of aggressive disease. The reactions with subclass antisera can be ascertained using four-fold dilutions of the specific antisera exactly as has already been described. The

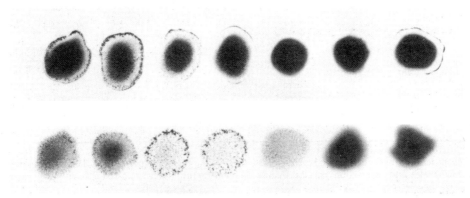

Fig. 29.2   Antiglobulin reactions carried out on a tile using various dilutions of an antiglobulin serum. *Upper series:* red cells coated by complement. *Lower series:* red cells sensitized with an IgG antibody. The dilutions of the antiglobulin serum ranged from 1 in 4 to 1 in 4096. The red cell suspension on the extreme right is the control with 9 g/l NaCl substituted for antiglobulin serum.

sera are unfortunately difficult to prepare. However, they are available commercially.*

SIGNIFICANCE OF POSITIVE DIRECT ANTIGLOBULIN TEST[40]

A positive DAT does not necessarily mean that the patient has auto-immune haemolytic anaemia.[6] However, it certainly calls attention to this possibility. The causes of a positive test include the following:

1. An auto-antibody on the red cell surface with or without haemolytic anaemia.

2. An allo-antibody on the red cell surface, as for example in haemolytic disease of the newborn or after an incompatible transfusion.

3. Antibodies provoked by drugs adsorbed to the red cell as the result of:
    a. Drug adsorption as in penicillin-induced immune haemolysis.
    b. Immune complex adsorption.

4. Normal globulins adsorbed to the red cell surface as the result of damage by drugs, e.g. cephalothin.

5. Interaction between the antiglobulin sera and anti-T, as with polyagglutinable red cells.

6. Anti-albumin and anti-transferrin antibodies in antiglobulin sera giving rise to false-positive reactions.

7. Adsorption of immune complexes to the red cell surface. This may be the mechanism of the (usually weak) reactions that are found in approximately 8% of hospital patients suffering from a wide variety of disorders (see p. 488).

8. Sensitization in vitro. If for instance, clotted or defibrinated normal blood is allowed to stand in a refrigerator at 4°C, or even at room temperature, and the antiglobulin test is subsequently carried out, the reaction may be positive due to the adsorption of incomplete cold antibodies and complement from normal sera.[4c] Samples of blood taken into EDTA or ACD and subsequently chilled do not give this type of false-positive result as the anticoagulant inhibits the complement reaction.

9. It is not unknown for the DAT to be positive with the blood of apparently perfectly healthy

individuals e.g. blood donors. Such occurrences are rare and have not been satisfactorily explained (see below). The possibility that α-methyldopa is being taken as an anti-hypertensive drug must not be overlooked: up to 20% of such patients on long-term therapy develop positive DATs—most show no signs of overt increased haemolysis.

In connection with positive reactions given by normal cells, it should be pointed out that slowly developing weak agglutination, occurring even in well diluted antiglobulin serum, is not uncommon. With suspensions on an opalescent tile, this is not, as a rule, evident to the naked eye under at least 5–7 min. However, this agglutination is probably real and appears to represent an interaction between globulins normally adsorbed to the red cell surface and the antiglobulin serum (see p. 488). Tests should normally be read before this type of false-positive agglutination occurs.

Stratton and Renton[35] emphasized yet another possible cause of false-positive agglutination. This is due to a silica gel derived from glass, and it is most commonly produced by using sodium citrate solutions autoclaved in glass bottles or in the case of tests carried out on glass tiles by scraping the surface of the tile in the course of mixing cells and serum with a corner of a microscope slide or glass rod.

Positive DATs in normal subjects

The occurrence of a clearly positive DAT in an apparently healthy subject is a rare but well known phenomenon. Worlledge[40] had reported an incidence in blood donors of approximately 1 in 9000. In a more recent report, Gorst et al[11] estimated that the incidence was approximately 1 in 14 000. 65 positive tests had been encountered in blood donors: of 59 samples that had been tested with anti-complement (anti-C) sera as well as with anti-IgG sera, 23 had been positive with anti-IgG sera alone, 28 by anti-C sera alone and eight by both anti-IgG and anti-C sera. 32 of the donors giving positive tests had been recalled for further study: none presented any abnormal clinical findings and all were fit and well. All except one (see below) remained healthy subsequently (for up to 18 years). The exception was a donor who, having had a positive DAT for 2 years, subsequently developed typical AIHA. It is interesting to note that the data of Gorst et al indicated an

---

*e.g. from the Central Laboratory of the Netherlands Red Cross Blood Transfusion Service, Amsterdam.

increasing likelihood of a positive test with increasing age. Their report, and other subsequent reports,[1,34] certainly suggests that the finding of a positive DAT, using an anti-IgG serum, in an apparently healthy person is usually of little clinical significance and that overt AIHA, although it may develop, hardly ever does. In some patients, too, the DAT eventually becomes negative!

Positive DATs in hospital patients

In contrast to the rarity of positive DATs in strictly healthy people, positive tests are much more frequent in hospital patients. Worlledge[40] reported that the red cells of 40 out of 489 blood samples (8.2%) submitted for routine tests had been agglutinated by anti-complement (anti-C sera). Only one sample was agglutinated by an anti-IgG serum and this had been obtained from a patient being treated with α-methyldopa. Freedman[8] reported a similar incidence—7.8% positive tests with anti-C sera. Lau et al[21] had used anti-IgG sera only. The tests were seldom positive (0.9% positive out of 4664 tests). The probable explanation for the relatively high incidence of positive tests with anti-C sera is that the reaction is between anti-complement antibodies and immune complexes adsorbed to the red cells.

Hypergammaglobulinaemia.

Another possible explanation for positive DATs in hospital patients is hypergammaglobulinaemia. Symanski et al[36] employed an AutoAnalyser and used Ficoll and PVP to enhance agglutination by an anti-IgG serum highly diluted (usually to 1 in 5 000) in 0.5% bovine serum albumin. In this sensitive system the strength of agglutination was clearly positively correlated with the serum γ-globulin concentration, being subnormal in hypogammaglobulinaemia and supranormal in hypergammaglobulinaemia.

It is typical to find in hypergammaglobulinaemic patients in whom the DAT is positive that attempts to demonstrate antibodies in eluates fail, i.e. that eluates are non-reactive.[12,15]

FALSE-NEGATIVE ANTIGLOBULIN TESTS

There are several causes:

1. Failure to wash the red cells properly—the antisera may then be neutralized by immunoglobulins or complement in the surrounding serum or plasma.

2. The use of impotent antisera so that weakly sensitized cells are not detected.

3. The use of incorrect dilutions of the anti-sera.

4. The use of antisera lacking the antibody corresponding to the subclass of immunoglobulin responsible for the red cell sensitization.

5. The antibody being readily dissociable and eluted in the washing process.

6. Excessive agitation at the reading stage may break up agglutinates leading to a false-negative result.

DAT-NEGATIVE AIHA

In approximately 2–6% of patients who present with the clinical and haematological features of AIHA the DAT is negative on repeated testing.[3,40,41]

In some of these patients auto-antibodies are being formed but they are of such a nature or present in such small amounts that routine testing fails to detect them. In such patients evidence for auto-antibody formation can often be obtained by careful screening of a concentrated ether eluate made from the patient's red cells or by the manual Polybrene test.

More complex techniques have, too, been used successfully to demonstrate low levels of immunoglobulin on the red cell surface in patients with a provisional diagnosis of DAT-negative AIHA. These methods include radio-immunoassay,[30] the use of the agglutination enhancers Polybrene and PVP in automated tests[13,19], the complement-fixing antibody consumption (CFAC) test[10] and enzyme-linked immunosorbent assays (ELISA) and enzyme-linked antiglobulin tests (ELAT).[2,32]

PREPARATION AND TESTING A CONCENTRATED ETHER ELUATE

This technique concentrates low levels of immunoglobulin present on the red cell surface so that antibody may then be detected by screening the eluate with enzyme-treated normal group-O red cells and by the IAT.

Method

1. Prepare a concentrated eluate by adding 1 volume of saline to 7 volumes of washed, packed

red cells. After this initial step the eluate is prepared by Rubin's method,[29] as described on p. 496.

2. Screen the eluate for the presence of antibody with the group-O red cells of three donors, using enzyme-treated cells and the IAT, as described on p. 490.

MANUAL DIRECT POLYBRENE TEST

The following method is modified from that described by Petz and Branch[24] who based their technique on that of Lalezari and Jiang.[18] Polybrene is a polyvalent cationic molecule, hexadimethrine bromide, which can overcome the electrostatic repulsive forces between adjacent red cells, bringing the cells closer together. When low levels of IgG are present on the red cell surface antibody linkage of adjacent red cells is enhanced. The Polybrene is then neutralized using a negatively charged molecule such as trisodium citrate. Sensitized red cells remain agglutinated after neutralization of the Polybrene. Unsensitized red cells will disaggregate after neutralization.

Reagents

Polybrene stock. 10% Polybrene in 9 g/l NaCl, pH 6.9 (saline).

Working Polybrene solution. Dilute the stock Polybrene solution 1 in 250 in saline.

Resuspending solution. 60 ml of 0.2 mol/l trisodium citrate added to 40 ml of 50 g/l dextrose.

Washing solution. 50 ml of 0.2 mol/l trisodium citrate in 950 ml of saline

Low ionic medium (LIM). 50 g/l dextrose containing 2 g/l disodium ethylenediamine tetraacetate. Adjust the pH of half the batch to 6.4. Store the remainder at the original pH (approx. 4.9); use this to repeat tests that are negative using LIM at pH 6.4.

Method

Ensure all reagents are at room temperature.

Positive control

Dilute an IgG anti-D in normal group-AB serum. Find a dilution which gives a positive result with papainized cells but is negative by the IAT on standard testing with group-O, D-positive red cells (a dilution of 1 in 10 000 is often suitable).

Negative control

Normal group-AB serum which fails to agglutinate papainized group-O, D-positive red cells.

1. Wash the cells four times in saline and make 3–5% suspensions of test and normal group-O Rh (D) red cells in saline.

2. Set up three 75 × 10 mm tubes as shown in Table 29.7. Incubate at room temperature for 1 min.

3. Add 1 drop of working Polybrene solution to each tube and mix gently. Reincubate for 15 s at room temperature.

4. Centrifuge for 10 s at 1000 g. Decant, taking care to remove all the supernatant.

5. Leave 3–5 min at room temperature before adding 2 drops of resuspending solution and mixing gently. Within 10 s aggregates will dissociate leaving true agglutination in the positive tubes.

6. Read macroscopically after 10–60 s. Check all negative results microscopically and compare with the negative control.

7. Repeat negative tests using LIM at the lower pH (approx 4.9).

If the direct Polybrene test is negative, a supplementary antiglobulin test may be performed by washing the cells twice in the washing solution, and testing with an anti-IgG antiglobulin reagent.

DETERMINATION OF THE BLOOD GROUP OF A PATIENT WITH AIHA

ABO grouping

No difficulty should be encountered in ABO grouping patients with warm-type AIHA, but the

Table 29.7 Setting up a direct manual Polybrene test

	Test	Positive control	Negative control
AB serum*	2	0	2
Dilute anti-D in AB serum*	0	2	0
2–3% test cells*	1	0	0
2–5% normal O Rh (D) cells*	0	1	1
LIM	0.6 ml	0.6 ml	0.6 ml

* drops

presence of cold agglutinins may well cause difficulties. The cells should in all cases be washed in warm (37°C) saline. They should then be groupable without trouble; the reactions must, however, be controlled with normal AB serum. Serum grouping should be performing strictly at 37°C or, in an emergency, on a warmed tile. Warm the known A_1, B and O cells to 37°C before adding them to the patient's serum at 37°C. Read the results on microscope slides warmed to 37°C.

Rh(D) grouping

When the DAT is positive only anti-sera active in saline should be used, as the cells will spontaneously agglutinate in the presence of albumin or other enhancing medium. Appropriate controls should be included. (See p. 462).

DEMONSTRATION OF FREE ANTIBODIES IN SERUM

The sera of patients suffering from AIHA often contain free auto-antibodies. This is the rule in cold-haemagglutinin disease, but in the warm-antibody type of disease IgG antibodies detectable by the indirect antiglobulin test (IAT) are usually only found free in the serum of patients who are suffering from a moderate or marked degree of haemolysis. Free warm antibodies detectable by the use of enzyme-treated cells are, on the other hand, not infrequently found and they may often be detected in patients in clinical and haematological remission.   In investigating a patient's serum for auto-antibodies a comprehensive screening procedure should be followed. If positive results are obtained, a more detailed quantitative assessment should be undertaken. If the results are negative, no further tests need to be carried out.

ROUTINE SCREENING TESTS FOR AUTO- (AND ALLO-) ANTIBODIES IN SERUM

The patient's serum is tested under optimal conditions for agglutination and lysis and by the IAT using two or three samples of group-O adult red cells (chosen to possess between them all the common red cell antigens) and the same cells enzyme-treated, e.g. pre-papainized.

The serum is tested undiluted and diluted 1 in 2 with fresh normal human ABO-compatible serum, both at the normal pH of the serum (pH 7.5–8.0) and acidified so that the pH of the cell-serum mixture is c 6.8. The pH of the serum should be checked before the cells are added; a pH of 6.0–6.5 is required. Fresh serum is added because the sera of some patients with AIHA may be deficient in complement. Acid is added because the pH optimum for the lytic activity of some types of antibodies is 6.5–6.8. Tests are carried out strictly at 37°C and at 20°C, the cells and serum being allowed to come to the chosen temperature before they are mixed and being centrifuged subsequently at that temperature. In tests at 37°C the tubes should be centrifuged at that temperature, e.g. in a centrifuge the buckets of which are surrounded by water warmed to 37–40°C. For the IAT the cells should be washed in saline at the appropriate temperature. The fresh normal serum used as complement must be tested against the same samples of test cells to ensure that it is free from antibody. Such sera should be separated immediately after collection and stored at − 70°C or below.

Method

Set up a series of 30 tubes (75 × 10 mm), as illustrated in Figure 29.3, the back row acting as master tubes. The master tubes contain the mixtures indicated A–F.

Pipette 9-drop samples from the master tubes A–F into each of four tubes. Incubate the first and third rows of tubes at 37°C, and the second and fourth rows of tubes at 20°C, as shown in the figure. Add 1 volume of 50% group-O normal cells

Tube No.	A	B	C	D	E	F
Patient's serum	40	36	20	20	0	0
Fresh normal serum (complement)	0	0	20	16	40	36
0.2 mol/l HCl	0	4	0	4	0	4

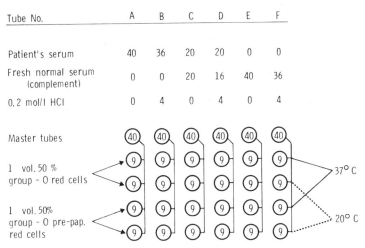

Master tubes

1 vol. 50 % group - O red cells

1 vol. 50% group - O pre-pap. red cells

37° C

20° C

Fig. 29.3 Suggested procedure for setting up a serum screening test for auto-immune haemolytic anaemia. The top row of circles represents the large master tubes in which the primary dilutions are made; the lower four rows of circles represent the tubes in which the tests are carried out. The figures represent drops or volumes.

to the first two rows of tubes, and 1 volume of 50% group-O pre-papainized cells to the other two rows. Mix and allow to stand for 1–1½h. Inspect all the tubes macroscopically for agglutination over a diffuse light source and then centrifuge at the temperature of the test and read for lysis by eye.

Wash the cells in the first row in warm saline at 37°C four times and carry out an IAT using anti-IgG and anti-C sera at their optimal dilutions. If the DAT had been positive with an anti-IgM or anti-IgA serum the cells should also be set up against the optimal dilution of the appropriate antiglobulin reagent.

Wash the cells in the second row at room temperature and carry out an IAT as described above.

By using this technique the serum has been screened to see whether:

1. Free antibody is present which agglutinates normal group-O red cells at 37°C (first row) or at 20°C (second row).
2. Free antibody is present which agglutinates enzyme-treated group-O red cells at 37°C (third row) or at 20°C (fourth row).
3. Free antibody is present which reacts in the IAT with normal group-O cells.
4. The group-O normal or enzyme-treated cells are lysed and whether this shows pH dependence.
5. There is evidence of a lack of complement,

lysis taking place in the presence of fresh normal serum but not without it (tubes 3 and 4, columns B and C).

If the screening test is positive, further tests are necessary to confirm the finding and demonstrate the antibody specificity.

Allo-antibodies will be detected by the screening procedure and will have to be carefully distinguished from auto-antibodies (see below). Representative examples of results of the screening tests in the different types of AIHA are shown in Table 29.8.

IDENTIFICATION BY ABSORPTION TECHNIQUES OF CO-EXISTING ALLO-ANTIBODIES IN THE PRESENCE OF WARM AUTO-ANTIBODIES.

Absorption techniques for the detection of allo-antibodies present in the sera or eluates of patients with suspected or proved AIHA can be helpful in the following situations:

1. In screening for co-exisiting serum allo-antibodies in patients with AIHA who have been pregnant or previously transfused and are found to have significant titres (>8) of a pan-reactive antibody in their serum.
2. In differentiating between auto- and allo-antibodies in the eluate of recently transfused

Table 29.8(1) Antibody screening test: typical result with IgG antibody (direct antiglobulin test positive with anti-IgG serum only).

Method		Red cells	Temperature (°C)	S	AS	S + C	AS + C	C	AC
Indirect antiglobulin test	anti-IgG	N	37	3+	4+	2+	3+	–	–
	anti-C	N	37	–	–	–	–	–	–
	anti-IgG	N	20	2+	3+	1+	2	–	–
	anti-C	N	20	–	–	–	–	–	–
Agglutination		N	37	–	–	–	–	–	–
		N	20	–	–	–	–	–	–
Lysis		N	37	–	–	–	–	–	–
		N	20	–	–	–	–	–	–
Agglutination		EN	37	3+	3+	3+	3+	–	–
		EN	20	2+	2+	2+	2+	–	–
Lysis		EN	37	–	–	–	–	–	–
		EN	20	–	–	–	–	–	–

Tables 29.8(2) Antibody screening test: typical result with antibody(ies) giving positive direct antiglobulin tests with anti-IgG and anti-C

Method		Red cells	Temperature (°C)	S	AS	S + C	AS + C	C	AC
Indirect antiglobulin test	anti-IgG	N	37	1+	2+	½+	1+	–	–
	anti-C	N	37	1+	2+	3+	3+	–	–
	anti-IgG	N	20	½+	–	–	–	–	–
	anti-C	N	20	1+	2+	2+	3+	–	–
Agglutination		N	37	–	–	–	–	–	–
		N	20	1+	1+	–	–	–	–
Lysis		N	37	–	–	–	–	–	–
		N	20	–	–	–	–	–	–
Agglutination		EN	37	1+	1+	–	–	–	–
		EN	20	2+	2+	1+	1+	–	–
Lysis		EN	37	1+	2+	3+	4+	–	–
		EN	20	–	–	1+	2+	–	–

Table 29.8(3) Antibody screening test: typical result with warm antibody giving positive direct antiglobulin test with anti-C only

Method		Red cells	Temperature (°C)	S	AS	S + C	AS + C	C	AC
Indirect antiglobulin test	anti-IgG	N	37	–	–	–	–	–	–
	anti-C	N	37	2+	3+	2+	2+	–	–
	anti-IgG	N	20	–	–	–	–	–	–
	anti-C	N	20	2+	3+	1+	2+	–	–
Agglutination		N	37	–	–	–	–	–	–
		N	20	–	–	–	–	–	–
Lysis		N	37	–	–	–	–	–	–
		N	20	–	–	–	–	–	–
Agglutination		EN	37	–	–	1+	1+	–	–
		N	20	1+	1+	2+	2+	–	–
Lysis		EN	37	3+	4+	1+	2+	–	–
		EN	20	1+	2+	–	–	–	–

Table 29.8(4) Antibody screening test: typical result in the cold-haemagglutinin disease (direct antiglobulin test positive with anti-C only)

Method		Red cells	Temperature (°C)	S	AS	S + C	AS + C	C	C
Indirect antiglobulin test	anti-IgG	N	37	−	−	−	−	−	−
	anti-C	N	37	−	−	−	−	−	−
	anti-IgG	N	20	} Cells too agglutinated to test					
	anti-C	N	20						
Agglutination		N	37	−	−	−	−	−	−
		N	20	4 +	4 +	4 +	2 +	−	+
Lysis		N	37	−	−	−	−	−	−
		N	20	−	−	−	2 +	−	−
Agglutination		EN	37	2 +	2 +	2 +	1 +	−	−
		EN	20	4 +	4 +	2 +	1 +	−	−
Lysis		EN	37	−	−	2 +	3 +	−	−
		EN	20	−	−	2 +	3 +	−	−

N = pooled normal adult group O red cells; EN = the same cells pre-treated with the enzyme papain; S = patient's undiluted serum; AS = patient's undiluted serum acidified to pH 6.0–6.5; C (complement) = fresh normal human compatible serum; AC = fresh normal human compatible serum acidified to pH 6.0–6.5; S + C = equal volumes of patient's serum and complement.

patients with AIHA.

3. In investigating haemolytic transfusion reactions due to red cell allo-antibodies in patients with AIHA.

In some cases of AIHA an underlying allo-antibody may be detected by titrating the patient's serum and eluate against a panel of phenotyped red cells from normal donors. However, a high-titre auto-antibody may mask the allo-antibody; hence the need for absorption techniques, especially in the situations outlined above. The techniques described are based on those of Petz and Branch.[24]

USE OF ZZAP REAGENT FOR USE IN AUTO-ABSORPTION TECHNIQUES

'ZZAP' reagent[24] is a mixture of dithiothreitol and papain. It dissociates an auto-antibody already coating the patient's red cells and enzyme-treats them, thus increasing the amount of auto-antibody that can subsequently be adsorbed onto the patient's cells in vitro.

Reagents

0.2 mol/l dithiothreitol (DTT).
1% papain.
Phosphate buffered saline (PBS), pH 6.8–7.2.

Prepare a suitable volume of ZZAP by making up the reagents in the following ratio: 0.2 mol/l DTT 5 volumes; 1% papain 1 volume.

Check the pH and adjust to pH 6.0–6.5 using one drop at a time of 0.2 mol/l HCl or 0.2 mol/l NaOH.

METHOD FOR AUTO-ABSORPTION USING ZZAP

1. Add 2 volumes of ZZAP to 1 volume of four-times-washed packed red cells. Incubate at 37°C for 30 min mixing occasionally.

2. After incubation, wash the cells four times in saline, packing hard after the last wash.

3. Divide the cells into two equal volumes. To one volume add an equal volume of the serum to be absorbed. Incubate at 37°C for 1 h.

4. Centrifuge at 1000 *g*. Remove the serum and add to the remaining volume of cells.

5. Repeat the absorption procedure.

6. Remove the absorbed serum and store at −20°C or below for allo-antibody screening or cross-matching, which may be performed by standard techniques.

Notes

The auto-absorption technique should only be used in the following circumstances:

1. When the patient has not been transfused in the previous 6 weeks, as the presence of transfused red cells may allow the absorption of allo-antibody as well as auto-antibody.

2. When at least 2–3 ml of packed red cells are available from the patient.

3. When the auto-antibodies present react well with enzyme-treated red cells.

If they do not, heat elution should be substituted for ZZAP treatment. Heat elution may be performed by shaking the washed cells for 5 min in a 56°C water-bath and then washing the cells.

ALLO-ABSORPTION USING PAPAINIZED R_1R_1, R_2R_2 AND rr CELLS

This method may be used when auto-absorption is not appropriate—for instance when the patient has been transfused in the previous 6 weeks or when at least 2–3 ml of patient's red cells are not available.

1. Select three normal group-O red cell samples, which undividually lack some of the blood-group antigens which commonly stimulate the production of clinically significant antibodies, e.g. C. E, K, Fy^a, Fy^b, Jk^a, Jk^b, S, s (Table 29.9).

2. Papainize 2 ml of packed cells from each sample after washing the cells in saline 4 times.

3. Add to 1 ml of each sample of washed, packed, papainized cells 1 ml of the patient's serum. Incubate for 1 h at 37°C.

4. Centrifuge to pack the cells. Remove the supernatant serum and add it to the second 1 ml volume of papainized cells. Incubate for 1 h at 37°C.

5. Centrifuge again to pack the cells. Remove the supernatant and store at $-20°C$ or below for further testing, e.g. allo-antibody screening and cross-matching.

Method for testing allo-absorbed sera

Allo-antibody screening. Each absorbed serum is tested against a panel of phenotyped red cells by the IAT, using undiluted serum and by a short titration, 1 in 2 to 1 in 16, against papainized cells.

Cross-matching. Each absorbed serum must be tested separately against the donor red cells by the IAT, using undiluted serum.

Example of allo-antibody detection using the allo-absorption technique in a recently transfused patient with AIHA

The patient's serum when first tested against a panel of group-O phenotyped red cells revealed only pan-reactive antibodies. In contrast, three absorbed sera, A, B and C, obtained by absorbing the patient's serum with three selected phenotyped samples of group-O cells, were shown to contain anti-E and anti-Jk^a when tested against a panel of phenotyped group-O cells using the IAT. The results of testing the absorbed sera, A, B and C, are shown in Table 29.9. The patient's red cell phenotype was R_1r, Jk(a – b –).

Explanation of the results of testing allo-absorbed sera, A, B and C

1. As the R_1R_1-absorbing cells were negative for the E and Jk^a antigens, absorbed serum A could contain

Table 29.9 Testing an allo-absorbed serum against a phenotyped panel of red cells

No.	Rh	M	N	S	s	P_1	Lu^a	Le^a	Le^b	K	Kp^a	Fy^a	Fy^b	Jk^a	Jk^b	Serum A	Serum B	Serum C
1.	R_1R_1	+	+	+	+	+	–	–	–	+	–	+	+	+	+	1+	1+	–
2.	R_1R_1	+	–	–	+	–	+	–	+	–	–	+	+	+	+	1+	3+	–
3.	R_2R_2	+	+	+	+	+++	+	+	–	–	–	–	+	–	+	1+	–	3+
4.	R_1R_2	+	+	+	–	+++	–	–	+	–	–	–	+	+	–	1+	4+	1+
5.	r'r	+	–	+	+	++	–	–	+	–	–	+	+	–	+	–	–	–
6.	r''r	+	+	+	–	++	–	–	+	–	–	+	–	+	+	2+	2+	2+
7.	rr	+	+	–	+	++	–	–	–	+	–	+	+	+	–	2+	2+	–
8.	rr	+	–	+	+	++	–	+	–	–	–	+	–	+	–	1+	2+	(+)
9.	rr	–	+	–	+	+	–	+	–	–	+	+	+	+	+	2+	2+	–
10.	R_1R_2	–	+	+	+	–	–	–	+	+	–	–	+	+	–	1+	3+	2+

Phenotype of cells selected for absorption of serum   Absorbed serum
1. R_1R_1, C^w+, K –, Fy(a + b –), Jk(a – b +), M +, N –, s –   Serum A
2. R_2R_2, C^w –, K –, Fy(a – b +), Jk(a – b +), M +, N +, s +   Serum B
3. rr, C^w –, K +, Fy(a + b –), Jk(a + b –), M +, N –, s –   Serum C

anti-E and anti-Jk^a. Testing the absorbed serum A against the panel of cells suggested that this was so.

2. As the R$_2$R$_2$-absorbing cells were positive for the E antigen but negative for the Jk^a antigen, absorbed serum B could contain anti-Jk^a but not anti-E. Testing absorbed serum B against the panel of cells confirmed the presence of anti-Jk^a.

3. As the rr-absorbing cells were negative for the E antigen but positive for the Jk^a antigen, absorbed serum C could contain anti-E but not anti-Jk^a. Testing absorbed serum C aginst the panel of cells confirmed the presence of anti-E.

4. As the phenotype of the patient's own red cells was R$_1$r, Jk(a – b –), the anti-E and anti-Jk^a detected in the allo-absorbed sera must be allo-antibodies. Blood for transfusion should be E-negative, Jk^a-negative.

Additional notes on absorption techniques

1. If the patient's serum contains a haemolytic antibody, EDTA should be added to prevent the uptake of complement and subsequent lysis of the cells used for absorption.

Add 1 volume of neutral EDTA (potassium salt) (see Appendix, p. 536) to 9 volumes of serum.

2. It is often useful to allo-absorb both serum and eluate to differentiate between auto- and allo-antibodies, particularly if the auto-antibody is the mimicking type described by Issitt.[16]

3. If the auto-antibody does not react with papainized cells, do *not* papainize the cells for absorption.

ELUTION OF ANTIBODIES FROM RED CELLS

The preparation of potent antibody-containing eluates from the red cells of patients with AIHA is essential in determining the specificity of the antibody.

Several methods are available for the preparation of eluates; each has advantages and disadvantages. The first step is to wash the red cells at least four times in a large volume of saline. At the last washing, centrifuge for 10 min at 1200–1500 *g* and save the supernatant. Ideally, 2–5 ml of packed red cells should be left at the end of this washing.

Landsteiner and Miller's method[20]

To the washed, packed cells add a suitable volume of saline containing 1% of human serum albumin or AB serum (see below). If the DAT gives a strong reaction (i.e. + + or + + +), add a volume of saline equal to the volume of the cells; if the reaction is a weak one (i.e. ± or +) , add only half the volume. Mix and agitate continuously in a water-bath at 56°C for 5 min. Centrifuge rapidly while still hot and remove the cherry-red supernatant at once—this is the eluate.

Eluates made into saline must be tested at once; those made into albumin-saline or AB serum will keep quite well at – 20°C, but the AB serum must be known to be free of any antibody.

Rubin's modification[29] of Vos and Kelsall's method[38]

To washed packed red cells in a glass tube add a suitable volume of saline (see above); then add a volume of ether twice that of the packed red cells. Stopper loosely, allowing release of vapour frequently and shake vigorously for 1 min. Place at 37°C for 30 min, mixing frequently; centrifuge at 1200–1500 *g* at 37°C for 10 min, after which, three layers will be found. The top layer is ether—this is discarded. The bottom haemoglobin-stained layer is the eluate. Collect this with a pipette passed through the middle layer of red cell stroma. Free the eluate of residual ether by leaving it at 37°C for 30–60 min. The smell of ether should have vanished before the eluate is tested or frozen for testing at a later date. Eluates prepared by Rubin's method into saline keep well if stored at – 20°C.

Hughes-Jones, Gardner and Telford[14] estimated that if the elution process is carried out as described above, 70% of antibody will be recovered, while Landsteiner and Miller's method[20] yields only a third as much antibody from the same volume of cells. For this reason, and because of the ease with which eluates can be prepared by Rubin's method, this is the method we recommend for use in the investigation of cases of AIHA.

SCREENING ELUATES

The eluate and the saline of the last wash (control) are first screened against two or three samples of washed normal group-O cells to see if they contain any antibodies:

1. *By titration against enzyme-treated group-O cells.* Prepare doubling dilutions of eluate and control in saline to give dilutions of 1 in 1 to 1 in 32. To 1 drop of eluate or dilution add 1 drop of 2% emzyme-treated cells. Incubate at 37°C for 1–1½ h and read microscopically.

2. *By the indirect antiglobulin test (IAT).* To 10 drops of eluate or control add 1 drop of a 50% suspension of group-O cells. Incubate for 1–½ h at 37°C. Wash four times and, using optimal dilutions of anti-IgG (and of anti-IgM and anti-IgA if these sera gave positive reactions in the DAT), carry out the IAT by either the tile or tube method.

If the control preparation (the supernatant saline from the last washing) gives positive reactions, the possibility that any eluate contains serum antibody has to be considered.

Determination of the specificity of warm auto-antibodies in eluates and sera.

When tested against a phenotyped panel, about two-thirds of auto-antibodies appear to have Rh specificity and in about half these cases specificity against a particular antigen can be demonstrated.[6,16,26]

The other one-third of auto-antibodies may show specificity against other very high incidence antigens, for example, Wr[b] and En[a], and rarely other blood-group specificities are involved. It is essential to differentiate between auto- and allo-antibodies, especially if transfusion is being considered. The presence of allo-antibodies in addition to auto-antibodies is suggested by any discrepancy between the serum and eluate results.

The ascertainment of specificity is not difficult but it is essential to have available a panel of normal red cells, the blood groups of which have been determined as completely as possible. Access to a source of $-D-/-D-$ or Rh[null] cells is a great advantage. Within the Rh system anti-e is the commonest specificity. This will be shown by R_2R_2 cells reacting much more weakly than do cells of the other common Rh genotypes. So-called 'Rh specificity' is demonstrated by Rh[null] cells reacting very weakly or failing to react while all the other cells on the panel react strongly.

As already mentioned, the presence of allo-antibodies in a serum complicates the determination of the specificity of an auto-antibody, and it can be argued that it would be better to test only the eluted auto-antibody and to leave the serum strictly alone. However, only a small volume of an eluate may be available, especially in anaemic patients, and it is generally wise to test both serum and eluate. The procedure is the same for both.

Titration of antibodies in eluates or sera

The methods used have already been described in Chapter 26, p. 437. The exact technique chosen, and the red cells used, should be those which have given the clearest results in the screening tests.

DEMONSTRATION OF LYSIS BY WARM AUTO-ANTIBODIES

As referred to on p. 479, auto-antibodies in serum capable of bringing about lysis in vitro of normal red cells at 37°C ('warm haemolysins') have rarely been demonstrated in cases of AIHA.[4b] In contrast, it is not rare for warm antibodies—presumably of the IgM variety—to bring about lysis, in the presence of complement, of enzyme-treated cells at 37°C, and it is significant that patients whose sera lyse these modified cells, but *not* normal cells, do not necessarily suffer from a serious degree of haemolysis.[37] PNH red cells, too, can be used, if available, as sensitive reagents for demonstrating the lytic potentiality of the antibodies (see p. 263).

Red cells which have been stored for several days at 4°C may occasionally undergo agglutination (or lysis) in certain pathological sera.[17] When this occurs at 37°C in the screening test, the preparation should be set up again with the same cells taken freshly from the donor. Not infrequently, lysis will not occur with perfectly fresh red cells even though sublytic amounts of complement may be bound. In all lysis tests using normal red cells the pH of the cell-serum mixtures should be adjusted to about 6.8, as this is the optimum pH for lysis. Adjustment of pH is less critical using enzyme-treated or PNH cells than when normal unmodified cells are used.[4b]

TITRATION OF COLD AGGLUTININS

While setting up screening procedures using serum, as described above, it is convenient to set up titrations for cold agglutinins in order to screen for their presence, and if present to obtain an indication of their specificity.

Prepare doubling dilutions of the serum in saline ranging from 1 in 1 to 1 in 512 and add 1 drop of each serum dilution into three series of small (e.g. 38 × 6.4 mm) glass tubes so that three replicate titrations can be made. Add 1 drop of a 2% suspension of saline-washed adult group-O (I) cells to the first row, 1 drop of enzyme-treated adult group-O cells to the second row and 1 drop of cord-blood group-O (i) cells to the third row. Mix and leave overnight at 4°C. Before reading place pipettes and a tray of slides at 4°C. Read microscopically at room temperature using the chilled slides.

Normal range. Using sera from normal adult Caucasians and normal adult I red cells, the cold-agglutinin titre at 4°C is from 1 to 32; using enzyme-treated I red cells the titre is from 1 to 64 and with cord-blood (i) cells 0 to 8. In cold-haemagglutinin disease (CHAD) the end-point may not have been reached at a dilution of 1 in 512; if so, further dilutions should be prepared and tested.

If a cold agglutinin is present at a raised titre, the presence of a cold allo-antibody has to be excluded. In this case the patient's own red cells will be found to react *much* less strongly than do normal adult I red cells. It should be noted that in CHAD the patient's cells commonly react rather less strongly than do normal adult I cells (see Table 29.10).

SPECIFICITY OF COLD ANTIBODIES

High-titre cold auto-antibodies have a well defined blood-group specificity which is almost invariably within the I/i system.[16,28,39] Since the I antigen is poorly developed in cord-blood red cells, whilst the i antigen is well developed, group-O cord-blood red cells should be included in the panel used to test for I/i specificity. Adult cells almost always have the I antigen well expressed but the strength of the antigen varies and it is of considerable advantage to have available adult cells known to possess strong I antigen. (The rare adult i cells, if available, are also a useful reagent.)

Cold agglutinin titration patterns

The presence of high-titre cold agglutinins in a patient's serum will be indicated by the screening procedure described above. To demonstrate that the agglutinins are auto-antibodies, it is necessary to show that the patient's own cells are also agglutinated. It is interesting to note that the titre using the patient's cells is usually less (one-half or one-quarter) than that of control normal adult red cells (Table 29.10)

In cold-haemagglutinin disease, whether 'idiopathic' or secondary to mycoplasma pneumonia or lymphoma, the auto-antibodies usually have anti-I specificity (Patient A.G. in Table 29.10).

In rare cases of haemolytic anaemia associated with infectious mononucleosis an auto-antibody of anti-i specificity has been demonstrated (Patient F.B. in Table 29.10), and this specificity, too, has been found in certain patients with lymphoma. Rarely, in chronic CHAD, the antibody has been shown to have anti-Pr or anti-M specificity; in

Table 29.10 Agglutination titres using various types of cold auto-antibodies and normal adult and normal cord red cells, the patient's red cells and enzyme-treated (papainized) normal adult red cells

Patient	Agglutination titre (4°C)			
	Adult (I) cells	Cord (i) cells	Patient's cells	Papainized adult (I) cells
A.G.	4000	512	2000	8000
F.B.	512	32000	128	8000
A.R.	2000	2000	2000	16

A.G. This patient had the cold-haemagglutinin disease. The antibody was of the common anti-I type.
F.B. This patient had a terminal haemolytic anaemia associated with a lymphoma. The antibody was of the anti-i type.
A.R. This patient had the cold-haemagglutinin disease. The antibody was of the rare anti-Pr type.

either type of case the antigen is destroyed by enzyme treatment (Patient A.R. in Tables 29.10).

DETERMINATION OF THE THERMAL RANGE OF COLD AGGLUTININS

From a series of master doubling dilutions of serum in saline place 1 drop of serum or serum dilution into four rows of small (38 × 6.4 mm) agglutinin tubes. Set them up at 30°C, 25°C and 20°C and to each tube add 1 drop of a 2% saline suspension of the following cells:

1. Pooled normal adult group-O (I) red cells.
2. Pooled enzyme-treated (e.g. pre-papainized) normal adult group-O (I) red cells.
3. Pooled cord-blood group-O (i) red cells.
4. Patient's red cells.

Titration should also be carried out at 37°C, if there had been agglutination at this temperature in the screening tests. After incubation at the appropriate temperature for $1\frac{1}{2}$–2 h, determine the presence or absence of agglutination macroscopically, using a concave mirror, as described on p. 431. It is hardly practical to read agglutination microscopically on slides warmed or cooled to the appropriate temperatures.

Alternatively, the thermal range of an antibody may be determined in the following simple way. Place three tubes each containing 10 drops of the patient's serum at 37°C. To each tube add 1 drop of a 50% saline suspension of pre-warmed red cells: to the first, normal adult group-O (I) red cells; to the second, normal cord-blood group O (i) red cells, and to the third, the patient's own red cells. Mix the contents of each tube and allow the red cells to sediment for about 1 h in a water-bath at 37°C. After this time, transfer the tubes to a beaker containing water at 37°C which is allowed to cool slowly and in which a thermometer records the fall in temperature. Inspect the three tubes visually for agglutination at 37°C by tipping them gently and watching the behaviour of the red cells, and re-inspect each time the temperature falls by 1°C until agglutination is unmistakeable. Results typical of a case of chronic cold-haemagglutinin disease are given in Table 29.11.

LYSIS BY COLD ANTIBODIES

If lysis is detected in the serum screening tests, the lysis titre and the thermal range for lysis should be determined and also the specificity of the antibody, e.g. anti-I, anti-i, anti-Pr or anti-M. To estimate the titre, dilutions of the patient's serum are made in fresh normal serum to provide a source of complement. Typically, although not invariably, more lysis takes places if the mixture of serum and complement is acidified.

Method

Prepare suitable dilutions of the patient's serum in fresh normal serum acidified to a pH of 6.0–6.5 (see p. 261). A series of master doubling dilutions should be set up initially,. If a high lysis titre is anticipated, it is convenient to prepare a 1 in 10 dilution initially and then set up doubling dilutions (1 in 10, 1 in 20 etc. to a dilution of 1 in 640).

To 5 drops of each dilution add 1 drop of a 25% saline suspension of red cells. The cells used in the test should be:

1. Adult group-O cells known to possess a strong I antigen.
2. The same cells after treatment with papain.
3. Group-O (i) cord-blood cells.

Table 29.11 Macroscopic agglutination at different temperatures of various red cell samples by the serum of a patient suffering from chronic cold-haemagglutinin disease

| Cells | Temperature (°C) | | | | | | | | | | |
	30	29	28	27	26	25	24	23	22	21	20
Patient (I)	—	—	½ +	1 +	2 +	2 +	3 +	3 +	3 +	3 +	3 +
Normal adult (I)	—	½ +	1 +	1 +	2 +	3 +	3 +	3 +	3 +	3 +	3 +
Normal cord (i)	—	—	—	—	—	—	—	—	—	?	½ +

Each test should be set up at 20°C, 30°C and 37°C, and it is most important that the cells and serum are brought to the correct temperature before they are mixed.

Optimum temperature for demonstrating lysis by a high-titre cold antibody

A temperature of 25°C is about optimum for the demonstration of lysis by high-titre (anti-I) antibodies. Below 15°C lysis will not take place because some complement components will not bind at a low temperature; above 30°C, depending on the thermal range of the antibody, lysis is prevented because antibody is not adsorbed. Lysis taking place in one phase at normal bench temperature without preliminary chilling has been referred to as monophasic (Fig. 29.4). This contrasts with lysis brought about by the Donath-Landsteiner (D-L) antibody which is typically described as biphasic. Preliminary chilling below normal bench temperature is usually necessary to bring about binding of the antibody, followed by warming for lysis to occur (see p. 500). It should

be noted that high-titre anti-I antibodies will often, too, bring about lysis when the red cell-serum suspension is treated biphasically, i.e. give a type of positive D-L antibody test. Conversely, but rarely, genuine D-L antibodies, if active at a sufficiently high temperature, can also give rise to lysis monophasically, e.g. at 20°C. Anti-I antibodies can be distinguished from D-L antibodies by virtue of their remarkable agglutinating properties at low temperatures and in other ways even if they give a positive D-L test.

It is particularly important that the concentrated cell suspension be delivered directly into the serum dilution without running down the side of the tube, for tightly agglutinated cells lyse extremely easily under these conditions, even in the absence of complement. Lysis is usually read visually after the red cells have sedimented for 2 h or, if practicable, after remixing and centrifuging at the appropriate temperature.

Enzyme-treated cells are typically much more sensitive to lysis by high-titre anti-I and anti-i antibodies than are normal red cells (Table 29.12) and they may even by lysed at 37°C. PNH cells are particularly easily lysed because of their remarkable sensitivity to complement (Table 29.12), and the lysis titre with these cells at 30°C is usually as great as or may exceed the agglutination titre. PNH cells can be used as a sensitive and reliable tool for the demonstration of the lytic potential of any antibody which fixes complement. However, when using PNH cells the serum must not be acidified, and the control tube, containing fresh normal serum but no patient's serum, must be carefully examined for lysis.

To ensure that lysis is easily visible a stronger cell-serum suspension should be used than that used for agglutination tests. A final concentration of about 5% is suitable and this is attained by the method described above. The lysis titre is given by the reciprocal of the highest serum dilution causing (+) lysis. It is convenient to score complete lysis as C ; (+) represents definite but weak lysis compared with the colour of the supernatant of the control, while +, + + and + + + represent intermediate degrees of lysis.

Typical results obtained in a patient with chronic cold-haemagglutinin disease due to anti-I antibody are shown in Table 29.12.

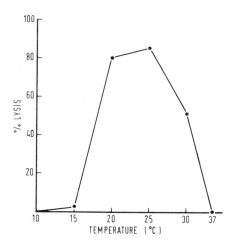

Fig. 29.4   Effect of temperature on lysis by a high-titre cold auto-antibody (anti-I). Chronic cold haemagglutinin disease. Normal group O (I) red cells in patient's serum. The serum was diluted with an equal volume of fresh normal serum and acidified by the addition of a one-tenth volume of 0.2 mol/l HCl. Incubation was carried out for 10 min at each temperature.

Table 29.12   Relative sensitivity of red cells to lysis by a high-titre cold antibody at 20°C

Type of cell	pH	Dilutions of serum								Control (normal serum diluent)
		1 in 1	1 in 4	1 in 16	1 in 64	1 in 256	1 in 1024	1 in 4096	1 in 16000	
Normal (I)	8.0	—	trace	—	—	—	—	—	—	—
Normal (1)	6.5	trace	+	(+)	trace	—	—	—	—	—
Trypsinized normal (I)	8.0	+	+ + +	+ +	+	(+)	—	—	—	—
PNH	8.0	+ + +	+ + +	+ + +	+ + +	+ + +	+ +	+ +	+	—

+ + + denotes marked lysis; + +, + and (+) denote lesser but definite degrees of lysis; — denotes no lysis.

DETECTION AND TITRATION OF THE DONATH-LANDSTEINER (D-L) ANTIBODY

The Donath-Landsteiner (D-L) antibody of paroxysmal cold haemoglobinuria differs from the high-titre cold antibodies referred to previously in that it is an IgG antibody and has a quite different specificity. It is, too, far more lytic to normal cells in relation to its titre than are anti-I or anti-i antibodies. Thus the lysis titre of a D-L, antibody may be the same or greater than its agglutination titre. Almost maximal lysis develops in unacidified serum.

DIRECT DONATH-LANDSTEINER TEST

Collect two samples of venous blood into glass tubes containing no anticoagulant, previously warmed at 37°C. Incubate the first sample at 37°C for $1\frac{1}{2}$ h. Put the second sample in a beaker packed with ice and allow to stand for 1 h; then place the tube at 37°C for a further 20 min. Centrifuge both tubes at 37°C and examine the supernatant serum for lysis. A positive test is indicated by lysis in the sample which had been chilled.

INDIRECT DONATH-LANDSTEINER TEST

Serum obtained from the patient's blood which has been allowed to clot at 37°C is used for this test.

Add 1 volume of a 50% suspension of washed normal group-O, P-positive red cells to 9 volumes of patient's unacidified serum in a glass tube.

Chill the suspension in crushed ice at 0°C for 1 h, then place the tube at 37°C for 30 min.

Centrifuge at 37°C and examine for lysis. Three controls should be set up at the same time:

1. A duplicate of the test cell-serum suspension, but kept strictly at 37°C for the duration of the test.

2. A duplicate of the test cell-serum suspension, except that an equal volume of ABO-compatible fresh normal serum is first added to the patient's serum as a source of complement. The same cells are added and the suspension is chilled and subsequently warmed in the same way as the test suspension. (This control excludes false-negative results due to the patient's serum being deficient in complement.)

3. A duplicate of the test cell-serum suspension, except that fresh normal serum is used in place of the patient's serum. This control, too, is chilled and subsequently warmed.

A positive test will be indicated by lysis in the test suspension and in control No. 2. If ABO compatible *pp* cells are available they should be used in a duplicate set of tubes. No lysis will develop—confirming the P specificity of the antibody.

Titration of a Donath-Landsteiner antibody

Prepare doubling or four-fold dilutions of the patient's serum in fresh normal human serum. To each tube add a one-tenth volume of a 50% suspension of washed group-O P-positive red cells and immerse each of the tubes in crushed ice at 0°C. After 1 h place at 37°C and incubate for a further 30 min. Then centrifuge and inspect for lysis.

Detection of a Donath-Landsteiner antibody by the indirect antiglobulin test

Since the D-L antibody is an IgG antibody, it can be detected by the indirect antiglobulin test (IAT) using an *anti-IgG* serum if the cells which have been exposed to the antibody in the cold are washed in cold (4°C) saline. At this temperature the antibody will not be eluted during washing. It should be noted, however, that exposing normal red cells at 4°C to many fresh normal sera results in a positive IAT with broad-spectrum antiglobulin sera because of the adsorption of incomplete anti-H (a normally-occurring cold antibody) on to the red cells. At a low temperature, complement is bound, too, and it is its adsorption which gives rise to the positive tests with broad-spectrum sera. The adsorption of complement can be prevented by adding an anticoagulant such as EDTA to the serum.

Method

Add a one-tenth volume of EDTA, buffered to pH 7.0 (see Appendix, p. 536) to the patient's serum. Prepare doubling dilutions in saline from 1 in 1 to 1 in 28.

Add 1 volume (drop) of a 50% suspension of group-O, P-positive red cells to 10 volumes (drops) of each dilution. Mix and incubate at 4°C (preferably in a cold room).

After 1 h wash the red cells four times in a large volume of cold (4°C) saline. Then carry out an antiglobulin test using an anti-IgG reagent, as described on p. 435, but keeping the red cell-antiglobulin serum suspension at 4°C.

As controls, set up a series of tests using a serum known to contain a D-L antibody and a normal serum, respectively.

This technique is the most sensitive way of detecting, especially in stored sera, the D-L antibody present in an amount insufficient to bring about actual lysis.

Thermal range of a Donath-Landsteiner (D-L) antibody

The highest temperature at which D-L antibodies are usually adsorbed to red cells is about 18°C. Hence little or no lysis can be expected unless the cell-serum suspension is cooled below this temperature. Chilling in crushed ice results in maximum adsorption of the antibody and leads to the binding of complement which brings about lysis when the cell suspension is subsequently warmed at 37°C. Hence the 'cold-warm' biphasic procedure necessary for lysis to be demonstrated by a typical D-L antibody.

Specificity of the Donath-Landsteiner antibody

The D-L antibody appears to have a well-defined specificity within the P blood-group system, namely, anti-P. However, in practice, almost all samples of red cells are acted upon, for the cells that will not react (P^k and *pp*) are extremely rare.[22,42] Cord-blood cells are lysed to about the same extent as are adult P_1 and P_2 cells.

TREATMENT OF SERUM WITH 2-MERCAPTO-ETHANOL (2-ME) OR DITHIOTHREITOL (DTT)

Weak solutions of 2-ME or DTT destroy the inter-chain sulphydryl bonds of gamma globulins. IgM antibodies treated in this way lose their ability to agglutinate red cells while IgG antibodies do not.[9,16] IgA antibodies may or may not be inhibited depending upon whether or not they are made up of polymers of IgA. Since almost all auto-antibodies are either IgM or IgG, treatment of serum or an eluate with 2-ME or DTT gives a reliable indication of the Ig class of auto-antibody under investigation.[9,16]

Method

(a) 2-MERCAPTO-ETHANOL (2-ME)

To 1 volume of undiluted serum add 1 volume of 0.1 mol/l 2-mercapto-ethanol in phosphate buffer, pH 7.2 (see p. 538).

As a control, add a volume of the serum to the phosphate buffer alone. Incubate both at 37°C for 2 h.

Then titrate the treated serum and its control with the appropriate red cells.

If IgG antibody is present, the antibody titration in the control serum will be the same as that of the treated serum. However, if the antibody is IgM, the treated serum will fail to agglutinate the test cells or agglutinate them to a much lower titre compared with the control untreated serum.

The control must remain active to show that the absence of agglutination is due to reduction of IgM antibody and not due to dilution.

(b) Dithiothreitol (DTT)

0.01 mol/l DTT can be used in place of 0.1 mol/l 2-ME in the above method.

DRUG-INDUCED HAEMOLYTIC ANAEMIAS OF IMMUNOLOGICAL ORIGIN

As already mentiond (p. 477), acquired haemolytic anaemias may develop as the result of immunological reactions consequent on the administration of certain drugs.[25,26] Clinically, they often closely mimic AIHA of 'idiopathic' origin and for this reason a careful enquiry into the taking of drugs is a necessary part of the interrogation of any patient suspected of having an acquired haemolytic anaemia. Two immunological mechanisms leading to a drug-induced haemolytic anaemia are recognized. These mechanisms are commonly referred to as 'drug-dependent immune' and 'drug-dependent auto-immune'. Similar mechanisms have been described for drug-induced immune thrombocytopenia and neutropenia of immunological origin (p. 443).

DRUG-DEPENDENT IMMUNE HAEMOLYTIC ANAEMIAS

In these cases antibodies are produced against a drug, and the drug is required in the in-vitro system for the antibodies to be detected. The red cells become damaged by one of two mechanisms:

1. The initial reaction is the production by the patient of antibodies against drug-protein complexes, the drug acting as a hapten. The antibodies fix complement and the resulting circulating immune complexes may attach themselves to the patient's red cells, and perhaps to platelets, too. This is the mechanism that has often been referred to as the 'innocent bystander' mechanism, the red cells (or platelets) being the 'bystanders'. A typical history is for haemolysis, which may be severe and intravascular, to follow the re-administration of a drug with which the patient has previously been treated, and for the haemolysis to subside when the offending drug has been identified and withdrawn. The DAT is likely to become strongly positive during the haemolytic phase, the patient's red cells being agglutinated by anti-C sera and sometimes by anti-IgG sera.

Drugs which have been shown to cause haemolysis by the above mechanism include quinine, quinidine and rifampicin, as well as chlorpropamide, hydrochlorothiazide, nomifensine, phenacetin, salicylazosulphapyridine, the sodium salt of p-aminosalicylic acid and stibophen. Petz and Branch[25] listed 25 drugs reported to have brought about haemolysis by the immune complex mechanism.

2. The drug or a metabolite of the drug is firmly bound to the red cell surface. Any antibodies the patient may form against the drug will be bound to the red cells, too. The DAT will be positive with broad-spectrum antiglobulin sera and with anti-IgG sera, and perhaps with anti-C sera and anti-IgM sera also.

The haemolytic anaemia associated with prolonged high-dose penicillin therapy is caused by the above mechanism, and other penicillin derivatives, as well as cephalosporins, and tetracycline may cause haemolysis in a similar fashion. As with the 'innocent-bystander' mechanism, haemolysis ceases when the offending drug has been identified and withdrawn.

Cephalosporins, in addition to causing the formation of specific antibodies, may alter the red cell surface so as to cause non-specific adherence of complement and immunoglobulins. This may lead to a positive DAT but is seldom associated with clinically apparent increased haemolysis.

DRUG-DEPENDENT AUTO-IMMUNE HAEMOLYTIC ANAEMIAS

In these cases the antibody is directed against the red cell, not the drug. The drug acts in some as yet ill-understood way to promote the development of anti-red cell auto-antibodies which seem serologically identical to those of 'idiopathic' warm-type AIHA. The great majority of cases have followed the use of the anti-hypertension drug α-methyldopa (Aldomet). The red cells are coated with IgG and the serum contains auto-antibodies which characteristically have Rh specificity.

Other drugs that have been reported to act in a similar fashion to α-methyldopa include chlordiazepoxide (Librium), mefenamic acid (Ponstam), flufenamic acid and indomethicine.[6]

Typical serological features of the different types of drug-induced haemolytic anaemia of immunological origin are summarized in Table 29.13.

PENICILLIN-INDUCED HAEMOLYTIC ANAEMIA

The characteristic features are:

1. Haemolysis occurs only in patients receiving large doses of a penicillin for long periods (e.g. weeks).

2. The DAT is strongly positive with anti-IgG reagents.

3. The patient's serum and antibody eluted from the patient's red cells react *only* with penicillin-treated red cells—they do not react with normal untreated red cells.

DETECTION OF ANTI-PENICILLIN ANTIBODIES

Reagents

Barbitone buffer. 0.14 mol/l, pH 9.5 (see p. 537).
Penicillin solution. 0.4 g of penicillin G dissolved in 6 ml of barbitone buffer.

Penicillin-coated normal red cells

Wash group-O normal red cells three times in saline and make a *c* 15% suspension in saline to which a one-tenth volume of barbitone buffer has been added. Add 2 ml of the red cell suspension to 6 ml of penicillin solution and incubate at 37°C for 1 h. Then wash 4 times in saline and make up 2% (for tube tests) and 20% (for tile tests) red cell suspension in saline.

Control normal red cells

These should be treated in exactly the same way as the penicillin-coated red cells except that the 6 ml of penicillin solution is replaced by 6 ml of barbitone buffer.

Method

Anti-penicillin antibodies can be detected by the IAT in the usual way using the penicillin-coated red cells in place of normal unmodified cells. However, three extra controls are necessary.

1. Red cells which have not been exposed to penicillin should be added to the patient's serum.

2. Penicillin-treated red cells should be added to two normal sera known not to contain anti-penicillin antibodies (*negative controls*).

Table 29.13 Serological features of the different types of drug-induced haemolytic anaemia of immunological origin

Mechanism	Prototype drug	DAT	IAT	IAT + Drug	
				Serum	Eluate
Drug-dependent antibody:					
(a) Drug adsorption	Penicillin	IgG	Neg	IgG	IgG
(b) Immune-complex	Quin(id)ine	C*	Neg	C*	Neg
Auto-antibody	α-methyldopa	IgG	IgG		

*Occasionally also IgG.

3. Penicillin-treated red cells should be added to a serum (if one is available) known to contain anti-penicillin antibodies (*positive control*).

Cephalosporin can be used in a similar way to sensitize red cells. Control (2) is particularly important when penicillin derivatives such as cephalosporin are used, since over-exposure in vitro to these drugs can lead to positive results with normal sera.

High-titre IgG anti-penicillin antibodies often cause direct agglutination of penicillin-treated red cells in low dilutions of serum. The antibodies can be differentiated from IgM-agglutinating antibodies by treatment with 2-ME or DTT (p. 501).

DETECTION OF ANTIBODIES AGAINST DRUGS OTHER THAN PENICILLIN

In a patient with an immune haemolytic anaemia whose serum and red cell eluate does *not* react with normal red cells and who is receiving a drug or drugs other than penicillin or a penicillin derivative, antibodies which react with red cells only in the presence of the suspect drugs or drugs should be looked for in the following way:

Table 29.14 Investigation of a suspected drug-induced haemolytic anaemia

Tube No.	1	2	3	4	5	6
Patient's serum volumes (drops)	10	10	5	5	0	0
Fresh normal serum volumes (drops)	0	0	5	5	10	10
Drug solution volumes (drops)	2	0	2	0	2	0
Saline volumes (drops)	0	2	0	2	0	2
50% normal group-O cells volumes (drops)	1	1	1	1	1	1

The patient's serum and red cell eluates should be tested with normal and enzyme-treated group-O red cells, carrying out the tests with and without the drug that the patient is receiving. The approach is essentially empirical. A saturated solution of the drug should be prepared in saline and the pH adjusted to 6.5–7.0.

Set up six tubes containing the patient's serum and the drug solution in the proportions shown in Table 29.14 and add one drop of a 50% saline suspension of group-O cells to each tube. Incubate at 37°C for 1 h and examine for agglutination and lysis. Wash the red cells four times in saline and carry out an IAT using a broad-spectrum antiglobulin serum or anti-IgG and anti-C sera separately.

REFERENCES

[1] BAREFORD, D., LONGSTER, G., GILKS, L. and TOVEY, L. A. D. (1985). Follow-up of normal individuals with a positive antiglobulin test. *Scandinavian Journal of Haematology*, **35**, 348.

[2] BODENSTEINER, D., BROWN, P., SKIKNE, B. and PLAPP, F. (1983). The enzyme-linked immunosorbent assay: accurate detection of red blood cell antibodies in autoimmune hemolytic anemia. *American Journal of Clinical Pathology*, **79**, 182.

[3] CHAPLIN, H. Jnr (1973). Clinical usefulness of specific antiglobulin reagents in autoimmune hemolytic anemia. *Progress in Hematology*, **8**, 25.

[4] DACIE, J. V. (1962). *The Haemolytic Anaemias: Congenital and Acquired. Part II: The Auto-Immune Haemolytic Anaemias*, 2nd edn, (a) p. 437, (b) p. 439, (c) p. 461, (d) p. 496. Churchill, London.

[5] DACIE, J. V. (1975). Auto-immune hemolytic anemias. *Archives of Internal Medicine*, **135**, 1293.

[6] DACIE, J. V. and WORLLEDGE, S. M. (1969). Auto-immune hemolytic anemias. *Progress in Hematology*, **6**, 82.

[7] ENGELFRIET, C. P., VON DEM BORNE, A. E. G., BECKERS, D. and VAN LOGHEM, J. J. (1974). Auto-immune haemolytic anaemia: serological and immunochemical characteristics of the auto-antibodies: mechanisms of cell destruction. *Series Haematologica*, **VII**, 328.

[8] FREEDMAN, J. (1979). False-positive antiglobulin tests in healthy subjects. *Journal of Clinical Pathology*, **32**, 1014.

[9] FREEDMAN, J., MASTERS, C. A., NEWLANDS, M. and MOLLISON, P. L. (1976). Optimal conditions for the use of sulphydryl compounds is dissociating red cell antibodies. *Vox Sanguinis*, **30**, 231.

[10] GILLILAND, B. C., BAXTER, E. and EVANS, R. S. (1971). Red-cell antibodies in acquired hemolytic anemia with negative antiglobulin serum test. *New England Journal of Medicine*, **285**, 252.

[11] GORST, D. W., RAWLINSON, V. I., MERRY, A. H. and STRATTON, F. (1980). Positive direct antiglobulin test in normal individuals. *Vox Sanguinis*, **38**, 99.

[12] HEDDLE, N. M., KELTON, J. G., TURCHYN, K. L. and ALI, M. A. M. (1988). Hypergammaglobulinemia can be associated with a positive direct antiglobulin test, a nonreactive eluate, and no evidence of hemolysis. *Transfusion*, **28**, 29.

[13] HSU, T. C. S., ROSENFIELD, R. E., BURKART, P., WONG, K. Y. and KOCKWA, S. (1974). Instrumental PVP augmented antiglobulin tests. II. Evaluation of acquired hemolytic anemia. *Vox Sanguinis*, **26**, 305.

[14] HUGHES-JONES, N. C., GARDNER, B. and TELFORD, R. (1963). Comparison of various methods of dissociation of anti-D, using ^{131}I-labelled antibody. *Vox Sanguinis*, **8**, 531.

[15] HUH, Y. O., LIU, F. J., ROGGE, K., CHAKRABARTY, L. and LICHTIGER, B. (1988). Positive direct antiglobulin test and high serum immunoglobulin G levels. *American Journal of Clinical Pathology*, **90**, 197.

[16] ISSITT, P. D. (1985). Serological diagnosis and characterization of the causative autoantibodies. *Methods in Hematology*, **12**, 1.

[17] JENKINS, W. J. and MARSH, W. L. (1961). Autoimmune haemolytic anaemia. Three cases with antibodies specifically active against stored red cells. *Lancet*, **ii**, 16.

[18] LALEZARI, P. and JIANG, A. C. (1980). The manual Polybrene test: a simple and rapid procedure for detection of red cell antibodies. *Transfusion*, **20**, 206.

[19] LALEZARI, P. and OBERHARDT, B. (1971). Temperature gradient dissociation of the red cell antigen–antibody complexes in the Polybrene technique. *British Journal of Haematology*, **21**, 131.

[20] LANDSTEINER, K. and MILLER. C. P. Jnr (1925). Serological studies on the blood of primates. II. The blood groups in anthropoid apes. *Journal of Experimental Medicine*, **42**, 853.

[21] LAU, P., HAESLER, W. E. and WURZEL, H. A. (1976). Positive direct antiglobulin reaction in a patient population. *American Journal of Clinical Pathology*, **65**, 368.

[22] LEVINE, P., CELANO, M. J. and FALKOWSKI, F. (1963). The specificity of the antibody in paroxysmal cold hemoglobinuria (P. C. H.). *Transfusion*, **3**, 278.

[23] MARSH, W. L. and JENKINS, W. J. (1960). Anti-i: a new cold antibody. *Nature* (London), **188**, 753.

[24] PETZ, L. D. and BRANCH, D. R. (1983). Serological tests for the diagnosis of immune hemolytic anemias. *Methods in Hematology*, **9**, 12.

[25] PETZ, L. D. and BRANCH, D. R. (1985). Drug-induced immune hemolytic anemias. *Methods in Hematology*, **12**, 47.

[26] PETZ, L. D. and GARRATTY, G. (1980). *Acquired Immune Hemolytic Anemias*. Churchill Livingstone, New York.

[27] PIROFSKY, B. (1969). *Autoimmunization and the Autoimmune Hemolytic Anemias*. Williams and Wilkins, Baltimore.

[28] ROELCKE, D. (1989). Cold agglutination. *Transfusion Medicine Reviews*, **3**, 140.

[29] RUBIN, H. (1963). Antibody elution from red blood cells. *Journal of Clinical Pathology*, **16**, 70.

[30] SCHMITZ, N., DJIBEY, T., KRETSCHMER, V., MAHN, I. and MUELLER-ECKHARDT, C. (1981). Assessment of red cell autoantibodies in autoimmune hemolytic anemia of warm type by radioactive anti-IgG test. *Vox Sanguinis*, **41**, 224.

[31] SOKOL, R. J. and HEWITT, S. (1985). Autoimmune hemolysis: a critical review. *CRC Critical Reviews in Oncology/Hematology*, **4**, 125.

[32] SOKOL, R. J., HEWITT, S., BOOKER, D. J. and STAMPS, R. (1985). Enzyme linked direct antiglobulin tests in patients with autoimmune haemolysis. *Journal of Clinical Pathology*, **38**, 912.

[33] SOKOL, R. J. HEWITT, S. and STAMPS, B. K. (1981). Autoimmune haemolysis: an 18-year study of 865 cases referred to a regional transfusion centre. *British Medical Journal*, **282**, 2023.

[34] STRATTON, F., RAWLINSON, V. I., MERRY, A. H. and THOMSON, E. E. (1983). Positive direct antiglobulin test in normal individuals. *Clinical and Laboratory Haematology*, **5**, 17.

[35] STRATTON, F. and RENTON, P. H. (1955). Effect of crystalloid solutions prepared in glass bottles on human red cells. *Nature* (London), **175**, 727.

[36] SZYMANSKI, I. O., ODGREN, P. R., FORTIER, N. L. and SNYDER, L. M. (1980). Red blood cell associated IgG in normal and pathologic states. *Blood*, **55**, 48.

[37] VON DEM BORNE, A. E. G. Kr., ENGELFRIET, C. P., BECKERS, D., VAN DER KORT-HENKES, G., VAN DER GIESSEN, M. and VAN LOGHEM, J. J. (1969). Autoimmune haemolytic anaemia. II. Warm haemolysins—serological and immunochemical investigations and ^{51}Cr studies. *Clinical and Experimental Immunology*, **4**, 333.

[38] VOS, G. H. and KELSALL, G. A. (1956). A new elution technique for the preparation of specific immune anti-Rh serum. *British Journal of Haematology*, **2**, 342.

[39] WIENER, A. S., UNGER, L. J., COHEN, L. and FELDMAN, J. (1956). Type-specific cold auto-antibodies as a cause of acquired hemolytic anemia and hemolytic transfusion reactions: biologic test with bovine red cells. *Annals of Internal Medicine*, **44**, 221.

[40] WORLLEDGE, S. M. (1978). The interpretation of a positive direct antiglobulin test. *British Journal of Haematology*, **39**, 157 (Annotation).

[41] WORLLEDGE, S. M. and BLAJCHMAN, M. A. (1972). The autoimmune haemolytic anaemias. *British Journal of Haematology*, **23** (Supplement), 61.

[42] WORLLEDGE, S. M. and ROUSSO, C. (1965). Studies on the serology of paroxysmal cold haemoglobinuria (P. C. H.) with special reference to a relationship with the P blood group system. *Vox Sanguinis*, **10**, 293.

30. The HLA system in bone marrow transplantation

(By E. H. Jones)

THE HLA SYSTEM

The major histocompatibility complex (MHC) in man is the HLA system which codes for cell membrane structures on cells of most tissues of the body including leucocytes, both granulocytes, lymphocytes and platelets. The MHC is coded by genes which have a crucial influence on allogeneic bone marrow transplantation. The antigenic specificities of the HLA system measure genetic disparity between the recipient and potential donor of a bone marrow graft.

SEROLOGY OF THE HLA SYSTEM

The antigens detected by serological techniques have been defined at a series of International Workshops which have taken place since 1965. The specificities defined at the Tenth International Histocompatibility Workshop 1987[5] are listed in Table 30.1. Well-defined antigens of the A, B, C and D locus are numbered and the designation of the prefix 'w' indicates that the specificity may be clearly identified but may not always be easily defined. Splits of previously defined antigens are indicated by parentheses and indentation, and, for example, both A23 and A24 have the broader specificity A9. The inclusion of the HLA-B locus specificities into broad specificities Bw4 and Bw6 are also listed. The HLA-DR specificities are found exclusively on B-lymphocytes and activated T-lymphocytes, but not on mature leucocytes or platelets. HLA-DP specificities are defined by Prime Lymphocyte Typing (PLT) and HLA-Dw specificities are defined by mixed lymphocyte culture (MLC) typing. Cross-reacting specificities associated with HLA-DQ and with HLA-DRw52 and HLA-DRw53 are shown in Table 30.2. At the Eighth Histocompatibility Workshop in 1980,[20] an association with a high level of statistical significance was demonstrated between D specificities and the correspondingly numbered DR specificities. Complex splits of DR and Dw antigens were recognised at the Ninth Histocompatibility Workshop in 1984,[19] and as there is a linkage disequilibrium between alleles at DR and DQ loci it is now difficult to maintain any relationship between the numbering of Dw and DR specificities.

The antigen distributions in different ethnic populations were first established at the Fifth Histocom-

Table 30.1   The HLA specificities (WHO nomenclature 1987)

A LOCUS	B LOCUS Bw4; Bw6		C LOCUS	DR	DQ	DP	DW
A1	B5		Cw1	DR1	DQw1	DP1	Dw1
A2		B51	Cw2	DR2	DQw2	DPw2	Dw2
A3		Bw52	Cw3	DRw15	DQw3	DPw3	Dw3
A9	B7		Cw4	DRw16	DQw4	DPw4	Dw4
A23	B8		Cw5	DR3	DQw5	DPw5	Dw5
A24	B12		Cw6	DRw17	DQw6	DPw6	Dw6
A10		B44	Cw7	DRw18	DQw7		Dw7
A25		B45	Cw8	DR4	DQw8		Dw8
A26	B13		Cw9	DR5	DQw9		Dw9
Aw34	B14		Cw10	DRw11			Dw10
Aw66		Bw64	Cw11	DRw12			Dw11
A11		Bw65		DRw6			Dw12
Aw19	B15			DRw13			Dw13
A29		Bw62		DRw14			Dw14
A30		Bw63		DR7			Dw15
A31		Bw75		DRw8			Dw16
A32		Bw76		DRw9			Dw17
Aw33		Bw77		DRw10			Dw18
Aw74	B16			DRw52			Dw19
A28		B38		DRw53			Dw20
Aw68		B39					Dw21
Aw69	B17						Dw22
Aw36		Bw57					Dw23
Aw43		Bw58					Dw24
	B18						Dw25
	B21						Dw26
		Bw49					
		Bw50					
	Bw22						
		Bw54					
		Bw55					
		Bw56					
	B27						
	B35						
	B37						
	B40						
		Bw60					
		Bw61					
	Bw41						
	Bw42						
	Bw46						
	Bw47						
	Bw48						
	Bw53						
	Bw59						
	Bw67						
	Bw70						
		Bw71					
		Bw72					
	Bw73						
	Bw4/Bw6						

The following are inclusions of HLA-B locus specificities into Bw4 and Bw6.
Bw4: B5, B44(12), B13, Bw63(15), Bw77, B38(16), B17, Bw49(21), B27, B37, Bw47, Bw53, Bw59. Bw6: B7, B8, B45(12), B14, Bw62(15), B39(16), B18, Bw50(21), Bw22, B35, B40, Bw41, Bw42, Bw46, Bw48, Bw67, Bw70, Bw73, Bw75, Bw76(15).

patibility Workshop 1972.[21] The frequency of serologically defined antigens in Caucasians defined at the Eighth Histocompatibility Workshop 1980[20] are listed in Table 30.3. The frequency of the antigens varies in different racial groups and the antigens A1 and B8 are predominantly characteristic of Caucasians. The A2 antigen is found with high frequency in all populations, but some antigens, for example Aw36 and Aw43, are found only in black populations. In the Ninth Histocompatibility Workshop

Table 30.2 Designations for HLA-DQ, DRw52 and DRw53 specificities

	Previous equivalent	Cross-reacting specificities
DQwl	MB1, MT1, DC1	DR1, DR2, DRw6, DRw10
DQw2	MB2, DC3	DR3, DR7
DQw3	MB3, MT4, DC4	DR4, DR5
DRw52	MT2	DR3, DR5, DRw6, DRw8
DRw53	MT3	DR4, DR7, DR9

1984[19] antigen frequency was estimated by serological analysis based on family studies.

The combination of alleles of the A, B, C and D loci present on one chromosome of an individual is known as a haplotype. In Caucasians, the most common A/B haplotype is A1/B8, the most common A/DR haplotype is A1/DR3, and the most common B/C haplotype is B14(Bw64,Bw65)/Cw8. All these haplotypes are rarely found in the Oriental or Negroid population. The most frequent three-locus haplotype found in the Caucasian and Negroid population is A1/B8/DR3 but this is not found in Orientals.

When family studies are made the haplotypes of an individual can be deduced as illustrated in Figure 30.1. Considering the A and B loci, any individual can express a maximum of four antigens, two controlled by each locus, and such a phenotype is described as a 'full house'. Each parent contributes one allele, from each locus, and the association between the alleles of the A and B loci is not random. This non-random association of antigens and haplotypes is termed genetic disequilibrium,

Table 30.3 HLA frequencies (%) in European Caucasians (Eighth Histocompatibility Workshop 1980)

A LOCUS	%	B LOCUS	%	C LOCUS	%	D LOCUS	%
A1	28	B5	17	Cwl	8	DR1	13
A2	45	B51	14	Cw2	10	DR2	25
A3	22	Bw52	3	Cw3	19	DR3	20
A9	23	B7	17	Cw4	23	DR4	18
A23	5	B8	16	Cw5	12	DR5	20
A24	18	B12	23	Cw6	15	DRw6	4
A10	11	B44	21	CW7	5	DR7	23
A25	4	B45	2	Cw8	4	DRw8	5
A26	7	B13	6			DRw9	2
A11	12	B14	6			DRw10	2
Aw19	31	B15	12				
A29	7	Bw62	11				
A30	9	Bw63	1				
A31	6	B16	9				
A32	5	B38	5				
Aw33	4	B39	4				
A28	8	B17	8				
Aw34	1	Bw57	6				
		Bw58	2				
		B18	11				
		B21	8				
		B49	5				
		Bw50	3				
		Bw22	5				
		Bw55	4				
		Bw56	1				
		B27	8				
		B35	18				
		B37	3				
		B40	10				
		Bw60	7				
		Bw61	3				
		Bw41	2				
		Bw42	1				
		Bw53	2				
		Bw47	1				
		Bw48	1				
		Bw59	1				

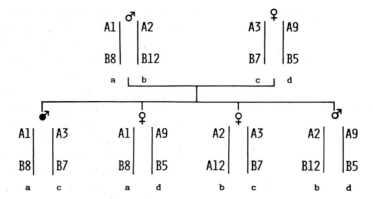

Fig. 30.1   HLA haplotypes. The paternal haplotypes are labelled a and b, the maternal c and d. There are four possible combinations amongst the offspring.

and is partially dependent on the racial origin of the individual. The A and B loci are thought to be very close together because the recombination frequency between them has been found to be 0.8% by family studies. A family with a recombinant is illustrated in Fig. 30.2. The second child has received paternal A1 antigen from the 'a' chromosome and the B44 antigen from the 'b' chromosome.

The complement marker system is useful in determining the haploytpe of the children, if one of the parents is homozygous for the HLA antigens. The family illustrated in Fig. 30.3 was typed to select a bone marrow transplant donor for the patient (♦). The mother had the phenotype A1, B8, and it was important to confirm whether the patient and sibling had a different A1, B8 maternal haplo-type. An analysis of C4 complement markers showed that the patient inherited the maternal 'c' haplotype HLA A1, B8, DR4, with C4 markers: A3, B2, and the sibling had inherited the 'd'

maternal haplotype HLA A1, B8, DR5 with C4 markers: A3, B1, and the father was used as a one haplotype matched donor. In this family segrega-tion of the maternal haplotypes was determined by DR typing and by complement markers, but con-firmation of haplotypes by complement markers in a patient and potential bone marrow donor may be particularly useful if typing for DR antigens of the patient proves difficult.

GENETICS OF THE HLA SYSTEM

The loci controlling the inheritance of the HLA system are located on the short arm of chromosome 6.[16] The control is mediated through four loci, A, B, C and D, each with multiple alleles, aligned on the chromosome so that the C locus lies between the A and B loci (Fig. 30.4). Class I genes control the HLA-A, B, C region, Class II genes control the HLA-D region (DR, DQ, DP). Class I antigens

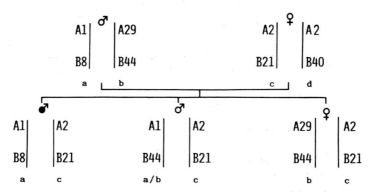

Fig. 30.2   HLA recombinant. The family was investigated to find a donor for patient (♦).

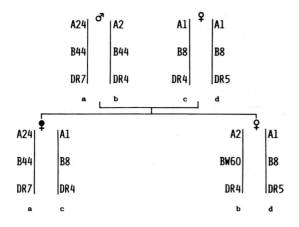

Complement (C4) markers on

Haplotype	a	A3, B1
	b	A3, B5
	c	A3, B2
	d	A3, B1

Fig. 30.3 HLA. The value of the complement marker system.

(HLA-A, B, C) are expressed on all somatic cells, and consist of a polymorphic glycoprotein heavy α chain (44kd) encoded by genes in the MHC on chromosome 6, associated non-covalently with a light β chain of B₂-microglobulin, encoded by a gene located on chromosome 15. Class I non-HLA differentiation antigens are expressed on activated T cells and are thought to be homologues of the murine Qa-Tla antigens.[17] Class II antigens (HLA-Dr, DQ and DP) are expressed mainly on macrophages, dendritic cells, B cells and activated T cells and consist of two non-covalently linked glycoprotein sub-units: an α heavy chain (32–35 kd) and a polymorphic β light chain (28–30 kd). Class I and II MHC antigens function as targets for T lymphocytes that regulate the immune response, and Class II antigens are restricting elements for regulator T cells. Class III antigens constitute the complement components.

(a) Molecular genetics of the MHC complex

Since the 1970s, progress in recombinant DNA technology has enabled the MHC complex to be studied in greater detail. In man, there are 20–40 genes for Class I antigens and for Class II antigens 5 or 6 α chain and 7 β chain genes are known to exist.[2] At least four Class III genes have been demonstrated.[9]

(b) The HLA-D region

Molecular studies of the HLA-D region together with conventional serology, monoclonal antibodies

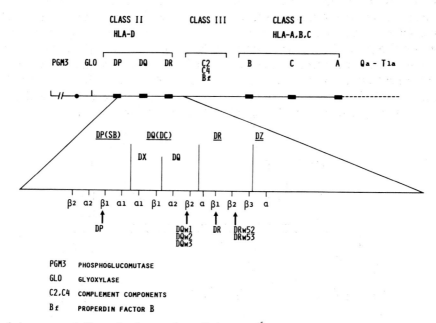

PGM3   PHOSPHOGLUCOMUTASE
GLO   GLYOXYLASE
C2,C4   COMPLEMENT COMPONENTS
Bf   PROPERDIN FACTOR B

Fig. 30.4 Map of chromosome 6. For updated map refer to Bodmer et al[5].

and biochemical analysis, have enabled the D locus to be subdivided into three clearly defined regions: DR, DQ (formerly DC) and DP (formerly SB)[4] and this is shown in Fig. 30.4. In the DR region, there is one polymorphic α gene and three polymorphic β genes (β_1, β_2, β_3). β_1 is thought to be associated with the DR specificities (DR1-w14) and β_2 codes for the DRw52 (MT1) and DRw53 (MT3) specificities. The DQ region contains two α genes (DXα and DQα), the latter being highly polymorphic. There are two β genes, DX β and DQ β and the latter gene codes for the recognized DQw specificities which have been identified serologically. The DP region contains 2 α and 2 β genes, and DP β_1 is polymorphic for the DP specificities. The position of the α gene in the DZ region has not been clearly defined.

(c) Recombinant DNA technology in HLA

Certain cloned pieces of DNA, when hybridized to human DNA that has been cut with a restriction enzyme and separated by electrophoresis, recognize fragments of varying length in different individuals. These variations in fragment length are referred to as restriction fragment length polymorphisms (RFLPs).

In monozygotic twins, hybridization of the HLA-DR cDNA probes to genomic DNA shows identical RFLPs. DNA of Dw homozygous-typing cells gives rise to unique RFLPs which correspond to the Dw type of the cell. In unrelated individuals, serologically typed as DR identical, genetic differences may occasionally be revealed, particularly with the DQβ cDNA probe.[1] Standardization of these polymorphisms has been aided by the use of EBV-transformed homozygous cell lines.

THE MIXED LYMPHOCYTE REACTION

The standard method for determining HLA-D compatibility is based on the mixed lymphocyte culture reaction (MLC), a functional assay that tests for T-cell recognition.[3] The D locus specificities, designated as Dw types (Table 30.1) are determined by using homozygous typing cells (HTC) in a primary MLC.[24] The main source of these cells is from the offspring of first cousin marriages, who have inherited an identical chromosome 6 from each parent. Genotypic identity for HLA-D in the

outbred human population exists only between siblings who have inherited the same parental HLA haplotypes and is demonstrated between HLA-identical siblings by non-reactivity in a one-way MLC. An increased MLC between HLA-identical patient and donor may predict rejection, but there is no correlation with graft-versus-host disease (GvHD) or with relapse.[12]

LEUCOCYTE ANTIBODIES

The first human leucocyte antigen was discovered in 1958 by Dausset, using an antibody produced in a multi-transfused patient.[11] The antigen was then called Mac and is now known to be the same as the antigen designated HLA-A2. The search for leucocyte antibodies in the sera of pregnant women was advocated by Payne[27] and van Rood.[29] During the late 1950s and early 1960s most of the work was performed using leucocyte agglutination tests, but after the lymphocyte microcytotoxicity test was introduced for HLA typing, lymphocyte suspensions were used in preference to leucocytes. Leucocyte antibodies are produced as a result of pregnancy, transfusion or by planned immunization and the majority of sera used for HLA typing are obtained from pregnant women. The chance of finding agglutinating antibodies in pregnancy increases with parity and the persistence of antibody after birth is variable.

MONOCLONAL ANTIBODIES

Monoclonal antibodies to the HLA antigens are now being used increasingly in the lymphocytotoxicity test, and antibodies can be selected for specificity against almost any antigenic determinant. Spleen cells (B lymphocytes) from immunized animals are fused with a neoplastic myeloma cell line using polyethylene glycol, by cell hybridization techniques.[22] The fusion products are grown in HAT medium (hypoxanthine, aminopterin and thymidine), and the resulting hybrids are cloned by limiting dilution. Hybrids inherit the capacity to secrete antibody against the immunizing antigen from a single clone of B cells, and the antibodies are therefore uniquely specific.

Monoclonal antibodies to many Class I HLA-A and B locus specificities have been produced and these have made a contribution in defining splits of recognized specificities, for example Aw69, a split of A28.[15] Monoclonal antibodies to class II antigens have helped in the identification of D locus products. Difficulties have been experienced in obtaining polymorphic Class I or Class II monoclonal antibodies for tissue typing. In particular many monomorphic Class II antibodies are not locus-specific and may detect shared determinants on DR, DQ and DP molecules.

BONE MARROW TRANSPLANTATION (BMT)

HLA typing has practical application in tissue matching for transplantation. Bone marrow transplantation (BMT) has come to play an increasingly important role in the treatment of certain potentially lethal congenital and acquired diseases, due in part to improved histocompatibility matching.

The most suitable donor for a patient is a monozygotic twin, genetically identical with the recipient. In the absence of an identical twin, the next donor in order of preference is an HLA-identical sib with the same maternal and paternal HLA haplotypes. Related donors, genotypically identical with the recipient for one pair of chromosomes (one haplotype match) are now generally used in BMT if an HLA-matched sibling is not available.

D locus compatibility is thought to be the single most important factor in selection of a donor and therefore the MLC reaction is an important test in donor selection. A negative reaction between donor and recipient lymphocytes is an essential prerequisite in the one-way MLC (one population of X-irradiated cells act as stimulator cells, and the other untreated population are the responder cells) and in the two-way MLC (both populations are viable, and act as both responder and stimulator cells). The MLC is generally performed when the patient is in remission, as it is difficult to interpret the MLC if the patient is in relapse as the cells from the patient will give a high background count.

The relationship between the size of an HLA-typed bone marrow pool and the chance of finding an unrelated donor for an individual patient has been estimated by a computer simulation[7] taking into consideration the known linkage disequilibrium between antigens of the HLA-A,B and D loci. For example, it has been calculated that 1 in 8 HLA-A,B,DR-identical donors will be MLC-negative and a pool of 10^5 volunteers will give HLA-A,B,DR and MLC-negative donors for 43% of the patients requiring BMT.

Use of DNA probes in bone marrow transplantation

Comparison of RFLPs in the donor and an HLA-identical recipient of an allogeneic BMT has detected genetic differences between them using DNA probes directed against HLA-DQ, DR and DP genes. In the two cases reported, there was fatal graft-versus-host disease, and disparities found at the molecular level may have some relevance in the clinical outcome of the transplant.[8] RFLPs have also been used to confirm donor cell engraftment in recipients of a BMT[18] and to evaluate the origin of leukaemic cells at relapse.[25]

GENERAL POINTS OF TECHNIQUE

CELL SEPARATION

(a) Collection of blood samples

For tissue typing by the lymphocytotoxicity method, and mixed lymphocyte cultures, blood is collected into an anticoagulant such as preservative-free heparin (10 iu/ml blood), ACD or EDTA. Blood may defibrinated to give a platelet-free suspension.

(b) Separation of blood components

Leucocytes can be separated from red cells with high molecular weight dextran (6%), gelatin (3%), polyvinyl pyrrolidone or polybrene.

Mix the anticoagulated blood with the sedimentation agent in a plastic tube. Place the tube at 37°C at an angle of 45° for 30 min. The leucocytes may be removed from the supernatant, centrifuged and washed with medium.

(c) Lymphocyte separation

The method of Boyum[6] or a modification is now most commonly used for cell separation.

Dilute heparinized blood with an equal volume of the tissue culture medium, RPMI 1640 medium. This contains 25 mmol/l Hepes with 10 mmol/l (0.85 g/l) sodium bicarbonate; it is used throughout for cell separation, typing and mixed lymphocyte cultures.

Layer 10 ml of diluted blood on to 4 ml of Lymphoprep (Nyegaard UK Ltd*) in a plastic centrifuge tube, and centrifuge at 400 g for 20 min at 4°C. Lymphocytes and platelets separate in a layer just below the interface of the plasma and Lymphoprep layer and red cells and granulocytes sediment through the Lymphoprep to the bottom of the tube.

Remove the lymphocyte layer with a pipette and wash the cells twice with RPMI, spinning at 70 g for 5 min at room temperature. Platelets can be removed from the cell suspension by spinning at 750 g for 1 min. Granulocytes can be removed by incubating the suspension with carbonyl iron and removing the granulocytes containing ingested particles using a magnet.[10]

(d) Separation of B and T lymphocytes

(i) By sheep erythrocytes

To prepare a B-lymphocyte-enriched suspension for DR typing, remove T cells from the mixture of T and B lymphocytes by rosetting the T lymphocytes with sheep erythrocytes. To ensure the rosettes are as stable as possible, treat the sheep erythrocytes with an enzyme such as neuraminidase, papain or AET (2-aminoethylisothiouronium bromide). Allow a centrifuged mixture of lymphocytes and treated sheep erythrocytes in RPMI containing 25% fetal calf serum (FCS) to stand at 4°C overnight; then centrifuge on a Lymphoprep gradient to obtain unrosetted B cells at the medium/Lymphoprep interface. Then wash the B cells in RPMI/FCS.

(ii) By magnetizable polymer beads

B and T lymphocyte populations may be separated from whole blood using magnetizable polymer beads of uniform size and shape coupled with monoclonal antibodies which separate T and B cells (Dynal A. S.*) Dynabeads HLA Class I will form rosettes with T cells (CD8 sub-type) and Dynabeads HLA Class II will form rosettes with DR positive B cells. Using this method, B cell separation from whole blood and DR typing may be completed in approximately 70 min.[31]

Collect 5 ml of blood in ACD in a plastic tube, cool to 2–8°C, add 100 µl of Dynabeads Class I or Class II and mix gently for 8 min. Apply a magnet to the outer wall of the test tube for 2 min to isolate the rosetted cells which attach to the wall. Discard the blood, resuspend and wash the rosetted cells four times in RPMI, and reapply the magnet to the tube wall before discarding the supernatant. Use the standard NIH method to HLA type the cell suspension with reduced incubation time.

Lymphocyte storage and cell recovery

Suspensions of lymphocytes can be distributed internationally in McCoy's 5A medium and remain in suitable condition for HLA typing.[26] Cells can also be stored in ampoules in liquid nitrogen tanks.

Lymphocytes are frozen at a concentration of 2×10^6 cells/ampoule in a mixture of RPMI medium containing 50% autologous plasma or AB serum, and 10–20% dimethyl sulphoxide (DMSO). The optimal rate of temperature decrease during lymphocyte freezing is 1°C/min to ensure adequate cell viability after subsequent thawing for the lymphocytotoxicity test. A machine with an automatically controlled rate of freezing can be used, or alternatively the ampoules containing the lymphocytes can be placed in the neck of a canister containing liquid nitrogen.[14] After a few hours the ampoules can be fixed to metal rods (cones) and stored in the liquid nitrogen.

---

*Nyegaard (UK Ltd), Nyegaard House, 2111 Coventry Road, Sheldon, Birmingham B26 3EA, UK.

* Dynal (AS), PO Box 158, Skøyen, N-0212, Oslo 2, Norway.

If cells stored in liquid nitrogen are to be used to respond to mitogens or allogeneic cells, the freezing process may be modified for optimal recovery of the lymphocyte mitotic function. Rapid cooling of small volumes of lymphocytes in 5% DMSO is interrupted with a timed exposure to a single sub-zero temperature.

Hold the cells at a temperature of −25°C to −26°C for at least 5 min in a deep freeze before immersion in liquid nitrogen. Thaw the cells rapidly by warming the ampoules with agitation in a water-bath at 37°C, and slowly suspend the cells by adding RPMI drop by drop up to a volume of approximately 1 ml. Check the viability of the cells by testing their capacity to exclude trypan blue. For a cytotoxicity test it is necessary that the cells have functionally intact membranes, and approximately 95% of the cells should be live and remain unstained in a lymphocyte suspension that has been frozen and thawed correctly.

LYMPHOCYTE CYTOTOXICITY TESTS

The principle of these tests is the demonstration of a cytotoxic effect of antibody on lymphocytes in the presence of complement.[13] The tests are set up in plastic Terasaki microplates with lids, containing 60 or 72 wells. Mineral oil may be dispensed into the plates using a Histo-Oiler (Dynatech Laboratories*), and sera may be automatically dispensed using a Seromat (Dynatech Laboratories). Single or multiple dispensing microlitre syringes (Hamilton Co**) are used to dispense cells and complement. Cells may be automatically dispensed using a Lamda Jet™ Dispenser, and antisera, cell suspensions, complement and dye may be added to Terasaki plates using the Lamda dot™ Multi reagent dispenser (One Lamda Inc***).

(a) Lymphocytotoxic sera

Sera for typing are obtained from individuals during pregnancy, and the sera are screened against a cell panel of known HLA type. If a useful specific

antibody is found, a larger donation of blood is requested from the individual.

Separate the serum from the blood by centrifugation and store in small aliquots at −70°C. Sera for DR typing may be absorbed with a platelet pool to remove contaminating HLA-ABC antibodies. For typing, dispense the sera in Terasaki plates under mineral oil and store at −70°C until required.

Sera for typing may be bought commercially (BioTest (UK) Ltd*), and monoclonal HLA antibodies are increasingly being used.

(b) Complement

Pool fresh sera from a number of rabbits, first determining that the individual sera are not cytotoxic in the absence of antibody. Store sera at −70°C. Lyophilized rabbit complement is commercially available (Buxted Rabbit Company**).

(c) Measurement of cytotoxicity

The cytotoxicity of the serum is measured as a percent kill using eosin or trypan blue. The dye is excluded from live cells with intact cell membranes, and is taken into dead cells which have been killed by the antibody. Phase contrast or direct illumination from an inverted microscope is used to read the plates. Alternatively, the cells may be labelled with fluorescein salts (fluorescein diacetate); the label is retained by live intact cells, which fluoresce in UV or blue light and this fluorescence is not retained by dead cells.

OFFICIAL NATIONAL INSTITUTES OF HEALTH CYTOTOXICITY TEST

This two-stage test is used at International Histocompatibility Workshops. Each well of a Terasaki plate contains 5 μl of mineral oil, 1 μl of HLA antiserum and 1 μl of lymphocyte suspension containing 3000 cells per μl in RPMI tissue culture medium.

---

*Dynatech Laboratories, Daux Road, Billingshurst, Sussex RH14 9SJ, UK.
**Hamilton Co, Reno, Nevada 89510, USA.
***One Lamda Inc, 2233 Corinth Avenue, Los Angeles, CA 90064, USA.

---

*Biotest (UK) Ltd, 171 Alcester Road, Birmingham B13 8JR, UK.
**Buxted Rabbit Company, Church Road, Buxted, E. Sussex TN22 4LP, UK.

Add the cells to the well, ensuring that the serum and cells are adequately mixed and that there is no contamination by serum from an adjacent well. This is important when monoclonal antibodies are used and it is often necessary to leave control wells of medium between sera.

Mix the suspension on a Vortex mixer, and incubate the plate at 20°C for 30 min (A, B and C antigens) or for 60 min (DR and DQ antigens). Add 5 μl of rabbit complement to each well; mix the suspension on a Vortex mixer and incubate the plate at 20°C for 60 min (A, B and C antigens) or 120 min (DR and DQ antigens). Add 3 μl of 5% eosin and 3 μl of formalin to each well and read the result under an inverted phase-contrast microscope at × 100 or × 250 magnification. Alternatively, remove oil and anti-sera by inverting the plate and tapping sharply several times on a paper towel or the bench. Add 1 μl of trypan blue and read on an inverted light microscope.

If cells separated with Dynabeads Class I and Class II are typed by the two-stage lymphocytotoxicity test, incubate the cells and anti-sera at 20°C for 20 min, and for an additional 20 min with complement, add acridine orange and ethidium bromide staining solution, incubate for 15 min at 20°C and read the plate using a fluorescence microscope. Dead cells stain red with ethidium bromide and live cells stain green with acridine orange.

DR TYPING BY THE TWO-COLOUR FLOURESCENCE METHOD

An enriched population of B lymphocytes is usually used for HLA-DR typing and if the sheep erythrocyte rosetting method is used, a large initial volume of peripheral blood is required. The two-colour fluorescence method enables DR typing to be performed on low concentrations of lymphocytes (B and T) and B cell separation is not necessary.[30]

Incubate at 37°C for 7 min lymphocytes in 0.5 ml of RPMI medium containing 20% decomplemented FCS with 0.05 ml of goat anti-human immunoglobulin IgG (Fab) conjugated with fluorescein isothiocyanate. Wash the cells three times with medium and resuspend in medium containing 20% FCS at a concentration of 10^6 cells/ml.

Add 0.5 μl of the cell suspension to 0.5 μl of DR anti-serum in flat bottom trays (Medicell International Ltd*) and incubate the plate at 20°C for 1 h in the dark. Add 2 μl of rabbit complement and continue the incubation for 2 h in the dark. Add 0.5 μl of ethidium bromide and examine using an inverted fluorescence microscope. Estimate the percentage of dead B cells which are identified by mixed green and red staining: live B cells stain green, dead T cells stain red and live T cells remain unstained.

In all these cytotoxicity tests, record the percentage of dead cells in each well and assign a score of 1, 2, 4, 6 or 8 as follows:

% Dead cells (score) : 0–10% (1) negative; 11–20% (2); 21–40% (4); 41–80% (6); 81–100% (8) strong positive.

Negative controls without antisera give the background kill and should not exceed 10%.

Comments

When typing cells it is desirable to have at least three different antisera representing each specificity, but tests in triplicate may not be possible due to scarcity of antisera for certain specificities.

Tissue-typing antisera are supplied to bona fide users in the United Kingdom from the National Tissue Typing Reference Laboratory, South Western Regional Transfusion Centre, Bristol BS10 5ND.

A stored panel of lymphocytes from individuals of known HLA type is essential in order to screen sera for antibodies. The lymphocytes from patients with chronic lymphocytic leukaemia, as well as normal B cells, are a convenient source of cells to screen for DR antibodies.

MIXED LYMPHOCYTE CULTURES

As already referred to (p. 513) patients with leukaemia or other haematological malignancies who require a bone marrow transplant (BMT) are tissue typed for HLA-ABC and DR antigens to select a donor of choice together with members of their

---

*Medicell International Ltd, 239 Liverpool Road, London N. 1.

family (parents and siblings). After HLA typing has been performed, mixed lymphocyte cultures are set up as a matrix between the patient, parents, siblings and an unrelated third party.

(a) Preparation of lymphocytes

30 ml of peripheral blood in preservative-free heparin (10 iu/ml) and 10 ml of clotted blood are collected from the patient, from all relevant family members and from an unrelated third party. The blood is treated under sterile precautions throughout, and lymphocyte separation and cell cultures are performed under a laminar flow hood.

Dilute the peripheral blood with an equal volume of RPMI 1646 medium containing preservative-free heparin, 25 mmol/l Hepes and 10 mmol/l sodium bicarbonate. This is used throughout. Separate lymphocytes by sedimentation through sterile Lymphoprep by centrifuging at 400 g at 4°C for 20 min. Remove the lymphocytes from the interface, wash twice with RPMI medium, and resuspend cells at a cell concentration of 10^6/ml in RPMI containing 20% heat-inactivated pooled human AB serum, and 2 mmol glutamine (Gibco$\star$) i.e. 1 ml of 200 mmol solution per 100 ml.

(b) Treatment of stimulators cells

Lymphocytes from each individual in the culture matrix are treated with mitomycin C, or irradiation, so that the cells only stimulate untreated cells of a different Dw type and are unable themselves to respond to other lymphocytes. Add 0.625 ml (25 μg) of mitomycin/10^6 lymphocytes (1 ml) and incubate the cell suspension at 37°C for 30 min. Centrifuge the cells, wash three times in RPMI medium and suspend in the culture medium described above or, alternatively, irradiate the cells using 4000 rads for 30 min.

(c) Mixed lymphocyte culture matrix

The one-way mixed lymphocyte culture (MLC) test consists of 50 μl (5 $\times$ 10^4) cells from a responder

and an equal concentration of cells from a stimulator. The two-way MLC consists of similar concentrations of the two cell populations, which have not been treated with X-rays or mitomycin C. For the one-way MLC, all possible combinations of responder and stimulator cells from all individuals (patient, parents, sibs) should be set up in culture as a matrix. Each combination should be set up at least in triplicate and the matrix should include controls of responder cells plus stimulator cells (treated by X-rays or mitomycin C) and untreated cells from the same individuals. Each cell in the matrix should be tested against an individual of unrelated HLA-DR specificity (a third party cell). A two-way MLC between cells from the patient and each potential donor should also be set up.

Set up the MLC in microtitre plates with U-shaped wells and incubate the cells at 37°C in an atmosphere of 5% CO_2 in air for 5 days. Then add 0.5 μCi of tritiated thymidine in a volume of 10 μl per well and reincubate at 37°C for a further 18 h.

(d) Termination of cultures

The cultures are terminated using a Titertek harvester (Flow$\star$). Cells from the microplates are washed, disrupted in the washing process and DNA is precipitated on to glass fibre sheets which are removed for scintillation counting.

Add 100 μl of water per well and leave for 10 min at room temperature. Wash the cells with water from off the plates on to glass fibre filters so the contents from each well form discrete areas on the glass fibre sheets. Dry the filters in an oven at 50°C for 2 h, place the glass fibre discs into counting vials, add 10 ml of phosphor scintillant and measure the activity in a liquid scintillation counter.

(e) Calculation of results

Record the results as counts per min (cpm) and use the mean of the triplicate counts to calculate the stimulation index and relative response.

1. Stimulator index $= \dfrac{\text{cpm ABX}}{\text{cpm AAX}}$

$\star$ Gibco BRL, PO Box 35, Trident House, Renfrew Road, Paisley PA3 4EN, Scotland.

$\star$ Flow Laboratories, Woodcock Hill, Harefield Road, Rickmansworth, Herts WD3 1PQ, UK.

2. *Relative response*

$$= \frac{\text{cpm ABX} - \text{cpm AAX}}{\text{cpm AUX} - \text{cpm AAX}} \times 100,$$

where A represents cells from the patient, B from the sibling and U from an unrelated third party control: X represents irradiated cells.

An HLA-identical pair should give a negative result in the two-way test, a stimulation index of not more than 2.0 and a relative response of less than 4%.

MOLECULAR STUDIES—AN OUTLINE

Isolate genomic DNA from peripheral blood by standard techniques of cell lysis. Remove high molecular weight protein by phenol-chloroform-isoamyl alcholol extraction, and recover DNA by ethanol precipitation. Digest genomic DNA with different restriction enzymes, separate the resulting DNA fragments on 0.5% agarose gels and transfer fragments to nitrocellulose filters.[28] Label chosen DNA probes by nick translation with [^{32}P] deoxynucleotide triphosphates. Prehybridize nitrocellulose filters and then hybridize filters with a ^{32}P-labelled probe. Expose X-ray film to the radioactive filter at $-70°C$ to detect the labelled fragments. These techniques are described in detail by Maniatis.[23]

ACKNOWLEDGEMENTS

I should like to thank Professor S. D. Lawler and Dr. W. F. Wakeling for their expert advice.

REFERENCES

[1] ANDERSSON, M., BOHME, J., ANDERSSON, G. et al (1984). Genomic hybridization with Class II transplantation antigen cDNA probes as a complementary technique in tissue typing. *Human Immunology*, **11**, 57.

[2] AUFFRAY, C. and STROMINGER, J. L. (1986). Molecular genetics of the human major histocompatibility complex. In *Advances in Human Genetics* 15. Eds. H. Harris and K. Hirschborn, p. 197. Plenum Press, New York.

[3] BACH, F. H. and HIRSCHHORN, K. (1964). Lymphocyte interaction: a potential histocompatibility test in vitro. *Science*, **143**, 813.

[4] BODMER, W. F. (1984). The HLA system. In *Histocompatibility Testing*, p. 11. Eds. E. D. Albert, M. P. Baur and W. R. Mayr. Springer-Verlag, Berlin.

[5] BODMER, W. F., ALBERT, E., BODMER, J. G. et al (1989). Immunobiology of HLA. Springer-Verlag, New York.

[6] BOYUM, A. (1978). Separation of leukocytes from blood and bone marrow. *Scandinavian Journal of Clinical and Laboratory Investigation*, **21**, Supplement 97.

[7] BRADLEY, B. A., GILKS, W. R., GORE, S. M. and KLOUDA, P. T. (1987). How many HLA-typed volunteer donors for bone marrow transplantation (BMT) are needed to provide an efficient service. *Bone Marrow Transplantation*, **2**, Supplement 1, 79.

[8] CARLSSON, J., BOHME, J., LUNDGREN, G. et al (1985) HLA Class II genes studied with genomic hybridisation in kidney and bone marrow transplantation donor-recipient pairs. *Transplantation Proceedings*, **17**, 952.

[9] CARROL, M. C., CAMPBELL, R. D., BENTLEY, D. R. and PORTER, R. P. (1984). A molecular map of the human major histocompatibility complex class II region linking complement genes C4, C2 and factor B. *Nature*, **307**, 237.

[10] COULSON, A. S. and CHALMERS, D. C. (1964). Separation of viable lymphocytes from human blood. *Lancet*, i, 468.

[11] DAUSSET, J. (1958) Iso-leuco-anticorps. Acta Haematologica, **20**, 156.

[12] deGAST, G. C., MICKELSON, E. M., BEATTY, P. G. et al (1987). Effect of mixed leukocyte culture reactivity on GVHD and relapse in HLA-matched BMT. *Bone Marrow Transplantation*, **2**, Supplement 1, 84.

[13] DICK, H. M. and CRICHTON, B. W. (1972). *Tissue Typing Techniques*. Churchill Livingstone, Edinburgh.

[14] FARRANT, J., KNIGHT, S. C., McGANN, L. E. and O'BRIEN J. (1974). Optimal recovery of lymphocytes and tissues following rapid cooling. *Nature*, **249**, 452.

[15] FAUCHET, R., BODMER, J. G., KENNEDY, L. J. et al (1984). In *Histocompatibility Testing*. Eds. E. D. Albert, M. P. Baur and W. R. Mayr, p. 211. Springer-Verlag, Berlin.

[16] FRANCKE, U. and PELLEGRINO, M. A. (1977). Assignment of the major histocompatibility complex to a region of the short arm of human chromosome 6. *Proceedings of the National Academy of Sciences USA*, **74**, 1147.

[17] GAZIT, E. GOTHELF, Y., GIL R. et al (1984). Alloantibodies to PHA activated lymphocytes detect human Qa-like antigens. *Journal of Immunology*, **132**, 165.

[18] GINSBURG, D., ANTIN, J. H., SMITH, B. R., ORKIN, S. H. and RAPPEPORT, J. M. (1985). Origin of cell populations after bone marrow transplantation. Analysis using DNA sequence polymorphisms. *Journal of Clinical Investigation*, **75**, 596.

[19] *Histocompatibility Testing 1984* (1984). Springer-Verlag, Berlin.

[20] *Histocompatibility Testing 1980* (1980). UCLA Tissue Typing Laboratory, Los Angeles, California.

[21] *Histocompatibility Testing 1972* (1972). Munksgaard, Copenhagen.

[22] KOHLER, G. and MILSTEIN, C. (1975). Continuous cultures of fused cells secreting antibody of predefined specificity. *Nature*, **256**, 495.

[23] MANIATIS, T., FRITSCH, E. F. and SAMBROOK, J. (1982). *Molecular Cloning: a Laboratory Manual*. Cold Spring Harbor Laboratory.

24 MEMPEL, W., GROSS-WILDE, H., BAUMAN, P., NETZEL, B. and STEINBAUER-ROSENTHAL, I. (1973). Population genetics of the MLC response: typing for MLC determinants using homozygous and heterozygous reference cells. *Transplantation Proceedings,* **V**, 1529.

25 MINDEN, M., CURTIS, C. and MESSNER, H. A. (1986). Origin of leukaemic relapse after bone marrow transplantation detected by restriction fragment-length polymorphisms. *International Journal of Cell Cloning,* **4**, **Supplement 1**, 194.

26 PARK, M. S. and TERASAKI, P. I. (1974) Storage of human lymphocytes at room temperature. *Transplantation,* **18**, 520.

27 PAYNE, R. and ROLFS, M. R. (1958). Fetomaternal leukocyte incompatibility. *Journal of Clinical Investigation,* **37**, 1756.

28 SOUTHERN, E. M. (1975). Detection of specific sequences among DNA fragments separated by gel electrophoresis. *Journal of Molecular Biology,* **98**, 503.

29 VAN ROOD, J. J., EERNISSE, J. G. and VAN LEEUWEN, A. (1958). Leucocyte antibodies in sera from pregnant women. *Nature,* **181**, 1735.

30 VAN ROOD, J. J., VAN LEEUWEN, A. and PLOEM, J. S. (1976). Simultaneous detection of two cell populations by two-colour fluorescence and application to the recognition of B-cell determinants. *Nature,* **262**, 795.

31 VARTDAL, F., GAUDERNACK, G., FUNDERUD, S. et al (1986). HLA Class I and II typing using cells positively selected from blood by immunomagnetic isolation—a fast and reliable technique. *Tissue Antigens,* **28**, 301.

31. Miscellaneous tests

TESTS FOR THE ACUTE PHASE RESPONSE

Inflammatory response to tissue injury (the acute phase response) includes alteration in serum protein concentration, especially increases in fibrinogen and C-reactive protein and decrease in albumin. The changes occur in both acute inflammation and during active phases of chronic inflammation.

Measurement of the acute phase response is a helpful indicator of the presence and extent of inflammation and its response to treatment. Useful tests include estimation of C-reactive protein, fibrinogen (see p. 316) and measurement of the erythrocyte sedimentation rate and plasma viscosity.

THE ERYTHROCYTE SEDIMENTATION RATE (ESR)

Estimation of the erythrocyte sedimentation rate has been widely used in clinical medicine. Two methods have been commonly used for measuring the ESR. In 1921 Westergren described a method using a long glass tube.[66] Wintrobe and Landsberg[69] proposed a modified method in which the ESR is measured on undiluted blood in a haematocrit tube. This was especially convenient as it was then possible to measure the PCV on the same sample after carrying out the ESR. However, with the advent of microhaematocrit and blood cell counters for measuring PCV Wintrobe's method has no practical advantage. Westergren's method has been selected as the recommended method by the International Committee for Standardization in Haematology[31,34] and also by various national organizations.[8,52] In the conventional Westergren method the blood sample is diluted. To make the test more reproducible a standardized method has been proposed in which the blood is not diluted but its PCV is adjusted to 0.30–0.36.[34,50] This is, however, too laborious for routine use.

Method of Westergren

The recommended tube is a straight glass tube 30 cm in length and 2.55 (± 0.15) mm in diameter. The bore must be uniform to 0.05 mm throughout. A scale graduated in mm extends over the lower 20 cm. The tube must be clean and dry and kept free from dust.

After use it should be thoroughly washed in tap water, then rinsed with acetone and allowed to dry before being reused. Specially made racks with adjustable levelling screws are available for holding the sedimentation tubes firmly in an exactly vertical position. The rack must be constructed so that there will be no leakage of the blood from the tube. It is conventional to set up sedimentation-rate tests at room temperature (18–25°C). Sedimentation is normally accelerated as the temperature rises[45] and if the tests is to be carried out at a higher ambient temperature, a normal range should be established for that temperature. Exceptionally, when high-thermal-amplitude cold agglutinins are present, sedimentation becomes noticeably less rapid as the temperature is raised towards 37°C.

109 mmol/l trisodium citrate (32 g/l $Na_3C_6H_5O_7.2H_2O$) is used as the anticoagulant diluent solution. It is filtered through a micropore filter (0.22 μm) into a sterile bottle. It can be stored for several months at 4°C but must be discarded if it becomes turbid through the growth of moulds. The test is performed on venous blood diluted accurately in the proportion of 1 volume of citrate to 4 volumes of blood. The usual practice is to collect the blood directly into the citrate solution. The test, however, can be carried out equally with blood anticoagulated with EDTA, provided that 1 volume of 109 mmol/l (32 g/l) trisodium citrate or 9 g/l NaCl (saline) is added to 4 volumes of blood immediately before the test is performed. The sedimentation rate is reduced in stored blood; the test should thus be carried out within 2 h of collecting the blood, although a delay of up to 6 h is permissible provided that the blood is kept at 4°C.

Mix the blood sample thoroughly and then draw it up into the Westergren tube to the 200 mm mark by means of a teat or a mechanical device; mouth suction should never be used. Place the tube exactly vertical and leave undisturbed for 60 min, free from vibrations and draughts, and not exposed to direct sunlight. Then read to the nearest 1 mm the height of the clear plasma above the upper limit of the column of sedimenting cells. This measurement in mm is the ESR (Westergren 1 h). A poor delineation of the upper layer of red cells, so called 'stratified sedimentation', has been attributed to the presence of many reticulocytes.[65]

Range in health

The mean values and the upper limit for 95% of normal subjects given in Table 31.1 are derived from several publications.

In the newborn the ESR is usually low. In childhood and adolescence it is the same as for normal men with no differences between boys and girls.[38,43]

Modified methods

A number of variations of the standard method have been developed. Whenever a different method is planned, a preliminary test should be carried out in order to compare results with those obtained by the standardized method as described below.

Plastic tubes. A number of plastic materials—for example, polypropylene and polycarbonate—are possible substitutes for glass in the Westergren tubes[61]. Nevertheless, not all plastics have similar properties and it must be demonstrated that the results with the chosen tubes are reproducible and comparable with those obtained with the standard method.

Disposable glass tubes. These should be supplied clean and dry and ready for use. It is necessary to show that neither the tube material nor the manufacturer's cleaning process affects the ESR.

Length of tube. To comply with standard specifications the tube should extend 100 mm beyond the calibrated length. This ensures that it fits correctly into the commonly available holding rack. However, the overall length is not a critical dimension for the test itself, and if the tube is designed for use with some other form of holding device the uncalibrated component may be shorter provided all other specifications are met.

Table 31.1   ESR ranges in health

	ESR (mm/1 h) Mean	95% upper limit
Men aged (years)		
17–50	4	10
51–60	6	12
>60	6	14
Women aged (years)		
17–50	6	12
51–60	9	19
>60	10	20

Capillary method. Short tubes of narrow bore are available mainly for tests on infants. Sedimentation is slower in these tubes and it is necessary to establish normal ranges or a correction factor to convert results to the equivalent ESR by the standard Westergren method.

Comparison with the standardized method[34]

Select 10 EDTA blood specimens the ESR of which by the routine method is in the range 15–100 mm/1 h and PCV is 0.30–0.36. If necessary adjust the PCV by centrifuging the specimens, remove an appropriate amount of plasma or red cells and then remix.

Measure the ESR on each specimen, *undiluted* by the standardized Westergren method.

Correct the reading for lack of dilution as follows:

Corrected Westergren ESR =
(Undiluted ESR × 0.86)−12.

If the routine method is performing satisfactorily the difference between it and the corrected Westergren ESR should not exceed 10 mm/1 h at any point in the range 15–105 mm/1 h.

Quality control

Perform a quality control check whenever routine ESR tests are performed. Select one blood sample with a PCV between 0.30 and 0.36 and perform the ESR by the routine method and by the undiluted Westergren ESR method as described above. Apply the formula to obtain the corrected ESR for the undiluted sample. The test is satisfactorily controlled if this result does not differ from that obtained by the routine method by more than 10 mm/1 h in the range 15–105 mm/1 h. A smaller difference would be expected for ESR values at the lower end of the range.

Mechanism of erythrocyte sedimentation

The phenomenon of erythrocyte sedimentation has been exhaustively investigated.[5,25,34,67]

The rate of fall of the red cells is influenced by a number of inter-reacting factors. Basically, it depends upon the difference in specific gravity between red cells and plasma, but it is influenced very greatly by the extent to which the red cells form rouleaux, which sediment more rapidly than single cells. Other factors which affect sedimentation include the ratio of red cells to plasma, i.e. the PCV, the plasma viscosity, the verticality or otherwise of the sedimentation tube, the bore of the tube and the dilution, if any, of the blood.

The all-important rouleaux formation and aggregation are mainly controlled by the concentrations of fibrinogen and other acute-phase proteins, e.g. haptoglobin, ceruloplasmin, $\alpha_1$acid-glycoprotein, α_1 antitrypsin and c-reactive protein. Rouleaux formation is also enhanced by the immunoglobulins. It is retarded by albumin. Defibrinated blood normally sediments extremely slowly, not more than 1 mm in 1 h, unless the serum-globulin concentration is raised or there is an unusually high globulin:albumin ratio.

Anaemia, by altering the ratio of red cells to plasma, encourages rouleaux formation and accelerates sedimentation. In anaemia, too, cellular factors may affect sedimentation. Thus in iron-deficiency anaemia a reduction in the intrinsic ability of the red cells to sediment may compensate for the accelerating effect of an increased proportion of plasma.[57]

Sedimentation can be observed to take place in three stages: a preliminary stage of at least a few minutes during which time rouleaux occur and aggregations form; then a period in which the sinking of the aggregates takes place at approximately a constant speed, and finally a phase during which the rate of sedimentation slows as the aggregated cells pack at the bottom of the tube. It is obvious that the longer the tube used the longer the second period can last and the greater the sedimentation rate may appear to be. This is an advantage of the Westergren tube. With a shorter tube, e.g. a Wintrobe tube, packing may start before an hour has elapsed.

The relative merits of the Westergren and Wintrobe methods have been investigated by Bull and his colleagues.[7,50] They concluded that the Wintrobe method is more sensitive when the ESR is low, whereas the Westergren method is a more reliable indicator of the patient's clinical state when the sedimentation rate is high. Using undiluted blood the PCV of which has been adjusted to 0.35

is thought to make the Westergren method more sensitive and more reproducible.[50] However, this makes the test more laborious and the virtue that ESR has of being a simple procedure is lost. Attempts have been made to correct for anaemia by means of a chart or nomogram; the results are, however, unsatisfactory.

Significance of the measurement of the erythrocyte sedimentation rate in clinical medicine

Although the ESR is a non-specific phenomenon, its measurement is clinically useful in disorders associated with an increased production of acute-phase proteins. In rheumatoid arthritis or tuberculosis it provides an index of progress of the disease, and it is also useful as a screening test in the routine examination of patients. An elevated ESR occurs as an early feature in myocardial infarction.[22] Although a normal ESR cannot be taken to exclude the presence of organic disease, the fact remains that the vast majority of acute or chronic infections and most neoplastic and degenerative diseases are associated with changes in the plasma proteins which lead to an acceleration of sedimentation. The ESR is higher in women than in men, and correlates with sex differences in fibrinogen levels.[2] An increase in fibrinogen occurs in normal pregnancy, resulting in increased red cell aggregation[76] and elevated sedimentation. The ESR is influenced by age, menstrual cycle and drugs (e.g. corticosteroids, contraceptive pills); it is especially low (0–1 mm) in polycythaemia, hypofibrinogenaemia and congestive cardiac failure, and when there are abnormalities of the red cells such as poikilocytosis, spherocytosis or sickle cells.[43]

Zeta sedimentation rate (ZSR)

To measure the ZSR EDTA blood is centrifuged in a special capillary tube in a Zetafuge (Coulter Electronics).[6,49] The advantages of the ZSR are that it eliminates the effect of anaemia, takes less than 5 min to carry out, requires only 0.2 ml of blood and obviates the need for dilution. It has been thought to be more sensitive than the Westergren ESR to minor rises in the acute-phase proteins[50]. But the need for special, relatively expensive apparatus is a limitation, and the ZSR test has not replaced the universally used ESR in routine practice.

PLASMA VISCOSITY

The ESR and plasma viscosity in general increase in parallel. Plasma viscosity is, however, primarily dependent on the concentration of plasma proteins, especially fibrinogen, and it is not affected by anaemia. Change in viscosity seems to reflect the clinical severity of disease more closely than does the ESR.[17,26] Also, changes in the ESR may lag behind changes in plasma viscosity by 24–48 h[17].

There are several types of viscometer; these are based on three principles:[26,34]

1. The rotational viscometer in which shear stress is determined at different shear rates.
2. The rolling ball viscometer in which the rate of rolling of a metal ball is measured in a tilted tube filled with plasma; and calibrated with fluids of known viscosity.
3. The capillary viscometer in which comparison is made of the flow rate of plasma and distilled water under equal pressure and constant temperature through capillary tubes of equal bore and length. The results are expressed as viscosity of plasma relative to that of water.

Most reports of clinical studies have been based on the capillary viscometer. It requires only 0.3–0.5 ml of plasma, obtained from EDTA blood. Results are highly reproducible (CV 1%); they are, however, very sensitive to changes in temperature. The test is usually performed at 25°C although some workers recommend 37°C;[32,55] in either case the temperature should be closely controlled, with a variation of less than ±0.5°C.

Precision is also affected by the way the plasma sample has been obtained and prepared; the formation of a fibrin clot will invalidate the test. Venous blood should be collected with minimum stasis into EDTA (1.2 mg/ml) and, as soon as possible, centrifuged in a stoppered tube at 3000 *g* for 5 min to obtain clear plasma. After separation, the plasma, if sterile, can be stored in a stoppered tube at room temperature (not in a refrigerator) for up to 1 week without change to its viscosity.

The actual test should be carried out as described in the instruction manual for the particular instrument used.

Reference values[32,34]

Normal plasma has a viscosity of 1.16–1.33 (mean 1.24) mPa/s* at 37°C; 1.50–1.72 (mean 1.60) mPa/s at 25°C. Plasma viscosity is lower in the newborn (0.98–1.25 mPa/s at 37°C), rising to adult values by the third year; it is slightly higher in old age. There are no significant differences in plasma viscosity between men and women, or in pregnancy. It is remarkably constant in health, with little or no diurnal variation, and it is not affected by exercise. A change of only 0.03–0.05 mPa/s is thus likely to be clinically significant.

WHOLE-BLOOD VISCOSITY

The viscosity of blood reflects its rheological properties; it is influenced by PCV, plasma viscosity, red cell aggregation and red cell deformability. It is especially sensitive to PCV, with which it is closely correlated. Its measurement has, however, limited clinical value as it does not take account of the interaction of the red cells with blood vessels which greatly influences blood flow in vivo. Guidelines for measuring blood viscosity and red cell deformability by standardized methods have been published.[33]

Rotational and capillary viscometers are suitable for measuring blood viscosity. Deformability can be measured by recording the rate at which red cells in suspension pass through a filter with pores 3–5 µm in diameter.

TESTS FOR HETEROPHILE ANTIBODIES IN HUMAN SERUM: THE PAUL-BUNNELL TEST FOR THE DIAGNOSIS OF INFECTIOUS MONONUCLEOSIS

The presence of anti-sheep-cell haemagglutinins at unusually high titres in the sera of patients suffering from infectious mononucleosis (glandular fever) was described in 1932 by Paul and Bunnell[53] and the demonstration of these antibodies is still widely used as a test—the Paul-Bunnell Test—for infectious mononucleosis. These (Paul-Bunnell) antibodies are immunologically related to but distinct from the type of anti-sheep red cell antibodies which may develop in serum sickness (see p. 528). The Paul-Bunnell antibodies are, however, not specific for sheep red cells. Thus, they react with horse red cells and ox red cells also; but they do not react with human red cells. They are known to be IgM (19S) globulins.[9,10]

For the diagnosis of infectious mononucleosis, it is necessary to demonstrate that the antibody present has the characters of the Paul-Bunnell antibody, i.e. it is absorbed by ox red cells but not by guinea-pig kidney. This is the basis of the absorption tests for infectious mononucleosis. Although sheep red cells have been widely used to demonstrate the Paul-Bunnell antibody, horse red cells give even better results.[40] Either type of cell, preserved by formalin, can be used in screening tests;[27] however, the preserved cells are less able to detect low-titre antibodies than are fresh horse cells.[39,64] The tests are usually carried out on serum, but plasma can be used equally well.[16]

A SLIDE SCREENING TEST FOR INFECTIOUS MONONUCLEOSIS

Reagents*

Sera. Patients' serum (fresh or inactivated by heating at 56°C for 30 min, and positive and negative control sera.

Red cell suspension. 20% suspension of horse blood in 109 mmol/l (32 g/l) trisodium citrate. Be-

---

*Previously measured in 'poise' (P); 1 cP = 1 mPa/s

---

*Available commercially, e.g. Monospot Slide Test (Ortho).

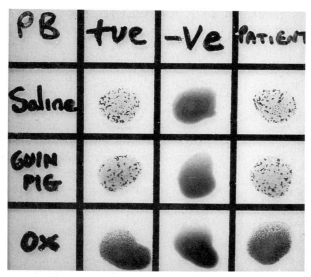

Fig. 31.1   Slide screening test for infectious mononucleosis. Upper: guinea pig kidney. Lower: ox cell suspension.

fore use the suspension must be well mixed by repeated inversion. For the screening test it is unnecessary to wash the cells.

Guinea-pig kidney emulsion. (See p. 529).

10% autoclaved ox red cell suspension. (See p. 529.)

Method[39]

Place 1 large drop (approximately 30 µl) of guinea-pig kidney emulsion and 1 large drop of ox-cell suspension on two adjacent squares on an opal glass tile. Add 1 drop of test serum adjacent to each. Deliver 10 µl of horse-blood suspension to the corner of each square, by means of a micropipette avoiding contact with the drops in the squares. With a wooden applicator stick, mix the reagents (guinea-pig kidney emulsion or ox-cell suspension, serum and horse-blood suspension) and then examine with the naked eye for agglutination, using oblique light at an angle over a dark background. Negative and positive serum controls should always be set up at the same time. The appearances are shown in Figure 31.1.

Interpretation

Positive. Agglutination is stronger in the square containing guinea-pig kidney emulsion.

Negative. Agglutination is absent in both squares or stronger in the square containing ox red cell suspension.

In one study on 500 students the test was shown to have a sensitivity of 86% and specificity of 99%[21] where the diagnosis was established by the presence of EBV-specific antibody. False positives have been reported in malignant lymphomas,[46] malaria,[59] rubella[54] and other diseases, and also occasionally without any apparent underlying disease.[29] A false negative is likely to occur with plasma.

Another slide screening test has been developed using aldehyde-treated horse red cell*[51]. It requires no absorption of serum. For the test 1 drop of serum and 1 drop of reagent are mixed on a slide with a rocking movement for 2 min. If agglutination occurs the test is positve. This test is said to have the same sensitivity and specificity as the Monospot slide test described above.

QUANTITATIVE PAUL-BUNNELL TEST

When the screening test is positive or doubtful a quantitative test with differential absorption should be carried out. The technique described below is based upon that of Barrett[3] and uses sheep red cells,

---

*Mono-check (Nyland).

but horse red cells, as recommended by Lee, Davidsohn and Slaby[40] can equally well be used.

Reagents

Patient's serum and positive control serum. 1 ml, previously inactivated by heating at 56°C for 30 min.

Guinea-pig kidney emulsion. (See p. 529.).

10% autoclaved ox red cell suspension. (See p. 529.)

Sheep red cells. 0.4 suspension in 9 g/l NaCl (saline). The sheep blood should preferably be not more than 7 days old. If stored red cells are used instead, they should be washed three times in saline immediately before the test.

Absorption of serum

Deliver three 0.25 ml volumes of patient's inactivated serum into three small glass or plastic tubes, A, B and C. Add 1.0 ml of saline to Tube A, 0.75 ml of saline and 0.3 ml of guinea-pig kidney emulsion to Tube B, and 0.75 ml of saline and 0.25 ml of 10% ox-cell suspension to Tube C. Mix the contents of the three tubes and place them at 4°C for at least 2 h or overnight. Then centrifuge the tubes and retain the supernatants. 1 in 5 dilutions in saline of unabsorbed serum and of the serum absorbed with guinea-pig kidney and ox red cells, respectively, are thus obtained.

Method

Make serial dilutions of the sera from Tubes A, B and C in saline; 0.15–0.2 ml volumes are suitable. Nine 75 × 8 mm tubes and a control tube to contain saline are usually sufficient. Add equal volumes of the 0.4% sheep (or horse) cell suspension to each tube, giving final serum dilutions of from 1 in 10 (Tube 1) to 1 in 2560 (Tube 9). After mixing their contents, incubate the tubes for 2 h at 37°C before reading the results. A standardized method of reading the end-point should be adopted. Macroscopic reading using a concave mirror is recommended (p. 431). The serum known to contain Paul-Bunnell antibody provides a control for the potency of the absorbents and the agglutinability of the red cells.

Interpretation

The following figures are given as examples of typical results with sheep cells:

1. Unabsorbed serum, end-point Tube 7; titre 640.
   Guinea-pig kidney absorbed serum, end-point Tube 7; titre 640.
   Ox-cell absorbed serum, end-point Tube 4; titre 80.

Such a result would be positive for infectious mononucleosis, the antibody being not absorbed by guinea-pig kidney and significantly absorbed by ox cells. Naturally occurring antibody is absorbed by guinea-pig kidney, but not by ox cells, and that of serum sickness is absorbed by both reagents.

2. Unabsorbed serum, end-point Tube 3; titre 40.
   Guinea-pig kidney absorbed serum, end-point Tube 3, titre 40.
   Ox-cell absorbed serum, no agglutination in Tube 1.

In spite of the low titre in the unabsorbed serum, this result would also be positive for infectious mononucleosis, the antibody being not absorbed by the guinea-pig kidney but absorbed by the ox cells.

3. Unabsorbed serum, end-point Tube 3; titre 40.
   Guinea-pig kidney absorbed serum, no agglutination in Tube 1.
   Ox-cell absorbed serum, end-point Tube 3; titre 40.

This is a normal result, and the screening test would have been negative. Caution is needed in interpreting the results when they are weakly positive or when there is only partial absorption by guinea-pig kidney.

Lack of complete absorption with guinea-pig kidney is not in itself diagnostic of infectious mononucleosis, as this may occasionally be observed with normal serum.[3] A positive test requires at least a two-tube difference in titre before and after absorption with ox cells.

The antibodies normally present in human sera which agglutinate sheep red cells are of the Forssman type, i.e. they react against an antigen widely spread in animal tissues. Antibodies of this type are formed by rabbits injected with an emulsion of guinea-pig kidney. The antibodies react with dog, cat and mouse tissues as well as with sheep and horse red cells, but not with the tissues of man, ox or rat[68]. The antibody formed in infectious mononucleosis is of a different nature and is not absorbed by red cells or tissues containing the Forssman antigen; hence the use, as absorbing agents, of guinea-pig kidney, rich in the antigen, and ox red cells, deficient in the antigen but capable of absorbing the Paul-Bunnell antibody.

The antibodies are lytic as well as agglutinating, and it is possible to read the results by recording lysis, if titrations are carried out in the presence of complement. Fresh ox red cells may be used instead of an autoclaved suspension, although less conveniently. It is remarkable that they may not be agglutinated although they absorb the antibody[23]; they will, however, regularly undergo lysis if complement is present. Leyton suggested that an ox red cell lytic test might prove to be a satisfactory substitute for the orthodox Paul-Bunnell agglutination test.[44] He stated that lysins for ox red cells develop sooner and persist longer than do agglutinins for sheep red cells. Other workers have subsequently advocated the lytic test using ox red cells on the grounds of its greater sensitivity[19,48]. The use of horse kidney instead of guinea-pig kidney as an absorbing agent has also been recommended because of the ease with which a large amount of a standard stable reagent can be prepared.[13]

The antigen on sheep red cells which reacts specifically with the Paul-Bunnell antibody is inactivated by papain and other proteolytic enzymes, and an enzyme test based on this has been proposed[71]. Davidsohn and Lee compared several serological tests and concluded that the differential absorption, enzyme and ox red-cell lysin tests were all equally valuable in the diagnosis of infectious mononucleosis.[14]

An immune-adherence haemagglutination test has been developed for assay of heterophile antibody. It has been reported to be as specific as other tests but to be more sensitive and to remain positive for a longer time.[20]

Technical factors affecting results

Temperature. The Paul-Bunnell antibody of infectious mononucleosis reacts well at 37°C; but agglutination is enhanced at lower temperatures and higher titres are obtained if the tests are carried out at 4°C. At this temperature, however, the test is less specific.[73] A cold agglutinin, anti-i, may appear transiently during the immunological response to infectious mononucleosis,[35,63] but as the antibody does not agglutinate sheep cells its presence does not affect the Paul-Bunnell test. It is usually present in a low titre but it may on rare occasions cause haemolytic anaemia if present at high titre.

Varying sensitivity of sheep red cells. A cause of difficulty in serial studies is the comparatively wide variation in sensitivity between one sample of sheep red cells and the next. Zarofonetis and Oster tested 24 sera with the red cells from 24 different sheep.[72] They found the titres given by the most sensitive cells to be from 4 to 16 times those given by the least sensitive cells. Comparable studies do not seem to have been carried out with horse red cells.

Clinical value of the Paul-Bunnell test

Infectious mononucleosis is caused by the Epstein-Barr virus (EBV). Tests for the heterophile antibody were developed before the EB virus was identified and they remain a useful aid to the diagnosis of the disease. However, the Paul-Bunnell test is not infallible. Most authors have reported 80–90% of positive results in patients thought to be suffering from infectious mononucleosis.[4,15,36] Antibodies are often present as early as the fourth to sixth day of the disease and are almost always found by the 21st day. They disappear as a rule within 4–5 months. There is no unanimity as to how frequently negative reactions are found in 'true' infectious mononucleosis. Occasionally, the characteristic antibodies develop very late in the course of the disease, perhaps weeks or even months after the patient becomes ill, and it is also known that a positive reaction may be transient and that the antibodies may be present at such low titres that they may be missed or may produce anomalous agglutination reactions when associated with the naturally occurring antibody at similar titres. For all the above reasons it is difficult to state categorically that any particular patient has not or will not produce antibodies. EBV-specific antibody has been demonstrated in the serum of 86% of patients with clinical and/or haematological features of infectious mononucleosis.[20]

As far as false-positive reactions are concerned, there is no substantial evidence that sera containing agglutinins in high concentration giving the typical reactions of infectious mononucleosis are ever found in other diseases uncomplicated by infectious mononucleosis. In particular, the heterophile-antibody titres in the lymphomas are similar to those found in unselected patients not suffering from infectious mononucleosis.[24] In virus hepatitis, although one-fifth of the patients in one series had antibody titres greater than normal, in only one patient did the result of absorption tests suggest the presence of the Paul-Bunnell antibody.[41]

Preparation of guinea-pig kidney suspension and heated ox red cell suspension (after Barrett[3])

Guinea-pig kidney suspension

Strip the capsules and perirenal fat from at least two pairs of kidneys. Then wash them well in running water. Homogenize the tissue in 9 g/l NaCl (saline) in a blender for 2 min, sterilize it at 121°C (by autoclaving at 15 lb pressure for 20 min) and blend it again so as to obtain a fine suspension. Then centrifuge the suspension in saline and wash the deposit in two changes of saline. Finally, add to the deposit about four times its volume of 5 g/l phenol in saline. After resuspension, centrifuge the sample in a haematocrit tube in order to estimate its concentration. Then add sufficient phenol-saline to the remainder to produce a 1 in 6 suspension. Use it without further dilution. Its absorbing power must be tested with known positive and negative sera. The reagent will remain potent for at least 1 yr if stored at 4°C.

Ox red cell suspension

Wash ox cells in several changes of 9 g/l NaCl (saline) and make a 30% suspension. Then sterilize it at 121°C (by autoclaving at 15 lb pressure for 20 min). When cool, adjust the PCV to 0.20 with saline and add an equal volume of 10 g/l phenol-saline to give a 10% suspension.

The ability of the suspension to absorb the infectious mononucleosis antibody must be tested with known positive sera. It should remain potent for several years if stored at 4°C.

DEMONSTRATION OF ANTINUCLEAR FACTORS

Antinuclear antibodies, or antinuclear factors (ANF), occur in the serum in a wide range of auto-immune disorders, including systemic lupus erythematosus (SLE), Sjögren's syndrome, rheumatoid arthritis, chronic hepatitis, thyroiditis, myasthenia gravis, pernicious anaemia, ulcerative colitis, red cell aplasia; they may be present, too, in cases of drug reactions. The antibodies may be specific for DNA, soluble nucleoprotein or an extract of cell nuclei (Sm antigen). There are also antibodies which react with cytoplasmic antigens (Ro antigen), and mixed nuclear and cytoplasmic antigens (La antigen). Several techniques for demonstrating the antibodies in patients with SLE and other disorders have been described.[60]

Immunofluorescence provides a sensitive method.[12] For this, the serum under investigation is added to a section of tissue (e.g. rat liver). Uptake of antinuclear factor (ANF) will be shown by fluorescence of cell nuclei when fluorescein-labelled rabbit anti-human-γ-globulin serum is subsequently added.[28] A characteristic of SLE is the presence of 7S IgG antibodies to double-stranded DNA (ds-DNA);[30] they can be detected and measured quantitatively by indirect immuno-fluorescence[56].

Radio-immunoassay also provides a sensitve and specific method for the detection of anti-DNA antibodies. Isotope-labelled antigen is added to the serum under test and the resultant mixture is then treated with 50%-saturated ammonium sulphate in order to precipitate immunoglobulins; the precipitate will contain radioactivity only if an antigen-antibody reaction has occurred, and the amount of antibody can be estimated from the radioactivity in the antigen-antibody complex.[70]

A rapid and simple qualitative method for detecting the presence of antinuclear antibodies is based on the ability of the serum to aggregate polystyrene latex particles coated with the appropriate nuclear components. Thus, the antinuclear antibody can be demonstrated fairly reliably with a reagent comprising latex and desoxyribonucleoprotein obtained from calf thymus.*[58]

Antinuclear antibodies can also be detected by the LE-cell test (see below). They have the property of causing in-vitro lysis of the nuclei of neutrophil polymorphonuclears and subsequent phagocytosis of the lysed nuclei by other neutrophils. The test requires four components: antinuclear antibody (the 'LE-cell' factor); nuclear protein material; complement, and actively phagocytic neutrophils. To provide access to the nuclear protein material the cell membranes must first be damaged by mechanical or chemical means.

DEMONSTRATION OF LE CELLS

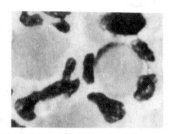

Fig. 31.2   Typical LE cells. The rounded amorphous LE body is well shown to the right of the picture with the segments of a neutrophil nucleus wrapped around it. Below and to the left is shown more amorphous nuclear material, but this is less obviously phagocytosed. × 1000.

In Romanowsky-stained preparations the LE cell appears as a neutrophil in the cytoplasm of which is a large spherical body (the LE body) which stains shades of pale purple. The nucleus of the ingesting leucocyte is usually displaced to one side and many appear to be wrapped around the ingested material (Fig. 31.2). The LE body, although derived from nuclear material, usually shows no evidence of nuclear structure and appears as an opaque homogenous mass. The ingesting leucocyte is almost invariably and characteristically a neutrophil polymorphonuclear, very rarely a monocyte or eosinophil.

The 'Tart'** cell is a monocyte—rarely a

neutrophil—which has phagocytosed another cell or the nucleus of another cell. The phagocytosed material most often resembles a lymphocyte nucleus, in which case a definite nuclear pattern can be seen (Fig. 31.3); a common alternative form is a pyknotic nucleus smaller than an LE body and staining far more intensely (Fig 31.4). Tart cells are often associated with leuco-agglutinins and may occur in drug reactions.[37] Such reactions have to be distinguised from the drug-induced lupus syndrome in which genuine LE cells occur.[18]

Many methods of demonstrating LE cells have been described. It seems clear that some degree of trauma to leucocytes is necessary for a successful preparation, for the LE factor does not appear to be capable of acting upon healthy living leucocytes. A good method of achieving the necessary degree of trauma is to rotate whole blood to which glass beads have been added before concentrating the leucocytes by centrifugation. The method described in

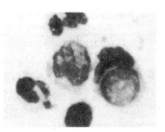

Fig. 31.3   'Tart' cell. A lymphocyte, with intact nuclear structure, has been engulfed by a monocyte, the nucleus of which has been compressed. × 1000.

---

*Available commercially as Hyland LE test (Travenol Laboratories Ltd.)
** 'Tart' apparently refers to the name of the patient in whom cells of this type were first seen.

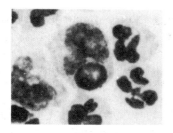

Fig. 31.4 'Tart' cell. A pyknotic (?) lymphocyte nucleus has been phagocytosed by a monocyte. × 1000.

the following section is based on that of Zinkham and Conley.[74]

I. METHOD USING THE PATIENT'S BLOOD

Blood to which the minimum amount of heparin has been added should be used. Transfer 1 ml of the blood into a 75 × 12mm glass test-tube; add four glass beads and seal the tube with a tightly fitting rubber bung. Rotate the preparation at c 33 rpm at c 20°C for 30 min; place it at 37°C for 10–15 min, and then transfer the contents of the tube to a Wintrobe haematocrit tube. Make buffy coat films after centrifuging for 10 min at 150–200 g. Allow the films to dry in the air, fix them in methanol and stain by a Romanowsky method in the usual way.

II. METHOD USING THE PATIENT'S SERUM AND NORMAL LEUCOCYTES

Patient's serum. Obtain this from blood allowed to clot undisturbed at room temperature or at 37°C or from defibrinated blood. It should be stored frozen at −20°C until used.

Normal leucocyte suspension. Deliver 5 ml of freshly drawn group-O blood into a container in which 1 mg of heparin has been dried. After mixing, centrifuge the blood at 1200–1500 g for 15 min. Remove the lower half of the column of packed red cells with a Pasteur pipette and discard it; remix the remaining red cells and the supernatant plasma, place in a tube of about 10 mm diameter and allow to sediment at 37°C. The removal of some of the red cells increases the rate of sedimentation.

Allow the blood to sediment until 1–2 ml of plasma are available. This usually takes 30–60 min. Place the supernatant plasma, which contains leucocytes, platelets and a small number of red cells, in a 75 × 12 mm tube and wash once in 9 g/l NaCl (saline). It is important to centrifuge the leucocyte suspension at a slow speed (150–200 g) and for no longer than 5 min. Before the saline is added, it is essential to resuspend, by tapping the tube, the button of leucocytes in the small volume of fluid that remains after the supernatant fluid has been poured off. After washing, remove the supernatant by pipette as completely as possible. Resuspend the leucocyte button in the fluid remaining in the tube; it is then ready for use.

Technique of test

Mix equal volumes (5–10 drops) of leucocyte suspension and patient's serum in a 75 × 12 mm tube and add three small glass beads. Fit the tube with a rubber bung and rotate it at c 33 rpm for 30 min at c 20°C, after which transfer its contents to a Wintrobe haematocrit tube. Make films of the deposited leucocytes after centrifuging at 150–200 g for 10 min. Dry them in the air, fix in methanol and stain by a Romanowsky method.

Examination of films

Slides should be examined for at least 10 min before a negative report is given. With practice it is possible to recognize LE cells using a 16 mm objective. In addition to intracellular LE bodies, extracellular material may also be seen. This consists of basophilic aggregations, either amorphous or in the form of round bodies. Extracellular material may be seen in SLE, but it may also be found in rheumatoid arthritis, discoid LE, cirrhosis of the liver, myelomatosis and possibly even in normal subjects.[1] The material should not be considered of significance unless the characteristic LE cells are also seen.

Interpretation

The number of LE cells found in cases of SLE varies within wide limits. Occasionally, large numbers are present; infrequently, particularly in patients who have received corticosteroid therapy, scattered cells are found only after a prolonged search. If sufficiently numerous, they may be reported as the number present per 1000 neutrophils. 'Tart' cells can usually be clearly differentiated from LE cells, but they are occasionally a source of difficulty, and, when LE cells are outnumbered by Tart cells, SLE should not be diagnosed.

Both the techniques described above are sensitive. That using the patient's whole blood is the simplest and should be used first, as positive results are more likely to be obtained in most instances than by the use of patient's serum. The chief value of the indirect method is in the retrospective assessment of the effect of the treatment on the LE-cell-forming activity of a sample of the patient's serum, when a stored sample of the patient's serum can be used as a control.

The LE-cell phenomenon, its relationship to SLE and other auto-immune disorders, and methods for its demonstration, have a large literature.[47] A positive LE-cell test is very suggestive of SLE and LE-cell demonstration is a useful diagnostic test. However, the test is positive in only *c* 75% of patients with SLE[30], and conversely, 'false' positive results have sometimes been found when immunofluorescence has failed to demonstrate antinuclear factor.[37] Moreover, clearly positive reactions have been reported in lupoid hepatitis, and in drug reactions.[11,18] Positive tests, too, have been found in 3.6% of patients with rheumatoid arthritis, especially when the disease is severe and highly active.[42]

REFERENCES

[1] ARTERBERRY, J. D., DREXLER, E. and DUBOIS, E. L. (1964). Significance of hematoxylin bodies in lupus erythematosus cell preparations. *Journal of American Medical Association*, **187**, 389.

[2] BAIN, B. J. (1983). Some influences on the ESR and the fibrinogen level in healthy subjects. *Clinical and Laboratory Haematology*, **5**, 45.

[3] BARRETT, A. M. (1941). The serological diagnosis of glandular fever (infectious mononucleosis): a new technique. *Journal of Hygiene* (Cambridge), **41**, 330.

[4] BERNSTEIN, A. (1940). Infectious mononucleosis. *Medicine* (Baltimore), **19**, 85.

[5] BULL, B. S. (1981). Clinical and laboratory implications of present ESR methodology. *Clinical and Laboratory Haematology*, **3**, 283.

[6] BULL, B. S. and BRAILSFORD, J. D. (1972). The zeta sedimentation ratio. *Blood*, **40**, 550.

[7] BULL, B. S. and BRECHER, G. (1974). An evaluation of the relative merits of the Wintrobe and Westergren sedimentation methods, including hematocrit correction. *American Journal of Clinical Pathology*, **62**, 502.

[8] British Standards Institution (1987). *Specification for Westergren Tube and Support for the Measurement of Erythrocyte Sedimentation Rate*. BS 1554. BSI, London.

[9] CARTER, R. L. (1966). Antibody formation in infectious mononucleosis. I. Some immunochemical properties of the Paul-Bunnell antibody. *British Journal of Haematology*, **12**, 259.

[10] CARTER, R. L. (1966). Antibody formation in infectious mononucleosis. II. Other 19 S antibodies and false-positive serology. *British Journal of Haematology*, **12**, 268.

[11] CONDEMI, J. J., BLOMGREN, S. E. and VAUGHAN, J. H. (1970). The procainamide induced lupus syndrome. *Bulletin on Rheumatic Diseases*, **20**, 604.

[12] COONS, A. H. and KAPLAN, M. H. (1950). Localization of antigen in tissue cells: II. Improvements in a method for the detection of antigen by means of fluorescent antibody. *Journal of Experimental Medicine*, **91**, 1.

[13] DAVIDSOHN, I. and GOLDIN, M. (1955). The use of horse kidney in the differential test for infectious mononucleosis. *Journal of Laboratory and Clinical Medicine*, **45**, 561.

[14] DAVIDSOHN, I. and LEE, C. L. (1964). Serologic diagnosis of infectious mononucleosis. A comparative study of five tests. *American Journal of Clinical Pathology*, **24**, 115.

[15] DAVIDSOHN, I., STERN, K. and KASHIWAGI, C. (1951). The differential test for infectious mononucleosis. *American Journal of Clinical Pathology*, **21**, 1101.

[16] DAVIDSON, R. J. L. and MAIN, S. R. (1971). Use of plasma instead of serum in laboratory tests for infectious mononucleosis. *Journal of Clinical Pathology*, **24**, 259.

[17] DINTENFASS, L. (1976). *Rheology of Blood in Diagnostic and Preventive Medicine*. Butterworth, London.

[18] DUBOIS, E. L. (1975). Serological abnormalities in spontaneous and drug-induced systemic lupus erythematosus, *Journal of Rheumatology*, **2**, 204.

[19] ERICSON, C. (1960). Sheep cell agglutinin and ox cell hemolysin in the serological diagnosis of mononucleosis infectiosa. *Acta Medica Scandinavica*, **166**, 225.

[20] EVANS, A. S. and NIEDERMAN, J. C. (1982). EBV-IgA and new heterophile antibody tests in diagnosis of infectious monocucleosis. *American Journal of Clinical Pathology*, **77**, 555.

[21] FLEISHER, G. R., COLLINS, M. and FARGER, S. (1983). Limitations of available tests for diagnosis of infectious mononucleosis. *Journal of Clinical Microbiology*, **17**, 619.

[22] FROOM, P., MARGALIOT, S., CAINE, Y. and BENBASSAT, J. (1984). Significance of erythrocyte sedimentation rate in young adults. *American Journal of Clinical Pathology*, **82**, 198.

[23] GLEESON-WHITE, M. H., HEARD, D. H., MYNORS, L. S. and COOMBS, R. R. A. (1950). Factors influencing the agglutinability of red cells: the demonstration of a variation in the susceptibility to agglutination exhibited by the red cells of individual oxen. *British Journal of Experimental Pathology*, **31**, 321.

[24] GOLDMAN, R., FISHKIN, B. G. and PETERSON, E. T. (1950). The value of the heterophile antibody reaction in the

lymphomatous diseases. *Journal of Laboratory and Clinical Medicine*, **35**, 681.

[25] HARDWICKE, J. and SQUIRE, J. R. (1952). The basis of the erythrocyte sedimentation rate. *Clinical Science*, **11**, 333.

[26] HARKNESS, J. (1971). The viscosity of human plasma; its measurement in health and disease. *Biorheology*, **8**, 171.

[27] HOFF, G. and BAUER, S. (1965). A new rapid slide test for infectious mononucleosis. *Journal of the American Medical Association*, **194**, 351.

[28] HOLBOROW, E. J., WEIR, D. M. and JOHNSON, G. D. (1957). A serum factor in lupus erythematosus with affinity for tissue nuclei. *British Medical Journal*, **ii**, 732.

[29] HORWITZ, C. A., HENLE, W., HENLE, G., PENN, G., HOFFMAN, N. and WARD, P. C. J. (1979). Persistent falsely positive rapid tests for infectious mononucleosis. Report of five cases with four–six year follow-up data. *American Journal of Clinical Pathology*, **72**, 807.

[30] HUGHES, G. R. V. (1973). The diagnosis of systemic lupus erythematosus (Annotation). *British Journal of Haematology*, **25**, 409.

[31] International Committee for Standardization in Haematology (1977). Recommendation for measurement of erythrocyte sedimentation rate of human blood. *American Journal of Clinical Pathology*, **68**, 505.

[32] International Committee for Standardization in Haematology (1984). Recommendation for selected method for the measurement of plasma viscosity. *Journal of Clinical Pathology*, **37**, 1147.

[33] International Committee for Standardization in Haematology (1986). Guidelines for measurement of blood viscosity and erythrocyte deformability. *Clinical Hemorheology*, **6**, 439.

[34] International Committee for Standardization in Haematology (1988). Guidelines on the selection of laboratory tests for monitoring the acute-phase response. *Journal of Clinical Pathology*, **41**, 1203.

[35] JENKINS, W. J., KOSTER, H. G., MARSH, W. L. and CARTER, R. L. (1965). Infectious mononucleosis: an unsuspected source of anti-i. *British Journal of Haematology*, **11**, 480.

[36] KAUFMAN, R. E. (1944). Heterophile antibody in infectious mononucleosis. *Annals of Internal Medicine*, **21**, 230.

[37] KOLLER, S. R., JOHNSTON, C. L., MONCURE, C. W. and WALLER, M. V. (1976). Lupus erythematosus cell preparation-antinuclear factor incongruity. A review of diagnostic tests for systemic lupus erythematosus. *American Journal of Clinical Pathology*, **66**, 495.

[38] LASCARI, A. D. (1972). The erythrocyte sedimentation rate. *Pediatric Clinics of North America*, **19**, 1113.

[39] LEE, C. L., DAVIDSOHN, I. and PANCZYSZYN, O. (1968). Horse agglutinins in infectious mononucleosis, II. The spot test. *American Journal of Clinical Pathology*, **49**, 12.

[40] LEE, C. L. DAVIDSOHN, I. and SLABY, R. (1968). Horse agglutinins in infectious mononucleosis. *American Journal of Clinical Pathology*, **49**, 3.

[41] LEIBOWITZ, S. (1951). Heterophile antibody in normal adults and in patients with virus hepatitis. *American Journal of Clinical Pathology*, **21**, 201.

[42] LENOCH, F. and VOJTÍŠEK O. (1967). The prevalence of LE cells in 1000 consecutive patients with active rheumatoid arthritis. *Acta Rheumatologica Scandinavica*, **13**, 313.

[43] LEWIS, S. M. (1980). Erythrocyte sedimentation rate and plasma viscosity. *ACP Broadsheet*, No. 94, BMA, London.

[44] LEYTON, G. B. (1952). Ox-cell haemolysins in human serum. *Journal of Clinical Pathology*, **5**, 324.

[45] MANLEY, R. W. (1957). The effect of room temperature on erythrocyte sedimentation rate and its correction. *Journal of Clinical Pathology*, **10**, 354.

[46] MERRILL, R. H. and BARRETT, O. (1976). Positive mono-spot test in histiocytic medullary reticulosis. *American Journal of Clinical Pathology*, **65**, 407.

[47] MIESCHER, P. W. and REITHMÜLLER, D. (1965). Diagnosis and treatment of systemic lupus erythematosus. *Seminars in Hematology*, **2**, 1.

[48] MIKKELSEN, W., TUPPER, C. J. and MURRAY, J. (1958). The ox cell hemolysin test as a diagnostic procedure in infectious mononucleosis. *Journal of Laboratory and Clinical Medicine*, **52**, 648.

[49] MORRIS, M. W., SKRODZSKI, Z. and NELSON, D. A. (1975). Zeta sedimentation rate (ZSR): a replacement for the erythrocyte sedimentation rate (ESR). *American Journal of Clinical Pathology*, **64**, 254.

[50] MOSELY, D. L. and BULL, B. S. (1981). A comparison of the Wintrobe, the Westergren and the ZSR erythrocyte sedimentation rate (ESR) methods to a candidate reference method. *Clinical and Laboratory Haematology*, **4**, 169.

[51] MYHRE, B. A. and NAKAYAMA, V. (1976). Serological evaluation of the Mono-Chek test. *American Journal of Clinical Pathology*, **65**, 987.

[52] National Committee for Clinical Laboratory Standards (1977). *Standardized Methods for the Human Erythrocyte Sedimentation Rate (ESR) Test (ASH-2)*. NCCLS, Villanova, Pa.

[53] PAUL, J. R. and BUNNELL, W. W. (1932). The presence of heterophile antibodies in infectious mononucleosis. *American Journal of Medical Sciences*, **183**, 90.

[54] PHILLIPS, G. M. (1972). False-positive monospot test in rubella. *Journal of American Medical Association*, **222**, 585.

[55] PHILLIPS, M. J. and HARKNESS, J. (1981). A study of plasma viscosity-temperature relationships. *Bibliotheca Anatomica*, **20**, 215.

[56] PINCUS, T., SCHUR, P. H. and TALAL, N. (1968). A diagnostic test for systemic lupus erythematosus using a DNA binding assay. *Arthritis and Rheumatism*, **11**, 837.

[57] POOLE, J. C. F. and SUMMERS, G. A. C. (1952). Correction of E.S.R. in anaemia. Experimental study based on interchange of cells and plasma between normal and anaemic subjects. *British Medical Journal*, **i**, 353.

[58] PULLUM, C. and KEECH, M. K. (1964). Evaluation of the Hyland LE-Test. *Acta Rheumatologica Scandinavica*, **10**, 165.

[59] REED, R. E. (1974). False-positive monospot tests in malaria. *American Journal of Clinical Pathology*, **61**, 173.

[60] REICHLIN, M. (1981). Current perspectives on serological reactions in SLE patients. *Clinical and Experimental Immunology*, **44**, 1.

[61] RODDIE, A. M. S. and POLLOCK, A. (1987). Plastic ESR tubes: does static electricity affect the results? *Clinical and Laboratory Haematology*, **9**, 175.

[62] ROSE, H. M., RAGAN, C., PEARCE, E. and LIPMAN, M. O. (1948). Differential agglutination of normal and sensitized sheep erythrocytes by sera of patients with rheumatoid arthritis. *Proceedings of the Society for Experimental Biology and Medicine*, **68**, 1.

[63] ROSENFELD, R. E., SCHMIDT, P. J., CALVO, R. C. and McGINNISS, M. H. (1965). Anti-i, a frequent cold agglutinin in infectious mononucleosis. *Vox Sanguinis*, **10**, 631.

[64] SCOTT, G. L. and PRIEST, C. J. (1972). An evaluation of the Monosticon rapid slide test diagnosis of infectious mononucleosis. *Journal of Clinical Pathology*, **25**, 783.

[65] STEPHENS, J. G. (1938). Stratified blood sedimentation —isolation of immature red cells. *Nature* (London), **141**, 1058.

[66] WESTERGREN, A. (1921). Studies of the suspension stability of the blood in pulmonary tuberculosis. *Acta Medica Scandinavica*, **54**, 247.

[67] WHICHER, J. T. and DIEPPE, P. A. (1985). Acute phase proteins. *Clinics in Immunology and Allergy*, **5**, 425.

[68] WILSON, C. S. and MILES, A. A. (1964). In *Topley and Wilson's Principles of Bacteriology and Immunity*, 5th edn., p. 1330. Arnold, London.

[69] WINTROBE, M. M. and LANDSBERG, J. W. (1935). A standardized technique for the blood sedimentation test. *American Journal of Medical Sciences*, **189**, 102.

[70] WOLD, R. T., YOUNG, F. E., TAN, E. M. and FARR, R. S. (1968). Desoxyribonucleic acid antibody: a method to detect its primary interaction with desoxyribonucleic acid. *Science*, **161**, 806.

[71] WÖLLNER, D. (1956). Differenzierungsmethoden zur serologishen Diagnose der infektiösen Mononucleose. II. Die differential-Agglutination mit nativem und papainisierten Hammelerythrozyten nach Absorption mit Meeschweinchennierenzellen und papainisierten Hammelblut. *Zeitschrift für Immunitätsforschung und experimentelle Therapie*, **113**, 301.

[72] ZAROFONETIS, C. J. D., and OSTER, H. L. (1950). Heterophile agglutination variability of erythrocytes from different sheep. *Journal of Laboratory and Clinical Medicine*, **36**, 283.

[73] ZAROFONETIS, C. J. D., OSTER, H. L. and COLVILLE, V. F. (1953). Cold agglutination of sheep erythrocytes as a factor in false positive heterophile agglutination tests. *Journal of Laboratory and Clinical Medicine*, **41**, 906.

[74] ZINKHAM, W. H. and CONLEY, C. L. (1956). Some factors influencing the formation of L. E. cells. A method for enhancing L. E. cell production. *Bulletin of the Johns Hopkins Hospital*, **98**, 102.

[75] FABRY, T. L. (1987). Mechanism of erythrocyte aggregation and sedimentation. *Blood*, **70**, 1572.

[76] HUISMAN, A., AARNOUDSE, J. G., KRANS, M., HUISJES, H. J. FIDLER, V. and ZIJLSTRA, W. G. (1988). Red cell aggregation during normal pregnancy. *British Journal of Haematology*, **68**, 121.

32. Appendices

1. PREPARATION OF CERTAIN REAGENTS, ANTICOAGULANTS AND PRESERVATIVE SOLUTIONS

Acid-citrate-dextrose (ACD) solution—'NIH-A'

Trisodium citrate, dihydrate (75 mmol/l)	22 g
Citric acid, monohydrate (42 mmol/l)	8 g
Dextrose (139 mmol/l)	25 g
Water	to 1 litre

Sterilize the solution by autoclaving at 121°C for 15 min. Its pH is 5.4. For use, add 10 volumes of blood to 1.5 volumes of solution.

Alsever's solution

Dextrose (114 mmol/l)	20.5 g
Trisodium citrate, dihydrate (27 mmol/l)	8.0 g
Sodium chloride (72 mmol/l)	4.2 g
Water	to 1 litre

Adjust the pH to 6.1 with citric acid (c 0.5 g) and then sterilize the solution by micropore filtration (0.22 μm) or by autoclaving at 121°C for 15 min. For use, add 4 volumes of blood to 1 volume of solution.

Citrate-phosphate-dextrose (CPD) solution, pH 6.9

Trisodium citrate, dihydrate (102 mmol/l)	30 g
Sodium dihydrogen phosphate, monohydrate (1.08 mmol/l)	0.15 g
Dextrose (11 mmol/l)	2 g
Water	to 1 litre

Sterilize the solution by autoclaving at 121°C for 15 min. After cooling to c 20°C, it should have a brown tinge and its pH should be 6.9. For use in red cell survival studies (see p. 382) add 1 volume of blood to 2 volumes of solution.

535

Citrate-phosphate-dextrose (CPD) solution, pH 5.6–5.8

Trisodium citrate, dihydrate (89 mmol/l)	26.30 g
Citric acid, monohydrate (17 mmol/l)	3.27 g
Sodium dihydrogen phosphate, monohydrate (16 mmol/l)	2.22 g
Dextrose (142 mmol/l)	25.50 g
Water	to 1 litre

Sterilize the solution by autoclaving at 121°C for 15 min. For use as an anticoagulant-preservative, add 7 volumes of blood to 1 volume of solution.

Citrate-phosphate-dextrose-adenine (CPD-A) solution, pH 5.6–5.8

Trisodium citrate, dihydrate (89 mmol/l)	26.30 g
Citric acid, monohydrate (17 mmol/l)	3.27 g
Sodium dihydrogen phosphate, monohydrate (16 mmol/l)	2.22 g
Dextrose (177 mmol/l)	31.8 g
Adenine (2.04 mmol/l)	0.275 g
Water	to 1 litre

Sterilize the solution by autoclaving at 121°C for 15 min. For use as an anticoagulant-preservative, add 7 volumes of blood to 1 volume of solution.

Low ionic strength solution

Sodium chloride (NaCl) (30.8 mmol/l)	1.8 g
Disodium hydrogen phosphate (Na_2HPO_4) (1.5 mmol/l)	0.21 g
Sodium dihydrogen phosphate (NaH_2PO_4) (1.5 mmol/l)	0.18 g
Glycine (NH_2CH_2COOH) (240 mmol/l)	18.0 g
Water	to 1 litre

Dissolve the sodium chloride and the two phosphate salts in c 400 ml of water; dissolve the glycine separately in c 400 ml of water; adjust the pH of each solution to 6.7 with 1 mol/l NaOH. Add the two solutions together and make up to 1 litre. Sterilize by Seitz filtration or autoclaving. The pH should be within the range of 6.65–6.85, the osmolality 270–285 mmol, and conductivity 3.5–3.8 mS/cm at 23°C.

EDTA

Ethylenediamine tetra-acetic acid, dipotassium or disodium salt	100 g
Water	to 1 litre

Allow apppropriate volumes to dry in bottles at c 20°C so as to give a concentration of 1.5 ± 0.25 mg/ml of blood.

Neutral EDTA, pH 7.0, 110 mmol/l

Ethylenediamine tetra-acetic acid, dipotassium salt	44.5 g
or disodium salt	41.0 g
1 mmol/l NaOH	75 ml
Water	to 1 litre

Neutral buffered EDTA, pH 7.0

Ethylenediamine tetra-acetic acid, disodium salt (9 mmol/l)	3.35 g
Disodium hydrogen phosphate (Na_2HPO_4) (26.4 mmol/l)	3.75 g
Sodium chloride (NaCl) (140 mmol/l)	8.18 g
Water	to 1 litre

Saline

Sodium chloride (NaCl) (154 mmol/l)	9.0 g
Water	to 1 litre

Trisodium citrate
($Na_3C_6H_5O_7.2H_2O$), 109 mmol/l

Dissolve 32 g in 1 litre of water. Distribute convenient volumes (e.g. 10 ml) into small bottles and sterilize by autoclaving at 121°C for 15 min.

Heparin

Powdered heparin (lithium salt) is available with an activity of *c* 160 iu/mg. Dissolve it in water at a concentration of 4 mg/ml. Sodium heparin is available in 5 ml ampoules with an activity of 1000 iu/ml. Add appropriate volumes of either solution to a series of containers and allow to dry at *c* 20°C so as to give a concentration not exceeding 15–20 iu/ml of blood.

Gibson and Harrison's artificial haemoglobin standard

Chromium potassium sulphate (CrK $(SO_4)_2.12H_2O$)	11.61 g
Cobaltous sulphate (anhydrous) ($CoSO_4$)	13.1 g
Potassium dichromate ($K_2Cr_2O_7$)	0.69 g
Water	to 500 ml

Add 1.8 ml of 1 mol/l sulphuric acid to the dissolved salts and heat the mixture to boiling. After boiling for 1 min, cool the solution and make up the volume to 1 litre with water. The chromium potassium sulphate crystals must be free from any signs of whitening due to efflorescence. The cobaltous sulphate must be anhydrous. Heat *c* 30 g of $CoSO_4.7H_2O$ for *c* 2 h in a small porcelain dish placed in an oven at a temperature just below its melting point (96°C). Then heat the coarser particles overnight in an electric muffle furnance kept at 400°C. The product should be a uniform lilac powder. Transfer while still hot to a stoppered bottle. As soon as it has cooled, weigh out 13.1 g and dissolve in 80 ml of water with the aid of heat. As the anhydrous salt is hygroscopic, seal in glass tubes immediately after preparation.

The undiluted standard is equivalent to 160 ± 2 g Hb per 1 (based on iron determinations) when used as described on p. 40.

WATER

For most purposes still-prepared distilled water or deionized water is equally suitable. Throughout this text this is implied when 'water' is referred to. When doubly-distilled or glass-distilled water is required this has been specially indicated, and when tap-water is satisfactory or indicated, this, too, has been stated.

---

2. BUFFERS*

Barbitone buffer, pH 7.4

Sodium diethyl barbiturate ($C_8H_{11}O_3N_2Na$) (57 mmol/l)	11.74 g
Hydrochloric acid (HCl) (100 mmol/l)	430 ml

Barbitone buffered saline, pH 7.4

NaCl	5.67 g
Barbitone buffer, pH 7.4	1 litre

Before use, dilute with an equal volume of 9 g/l NaCl.

Barbitone-buffered saline, pH 9.5

Sodium diethyl barbiturate ($C_8H_{11}O_3N_2Na$) (98 mmol/l)	20.2 g
Hydrochloric acid (HCl) (100 mmol/l)	20 ml
NaCl	5.67g

Before use, dilute the buffer with an equal volume of 9 g/l NaCl.

---

*Other buffers which are used for specific purposes are described under the appropriate tests.

Barbitone-bovine serum albumin (BSA) buffer, pH 9.8

Sodium diethyl barbiturate $(C_8H_{11}O_3N_2Na)$ (54 mmol/l)	10.3 g
NaCl (102 mmol/l)	6.0 g
Sodium azide (31 mmol/l)	2.0 g
Bovine serum albumin (e.g. Sigma)	5.0 g
Water	to 1 litre

Dissolve the reagents in c 900 ml of water. Adjust the pH to 9.8 with 5 mol/l HCl. Make up the volume to 1 litre with water. Store at 4°C.

Citrate-saline buffer

Trisodium citrate $(Na_3C_6H_5O_7.2H_2O)$ (5 mmol/l)	1.5 g
NaCl (96 mmol/l)	5.6 g
Barbitone buffer, pH 7.4	200 ml
Water	800 ml

Glycine buffer, pH 3.0

Glycine (NH_2CH_2COOH) (82 mmol/l)	6.15 g
NaCl (82 mmol/l)	4.80 g
Water	820 ml
0.1 mol/l HCl	180 ml

HEPES buffer, pH 6.5

4-(2-hydroxyethyl)-1-piperazineethane sulphonic acid (100 mmol/l)	23.83 g.

Dissolve in c 100 ml of water. Add a sufficient volume of 1 mol/l NaOH (c 1 ml) to adjust the pH to 6.5. If the buffer is intended for use with Romanowsky staining (p. 79), then add 25 ml of dimethyl sulphoxide (DMSO). Make up the volume to 1 litre with water.

HEPES-saline buffer, pH 7.6

HEPES (4-(2-hydroxyethyl)-1-piperazineethane sulphonic acid (20 mmol/l)	4.76 g
NaCl	8.0 g

Dissolve in c 100 ml of water. Add a sufficient volume of 1 mol/l NaOH to adjust the pH to 7.6. Make up volume to 1 litre with water.

Imidazole-buffered saline, pH 7.4

Imidazole (50 mmol/l)	3.4 g
NaCl (100 mmol/l)	5.85 g

Dissolve in c 500 ml of water. Add 18.6 ml of 1 mol/l HCl and make up the volume to 1 litre with water. Store at room temperature (18–25°C).

Phosphate buffer, iso-osmotic

(A) $NaH_2PO_4.2H_2O$ (150 mmol/l)	23.4 g/l	
(B) Na_2HPO_4 (150 mmol/l)	21.3 g/l	

pH	Solution A	Solution B
5.8	87 ml	13 ml
6.0	83 ml	17 ml
6.2	75 ml	25 ml
6.4	66 ml	34 ml
6.6	56 ml	44 ml
6.8	46 ml	54 ml
7.0	32 ml	68 ml
7.2	24 ml	76 ml
7.4	18 ml	82 ml
7.6	13 ml	87 ml
7.7	9.5 ml	90.5 ml

Normal human serum has an osmolality of 289 ± 4 mmol. Hendry[1] recommended slightly different concentrations of the stock solution, namely, 25.05 g/l $NaH_2PO_4.2H_2O$ and 17.92 g/l Na_2HPO_4 for an iso-osmotic buffer.

Phosphate-buffered saline

Equal volumes of iso-osmotic phosphate buffer and 9 g/l NaCl.

Phosphate buffer, Sörensen's

66 mmol/l stock solutions:
- (A) KH_2PO_4 9.1 g/l
- (B) Na_2HPO_4 9.5 g/l or
-     $Na_2HPO_4.2H_2O$ 11.9 g/l

100 mml/l and 150 mmol/l stock solutions may be similarly prepared. To obtain a solution of the required pH, add A and B in the indicated proportions:

pH	A	B
5.4	97.0	3.0
5.6	95.0	5.0
5.8	92.2	7.8
6.0	88.0	12.0
6.2	81.0	19.0
6.4	73.0	27.0
6.6	63.0	37.0
6.8	50.8	49.2
7.0	38.9	61.1
7.2	28.0	72.0
7.4	19.2	80.8
7.6	13.0	87.0
7.8	8.5	91.5
8.0	5.5	94.5

This buffer is not iso-osmotic with normal plasma (see above).

Tris-HCl buffer (200 mmol/l)

Tris (hydroxymethyl) aminomethane
(24.23 g/l)   250 ml

To obtain a solution of the required pH add the appropriate volume of 1 mol/lHCl and then make up the volume to 1 litre with water:

pH	Volume
7.2	44.5 ml
7.4	42.0 ml
7.6	39.0 ml
7.8	33.5 ml
8.0	28.0 ml
8.2	23.0 ml
8.4	17.5 ml
8.6	13.0 ml

pH	Volume
8.8	9.0 ml
9.0	5.0 ml

100 mmol/l, 150 mmol/l, 300 mmol/l and 750 mmol/l stock solutions may be similarly prepared with an appropriate weight of tris and volume of acid.

Tris-HCl bovine serum albumin (BSA) buffer, pH 7.6, 20 mmol/l

Tris (hydroxymethyl) aminomethane
(20 mmol/l)   2.42 g
EDTA, disodium salt (10 mmol/l)   3.72 g
NaCl (100 mmol/l)   5.85 g
Sodium azide (3 mmol/l)   0.2 g

Dissolve the reagents in c 800 ml of water. Adjust the pH to 7.6 with 10 mol/l HCl. Add 10 g of bovine serum albumin (e.g. Sigma) and make up to 1 litre with water.

3.   PREPARATION OF GLASSWARE

FLASK FOR THE DEFIBRINATION OF BLOOD

Provide a 100 ml conical flask with a central glass rod to the bottom end of which are fused pieces of glass capillary (Fig. 1.1, p. 3). The rod is kept in position with a cotton-wool plug. Deliver 10–50 ml of blood into the flask and, after re-inserting the central rod, hold the flask by the neck and rotate it by hand. The blood is usually successfully defibrinated within 5 min, the fibrin forming on the glass rod, usually in one piece. Little or no lysis is caused, and the blood is as a rule completely free from small clots.

SILICONIZED GLASSWARE

Use *c* 2% solution of silicone (dimethyldichlorosilane) in solvent. This is available commercially.* Immerse the clean glassware or syringes to be coated in the fluid and allow to drain dry. (It is advisable to wear rubber gloves and to prepare the apparatus in a fume cupboard provided with an exhaust fan.) Then rinse the coated glassware thoroughly in water, and allow to dry in an oven at 100°C for 10 min or overnight in an incubator.

4.   METHODS OF CLEANING SLIDES AND APPARATUS

New slides

Place them in 3 mol/l HCl for at least 48 h. Wash the treated slides well in running tap-water, rinse in water and store in 95% ethanol until used. Dry with a clean linen cloth and carefully wipe free from dust before they are used.

Dirty slides

When discarded, place in a detergent solution, heat to 60°C for 20 min and then wash in hot running tap-water. Finally, rinse in water before being dried with a clean linen cloth.

Chemical apparatus and glassware

Wash in running tap-water and then boil in a detergent solution, rinse in acid and wash in hot running tap-water, as described above. Alternatively, the apparatus can be soaked in 3 mol/l HCl.

For the removal of deposits of protein and other organic matter, 'biodegradable' detergents are recommended. Decon 90 (Decon Laboratories Ltd., Hove BN3 3LY, UK) is suitable but a number of similar preparations are also available.

Iron-free glassware

Wash in a detergent solution, then soak in 3 mol/l HCl for 24 h and finally rinse in de-ionized, double-distilled water.

---

* e.g. BDH Silicone solution; Sigmacote (Sigma).

5. SIZES OF TUBES

The sizes of tubes recommended in the text have been chosen as being appropriate for the tests described. The dimensions given are the length and external diameter (in mm). The equivalent in inches, as given in some catalogues, and certain corresponding internal diameters, are as follows:

75 × 10 mm (internal
  diameter 8 mm)   = 3 × $\frac{3}{8}$″

75 × 12 mm (internal
  diameter 10 mm)   = 3 × $\frac{1}{2}$″

65 × 10 mm   = $2\frac{1}{2}$ × $\frac{3}{8}$″

38 × 6.4 mm   = $1\frac{1}{2}$ × $\frac{1}{4}$″ ('precipitin tubes')

100 × 12 mm   = 4 × $\frac{1}{2}$″

150 × 16 mm   = 6 × $\frac{5}{8}$″

150 × 19 mm   = 6 × $\frac{3}{4}$″

6. SPEED OF CENTRIFUGING

Throughout the book the unit given is the relative centrifugal force (*g*). Conversion of this figure to rpm depends upon the radius of the centrifuge; it can be calculated by reference to the nomogram illustrated in Fig. 32.1 (see p. 545), or from the formula: Relative centrifugal force (RCF)

$$= 118 \times 10^{-7} \times r \times N^2,$$

where *r* = radius (cm) and *N* = speed of rotation (rpm).

The following centrifugal forces are recommended:

'Low-spun' platelet-
  rich plasma   150–200 *g* (for 10–15 min).
'High-spun' plasma 1200–1500 *g* (for 15 min).
Packing of red cells 2000–2300 *g* (for 30 min).

7. UNITS OF WEIGHT AND MEASUREMENT IN COMMON USE IN HAEMATOLOGY

Throughout the book measurements have been expressed in SI units, in accordance with international recommendations. These units are derived from the metric system. The base units are shown below and the abbreviated forms are indicated alongside.

Weight (unit: gram [g])
  × 10^3 kilogram (kg)
  × 10^{-3} milligram (mg)
  × 10^{-6} microgram (μg) (formerly γ)
  × 10^{-9} nanogram (ng) (formerly μmg)
  × 10^{-12} picogram (pg) (formerly μμg)

Length (unit: metre [m])
  × 10^{-1} decimetre (dm)
  × 10^{-2} centimetre (cm)
  × 10^{-3} millimetre (mm)
  × 10^{-6} micrometre (μm) (formerly μ)
  × 10^{-9} nanometre (nm) (formerly mμ)

Volume (unit: litre [l] = dm^3)
  × 10^{-1} decilitre (dl) (formerly 100 ml)
  × 10^{-3} millilitre (ml) = cm^3 (formerly cc)
  × 10^{-6} microlitre (μl) = mm^3
  × 10^{-9} nanolitre (nl)
  × 10^{-12} picolitre (pl) (formerly μμl)
  × 10^{-15} femtolitre (fl) = μm^3

Amount of substance (unit: mole [mol])
$\times 10^{-3}$ millimole (mmol)
$\times 10^{-6}$ micromole (μmol)
Substance concentration (unit: moles per litre [mol/l]) (formerly M)
$\times 10^{-3}$ millimole per litre (mmol/l)
$\times 10^{-6}$ micromole per litre (μmol/l)

Mass concentration (unit: gram per litre [g/l])
$\times 10^{-3}$ milligram per litre (mg/l)
$\times 10^{-6}$ microgram per litre (μg/l)

When preparing a small amount of a reagent, it is more appropriate to express its concentration per ml or dl.

---

8. MICROSCOPE MAGNIFICATION

It has become customary for the objective lenses of microscopes to be marked with their magnifying power rather than their focal length. The approximate equivalents are as follows:

Focal length (mm)	*Magnification*
2	× 100
4	× 40
16	× 10
40	× 4

---

9. ATOMIC WEIGHTS AND MOLECULAR CONCENTRATIONS

The concentration of a substance in solution can be expressed either in g/l or in mol/l. The molecular weight of the substance (including water of crystallisation if present in the chemical form) expressed as g/l is equivalent to 1 mol (or 1000 mmol)/l. Thus, e.g.

Mol wt of NaCl   = 58.5
∴ 1 mol/l   = 58.5 g/l
9 g/l   = 9 ÷ 58.5   = 0.154 mol/l
= 154 mmol/l

The atomic weights of some chemicals which are commonly used in preparation of reagents are as follows:

Calcium	40
Carbon	12
Chlorine	35
Chromium	52
Hydrogen	1
Iron	56
Magnesium	24
Nitrogen	14
Oxygen	16
Phosphorus	31
Potassium	39
Sodium	23
Sulphur	32

10.   STATISTICAL PROCEDURES

Mean ($\bar{x}$) is the sum of all the measurements (Σ) divided by the number of measurements (n).

Median (m) is the point on the scale that has an equal number of observations above and below.

Mode is the most frequently occurring result.

Gaussian distribution describes events or data which occur symetrically about the mean (see Fig. 2.1); with this type of distribution mean, median and mode will be approximately equal. The extent of spread of measurements about the mean is expressed as the standard deviation (SD). Its calculation is described below. 68% of all the measurements will be within the ± 1 SD range, 95% within ± 2 SD and 99% within ± 3 SD.

Log normal distribution describes events which are asymetrical (skewed) with a larger number of observations towards one end. The mean will thus be nearer that end; the mean, median and mode may differ from each other. To calculate geometric mean and SD the data are first converted to their logarithms and after calculating the mean and SD of the logarithm, the results are reconverted to the antilog.

Poisson distribution describes events which are random in their occurence. This will be the case, for example, when blood cells are counted in a diluted suspension. The number of cells which are counted in a given volume will vary on each occasion; this count variation (σ) is $0.92\sqrt{\lambda}$, where $\lambda = $ the total number of cells counted (see p. 48). It is an estimate of the standard deviation of the entire population whereas SD denotes the standard deviation of the items that were actually measured.

Coefficient of variation (CV) is another way of indicating standard deviation, related to the actual measurement so that variation at different levels can be compared. It is expressed as a percentage.

Standard error of mean (SEM) is a measure of dispersion of the mean of a set of measurements. It is used to compare means of two sets of data.

CALCULATIONS

Variance $(s^2) = \dfrac{\Sigma(x - \bar{x})^2}{n - 1}$

Standard Deviation (SD) $= \sqrt{s^2}$

Coefficient of variation (CV) $= \dfrac{SD}{\bar{x}} \times 100\%$

Standard error of mean (SEM) $= \dfrac{SD}{\sqrt{n}}$

Standard deviation of paired (duplicate)

results $= \sqrt{\dfrac{\Sigma d^2}{2n}}$

where d = difference between duplicates,
    n = number of duplicate measurements.

ANALYSIS OF DIFFERENCES BY t-TEST

This is a method for comparing two sets of data.

Calculation

(1) Variance $(s^2) = \dfrac{\Sigma(d - \bar{d})^2}{n - 1}$,

where d = differences between paired measurements

$\bar{d}$ = mean of the differences

n = number of paired measurements

(2) $t = \bar{d} \div \sqrt{\dfrac{s^2}{n}}$

From the t-test chart (Table 32.1 p. 546) read the value of t for the appropriate degree of freedom (i.e. n − 1). Express results as the level of probability (p) that there is *no* significant difference between the sets of data that are being compared.

11. RABBIT BRAIN THROMBOPLASTIN

Freeze-dried rabbit brain thromboplastins are now widely available commercially with a shelf life of at least 2–5 years. Usually, they are calibrated against the WHO International Reference Preparation of thromboplastin and are supplied with an International Sensitivity Index (ISI) and a table converting prothrombin times to International Normalized Ratios (INR).

If a commercial preparation is not available it is possible to prepare a home-made substitute using rabbit brain which does not require freeze drying and which is relatively stable.

ACETONE-DRIED BRAIN POWDER

Strip the membrane off freshly collected rabbit brain, wash free from blood and place in *c* three times its volume of cold acetone. Macerate for 2–3 min and then filter through absorbent lint (BP or USP grade) on a Büchner funnel. Repeat the extraction 7 times; after two extractions increase the time of exposure to acetone to *c* 20 min for each subsequent extraction. The material should become 'gritty' by the fourth or fifth extraction. After the last extraction spread the acetone-dried brain on a piece of paper and allow to dry in air for 30 min. Rub through a 1 mm mesh nylon sieve to produce a coarse powder. Dispense into a batch of screw-capped bottles and dry over phosphorus pentoxide in a vacuum desiccator. After drying, screw down the caps tightly and store at 4°C or – 20°C. At – 20°C the material should be stable for at least 5 yr. 100 g of whole brain yield *c* 15 g of dried powder.

Preparation of liquid suspension

Dissolve 0.9 g of NaCl and 0.9 g of phenol in 100 ml of water. Suspend 3.6 g of the acetone-dried brain in 100 ml of this phenol-saline solution at 15–20°C and allow to stand at this temperature for 4–5 h, mixing at 30 min intervals. Transfer to a 4°C refrigerator for 24 h with occasional mixing. Thereafter, leave undisturbed at 4°C for 3 h and then decant the supernatant carefully through fine muslin or similar material. The ISI should be not more than 1.4 (see p. 337) and the mean normal prothrombin time 12–13 s. Store the suspension at 4°C. At this temperature it will be stable for at least 6 months, and for at least 7 days at 37°C. It must not be allowed to freeze as freezing results in flocculation of the smooth suspension with deterioration of thromboplastic activity.

12. PTT PHOSPHOLIPID REAGENT

Acetone-dried rabbit brain is suitable for preparing a PTT reagent. Bovine brain may also be used for the PTT reagent, but not for thromboplastin.

Prepare acetone-dried brain powder as described above. Suspend 5 g of the powder in 20 ml of chloroform (analytic grade) in a covered beaker for 1–2 h. Filter through filter paper to obtain a clear filtrate. Wash the brain deposit on the filter paper with 20 ml of chloroform and pool the clear filtrate with the previous filtrate. Evaporate the filtrate to dryness in a beaker of known weight in a water-bath at 60–70°C and weigh the residual deposit: 5 g of dried brain should yield *c* 1.5 g of phospholipid deposit. Emulsify in saline to give a 5% emulsion; 1.5 g of deposit should provide 30 ml of emulsion. Distribute the emulsion in small volumes in stoppered tubes. At – 20°C it should be stable for at least 1 yr.

For use dilute 1 in 100 in saline. For the APTT (PTTK) test (p. 282) mix with an equal volume of 2.5 mg/ml kaolin suspension in imidazole buffer.

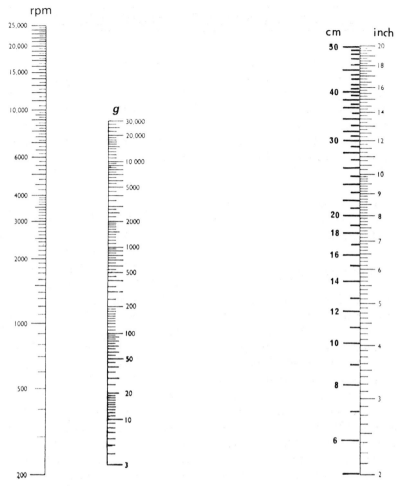

Fig. 32.1 Nomogram for computing relative centrifugal forces. (By courtesy of MSE Ltd).

Table 32.1   *t*-Test table

d.f.	Probability					
	>0.5<	>0.1<	>0.05<	>0.02<	>0.01<	>0.001<
1	1.000	6.314	12.706	31.821	63.657	636.619
2	0.816	2.920	4.303	6.965	9.925	31.598
3	0.765	2.353	3.182	4.541	5.841	12.941
4	0.741	2.132	2.776	3.747	4.604	8.610
5	0.727	2.015	2.571	3.365	4.032	6.859
6	0.718	1.943	2.447	3.143	3.707	5.959
7	0.711	1.895	2.365	2.998	3.499	5.405
8	0.706	1.860	2.306	2.896	3.355	5.041
9	0.703	1.833	2.262	2.821	3.250	4.781
10	0.700	1.812	2.228	2.764	3.169	4.587
11	0.697	1.796	2.201	2.718	3.106	4.437
12	0.695	1.782	2.179	2.681	3.055	4.318
13	0.694	1.771	2.160	2.650	3.012	4.221
14	0.692	1.761	2.145	2.624	2.977	4.140
15	0.691	1.753	2.131	2.602	2.947	4.073
16	0.690	1.746	2.120	2.583	2.921	4.015
17	0.689	1.740	2.110	2.567	2.898	3.965
18	0.688	1.734	2.101	2.552	2.878	3.922
19	0.688	1.729	2.093	2.539	2.861	3.883
20	0.687	1.725	2.086	2.528	2.845	3.850
21	0.686	1.721	2.080	2.518	2.831	3.819
22	0.686	1.717	2.074	2.508	2.819	3.792
23	0.685	1.714	2.069	2.500	2.807	3.767
24	0.685	1.711	2.064	2.492	2.797	3.745
25	0.684	1.708	2.060	2.485	2.787	3.725
26	0.684	1.706	2.056	2.479	2.779	3.707
27	0.684	1.703	2.052	2.473	2.771	3.690
28	0.683	1.701	2.048	2.467	2.763	3.674
29	0.683	1.699	2.045	2.462	2.756	3.659
30	0.683	1.697	2.042	2.457	2.750	3.646
40	0.681	1.684	2.021	2.423	2.704	3.551
60	0.679	1.671	2.000	2.390	2.660	3.460
120	0.677	1.658	1.980	2.358	2.617	3.373
∞	0.674	1.645	1.960	2.326	2.576	3.291

REFERENCES

[1] HENDRY, E. B. (1961). Osmolarity of human serum and of chemical solutions of biological importance. *Clinical Chemistry*, **7**, 156.

[2] KABAT, E. A. and MAYER, M. M. (1961). *Experimental Immunochemistry*, 2nd edn., p. 149. Thomas, Springfield, Ill.

[3] MOORE, H. C. and MOLLISON, P. L. (1976). Use of a low-ionic-strength medium in manual tests for antibody detection. *Transfusion*, **16**, 291.

[4] World Health Organization (1977). *The SI for the Health Professions*. WHO, Geneva.

Index